Oxford Textbook of
Vertigo and Imbalance

Start using the online version today at www.oxfordmedicine.com

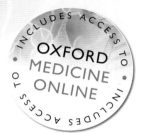

INCLUDES ACCESS TO · OXFORD MEDICINE ONLINE · INCLUDES ACCESS TO

Thank you for purchasing this work from Oxford University Press. The purchase price includes twelve months' access to the online version. To get started, register your access token, which you'll find bound into the front of this book, at https://subscriberservices.sams.oup.com/token

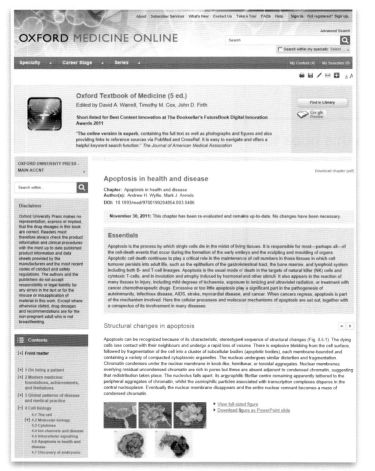

THE ONLINE VERSION ENABLES YOU TO:

- Find exactly what you're looking for, using the 'quick search' and advanced search functions
- Navigate around the content quickly and easily
- Share content with colleagues using integrated tools including social bookmarking, email and citation export
- Return to frequently-used content by saving searches and favourite chapters
- Enlarge images and charts, or download them to PDF or PowerPoint
- Access the content wherever you are, from your desktop, mobile device or tablet

Once your twelve months' access has expired, you can extend your online access by taking out a subscription, and take advantage of our renewal discounts for book purchasers.

Start using your online access today.

Visit https://subscriberservices.sams.oup.com/token and register your access code

(Inclusive online access is only available to individuals.)

And why not recommend Oxford Medicine Online to your librarian?

Free trials are available for institutions, simply visit www.oup.com/online/freetrials/

Oxford Textbook of
Vertigo and Imbalance

Edited by

Adolfo M. Bronstein

Neuro-otology Unit (Centre for Neuroscience)
Imperial College London
Charing Cross Hospital
London, UK

Series Editor
Christopher Kennard

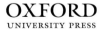

OXFORD
UNIVERSITY PRESS

OXFORD
UNIVERSITY PRESS

Great Clarendon Street, Oxford, OX2 6DP,
United Kingdom

Oxford University Press is a department of the University of Oxford.
It furthers the University's objective of excellence in research, scholarship,
and education by publishing worldwide. Oxford is a registered trade mark of
Oxford University Press in the UK and in certain other countries

British Library Cataloguing in Publication Data
Data available

Library of Congress Cataloguing in Publication Data
Data available

ISBN 978-0-19-960899-7

Printed in Spain by
Grafos, Barcelona

Preface

When grouped together, symptoms of dizziness, vertigo, and off-balance feelings make up to 30% of all consultations in neurology, otorhinolaryngology, and old age medicine. Many of these symptoms do arise from dysfunction of the vestibular system in the inner ear—but many or even most don't. In this book we try to keep the differential diagnoses as wide as possible and present well-established vestibular syndromes like Ménière's disease alongside new disorders like small-vessel white matter disease or conditions not fully established, such as psychogenic dizzy syndromes. We also try to subvert traditional clinical thinking, not shying away from the fact that despite being 'well established', Ménière's disease is rare but white matter disease and psychogenic presentations are common. In order to promote the viewing of the same topic from different angles, we have encouraged what we think is a healthy degree of overlap amongst the different chapters.

This book is conceptually divided into an introductory section (Chapters 1–8), aiming to provide the scientific basis of clinical practice, a general clinical section, syndrome-based (Chapters 9–18), and a final section detailing the specific diseases responsible for complaints of dizziness and unsteadiness (Chapters 19–30).

The book starts with the biophysics and the physiology of the vestibular system but, with the clear remit that these chapters are introductions for an essentially very practical clinical book (Chapters 1–3). You will understand the basic functioning of the vestibulo-ocular reflex—the reflex that allows you to read this page even if you are wobbling your head. And why, when a lesion damages the labyrinth on one side, the world spins around—vertigo, a cardinal sign in acute unilateral vestibular lesions. Indeed the process of recovery of such peripheral vestibular lesions rests on a fascinating process of central compensation, where the central nervous system presides over significant multisensory rearrangements and complex neural plasticity (Chapter 6). But the vestibular system is much more than the vestibulo-ocular reflex and we provide introductory chapters on the vestibular (and proprioceptive) contribution to postural stability (Chapter 4) and vestibulo-autonomic function (Chapter 5). Some of you will be surprised to learn that the vestibular contribution to autonomic function is much more than the nausea that accompanies any vertigo and it expands to the

control of heart, lung, and blood pressure regulation. Chapter 7 on the emerging field of functional neuroimaging of the vestibular system, provides insight into the functional relationship between vestibular and visual areas of the brain and how these interact in health, disease, and during the central compensation process.

In the general clinical section you will find a chapter devoted to otologists (written by a neurologist) and a chapter devoted to neurologists (written by otologists) (Chapters 9 and 10). The aim is to provide the complementary 'missing information' required to practise medicine in the area of balance disorders. If the otologist is not prepared to practise a bit of neurology and the neurologist is not prepared to practise a bit of otology many patients will fall in the gap left between these two specialities. Indeed both need to practise ophthalmology as well since the clinical assessment of the patient with a balance disorder relies heavily on the examination of the eye movements (Chapter 12). This is not only to elicit vestibulo-ocular signs such as a positive head impulse test in vestibular neuritis or a positional Hallpike manoeuvre in positional vertigo. Abnormalities of non-vestibularly elicited eye movements will move the diagnosis in the direction of a brainstem, cerebellar, or cerebral hemisphere disorder and away from the labyrinth. The chapter on functional investigations (Chapter 14) asks if laboratory vestibular tests are necessary. The reader should not be surprised to see that the answer to this question often is 'No, actually, tests are not always necessary', as in many conditions they can be superfluous (vestibular neuritis, benign paroxysmal positional vertigo (BPPV), cerebellar disorders) or normal (vestibular migraine or some gait disorders). We summarize the vertigo syndromes along three main presentations and briefly mention the main diagnoses: the single acute vertigo attack (vertebro-basilar stroke, vestibular neuritis), episodic or recurrent vertigo/dizziness (BPPV, migraine, Ménière's disease, postural hypotension, vestibular paroxysmia) and chronic dizziness/unsteadiness (bilateral vestibular failure, neurological gait disorders, psychogenic dizziness) (Chapter 11). An additional chapter (Chapter 15) summarizes the main advances and uses of structural imaging procedures as an important aid to diagnosis. Given that many patients with acute and recurrent dizziness, and probably all with chronic dizziness, require physiotherapy input, the principles of rehabilitative treatment for vestibular and balance disorders are included in Chapter 17. The epidemiology chapter (Chapter 18) provides an indication of the size of the problem—recent research suggests that dizziness affects about one in three people every year.

Although the third section of this book is dedicated to the specific diseases diagnosed in clinical practice (a chapter each for BPPV, vestibular migraine, vestibular neuritis, stroke, Ménière's disease) we have kept a syndrome-based approach for a number of conditions. These include cerebellar disorders affecting balance, bilateral vestibular failure, general medical conditions affecting balance, gait disorders and psychological disorders, all syndromes in which patients can present with dizzy or off-balance symptoms. Chapter 29 discusses the patient with 'funny turns' and falls, a difficult clinical scenario in which diagnoses range from BPPV to epilepsy, syncope, autonomic disorders, and vascular disease (transient ischaemic attacks and heart dysrhythmia). In Chapter 28 the scenarios and scientific bases of symptoms created by motion (motion sickness) and disorientating vehicular conditions are discussed.

This is not a neuro-otology or audiology book, and we have deliberately left out conditions such as the cerebellopontine angle lesion, acoustic neuroma in particular, as they rarely present in clinic as a balance disorder. We have tried to provide a comprehensive, but not necessarily scholarly or exhaustive, view of the syndromes encountered when dealing with the dizzy or unsteady patient. As the underdeveloped world develops and the population in industrialized societies ages gracefully all doctors will be exposed to more and more patients reporting dizziness and problems with their balance.

Adolfo M. Bronstein
London, January 2013

Contents

List of Contributors

Yuri Agrawal
Department of Otolaryngology-Head and Neck Surgery,
The Johns Hopkins University School of Medicine,
Baltimore, MD, USA

John H. J. Allum
Department of ORL, University Hospital, Basel, Switzerland

Kevin Barraclough
General Practitioner, Hoyland House,
Painswick, Gloucestershire, UK

Alexandre R. Bisdorff
Department of Neurology, Centre Hospitalier Emile Mayrisch,
Luxembourg

Thomas Brandt
Institute for Clinical Neurosciences, Ludwig-Maximilians-University;
and Integrated Center for Research and Treatment of
Vertigo, Balance and Ocular Motor Disorders (IFB^{LMU}),
Ludwig-Maximilians-University, Munich, Germany

Adolfo M. Bronstein
Neuro-otology Unit (Centre for Neuroscience), Imperial College
London, and Charing Cross Hospital, London, UK

Mark G. Carpenter
School of Kinesiology, University of British Columbia,
Vancouver, BC, Canada

Ian S. Curthoys
Neurology Department, Royal Prince Alfred Hospital, Sydney;
and Vestibular Research Laboratory, School of Psychology,
University of Sydney, Sydney, Australia

Rosalyn A. Davies
Department of Neuro-otology, The National Hospital for
Neurology and Neurosurgery, London

Marianne Dieterich
Department of Neurology, Ludwig-Maximilians-University and
Integrated Center for Research and Treatment of Vertigo, Balance
and Ocular Motor Disorders (IFB^{LMU}), Ludwig-Maximilians-
University, Munich, Germany

Scott Eggers
Department of Neurology, Mayo Clinic, Rochester, MN, USA

John F. Golding
Department of Psychology, University of Westminster,
London, UK

Tracey D. Graves
Department of Neurology, Hinchingbrooke Hospital, Huntingdon
and Addenbrooke's Hospital, Cambridge, UK

Michael A. Gresty
Neuro-otology Unit (Centre for Neuroscience), Imperial College
London and Charing Cross Hospital, London, UK

G. Michael Halmagyi
Neurology Department, Royal Prince Alfred Hospital,
Sydney, Australia

Kristen Janky
Department of Audiology, Boys Town National Research Hospital,
Omaha, NE, USA

Maurice Janssen
Department of ORL and Head and Neck Surgery, Division
of Balance Disorders, Maastricht University Medical Centre,
Maastricht, the Netherlands

Joanna C. Jen
Department of Neurology, UCLA School of Medicine,
Los Angeles, CA, USA

Brian J. Jian
Department of Neurosurgery, University of California at
San Francisco, San Francisco, CA, USA

Ilan A. Kerman
Department of Psychiatry and Behavioral Neurobiology, University of Alabama at Birmingham, Birmingham, AL, USA

Amir Kheradmand
Department of Neurology, The Johns Hopkins Hospital, Baltimore, MD, USA

Ji Soo Kim
Department of Neurology, College of Medicine, Seoul National University, Seoul National University Bundang Hospital, Gyeonggi-do, South Korea

T. E. Kimber
Department of Neurology, Royal Adelaide Hospital; and University Department of Medicine, University of Adelaide, Adelaide, Australia

Herman Kingma
Department of ORL and Head and Neck Surgery, Division of Balance Disorders, Maastricht University Medical Centre, Maastricht, the Netherlands

Hyung Lee
Department of Neurology, Keimyung University School of Medicine, Daegu, South Korea

R. John Leigh
Neurology Service, Veterans Affairs Medical Center and Case Medical Center, Cleveland, OH, USA

Thomas Lempert
Department of Neurology, Schlosspark-Klinik, Berlin; and Vestibular Research Group, Charité University Hospital, Berlin, Germany

Ke Liao
Neurology Service, Veterans Affairs Medical Center and Case Medical Center, Cleveland, OH, USA

Lloyd B. Minor
Department of Otolaryngology-Head and Neck Surgery, The Johns Hopkins University School of Medicine, Baltimore, MD, USA

Louisa J. Murdin
National Hospital for Neurology and Neurosurgery and UCL Ear Institute, London

Hannelore K. Neuhauser
Department of Epidemiology, Robert Koch Institute, Berlin; and Vestibular Research Group, Department of Neurology, Charité University Hospital, Berlin, Germany

Di Newham
Centre of Human and Aerospace Physiological Sciences, King's College London, London, UK

David E. Newman-Toker
Department of Neurology, Johns Hopkins University School of Medicine, Baltimore, MD, USA

Daniele Nuti
Department of Human Pathology and Oncology, Section of Otolaryngology, Siena Medical School, Siena, Italy

Marousa Pavlou
Centre of Human and Aerospace Physiological Sciences, King's College London, London, UK

M. Radon
Consultant Neuroradiologist, The Walton Centre Foundation Trust, Liverpool, UK

Karim Salame
Neurology Service, Veterans Affairs Medical Center and Case Medical Center, Cleveland, OH, USA

Barry Seemungal
Neuro-otology Unit (Centre for Neuroscience), Imperial College London and Charing Cross Hospital, London, UK

Alessandro Serra
Neurology Service, Veterans Affairs Medical Center and Case Medical Center, Cleveland, OH, USA

Neil Shepard
Department of Otolaryngology, Mayo Clinic, Rochester, MN, USA

Jeffrey P. Staab
Department of Psychiatry and Psychology, Mayo Clinic, Rochester, MN, USA

Dominik Straumann
Department of Neurology, University Hospital Zurich, Zurich, Switzerland

Michael Strupp
Department of Neurology, Ludwig-Maximilians-University; and Integrated Center for Research and Treatment of Vertigo, Balance and Ocular Motor Disorders (IFB[LMU]), Ludwig-Maximilians-University, Munich, Germany

Alexander A. Tarnutzer
Department of Neurology, University Hospital Zurich, Zurich, Switzerland

P. D. Thompson
Department of Neurology, Royal Adelaide Hospital; and University Department of Medicine, University of Adelaide, Adelaide, Australia

Michael von Brevern
Department of Neurology, Park-Klinik Weissensee, Berlin, Germany

Timothy D. Wilson
Department of Anatomy and Cell Biology, University of Western Ontario, London, ON, Canada

Bill J. Yates
Departments of Otolaryngology and Neuroscience, University of Pittsburgh, Pittsburgh, PA, USA

T. A. Yousry
Lysholm Department of Neuroradiology, Division of Neuroradiology and Neurophysics, UCL Institute of Neurology, London, UK

David S. Zee
Department of Neurology, The Johns Hopkins Hospital, Baltimore, MD, USA

List of Abbreviations

3D	three-dimensional	DLPN	dorsolateral pontine nuclei
AAO-HNS	American Academy of Otolaryngology-Head and Neck Surgery	DSM	Diagnostic and Statistical Manual of Mental Disorders
AC	anterior canal	DVA	dynamic visual acuity
AC	air conduction	DVA	dynamic visual acuity
ADL	activity of daily living	EA	episodic ataxia
AED	antiepileptic drug	EAAT	excitatory amino acid transporter
AICA	anterior inferior cerebellar artery	EAM	external auditory meatus
AN/AD	auditory neuropathy/auditory dys-synchrony	ECG	electrocardiography
AP	action potential	ED	emergency department
APV	acute peripheral vestibulopathy	EEG	electroencephalography
AVA	anterior vestibular artery	ENG	electronystagmography
aVOR	angular vestibulo-ocular reflex	FDG	fluorodeoxyglucose
BA	Brodmann area	FHM	familial hemiplegic migraine
BC	bone conduction	fMRI	functional magnetic resonance imaging
BCV	bone-conducted vibration	FNL	flocculonodular lobe
BOLD	blood oxygen-level-dependent	GABA	gamma-aminobutyric acid
BOS	base of support	GIF	gravitoinertial force
BPPV	benign paroxysmal positional vertigo	GST	gaze stabilization test
BRV	benign recurrent vertigo	HDNE	head-down neck extension
BVF	bilateral vestibular failure	HDNF	head-down neck flexion
BVL	bilateral vestibular loss	HIS	International Headache Society
CAPD	central auditory processing disorder	HIT	head impulse test
CBT	cognitive behaviour therapy	HL	hearing level
CISS	constructive interference in the steady state	HSMN	hereditary sensorimotor neuropathy
CMT	Charcot–Marie–Tooth	HSN	head-shaking induced nystagmus
CNS	central nervous system	HSN	head-shaking nystagmus
COM	centre of mass	IAA	internal auditory artery
CoM	centre of mass	IAC	internal auditory canal
CPA	cerebellopontine angle	ICHD	International Classification of Headache Disorders
CRP	canalith repositioning procedure	ICVD	International Classification of Vestibular Disorders
CSD	chronic subjective dizziness	INC	interstitial nucleus of Cajal
CSF	cerebrospinal fluid	INO	internuclear ophthalmoplegia
cVEMP	cervical vestibular evoked myogenic potential	IPL	inferior parietal lobule
dB	decibel	LARP	left anterior, right posterior
DBN	downbeat nystagmus	LC	lateral canal
DBS	deep-brain stimulation	LGN	lateral geniculate nucleus
dePa	dekapascal	LMI	lateral medullary infarction

MARD	migraine-anxiety dizziness	RIS	retinal image speed
MD	Ménière's disease	RVLM	rostral ventrolateral medulla
MLF	medical longitudinal fasciculus	SCA	spinocerebellar ataxia
MMI	medial medullary infarction	SCC	semicircular canal
MRA	magnetic resonance angiography	SD	standard deviation
MS	multiple sclerosis	SNHL	sensorineural hearing loss
MVC	muscle vasoconstrictor	SOT	Sensory Organization Test
NMDA	N-methyl-D-aspartate	SP	summating potential
NPH	nucleus prepositus hypoglossi	SPV	slow-phase velocity
NRTP	nucleus reticularis tegmenti pontis	SRO	Steele–Richardson–Olszewski [syndrome]
NTS	nucleus tractus solitarius	STG	superior temporal gyrus
OAE	otoacoustic emission	SVV	subjective visual vertical
OKN	optokinetic nystagmus	TBI	traumatic brain injury
OTR	ocular tilt response	TEOAE	transient-evoked otoacoustic emission
OVAR	off-vertical axis rotation	TIA	transient ischaemic attack
oVEMP	ocular vestibular evoked myogenic potential	TM	tympanic membrane
PC	posterior canal	TND	transient neurological deficit
PD	Parkinson's disease	tVOR	translational vestibulo-ocular reflex
PET	positron emission tomography	uVD	unilateral vestibular deafferentation
PICA	posterior inferior cerebellar artery	UVL	unilateral vestibular loss
PIVC	parieto-insular vestibular cortex	VBRT	vestibular and balance rehabilitation therapy
PL	proprioceptive loss	VEMP	vestibular-evoked myogenic potential
PMT	paramedian tract	Vim	ventro-oralis intermedius
PN	peripheral neuropathy	VIP	ventral-intraparietal area
PONV	postoperative nausea and vomiting	VL	vestibular loss
PPN	paroxysmal positional nystagmus	VM	vestibular migraine
PPRF	paramedian pontine reticular formation	VN	voluntary nystagmus
PPV	phobic postural vertigo	VNG	videonystagmography
PSP	progressive supranuclear palsy	VOR	vestibulo-ocular reflex
PTA	pure tone audiometry	VS	vestibulospinal
RALP	right anterior, left posterior	VSR	vestibulospinal reflex
rCGM	regional cerebral glucose metabolism	VTS	visual temporal sylvian
riMLF	rostral interstitial nucleus of the medial longitudinal fasciculus	WBV	whole-body vibration
		WHO	World Health Organization

CHAPTER 1

Biophysics of the Vestibular System

Herman Kingma and Maurice Janssen

Aim

In contrast to the impact of diseases of the eye and ear upon vision and hearing respectively, many patients and doctors find it much more difficult to understand which complaints and impairments are exclusively associated with a dysfunction of the vestibular labyrinth or central vestibular pathways. The often propagated classical idea that *vertigo* is the major vestibular symptom of a peripheral vestibular function disturbance only holds for abrupt changes of vestibular function in one labyrinth. Vertigo is very rare in a slowly changing peripheral vestibular function or any function loss that affects both labyrinths simultaneously and equally. A relatively stable but permanent function loss is much more frequent and—despite central compensation—leads to a diversity of persistent complaints due to a decrease in the sensitivity and accuracy of the labyrinthine sensors to detect head motion and head orientation in space: a permanent loss of automatization of balance, loss of image stabilization (decrease of dynamic visual acuity), and loss of automatization of spatial orientation. The aim of this chapter is to provide the reader with the basic knowledge of the physics and function of the vestibular labyrinth for a better understanding of the diversity of these permanent problems that a patient with a vestibular function loss experiences and to encourage us to develop vestibular prostheses (1–6).

General introduction to the labyrinth

The two balance organs located in the left and right temporal bone, the vestibular nerves, the vestibular nuclei, the vestibulo-cerebellum, and the vestibular cortex are the major structures that together form the vestibular system. In this chapter we will focus on the balance organs themselves, providing the sensory input to the central vestibular system.

To allow detection of body movement and orientation in space we use vision, proprioception (including gravitoreceptors along the large blood vessels), hearing, and the vestibular system. The latter makes use of specialized sensor systems located in the head to monitor the angular accelerations (rotations in three dimensions (3D)) and linear accelerations (translations in 3D and tilt relative to the gravity vector) of the head in space. During head movements many forces act upon these sensors and often all sensors are stimulated simultaneously: on earth, head movements always occur within the gravitational field and are often composed of both rotations and translations. Physical principles imply that the position and orientation of the sensors in the head is irrelevant for the precise detection of head rotations (Figure 1.1A) but crucial for detection of additional translational components and centrifugal forces (Figure 1.1B).

In each temporal bone, on either side (Figure 1.2A), we find a bony labyrinth, composed of cavities and tubes. The membranous labyrinth lies inside the bony labyrinth (Figure 1.2B) surrounded by perilymph that via the ductus perilymphaticus is supplied from the arachnoidal space. The membranous labyrinth is filled with endolymph. The endolymph is a secretion product of the dark cells in the vestibular part of the labyrinth and the stria vascularis in the cochlear part of the labyrinth. The resorption of the endolymph takes place in the saccus endolymphaticus. The membranous labyrinth is kept in position within the bony labyrinth by a fine network of connective fibres.

Within the membranous labyrinth we can distinguish three functional entities: the semicircular canals, the vestibule, and the cochlea (Figure 1.2B). The semicircular canals and vestibule form the vestibular part of the labyrinth. The vestibule hosts the otolith organs, the utriculus and sacculus. Together, the canals and otolith organs are optimally sensitive for relatively low-frequency head movements and head tilt. The auditory part, the cochlea, can be considered as a phylogenetically later developed extension of the vestibular vestibule allowing the perception of high-frequency movements and vibrations (sound) but of which a further description is out of the scope of this chapter. The semicircular canals and otolith organs have a complementary functionality. The three mutual orthogonal oriented canals (Figure 1.2C, D) sense angular accelerations whereas the otolith system senses linear accelerations of the head including head tilt.

The actual primary motion sensors in the labyrinth, the so-called hair cells, are mechanoreceptor cells that transform a mechanical displacement into electrical energy. In line with this phylogenetic

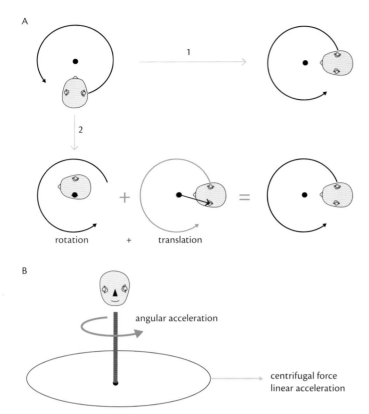

A

1

2

rotation   +   translation

B

angular acceleration

centrifugal force
linear acceleration

Fig. 1.1 A movement of an object is generally the sum of rotations and translations. Any movement can be divided into a rotation around a freely chosen rotation axis combined with an appropriate translation. For example, when the head rotates around an axis in the middle of the head, the labyrinth will be subject to a simultaneous translation and rotation (A: arrow 1). But the same result can be obtained by first rotating the labyrinth around an axis positioned in the labyrinth, followed by a separate translation (A: arrow 2). So, the rotation component of the labyrinth is always the same irrespective the position of the rotation axis relative to the labyrinth and always similar for both labyrinths: only the additional translation component depends on the eccentricity (A). Rotation induces always additional radial (centrifugal) and tangential forces of any structure not on the rotation axis (B). So during rotation the centrifugal forces acting on the labyrinths will always be different for the left and right labyrinths (different stimulation of the left and right utriculus and sacculus).

aspect they are to some extent similar in both the vestibular and the auditory organs. The sensitivity of the three functional entities in the labyrinth for translations, rotations, tilts, and sounds does not depend so much on the type of hair cell, but much more on the specific place and way the hair cells are built in dedicated structures: the cupula in the canals, the macula in the vestibule, and the organ of Corti in the cochlea.

The vestibular hair cells (Figure 1.3) are composed of a cell body and a bundle of cilia on top of them, on average about 50 stereocilia and 1 kinocilium (7; frog's sacculus). The stereocilia form a bundle of cilia that increase in length the closer they are to the kinocilium. On their top, the cilia are mechanically interconnected by elastic tip links. The tip links make the cilia of one hair cell all move together upon acceleration and are also thought to mechanically open and close ion channels positioned on top of the stereocilia. The kinocilium as the longest cilium, is the cilium that will be deflected the most by small movements of the cupula in the canals and macula in the vestibule, but thanks to the tip

links all cilia will move in synchrony with the kinocilium, leading to a high sensitivity.

The hair-cell receptor potential at rest is about −60 mV and changes about 20 mV per micron lateral shift of the cilia. Afferent nerve fibres to the hair cells show a spontaneous firing rate in the range of about 100 spikes per second (3, 7). The receptor potential decreases and nerve fibre spike rate increases when the stereocilia move towards the kinocilium and vice versa. The maximum change in receptor potential due to a deflection of cilia in the direction of the kinocilia is in the hair cell of the frog's sacculus, the maxima differs by a factor of about 4: a change of −1.8 mV versus +7.0 mV in case of a cilia deflection away from or towards the kinocilia, making the hair cell an *asymmetric* sensitive mechanoreceptor cell (7; second law of Ewald).

The two balance organs that make use of hair cells as mechanoreceptors each host five primary sensors for the detection of movements and orientation of the head in space. Three semicircular canals detect angular acceleration in 3D (rotations). Two otolith organs, the utriculus and sacculus, detect linear accelerations in 3D (translations) and head orientation (tilt) relative to the gravity vector. During rotations the head also undergoes centrifugal forces directed away from the rotation axis; these forces are also detected by the utriculus and sacculus. The canals are able to detect angular accelerations exceeding $0.5°/s^2$. The otolith organs detect linear accelerations exceeding 2 cm/s^2 and head tilts relative to gravity with an accuracy of about 0.5°.

The specific difference in sensitivity for rotations, translations, and tilt of the vestibule is explained solely by the specific anatomical shape and structure of the canals and statolith organs, and is not due to any differences in hair-cell structure.

Semicircular canals

As shown in Figure 1.2, three semicircular canals can be identified in the vestibular labyrinth: the lateral, posterior, and anterior canal which differ slightly in size—the lateral canal has a diameter of about 2.3 mm (standard deviation (SD) 0.21), the posterior canal of 3.1 mm (SD 0.30), and the anterior canal of 3.2 mm (SD 0.24). The canals are oriented more or less mutually orthogonal (Figure 1.4) to each other; the orientation of all canals vary among healthy subjects (SD between 4.1–5.4°). The inner diameter of the canals is estimated to vary between 0.2–0.3 mm (8, 9).

The hair cells of the canals are located in the cupula, a basal part of a gelatinous mass, which extends from the ampulla of each canal and forms a flap that closes the semicircular canal, preventing endolymph from passing the ampulla (Figure 1.4). The cilia extend into the cupula.

As indicated earlier, the hair cells have the highest sensitivity for deflections to the kinocilium: the polarization direction. In the cupula all hair cells are arranged with the same polarization direction. As a consequence the receptor potential of all hair cells in a cupula decreases or increases in synchrony upon a cupula deflection. But again, as the maximum sensitivity is in the polarization direction, there is also a preferred direction of a cupula deflection, explaining an asymmetric sensitivity for each semicircular canal: in fact, each canal is most sensitive for rotations in the direction of that specific canal (Figure 1.4).

The polarization direction of the hair cells in the cupula of the *horizontal* canals is such that the canal is more sensitive for a cupula

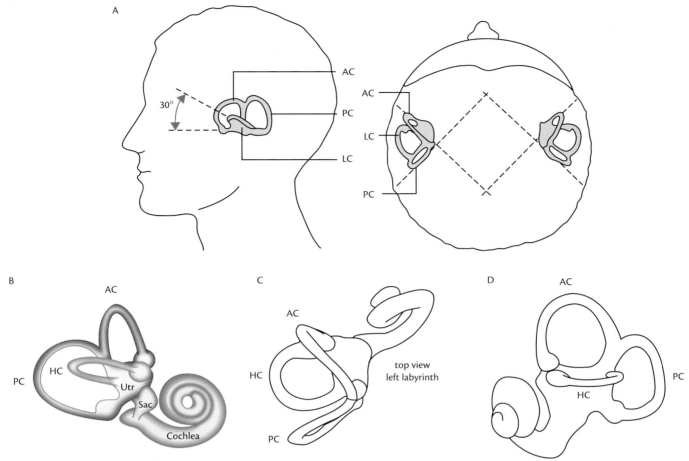

Fig. 1.2 (A) Schematic drawing of the orientation of the two labyrinths in the skull. (B) Schematic drawing of the right membranous labyrinth. (C) Top view left labyrinth. Schematic drawing slightly modified after Jeffrey and Spoor (8). The vestibular labyrinth reaches its mature size between 17–19 weeks of gestational age. A detailed quantitative description of the dimensions of the human labyrinth is given by Jeffery (8). (D) Frontal view left labyrinth with the head 45° degrees rotated to the left. AC: anterior (or superior) canal; HC, horizontal (or lateral) canal; PC, posterior canal; Sac: sacculus; Utr: utriculus.

deflection towards the ampulla (ampullopetal), which corresponds to an opposite head rotation (Figure 1.4, arrow; see later explanation on the physics behind the mechanism of cupula deflection). The polarization direction of the hair cells in the cupula of the *vertical* canals is such that the canal is more sensitive for a cupula deflection away from the ampulla (ampullofugal), which again corresponds to an opposite head rotation (Figure 1.4, arrow). As a rule of thumb, each canal is maximally sensitive for rotations around an axis orthogonal to the plane of that canal and in the direction of that canal (e.g. the right horizontal canal is most sensitive for head rotations to the right).

Through this orientation we are supplied with three pairs of canals with a complementary opposite optimal sensitivity (Figure 1.4: 1) the left and right horizontal canal (HC); 2) the left anterior (AC) and right posterior canal (PC); 3) the right AC and left posterior canal (PC). The sensitivity (gain) of the semicircular canal is such that it generates close to 1 spike/s per °/s at 0.5 Hz in the afferent nerve fibres (10).

When the head is rotated, the endolymph fluid lags behind due to mass inertia and exerts a force against the cupula (Figure 1.5A, B) causing the cupula to bend. The endolymph will move maximally when the rotation axis is orthogonal to the plane in which the canal is oriented (Figure 1.6; the endolymph and cupula will not move when the rotation axis is in the plane of the canal: Ewald's

first law). As mentioned previously (see Figure 1.1), the impact of rotation of an individual canal does not depend on the distance between the axis of rotation and the centre of the canal–parallel axis theorem (11): the position of the canals in the head is irrelevant for the sensitivity for rotations.

Physics of the canals

An analogue of a canal without a cupula is a closed bottle completely filled with water (without any air on top) fixed on a turntable. As soon as the turntable starts to rotate the bottle will follow the rotation immediately. However, due to the inertia of mass the water will lag behind and only after a while—due to the adhesion of the water to the bottle wall and the internal cohesion of the water molecules—the water will start to rotate until it reaches the same angular velocity as the bottle and turntable. Without this friction (adhesion) and viscosity (cohesion) the water would not move at all; with more friction and viscosity the water will follow the bottle movement faster. Besides friction and viscosity the total mass and specific mass of the fluid or inertia also plays a crucial role: the more fluid mass the more force (acceleration) is needed in order to move the water. Friction, viscosity, mass, and acceleration all determine how much the water will lag behind the bottle movement and

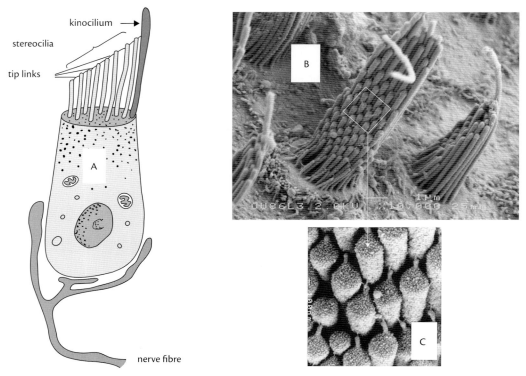

Fig. 1.3 (A) Schematic drawing of a hair cell. (B) and (C) Scanning electron-microscopic photo of vestibular hair cells with tip links. Figures combined and modified after Valk (32).

over which angle it will be displaced until the water has reached the same angular velocity as the bottle. As long as the turntable, bottle, and water rotate at a constant velocity nothing happens anymore. The angle over which the water is rotated compared to bottle is proportional to the applied angular acceleration to the bottle. As soon as the turntable stops, the bottle will stop as well, but now the water will still rotate in the bottle. The velocity of the water will decrease in time due to the friction between bottle and water and ultimately also the water comes to a complete standstill. If the deceleration is the same as the acceleration, the same time will be needed for

the water to come to a standstill and the water will have rotated to exactly the same position as in the beginning of the experiment: no net relative angular displacement is left. In fact, deceleration and acceleration need not be the same: the same position is always reached when the steps in velocity during acceleration and deceleration are opposite but have the same magnitude. For example, the velocity step is the same but opposite (120°/s and −120°/s), when we accelerate in 12 s with 10°/s^2 to 120°/s and the bottle stops when we decelerate in 2 s by 60°/s^2 from 120°/s to stand still. So the relative displacement is proportional to the velocity step: = acceleration

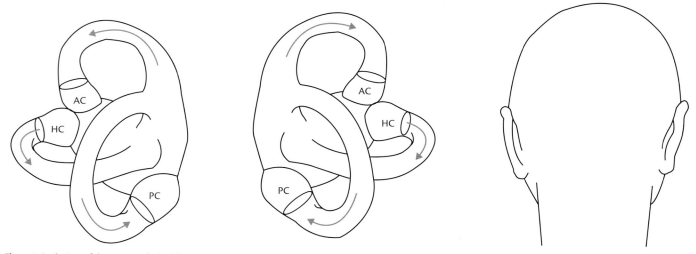

Fig. 1.4 Back view of the two vestibular labyrinths modified after Jeffery (8). The arrows indicate the preferred rotation direction in each canal. AC, anterior canal; HC, horizontal canal; PC, posterior canal.

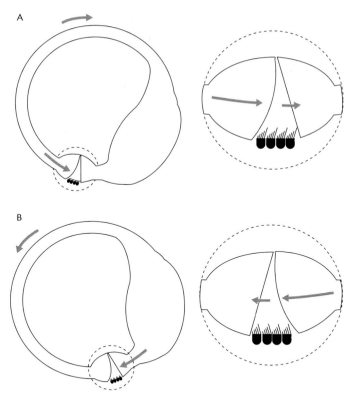

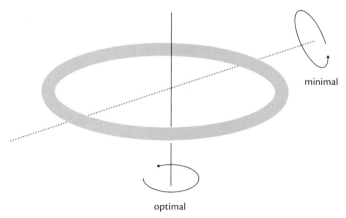

Fig. 1.6 First law of Ewald: cupula deflection will be maximal for rotations around an axis orthogonal to the plane in which the canal is situated; cupula deflection will be minimal for rotations around an axis in the plane in which the canal is situated.

Fig. 1.5 Clockwise angular acceleration of the canals leads to a ampullopetal endolymphatic flow and a deflection of the cupula and hair cells that all have the same polarization. (A). Clockwise angular acceleration leads to cupula deflection in the opposite direction (B).

× T$_{acceleration}$. This has a direct clinical application: velocity steps are used widely in vestibular diagnostics using rotatory chairs.

When we put a very light fluid or gas (low specific mass) in the bottle (decreasing the mass inertia) or a very viscous fluid that has a strong adherence (high friction) to the bottle wall, the displacement of the content relative to the bottle will be almost negligible.

So, the relative displacement will increase with mass, decrease with friction (adhesion and cohesion), and increase with the magnitude of the step in velocity. Any translation of the turntable and bottle on top will not lead to any movement of the water as the water cannot be compressed. The water will only start to move by rotations.

The situation is slightly more complex in the semicircular canal: here the cupula prevents the endolymph freely rotating in the canal (Figure 1.5A, B). The cupula can be considered as an elastic membrane that can slightly bend in both directions. As soon as the canal starts rotating the endolymph will lag behind due to the inertia of mass. Again, the less friction and the more endolymph mass are in the canal the more the fluid will tend to lag behind and the stronger will be the force acting upon the cupula. The stiffness of the cupula will, however, prevent a large deflection: within milliseconds equilibrium will be reached between the inertial force acting upon cupula and the elastic force from the cupula. As long as the acceleration continues, this equilibrium will remain, resulting in a persisting deflection that stimulates the hair cells in the cupula. The stronger the acceleration the more the cupula will bend: the constant deflection of the cupula will be proportional to the actual acceleration. Low

cupula stiffness (high elasticity), a high endolymph mass, and a low friction will all result in a larger cupula deflection (higher sensitivity). When constant angular velocity is reached, the cupula will start to bend back to its neutral position as there is no driving force (acceleration) anymore to maintain the cupula deflection. However, the return time is quite long, as now the elastic force of the cupula alone will have to move the endolymph mass against friction. A low cupula stiffness (high elasticity = small elastic force), a high endolymph mass, and strong friction will result in a slower return of the cupula to its neutral position. In pathology and ageing, endolymph viscosity (friction) and cupula stiffness could change; in benign paroxysmal positional vertigo (BPPV), endolymph (specific) mass could be assumed to increase. In summary:

◆ Increase of cupula stiffness or increase of endolymph viscosity: lower canal sensitivity and shorter postrotatory sensations.

◆ Increase of absolute endolymph mass: higher canal sensitivity and longer postrotatory sensations.

◆ Change of endolymph specific mass compared to that of the cupula: sensitivity canals for gravity and linear accelerations are induced. A canal is insensitive to (coincidental) linear accelerations (9) because the cupula and endolymph have the same density. If differences in densities occur the canal dynamics will be more complex, and would lead to a dependency on the orientation of both the gravity vector relative to the canal plane and the axis of rotation, as well as on the distance between the axis of rotation and the centre of the semicircular canal (12). This is the effect most people experience after alcohol intake, resulting in sensations of rotation when lying in bed and can even induce eye movements known as positional alcohol nystagmus (13). This is also the effect experienced in the common vestibular disorder BPPV. In BPPV, otoconia particles are present in the semicircular canals. These particles make the semicircular canal system sensitive to the orientation of gravity and increase the sensitivity to accelerations (more mass). The particles are supposed to be able to become attached to the cupula, which is called cupulolithiasis (14), or remain free floating and clump together in the canal, which is called canalithiasis (15, 16).

Theoretical model of the semicircular canals

Some years ago Melvill-Jones (9) and Groen (17) presented a second-order mathematical model that could explain the precise working of the semicircular canal. We refer to this excellent paper for a more detailed description.

During head rotation the endolymph lags behind the movement of the semicircular canals due to mass inertia, causing viscous friction. Additionally, the deflected cupula has elastic properties. Therefore the semicircular canals can be modelled with a mechanical analogue, using inertia (I), viscosity (B), and elasticity/stiffness (K) as physical quantities (see Figure 1.7). The following assumptions are made. The fluid flow in the semicircular canal is assumed to be laminar as the Reynolds number is below 1. The density of the endolymph is extremely close to 1 and considered similar to the density of the cupula. This similarity makes the canals insensitive for linear accelerations. The endolymph dynamic viscosity is estimated to be 0.001 Pa/s, the inner radius of the membranous tube 0.163 mm (e.g. see (9)), Young's elasticity modulus of the cupula is estimated to be 5.4 Pa (18).

The moment of inertia is given by $l \cdot \overline{P}$, the moment of viscous friction by $B \cdot v$ and the moment of elasticity by $k \cdot v$, which leads to a second-order differential equation:

$$l \cdot \overline{p} = B \cdot v + K \cdot v \qquad (1)$$

with $\overline{P}$ angular endolymph acceleration, $\dot{q}$ angular head velocity, and v cupula angle. Using $v = q - p$ and the fact that l/B ($T_1 \approx 3$ ms) is much smaller than B/K ($T_2 \approx 10$ s) (9), the transfer function can be written as

$$\frac{v}{\dot{q}}(s) = T_1 \cdot T_2 \cdot \frac{s}{(T_1 \cdot s + 1)(T_2 \cdot s + 1)} \qquad (2)$$

with angular head velocity $\dot{q}$ as input and cupula angle v as output. The shape of this transfer function is shown in Figure 1.8.

The model predicts a maximum endolymph movement in the order of magnitude of 1° at velocity steps of 500°/s. Grabherr (19) reported a perception threshold for angular velocity steps in young adults from 0.4–2.8°/s (at 0.05–5 Hz, lowest threshold of 0.4°/s at 2 Hz). Using a different stimulus conditions, Janssen found a 95% confidence interval between 1–5.5°/s (1). This order of magnitude implies that the mechanoreceptors are stimulated already by an endolymph displacement of about 0.002°. The semicircular canals sense angular acceleration because the endolymph mass inertia is the driving force, but at physiological frequencies of head movements (about 0.5–5 Hz) the semicircular canal works as integrating angular accelerometer (20): the cupula afferent signals are proportional to angular head velocity as indicated by the flat response of the transfer function between 0.5–10 Hz (see Figure 1.8). Additionally, as shown in Figure 1.9, compensatory eye velocity is proportional to and in antiphase with head velocity (21). Two commonly applied paradigms in vestibular tests using a rotational chair are: 1) a constant angular acceleration and 2) a very short angular acceleration (velocity step). Figure 1.10 shows the cupula response to these stimuli.

Clinical interpretation of the theoretical model

The gain in the curves reflects the sensitivity of the canal for rotations. The phase in the curves reflects the timing: the synchronization

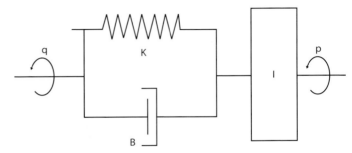

Fig. 1.7 Mechanical analogue of the semicircular canal. B, viscous friction; I, endolymph mass inertia; K, cupula restoring force, p, angular position of the endolymph; q, angular position of the head; q–p, deflection angle of the cupula.

between head and cupula movement. Both need to be optimal for an accurate detection of the actual head rotation.

In the graphs in Figure 1.11A, B, the gain and phase of the cupula deflection is plotted as a function of head *acceleration*. For all frequencies below 0.1 Hz, the cupula deflection is clearly proportional and in phase with the head acceleration (upper two graphs); the curves are flat up to about 0.1 Hz. However, at higher frequencies the sensitivity (gain) rapidly decreases and the response starts to lag behind (phase).

When we plot the gain and phase of the cupula deflection as a function of head *velocity* (Figure 1.11C, D), the curves become flat between the middle to higher frequencies (0.1–10 Hz): the cupula deflection is proportional and in phase with the head velocity (lower two graphs).

The frequency dependence of the canal is not so easily objectified and quantified in clinical practise. The caloric test can be considered as a low-frequency test, so evaluating the low-frequency part of the function of the horizontal canal as depicted in Figure 1.11A, B. Sinusoidal rotatory tests (torsion swing, sinusoidal harmonic acceleration tests) evaluate the low and middle frequency range (0.01–1 Hz) of the canal function.

When we use a velocity step stimulus in the clinic (velocity step), the decay of the eye velocity in time reflects the time constant T2 of the earlier described mathematical model. When we apply a sinusoidal rotational stimulus, we can quantify the phase shift between head and eye velocity. This time constant T is in the velocity domain physically related to the phase shift detected by sinusoidal stimulation (stimulation frequency f Hz) by the formula: $\phi = 90° - \tan^{-1}([2\pi fT])$.

As a rule of thumb for clinicians: the time constant is defined as the time it takes before the gain decreases down to about 37% (= 1/e where e is Euler's constant); this implies that it takes at least three times longer before the cupula deflection is less than 5% (e.g. the typical time constant of the cupula is about 6 s which means that it takes a minimum of 18 s before the cupula deflection is less than 5% and almost no rotation is detected anymore by the labyrinth anymore).

So, the velocity step tests (= acceleration impulse response test) allow in theory a direct quantification of the gain and time constant T2 of the canals via measurement of the vestibulo-ocular reflex (22, 23). However, central processing and cognitive processes also modify both gain and phase considerable. Due to storage of the signal in the brain during acceleration, the response to a velocity step (postrotatory nystagmus and rotation sensation) lasts much longer than the mechanical response of the labyrinth, namely 30–60 seconds (time constant between 11–26

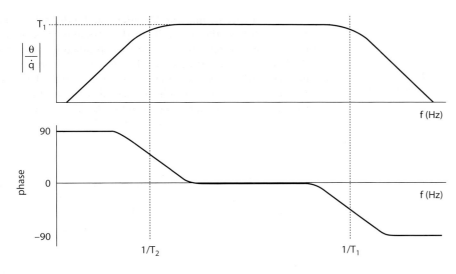

Fig. 1.8 Bode plot of the frequency response of the transfer function equation 2, representing the dynamic response of the mechanical analogue of the semicircular canals. Upper trace: amplitude spectrum (gain = sensitivity). Lower trace: phase as a function of frequency.

seconds in healthy subjects); this limits a direct interpretation of the function of the peripheral canal based upon any rotatory test. Also, due to the simultaneous stimulation of both labyrinths and because central compensation of peripheral lesions is quite effective after a few months, it often remains difficult to find out by use of a rotational test which canal is affected.

In the past, a discrepancy between the duration of the postrotatory nystagmus and rotation sensation was suggested to allow identification of certain vestibular pathologies (cupulometry; 24). Many attempts have been made to develop high-frequency tests (vestibular autorotation test, head shakers, high-frequency (hydraulic) torsion swing chair

tests). None of these obtained a widespread application comparable to the caloric test due to too many practical limitations, limited sensitivity, and reproducibility. Passive head impulse tests, fast small-amplitude head rotations, can also be considered as evaluating the high-frequency function of the canals. Meanwhile this test, especially when detection of the induced eye and head movement is quantified, has become a very important clinical tool, allowing quantification of the gain and detection of overt and covert saccades in cases of pathology, but unfortunately not allowing both time constants described earlier. Alternatively, the impact of the labyrinth upon image stabilization, i.e. visual acuity during head movements, can also be quantified (6) but

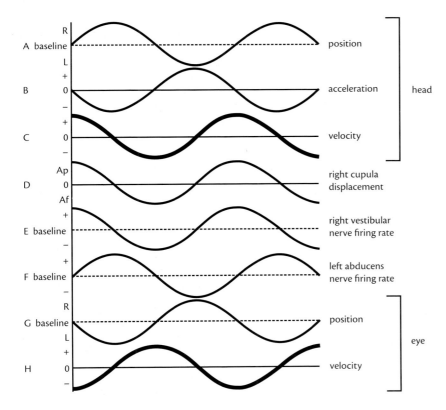

Fig. 1.9 Mechanism by which a sinusoidal change in head position (A) is converted to an equal and opposite eye position (G) (see also (33)). Cupula deflection (D) and vestibular nerve firing rate (E) are proportional and in phase with head velocity (C). The abducens nerve firing rate (F) lags the cupula deflection (D) by 90°, caused by an oculomotor integrator, because the lateral rectus muscle contraction needs position-coded information, which is superimposed on the baseline contraction (voluntary eye position). Compensatory eye velocity (H) is then proportional to and in antiphase with head velocity (C). Ap, ampullopetal; Af, ampullofugal.

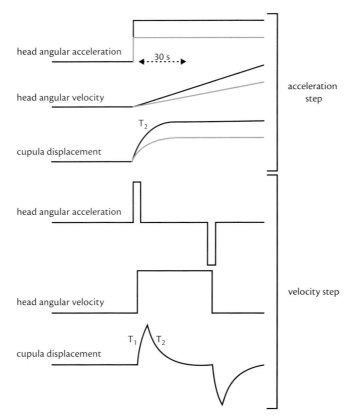

Fig. 1.10 Cupula response to constant angular acceleration and to velocity steps.

such approaches do not allow assessment of the physical parameters of the labyrinth, though are highly clinically relevant.

A more detailed mathematical treatment of the flow inside the vertebrate labyrinth is given by Muller (25). The main difference to the earlier described simple 'torsion pendulum' theory is that the entire system formed by the three semicircular ducts, interconnected by the crus commune and the utriculus, is considered, instead of a single duct circuit. Currently a new mathematical approach incorporating a specific shape of the cupula membrane, and the shape and orientation of the semicircular canals is being studied, which suggests that the relation between shape, orientation, and size of the canals and sensitivity for angular accelerations is more complex than suggested by the basic second-order model presented here (26).

The otolith (synonym: statolith) organs

There are two otolith organs in each labyrinth: the utriculus and sacculus which are located in the membranous labyrinth, in the vestibule (see Figure 1.2B). Both organs contain a sensory epithelium, the macula utriculus, and macula sacculus. When we keep our head upright, the surface of the macula utriculus is oriented in the horizontal plane and towards anterior slightly curved upward for about 20–30°. The macula sacculus is oriented against the medial wall of the sacculus, parallel to the sagittal plane, orthogonal to the macula utriculus. The stereocilia of the hair cells expand into a gelatinous, deformable, elastic mass (Figure 1.12A). Relatively heavy calcium carbonate crystals or otoconia are attached on the top of this gelatinous mass by fine collagen connective fibres. These mostly hexagonally-shaped crystals have a specific mass of 2.95 g/cm³ and a diameter varying from 3–30 μm. The hair cells in the utriculus are oriented with their polarization direction towards an imaginary line, the striola, in the middle of the surface (Figure 1.12B). At the level of the utricular striola, the membrane is very thin and the hair cells have short cilia. The hair cells in the sacculus are oriented with their polarization direction away from the striola. At the level of the saccular striola, the membrane is relatively thick and the hair cells have long cilia.

Physics of the otolith system

An analogue of the otoconia membrane is a car with an antenna on which an orange is pierced (air friction is neglected). Due to the inertia of mass the orange will bend backwards as soon as the car accelerates. The antenna will bend backwards and remain deflected over an angle proportional to the car acceleration. Due to its elasticity, the antenna will start to return to its vertical orientation as soon as the car reaches constant velocity. Now the erect position of the antenna indicates constant velocity or stand still. Upon deceleration of the car, due to the inertia of the orange, the antenna will bend forwards. Now the inclination of the antenna is proportional to the deceleration. Due to its elasticity, the antenna will return to its vertical orientation as soon as the car stops. When we tilt the car, the antenna will deflect in the direction of tilt over an angle proportional to the tilt angle relative to the gravity vector. No distinction is possible between tilt and translation (compare with Figure 1.12C).

Also the otolith system is sensitive to linear accelerations and tilt thanks to the principle of inertia of mass. Assume that the head undergoes linear accelerations (Figure 1.12C). The lower part of the utricular membrane immediately follows the head movement (Figure 1.12A), but the otoconia on the top of the membrane will lack behind which results in a deflection of the cilia. This bending causes depolarization or hyperpolarization of the hair cells depending on the direction of deflection of the cilia. The hair cells of the macula are polarized in all directions, in contrast to the semicircular canals. A tilt relative to the gravity vector also induces a shear force in the plane of the otoconia membrane and a deflection of the cilia. The otolith organs cannot distinguish between head tilt and head translation (for example, an acceleration forwards leads to a similar deflection of the cilia as a backward tilt of the head; Figure 1.12C). Jongkees and Groen made this ambiguity very clear in their 1946 paper (27):

Let a well-known example of Einstein make this clear. Suppose a person finds himself in a cage somewhere in our universe, beyond the gravitational range of influence of any celestial body. The cage is supposed to possess no acceleration relative to the average stellar matter. Then for him no gravity will exist. In this cage everything will float, the otoliths will not exert any pressure on the maculae. Now suppose we give to this cage an acceleration of 9.8 m/sec². From this moment in a mechanical way everything is for the inhabitant of the cage as if he were back on earth. The objects will fall, the test person will stay on the floor (that is that wall of the cage which lies at the side from which the acceleration is pointed within the cage) and the otoliths will again press on their bottom layer. In this way Einstein elucidates the meaning of his statement, that a body in the field of gravity of the earth finds itself in a field of acceleration of 9.8 m/sec². It is absolutely the same for this body from a mechanical point of view to be either in the field of gravity of the earth or to be moved outside this field with a linear acceleration of the magnitude of the

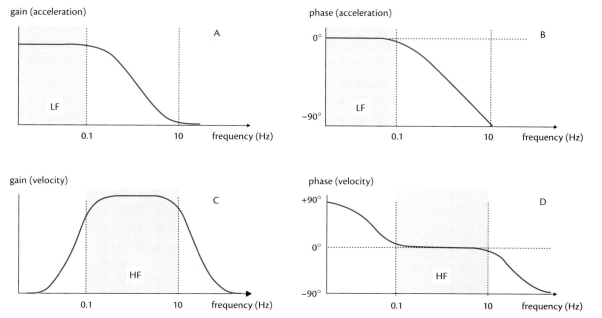

Fig. 1.11 Figure shows gain (sensitivity) and phase (timing) of the canals as a function of the frequency of head rotations. Based upon the second-order model and the various known or estimated constants of the canals, the canals behave differently for low versus high rotation frequencies. For low frequencies the cupula deflection is proportional to head acceleration; for high frequencies the cupula deflection is proportional to head velocity.

acceleration of gravity. The centrifugal force has just the same character. The action of an accelerated movement in which the acceleration is as great as the acceleration of the centrifugal force is mechanically identical with the action of this force. It must be kept in mind however that the direction of the replacing gravitation or centrifugal force is just opposite to the direction of the replaced acceleration. Already Newton in his law of inertia expressed the same idea about the relationship of force and acceleration. No measuring instrument, however fine, can distinguish between a field of gravitation (i.e. a field of forces caused by gravity) or a field of forces caused by centrifugal force and a field of forces (of inertia) caused by an accelerated movement of the same magnitude and opposite direction. This is not a result of the practical inadequacy of the instruments, but of the essential identity of all three. In the same way it must be impossible for the measuring device in the human body, wherever this organ may be located, to distinguish between the action of gravity, of the centrifugal force, or of the force of inertia caused by a linear accelerated movement.

At constant rotational head velocity, the canals are not stimulated. However, during both constant and changing rotational head velocity the otolith system is still stimulated due to the centrifugal force, probably having a supporting and regulatory function for the canals.

Theoretical model of the otolith system

During a linear head acceleration or head tilt the otoconia mass shifts relative to the macula due to the otoconia mass inertia, causing opposing viscous friction and an elastic force. Therefore the otolith organ semicircular canals can be modelled in a similar way to the semicircular canals with a simple mechanical analogue, using inertia (I), viscosity (B), and elasticity (K) as physical quantities (see Figure 1.13). The moment of inertia is given by $I \cdot \ddot{y}$, the moment of viscous friction by $B \cdot \dot{\delta}$, and the moment of elasticity by $K \cdot \delta$, which would lead to a second-order differential equation similar to that of the semicircular canals. In the case of the otolith

organ, however, since the otoconia mass is immersed in endolymph fluid of density ρ_e, any linear acceleration will generate a buoyancy force acting according to Archimedes' principle in the direction of imposed acceleration and equal to $(\rho_e / \rho_o) \cdot I \cdot \ddot{x}$, with ρ_o the density of the otoconial mass. Therefore the second-order differential equation of the otolith organ is:

$$\left(1 - \frac{\rho_e}{\rho_o}\right) I \cdot \ddot{x} = I \cdot \ddot{\delta} + B \cdot \dot{\delta} + K \cdot \delta \tag{3}$$

with $\ddot{x}$ linear head acceleration, $\ddot{y}$ linear otoconia acceleration, and δ relative displacement of the otolithic membrane, using $\delta = x - y$ (9). The transfer function can be written as

$$\frac{\delta}{\ddot{x}}(s) = \left(1 - \frac{\rho_e}{\rho_o}\right) \cdot \frac{I}{I \cdot s^2 + B \cdot s + K} \tag{4}$$

with linear head acceleration $\ddot{x}$ as input and relative otolithic membrane displacement δ as output. The form of this transfer function is shown in Figure 1.14, using the fact that $1/B (T_1 \approx 0.1$ s) is smaller than $B/K (T_2 \approx 1$ s).

The otolith organ is sensitive for constant (0 Hz) and low-frequency linear accelerations. Because a gravitational acceleration and a corresponding linear acceleration of the system are physically equivalent as cited from Groen earlier (Einstein's equivalence principle; 27), the otolith organs cannot distinguish between pure head translations and static head tilts. The relative otolith membrane displacement δ in response to a constant linear acceleration is similar to the cupula displacement in response to an angular acceleration as shown in Figure 1.12C.

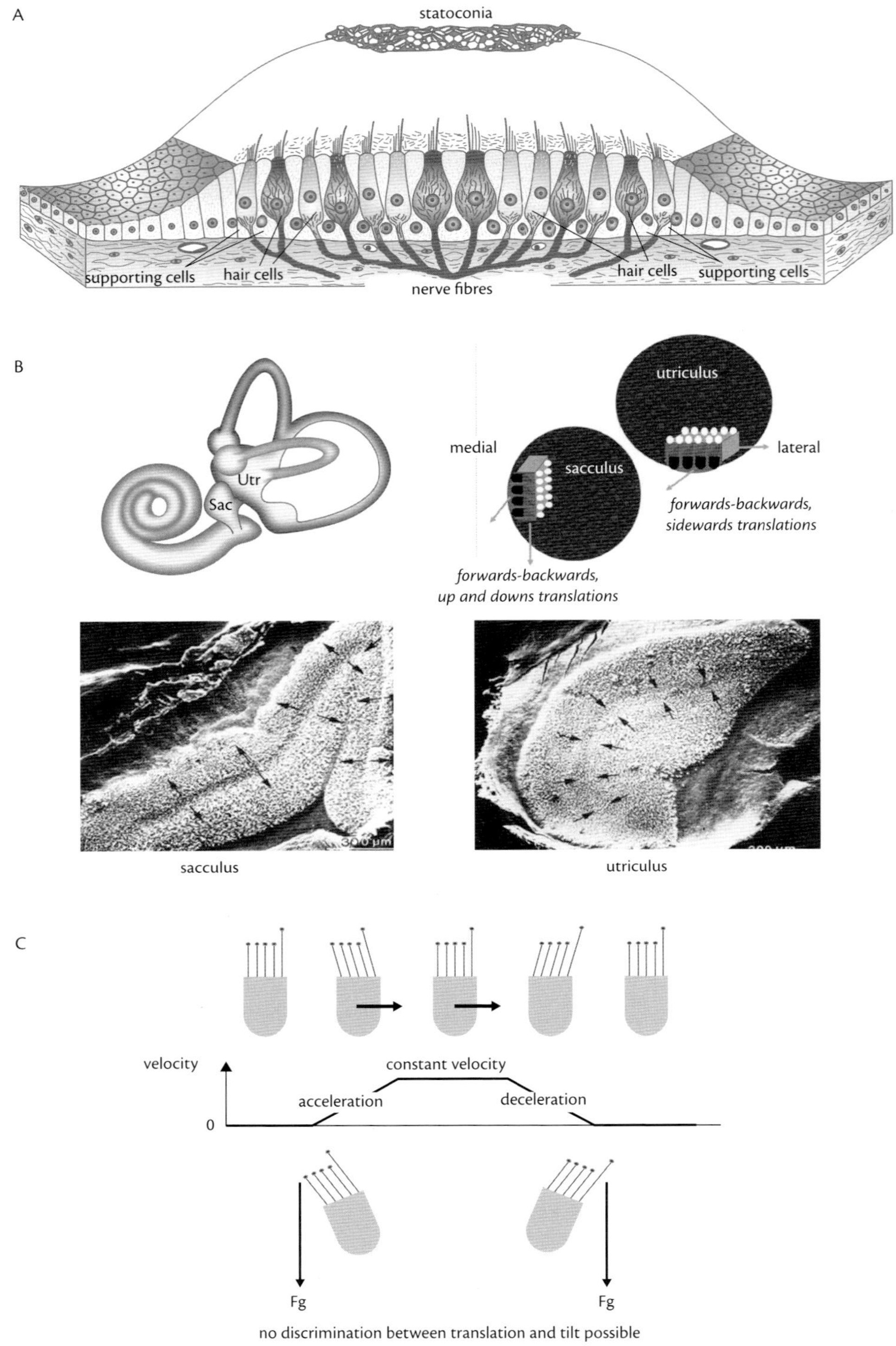

Fig. 1.12 (A) Schematic representation of the otolith organ, with the macula as sensory epithelium, the otolith membrane. (B) Orientation of the sacculus and utriculus in the labyrinth (upper left figure) and head (upper right figure); polarization direction of the hair cells in the sacculus (lower left figure) and utriculus (lower right figure). (C) Schematic deflection pattern of the cilia of the hair cells upon translation and tilt.

As indicated earlier, the sudden stopping of a rotating chair gives rise to after-sensations of a duration of 30–60 s due to the specific cupula mechanics and the velocity storage memory in the brain. In contrast, the otolith mechanics in combination with the lack of a specific related memory in the brain, explains that the sudden stopping of a long lasting linear movement only gives rise to a very short after movement sensation of less than a second. Based on delicate centrifuge experiments, masking any non-vestibular cues for tilt perception as much as possible, we observed that the static vestibular threshold for perception of tilt estimates about 2° which corresponds well with the linear deceleration thresholds of 10–20 cm/s² for perception of fore-aft

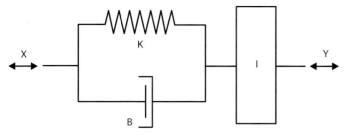

Fig. 1.13 Mechanical analogue of the otolith organ. B, viscous friction; I, otoconia mass inertia; K, elastic restoring force; x, position of the head; y, position of the otoconia; δ, x − y = relative displacement of the otolith membrane.

decelerations to the actual linear velocity direction using a linear sled (21).

Integration of canal and otolith sensitivity to detect rotation, translation, and tilt: multisensory aspects

Canals, maculae, vision, and propriocepsis all contribute to motion and tilt perception. Both the visual and somatosensory system can only process relatively slow body movements, and can be modelled with a low pass transfer function with a cut-off frequency of about 0.2 Hz. The otolith organs detect low-frequency linear accelerations (translations and tilt) up to about 1 Hz, the semicircular canals (semicircular canals) detect angular velocity between 0.1–10 Hz. Based on the physics already described we can estimate the frequency dependence of human canals and statolith organs as is depicted in Figure 1.15, but the reader should realize that this is more a speculation than even an

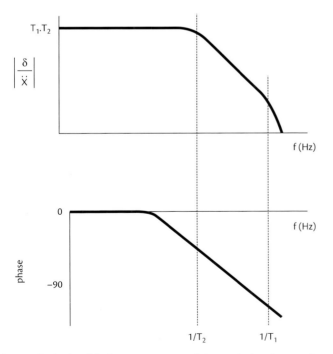

Fig. 1.14 Bode plot of the frequency response of the transfer function equation 4, representing the dynamic response of the mechanical analogue of the otolith organ. Upper trace: amplitude spectrum (gain = sensitivity). Lower trace: phase as a function of frequency.

estimation! At present these curves cannot be verified in detail due to limits of the diagnostic tests, in particular as it is still not possible to separately stimulate any of the five vestibular sensor systems per labyrinth. Also the vestibular responses quantified depend on many factors, including several cognitive factors (alertness, instruction) and the precise stimulus conditions used (in darkness versus in the light). The visual and somatosensory system support the otolith organs for detection of constant linear accelerations (28) and tilt perception at low frequencies, whereas the semicircular canals support the otolith organs in distinguishing true body tilt from translations at frequencies above 0.1 Hz (29, 30). If different sensory systems give conflicting or insufficient information, hindering the determination of the direction of gravity or distinguishing correctly between environmental and self-motion, motion sickness is quite common (31), especially in those individuals with substantial active vestibular projections to the autonomic nervous system (neuro-vegetative sensitivity). It has been hypothesized that a low sensitivity for motion sickness in specific individuals is much more correlated to less active or developed vestibular-autonomic projections than to better spatial orientation abilities.

Divers in deep unclear water or mountaineers covered by an avalanche (deprived from visual and proprioceptive cues), are unable to perceive their orientation, up or down, despite the fact that the physical principles under water still allow the otolith system to detect the orientation relative to gravitation vector. It is hypothesized that under these conditions, the perception of tilt angle or constant acceleration by the otolith system is neglected unless confirmed to full awareness by vision or proprioception to lead to an unambiguous perception. If not, tilt angles could lead to the perception of constant falling at different accelerations, as sometimes perceived as alertness decreases when falling asleep.

Pathology

Losing sensors for motion and tilt detection leads unavoidably to a loss of functionality and cannot be compensated for by other sensory systems which do not have sufficient sensitivity for the higher frequencies (Figure 1.15). Indeed, a permanent unilateral or bilateral peripheral loss leads to a permanent reduction of automation of image stabilization during head movement (oscillopsia, reduction of dynamic visual acuity (DVA)), a permanent loss of automation of balance ('no more talking while walking'), and a permanent loss of automation of spatial orientation (feeling insecure in situations with strong optokinetic stimuli such as busy traffic and supermarkets). The continuous and intense extra cognitive load needed for vision, balance, and orientation lead to fast fatigue as a major problem secondary to the permanent vestibular deficit.

A decrease in vestibular sensitivity with ageing, similar to perceptive hearing loss (presbycusis), is a likely to be a major cause of a decrease of DVA, reduced balance, and high incidence of falls in the elderly. Besides hair-cell degeneration, aging might also affect the body's stiffness and hydration, and thus also affects the vestibular physical quantities of both the semicircular canals and otolith organs:

- An increasing stiffness K increases the lower cut-off frequency (K/B) and decreases the gain (I/K) below this cut-off frequency.

- An increasing viscosity B decreases the higher cut-off frequency (B/I) and decreases the gain (I/B) below this cut-off frequency.

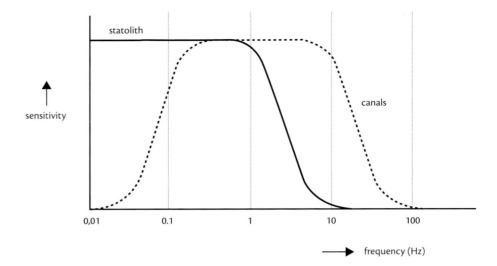

Fig. 1.15 Schematic representation of the different transfer functions of vision, somatosensory, and vestibular organs.

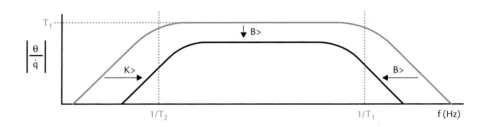

Fig. 1.16 Effect of increasing stiffness K and increasing viscosity on the transfer functions equations 2 and 4 of the semicircular canals.

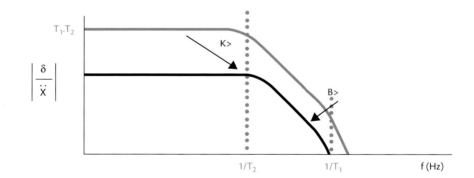

Fig. 1.17 Effect of increasing stiffness K and increasing viscosity on the transfer functions equations 2 and 4 of the otolith organs.

These effects are schematically shown in Figures 1.16 and 1.17. The vestibular system as a whole is thus disturbed as well, affecting the distinction between tilt and translation, because the semicircular canals' optimal range shifts to higher frequencies.

References

1. Janssen M (2011). *Vestibular exploration on advanced diagnostics and therapy*. Thesis, Maastricht University, the Netherlands.
2. Janssen M, Pas R, Aarts J, *et al.* (2012). Clinical observational gait analysis to evaluate improvement of balance during gait with vibrotactile biofeedback. *Physiother Res Int*, 17(1), 4–11.
3. van der Berg R, Guinand N, Stokroos RJ, Guyot JP, Kingma H (2011). The vestibular implant: quo vadis? *Front Neurol*, 2, 47.
4. van der Berg R, Guinand N, Guyot JP, Kingma H, Stokroos RJ (2012). The modified ampullar approach for vestibular implant surgery: feasibility and its first application in a human with a long-term vestibular loss. *Front Neurol*, 3, 18.
5. Guinand N, Guyot JP, Kingma H, Kos I, Pelizzone M (2011). Vestibular implants: the first steps in humans. *Conf Proc IEEE Eng Med Biol Soc*, 2011, 2262–4.
6. Guinand N, Pijnenburg M, Janssen M, Kingma H (2012). Visual acuity while walking and oscillopsia severity in healthy subjects and patients with unilateral and bilateral vestibular function loss. *Arch Otolaryngol Head Neck Surg*, 138(3), 301–6.
7. Hudspeth AJ, Corey DP (1977). Sensitivity, polarity, and conductance change in the response of vertebrate hair cells (the frog's sacculus) to controlled mechanical stimuli. *Proc Natl Acad Sci U S A*, 74(6), 2407–11.

8. Jeffery N, Spoor F (2004). Prenatal growth and development of the modern human labyrinth. *J Anat*, 71–92.

9. Melvill Jones G (1979). Biophysics of the peripheral end organs. In Wilson VJ, Melvill-Jones G (Eds) *Mammalian Vestibular Physiology*, pp. 41–76. New York: Plenum Press.

10. Yang A, Hullar TE (2007). Relationship of semicircular canal size to vestibular-nerve afferent sensitivity in mammals. *J Neurophysiol*, 98(6), 3197–205.

11. Feynman RP, Leighton RB, Sands ML (1989). *The Feynman lectures on Physics* (Commemorative ed). London: Addison Wesley Longman.

12. Kondrachuk AV, Sirenko SP, Boyle R (2008). Effect of difference of cupula and endolymph densities on the dynamics of semicircular canal. *J Vestib Res*, 18, 69–88.

13. Goldberg L (1966). Behavioral and physiological effects of alcohol on man. *Psychosom Med*, 28, 570–95.

14. Schuknecht HF (1962). Positional vertigo: clinical and experimental observations. *Trans Am Acad Opthalmol Otol*, 66, 319–31.

15. Rajguru SM, Ifediba MA, Rabbitt, RD (2004). Three-dimensional biomechanical model of benign paroxysmal positional vertigo. *Ann Biomed Eng*, 32, 831–46.

16. Rajguru SM, Ifediba MA, Rabbitt RD (2005). Biomechanics of horizontal canal benign paroxysmal positional vertigo. *J Vestib Res*, 15, 203–14.

17. Groen JJ, Lowenstein O, Vendrik AJH (1952). The mechanical analysis of the responses from the end-organs of the horizontal semicircular canal in the isolated elasmobranch labyrinth. *J Physiol*, 117, 329–46.

18. Selva P, Oman CM, Stone HA (2009). Mechanical properties and motion of the cupula of the human semicircular canal. *J Vestib Res*, 19(3–4), 95–110.

19. Grabherr L, Nicoucar K, Mast FW, Merfeld DM (2008). Vestibular thresholds for yaw rotation about an earth-vertical axis as a function of frequency. *Exp Brain Res*, 186(4), 677–81.

20. Goldberg JM, Fernandez C (1971). Physiology of peripheral neurons innervating semicircular canals of the squirrel monkey. I. Resting discharge and response to constant angular accelerations. *J Neurophysiol*, 34, 635–60.

21. Janssen M, Lauvenberg M, van der Ven W, Bloebaum T, Kingma H (2011). Perception threshold for tilt. *Otol Neurotol*, 32(5), 818–25.

22. Boumans LJ, Rodenburg M, Maas AJ (1980). Statistical evaluation of nystagmus in cupulometry. *ORL J Otorhinolaryngol Relat Spec*, 42(5), 292–303.

23. Huygen PL, Nicolasen MG (1985). Diagnostic value of velocity-step responses. *ORL J Otorhinolaryngol Relat Spec*, 47(5), 249–61.

24. Egmond AA van, Groen JJ, Hulk J, Jongkees LBW (1949). The turning test with small regulable stimuli; deviations in the cupulogram; preliminary note on the pathology of cupulometry. *J Laryngol Otol*, 63(5), 306–10.

25. Muller M, Verhagen JH (1988). A mathematical approach enabling the calculation of the total endolymph flow in the semicircular ducts. *J Theor Biol*, 134(4), 503–29.

26. David R, Berthoz A, Bennequin D (2011). Secret laws of the labyrinth. *Conf Proc IEEE Eng Med Biol Soc*, 2011, 2269–72.

27. Jongkees LBW, Groen JJ. (1946). The nature of the vestibular stimulus. *J Laryngol Otol*, 38, 529–41.

28. Vaugoyeau M, Viel S, Amblard B, Azulay JP, Assaiante C (2008). Proprioceptive contribution of postural control as assessed from very slow oscillations of the support in healthy humans. *Gait Posture*, 27, 294–302.

29. Green AM, Shaikh AG, Angelaki DE (2005). Sensory vestibular contributions to constructing internal models of self-motion. *J Neural Eng*, 2, S164–79.

30. Merfeld DM, Park S, Gianna-Poulin C, Black FO, Wood S (2005). Vestibular perception and action employ qualitatively different mechanisms. I. Frequency response of VOR and perceptual responses during translation and tilt. *J Neurophysiol*, 94, 186–98.

31. Bles W, Bos JE, de Graaf B, Groen E, Wertheim AH (1998). Motion sickness: only one provocative conflict? *Brain Res Bull*, 47, 481–7.

32. Valk WL, Oei ML, Segenhout JM, Dijk F, Stokroos I, Albers FW (2002). The glycocalyx and stereociliary interconnections of the vestibular sensory epithelia of the guinea pig. A freeze-fracture, low-voltage cryo-SEM, SEM and TEM study. *ORL J Otorhinolaryngol Relat Spec*, 64(4), 242–6.

33. Baloh RW, Honrubia V (2001). *Clinical Neurophysiology of the Vestibular System* (3rd ed). New York: Oxford University Press.

CHAPTER 2

Vestibular Physiology: How to be a Clinician and Yet Think Physiologically

Dominik Straumann

Introduction

One of the most gratifying aspects of neuro-otology derives from the fact that, based on a fine clinical analysis of eye movements, one can accurately infer the pathological mechanism and anatomical localization of a vestibular disorder. The reason for this 'diagnostic privilege' of neuro-otology is the existence of the vestibulo-ocular reflex (VOR), which connects the labyrinths with the eye muscles via extremely fast oligosynaptic brainstem pathways and somewhat slower multisynaptic pathways comprising the vestibulo-cerebellum.

Normal ocular motor behaviour is relatively stereotypic and therefore can be well described by 'laws' that govern the dynamic and kinematic properties of eye movements. By knowing these laws or stereotypic properties, the clinician can easily detect aberrations and also deduce what and where the underlying problem is located within the vestibular and ocular motor systems. Not all of these laws, however, are clinically relevant. Ewald's second law, for instance, is indispensable to understand the diagnostic value of the head impulse test, while Listing's law might be not be of great importance for distinguishing skew deviation from central trochlear nerve palsy.

Neurologists and otorhinolaryngologists who want to gain more insight in the subspecialty of neuro-otology often assume that they first should learn the functions of the different peripheral and central neuroanatomical structures and then try to relate the signs and symptoms gathered at the bedside to these structures. With this approach, the clinicians often lose sight of the wood for the trees and become frustrated. A more successful road to neuro-otology is based on phenomenology, in particular the movements of the eyes. First, one needs to become confident in estimating whether ocular motor behaviour ranges within normal limits, i.e. accords with the 'biological laws'. Second, with this knowledge, one can easily identify behaviour that violates these laws. Finally, being familiar with the mechanisms and neuroanatomical structures underlying the laws, one can make accurate diagnoses.

This chapter aims to discuss a potpourri of clinically relevant normal features, i.e. 'laws' or stereotypic properties, of vestibular-evoked eye movements. The choice of topics, which might appear rather arbitrary, was driven by the question to myself, what I should have comprehended before seeing my first dizzy patient as a resident (without first reading too many books and papers). Hopefully, this will help the clinician to think physiologically while he/she is investigating the patient with vertigo or balance disorders at the bedside and with vestibular tests. The neuroanatomical structures are only touched on in this chapter since they are delineated in different chapters throughout this book.

Frequency-dependence of the angular VOR

The VOR serves to stabilize the position of the eyes in space (Figure 2.1) (1). This mechanism in turn, leads to a stable projection of the visual world on the retina. During a head rotation of 15° to the right, the VOR ideally leads to a rotation of the eyes 15° to the left for fixation upon visual targets at infinity (Figure 2.2). In other words, gaze, i.e. eye position in space, remains unchanged when eye position relative to head mirrors head positions relative to space (Figure 2.3).

The relation between eye movements and head movements during head rotations is best described in the velocity domain, because the rotatory or angular VOR does not control absolute eye position but eye displacement as the critical factor for stabilizing the visual world on the retina. The so-called gain g is defined by coefficient of eye velocity $\dot{E}$ divided by head velocity $\dot{H}$. Since eye and head movements during the VOR are oppositely directed, head velocity is multiplied by (-1).

$$g = \frac{\dot{E}}{-\dot{H}}$$

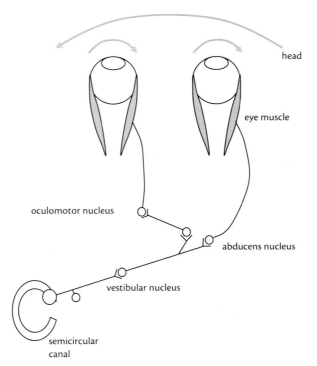

Fig. 2.1 Basic excitatory reflex arc from the left horizontal semicircular canal to the right lateral rectus muscle (3 neurons) and to left medial rectus muscle (4 neurons) when the head rotates to the left. The eyes move in the opposite direction to the head.

If eye velocity exactly mirrors head velocity, the gain remains at 1 during the entire head movement (Figure 2.4). This, however, is only true, if one assumes zero latency between head and eye movements. In fact, the latency of the VOR ranges around 10 ms (2, 3).

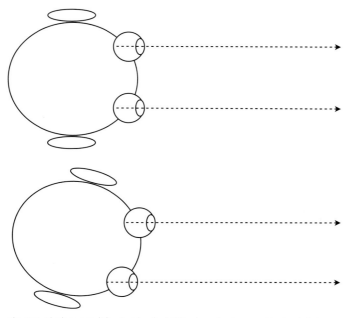

Fig. 2.2 Ideal gaze stabilization by the VOR when viewing an object at infinity. The line of sight is independent of head position.

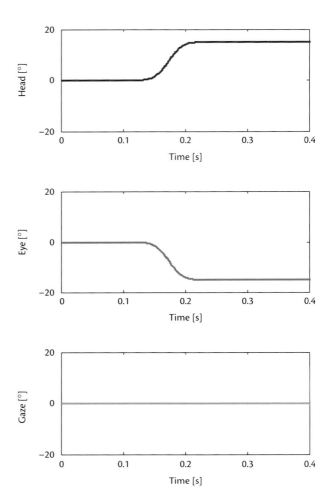

Fig. 2.3 Schematic position traces of head in space (top row), eye in head (middle row), and gaze, i.e. eye in space (bottom row) with ideal performance of the VOR and no latency.

The gain of the VOR is different during fast and slow head rotations: The higher the frequency of the head rotation, the higher the VOR gain (4). Only at very high head accelerations can a slight, but significant decrease of the VOR gain be measured (5). The low VOR gain at low frequencies can only be appreciated if head movements occur in total darkness or if subjects are wearing Frenzel glasses. In the light, the low VOR gain during slow head movements leads to slippage of the visual world on the retina. This signal is used by the smooth pursuit and optokinetic systems to increase the velocity of the eyes for almost complete stabilization of the eyes relative to space.

Using oscillations of a turntable about an earth-vertical axis in total darkness one can demonstrate the frequency-dependence of the VOR gain (Figure 2.5). The subject is seated on the turntable such that the rotation axis passes through the centre of the interaural line. Besides the decreasing gain, one observes an additional phenomenon with decreasing frequency: eye velocity increasingly leads head velocity. This can best be seen if one compares the moments when eye and head velocities peak. Thus, decreasing the frequency of the vestibular stimulus increases the phase lead.

This dependence of VOR gain and phase can be visualized by Bode plots (Figure 2.6), named after their inventor Henrik W.

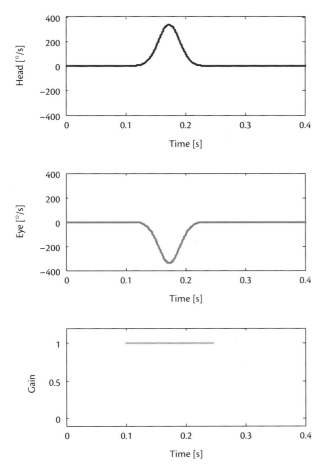

Fig. 2.4 Schematic velocity traces of the same movements as in Figure 2.3. The gain of the ideal VOR is 1.

Bode (1905–1985) (6). For each set of oscillations with a fixed frequency, one determines the gain (amplitude of eye velocity divided by amplitude of turntable velocity) and the phase (difference of between peaks of eye and head velocities in radian coordinates). Note that the turntable oscillations not only evoke the VOR, but also rapid eye movements that re-centre the eye, which results in nystagmus. Before analysing the VOR it is therefore indispensable to separate the quick phases of nystagmus (re-centring saccades) from the slow phases (VOR) and fill the missing gaps by interpolation or by overlaying multiple cycles of eye movements. Typically, gain g, phase φ (in degrees) and offset $\dot{E}_D$ are determined for every frequency f, by fitting a sine function to the data cloud of eye velocities $\dot{E}$ as a function of time:

$$\dot{E}(t) = g \bullet \sin\left(f \cdot 2\pi \cdot t + \varphi \cdot \frac{\pi}{180} \right) + \dot{E}_I$$

Angular velocity steps

To map out Bode plots for individual patients by turntable testing is too time-consuming as routine, since it requires oscillations at a minimum of 4–6 frequencies with enough cycles at each frequency to ensure stable sinusoidal fits. An elegant way to assess the effectiveness (gain and phase) of the angular VOR at a

wide range of frequencies with a single trial is by using velocity steps (7), e.g. by accelerating the turntable quickly (e.g. within 1 s) from 0°/s to 100°/s and then continue rotating at 100°/s (Figure 2.7).

If a velocity step were infinitely short, it would drive the VOR at all frequencies. With increasing duration of the acceleration phase, the upper range of tested frequencies decreases. But since another test, the head impulse test, assesses the high-acceleration VOR, the exact duration of the acceleration period of velocity steps on the turntable is less critical.

The slow-phases of vestibular nystagmus evoked by an angular velocity step reach their maximal velocity immediately after the turntable has completed the velocity step. Thereafter, sometimes after a short plateau, velocities decay exponentially from a maximal value $\dot{E}_0$ with a time constant T to zero or to an offset velocity $\dot{E}_D$ that represents the drift during spontaneous nystagmus.

$$\dot{E}(t) = \dot{E}_0 \cdot e^{-\frac{t}{T}} + \dot{E}_D$$

The gain g of the vestibular step response is defined by the maximal eye velocity $\dot{E}_0$ and the turntable velocity step $\dot{T}_{step}$:

$$g = \frac{\dot{E}_0}{-\dot{T}_{step}}$$

After the time constant T, eye velocity evoked by vestibular stimulation has decreased by 63.2%. The time for this eye velocity to decrease by 50%, the so-called half-life $t_{1/2}$, is computed by:

$$t_{1/2} = \ln(2) \cdot T$$

Since during constant rotation of the turntable, artefacts (e.g. signal noise by turntable slip-rings) may occur, many laboratories prefer to analyse the postrotatory nystagmus, i.e. the nystagmus that is evoked by stopping the turntable from a constant velocity. This deceleration, which can be enhanced by using turntable breaks, is equivalent to acceleration, if the period of constant turntable velocity in the dark is long enough to let nystagmus decay to its offset-level, which takes about 2 min.

Note again that vestibular turntable testing is always performed in total darkness. The completeness of darkness has to be checked regularly by sitting inside the setup and dark-adapt the eyes for at least 10 min. If then the examiner cannot see any light, the darkness in the setup is good enough for vestibular testing.

A time constant that is greater than the time constant given by the mechanical properties of the cupula (around 4 s) (8) indicates the presence of the a central neural mechanism in the brainstem and cerebellum, called velocity-storage mechanism (9), which integrates the velocity signals from the semicircular canals (Figure 2.8). The time constant of normal velocity storage for horizontal vestibular nystagmus ranges around 10–15 s. Absent (short time constant) or unusually strong (very long time constant) velocity storage is abnormal, but there are large interindividual differences. On Bode plots, velocity storage improves the gain and reduces the phase lead at 0.1 Hz and frequencies below (Figure 2.9).

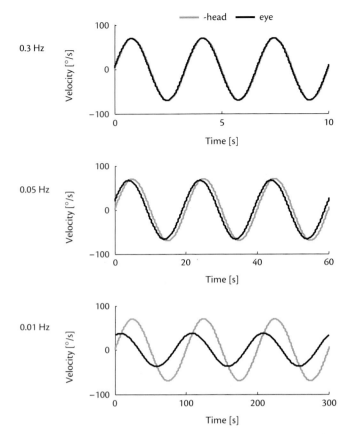

Fig. 2.5 Schematic velocity traces during whole-body turntable oscillation about an earth-vertical axis. Head velocity (= turntable velocity) is multiplied by (−1) for better visualization. Decreasing frequency leads to decreasing gain and increasing phase lead.

On a mathematical level, velocity storage can be achieved by either a feedforward leaky integrator (9) or by negative feedback (10) (Figure 2.10). The exact implementation of velocity storage in the brainstem and cerebellum, however, is still unknown. Not included in these original models is the fact that velocity storage depends on vestibular signals from both labyrinths. A total or partial peripheral vestibular loss results in a reduction of the vestibular time constant (11, 12), while lesions of the cerebellar nodulus and uvula may lead to an increase of the time constant (13).

Vestibular resting rate

A sudden peripheral vestibular loss leads to spontaneous nystagmus, which is predominantly horizontal, and to a turning sensation. These phenomena can be explained by the fact that there is tonic firing of vestibular neurons on both sides when the head is not moving (14). The so-called vestibular resting rates from both sides are centrally subtracted and the net resting rate is zero in the absence of head movements (Figure 2.11). If the tonic vestibular signal from one side is abruptly lost, the net resting rate becomes different from zero (Figure 2.12). This vestibular tone asymmetry is perceived as an ongoing head rotation to the intact side, which leads to compensatory eye drift to the affected side. Resetting saccades, in turn, are directed to the intact side, which leads to a spontaneous nystagmus in this direction. Central compensation mechanisms

lead to a decrease of spontaneous nystagmus over days (11). After 1–2 weeks most patients can suppress the remaining spontaneous nystagmus by visual fixation.

Alexander's law

Spontaneous nystagmus as a result of an acute peripheral vestibular loss regularly follows Alexander's law (15). This law describes the phenomenon that the slow-phase velocity of the nystagmus increases when gaze is moved in the direction of the quick phases. The exact mechanism of this phenomenon is not known; however, an explanation that postulates a change of the velocity-to-position integrator in the presence of a vestibular velocity bias is plausible (16).

To understand the function of the velocity-to-position integrator in eye movement control, one has to consider the two most relevant physical properties of the eye plant. These are elasticity and viscosity (17). In order to make a rapid eye movement and keep the eye in the new eccentric position, the neural signals to the contracting eye muscles must include a pulse to reach a high velocity against the viscosity and a step to counteract the elasticity that pulls the eye back to the straight-ahead position (Figures 2.13 and 2.14) (18). Neurally, the step signal is computed by mathematical integration of the pulse signal, thus the name velocity-to-position integrator (Figure 2.15) (19).

This integrator is not perfect, but its time constant, which is around 20 s, is sufficient to keep the eyes stable in eccentric positions. Reduction of the velocity-to-position integrator time constant leads to gaze-evoked nystagmus, i.e. the eyes drift back to their straight-ahead position and repetitive saccades bring the eyes back to their eccentric position (20). Usually, gaze-evoked nystagmus are caused pharmacologically (alcohol, medications, etc.) or by neural lesions in the brainstem or cerebellum, but the reduction of the reduction of the velocity-to-position integrator time constant may also be adaptive in the presence an eye drift due to an acute one-sided vestibular lesion (16, 21). Summing a vestibular eye drift, which is eye position independent, with a gaze-evoked centripetal drift results in Alexander's law (Figure 2.16). The benefit of Alexander's law for the patient is that the ocular drift becomes minimal when gaze is directed to the side of the vestibular lesion. If the ocular drift changes the direction with gaze directed opposite to the quick phases, the velocity-to-position integrator appears leakier than necessary for Alexander's law. In this case, one has to assume a lesion of the integrator itself, i.e. the horizontal spontaneous nystagmus is most likely central (22).

Alexander's law is not restricted to horizontal spontaneous nystagmus due to acute one-sided peripheral or central vestibular lesions, but also is found in the majority of patients with downbeat nystagmus (23), which is always central (see following section).

Mechanisms of downbeat and upbeat nystagmus

The most common central spontaneous nystagmus is downbeat nystagmus, which is usually chronic and due to degeneration of the cerebellar flocculi (24, 25). Conceptually, we may assume that the major projection to the pool of vertical motoneurons originates from neurons in the y-group and superior vestibular nucleus.

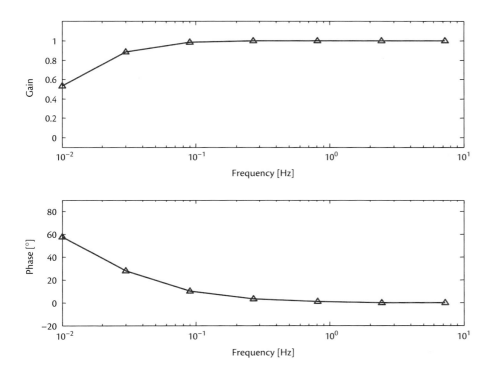

Fig. 2.6 Schematic Bode plot of a normal VOR. Gain (upper row) and phase (lower row) of elicited eye movements are plotted as a function of logarithmic head (= turntable) frequency. Decreasing frequency leads to decreasing gain and increasing phase lead.

These neurons fire predominantly when the eyes move upward; their activity is inhibited by neurons in the cerebellar flocculus, which fire predominantly when the eyes move downward (Figure 2.17A). Consequently, degeneration of floccular neurons leads to a disinhibition of neurons in the y-group and superior vestibular nucleus, which leads to upward ocular drift and hence downbeat nystagmus (Figure 2.17B) (26). Typically, downbeat nystagmus also follows Alexander's law since the degeneration of the floccular

neurons also affects the velocity-to-position integrator (23, 27). The upward velocity bias together with a vertical centripetal drift results in nystagmus slow-phase velocity that increases with increasing downgaze. Why drift velocity also increases with horizontal gaze eccentricity, is not known.

This scheme alone can not explain the occurrence of upbeat nystagmus if the pool of vertical motoneurons is disconnected from the y-group and superior vestibular nucleus due to a bilateral tegmental

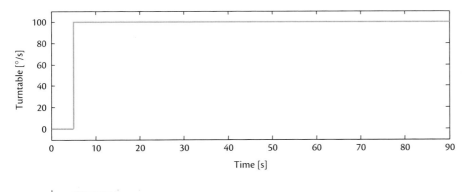

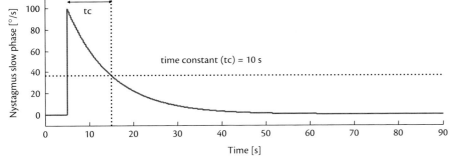

Fig. 2.7 Schematic velocity traces of turntable and ocular slow phases during a velocity step paradigm. During constant turntable velocity, slow-phase eye velocity decays exponentially with a time constant that is greater than the time constant of the semicircular canal cupula.

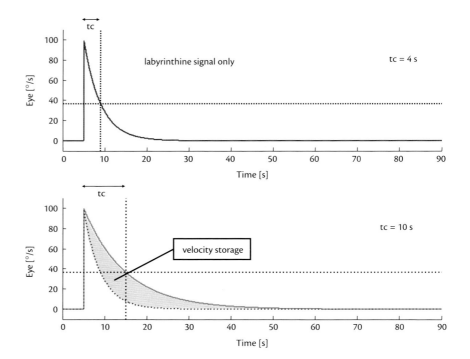

Fig. 2.8 Schematic slow-phase velocity decays after a turntable velocity step. In the absence of a velocity storage mechanism, the nystagmus fades away within a few seconds.

pontine lesion (Figure 2.17C). One needs to assume an additional relative hypoactivity of the elevator muscle motoneurons in the absence of these projections (28). This, in turn, causes the eyes to drift downward, which elicits upbeat nystagmus.

Upbeat nystagmus is also observed due to lesions in the caudal medulla oblongata. If one postulates an inhibitory pathway from the y-group and superior vestibular nucleus to the cerebellar flocculus, a disconnection of this pathway would disinhibit the floccu-

lar neurons and lead also to downward drift and upbeat nystagmus (Figure 2.17D).

Generally, upbeat nystagmus is transient, while downbeat nystagmus is chronic. Adaptive mechanisms of an intact cerebellar flocculus usually lead to a gradual decrease of downward drift (i.e. upbeat nystagmus), while no other adaptive mechanisms against upward drift (i.e. downbeat nystagmus) are available if the cerebellar flocculus itself is deficient.

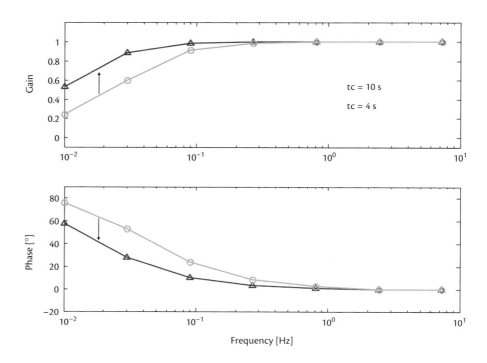

Fig. 2.9 Schematic Bode plots from turntable oscillation. At low frequencies, velocity storage increases the gain and reduces the phase lead of the VOR.

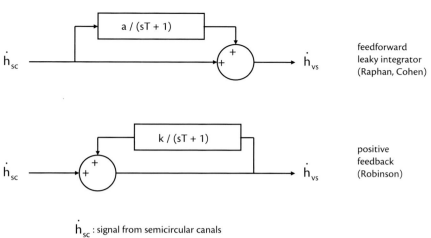

$\dot{h}_{sc}$: signal from semicircular canals

$\dot{h}_{vs}$: signal from velocity storage

Fig. 2.10 Simplified versions of the two models representing velocity storage. Mathematically the two models are equivalent.

Push–pull configuration of semicircular canals

The six labyrinthine semicircular canals form three pairs of angular acceleration sensors (Figure 2.18): 1) the right lateral canal and the left lateral canal; 2) the right anterior canal and the left posterior canal; 3) the right posterior canal and the left anterior canal. These pairs work in a push–pull fashion, that is, if one semicircular canal is excited, the corresponding canal in the contralateral labyrinth is inhibited (29). Both the excited ('pull') and the inhibited ('push') canals contribute to the overall vestibular signal, which represents approximately the difference of vestibular signals from the two labyrinths in semicircular canal coordinates; these approximately match the coordinates of extraocular muscle pulling directions (30). As a consequence, three-dimensional testing of the VOR in semicircular canal coordinates includes three principal planes: 1)

horizontal plane; 2) right-anterior-left-posterior plane (RALP); 3) left-anterior-right-posterior plane (LARP). In the Far East, RALP and LARP are usually replaced by other terms to rule out verbal misunderstandings.

Ewald's second law

To understand why it is possible to identify the side of a unilateral peripheral vestibular lesion at the bedside, one has to consider Ewald's second law (31). This law describes the phenomenon that excitation ('pull') of a vestibular semicircular canal is more effective than its inhibition ('push'). Thus, a hypofunction of a semicircular canal or the vestibular nerve not only decreases the overall vestibular signal during head rotation to both sides, it also causes a asymmetry of the response, such the response is more decreased during ipsilesional than during contralesional head rotation (Figure 2.19) (32).

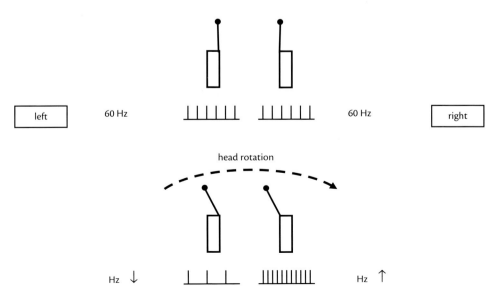

Fig. 2.11 Firing rate of vestibular neurons from the horizontal semicircular canals with the head not moving (upper panel) and during head rotation to the right. Relative to the resting rate, the head rotation causes an ipsilateral increase and a contralateral decrease of firing rate.

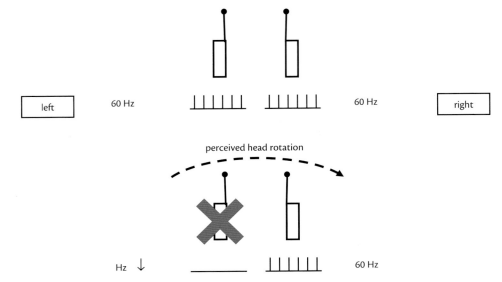

Fig. 2.12 Unilateral destruction of the labyrinth or the vestibular nerve causes leads to a reduction of the ipsilateral resting rate. The resulting asymmetry of firing rates leads to the misperception of a rotation to the contralateral side and ocular drift to the ipsilateral side (with contralateral quick-phases of nystagmus).

This asymmetry becomes greater the more the head accelerates (5, 33). Therefore, the most effective way to detect peripheral vestibular lesions is head thrusts, i.e. the head impulse test (see Chapter 8) (34). At the bedside, the clinician observes catch-up saccades after the head thrust. These catch-up saccades are larger after head thrusts towards the side of the lesion than after head thrusts to the other side. With a laboratory head impulse test, however, the gain of the VOR can be measured based on recorded velocity signals from the eye (search coil or video) and the head (search coil or accelerometer) (35, 36).

Some patients, probably those with excellent clinical recovery after a one-sided vestibular lesion, produce catch-up saccades that already occur during the head thrust. As a consequence, the head impulse test appears normal at the bedside and the gain of the VOR is only measurable during the early phase of the head movements applied in the laboratory test (5).

On a neurophysiological basis, Ewald's second law can be explained by the coexistence of two vestibular pathways: one pathway is linear in which excitation and inhibition is equally strong and firing rates of the inhibited sensor never reaches zero (inhibitory cut-off). The other pathway is non-linear, i.e. is more sensitive to high accelerations and shows only minimal contribution when inhibited (33).

Ewald's first law, by the way, describes the phenomenon that the eye moves approximately in the plane of a stimulated semicircular canal (31).

Tilt-translation dilemma

A linear movement of the head parallel to the interaural line with the subject in upright position (sitting or standing), so-called sway, has two effects on the position of the eyes. First, a horizontal rotation

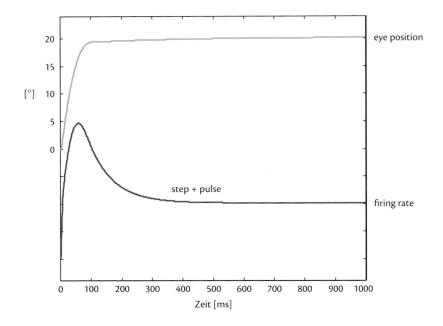

Fig. 2.13 Computer simulation of saccade. To speed up the eye despite the viscosity of the eye plant, the step of firing rate needs to be supplemented by a pulse of firing rate.

Superior rectus
motoneuron

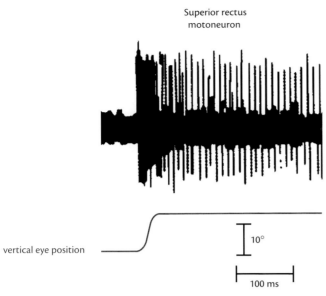

vertical eye position

10°

100 ms

Fig. 2.14 Single-unit recording of superior rectus neuron before, during, and after a saccade (juvenile rhesus monkey). The density of spikes during the saccade is higher than after the saccade.

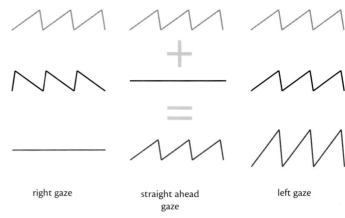

right gaze   straight ahead   left gaze
gaze

Fig. 2.16 Schematic eye position traces at right, straight-ahead, and left gaze. The ocular drift to the right as a result of the tonic vestibular asymmetry is eye-position independent (first row). Reduction of the velocity-to-position integrator time constant leads to a gaze-evoked centripetal drift (middle row). The summation of vestibular and gaze-evoked nystagmus leads to nystagmus obeying Alexander's law.

of the eyes in the opposite direction of the linear head displacement to keep a visual target stable on the retina; this response of the linear VOR depends on the distance of the target (no response for target at infinity, increasing response with decreasing distance) (37) and is enhanced by catch-up saccades in the light (38). Second, a binocular torsion that is a function of the inter-aural acceleration, whereby the upper poles of the eyes move in the direction of the acceleration vector (39). This latter ocular motor response is the same response that one observes when the head is kept in an opposite roll-tilted position (40). In this case, binocular torsion is called ocular counter-roll.

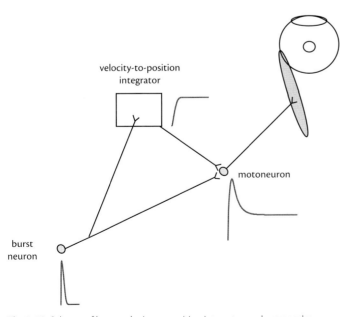

velocity-to-position
integrator

motoneuron

burst
neuron

Fig. 2.15 Scheme of burst, velocity-to-position integrator, and extraocular motoneurons.

According to Albert Einstein, linear accelerometers, such as the otolith organs, can not distinguish between gravity and linear acceleration (41). The brain, however, by processing the signals from the semicircular canals, is able to construct the appropriate self-motion perception even in total darkness (42), e.g. the appearance of a linear acceleration signal to the left together with a transient rotation signal to the right is correctly interpreted as a head roll-tilt to the right. Of course, this mechanism not only applies to this distinction between sway (interaural acceleration, also called heave by some authors) and roll-tilt (rotation about the earth-horizontal naso-occipital axis), but also to the distinction between surge (naso-occipital acceleration) and pitch-tilt (rotation about the earth-horizontal inter-aural axis). Heave (up-down) accelerations, however, cause no dilemma since during this movement the gravitoinertial vector is only changing its magnitude and not its orientation relative to the head. Sway and surge movements modulate mainly the utricular sensors (macula-orientated approximately horizontal in the head), while heave movements modulate mainly saccular sensors (macula-oriented approximately vertical the head). These otolith structures are both not planar, but curved (43).

The definition of linear VOR gain is not as straightforward as the definition of angular VOR gain, in which eye rotation is compared with head rotation. For quantifying the linear VOR, eye rotation has to be compared with head translation. This is typically done by computing the so-called ideal eye velocity $\dot{E}_i$, which is the derivative of the virtual trace of eye position necessary to keep a visual target on the fovea (44). Ideal angular eye velocity depends on the distance of the fixation target from the eye and the head movement. The gain g of the linear VOR is defined by coefficient of actual eye velocity $\dot{E}$ divided by ideal eye velocity $\dot{E}_i$:

$$g = \frac{\dot{E}}{\dot{E}_i}$$

If eye velocity coincides with ideal eye velocity, the gain remains at 1 during the entire linear displacement of the head,

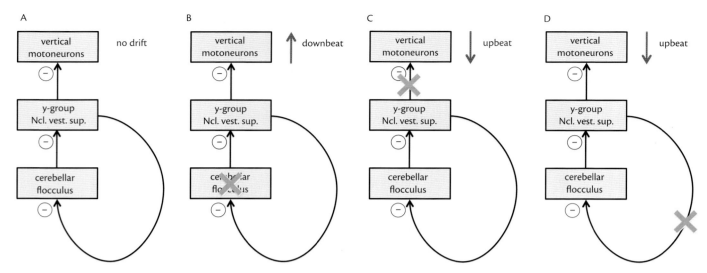

Figure 2.17 Schematic explanation of stable vertical eye position (A), downbeat (B), und upbeat (C, D) nystagmus. For details, see text.

if one shifts the eye trace backward in time by the latency. In humans, the latency of the linear VOR has been reported to be somewhat longer than the latency of the angular VOR (38, 45), but it is still unclear whether this difference is real or an artefact of computational methods used to determine onsets of head and eye movements. The gain of the linear VOR is usually around 0.5, i.e. for foveation of a visual target, the ocular motor system relies on enhancing smooth pursuit and catch-up saccades (Figure 2.19).

Multiaxis rotations

The vestibular system is not capable of correctly sensing rotations about more than one axis at the same time (46). This can easily be demonstrated by letting a subject rotate on an office chair with approximately constant angular velocity while the head is pitched back and forth (so-called pitch-while-rotating) (47). The subject becomes quickly nauseated and, if the eyes are closed, disoriented. The reason for this phenomenon can be demonstrated with the following experiment, which takes place in total darkness (48): a subject lying on the side in a turntable is rotated about the earth-vertical axis with constant velocity. After 1–2 min, the vestibular signal has faded away and the subject feels stationary. Then, the subject is rotated about the naso-occipital axis to the upright position, while the turntable is continuing to rotate about the earth-vertical axis. Thus, relative to the head of subject, the orientation of the rotation axis moves from interaural to head-vertical. This manoeuvre

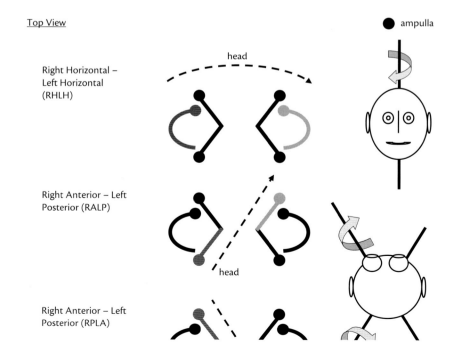

Fig. 2.18 Schematic push–pull configurations of the horizontal, anterior, and posterior semicircular canals.

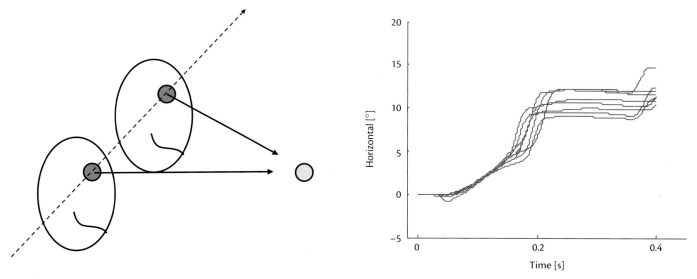

Fig. 2.19 Horizontal eye movements to the right elicited by translational head impulses to the left. Catch-up saccades are needed to refixate the space-fixed visual target after each head displacement.

represents an acceleration about the head's vertical axis and a deceleration about the head's interaural axis. These two signals are centrally summed to provide a perception of self-rotation (Figure 2.20) and a corresponding nystagmus about an oblique axis in the head's coronal plane. While this oblique rotation signal is still ongoing due to velocity storage, the otolith organs indicate stationary upright position. So the subject feels rotated about an off-earth-vertical oblique axis, but upright. This mismatch of signals causes nausea and disorientation. Multiaxis stimulation is sometimes also called Coriolis stimulation, although Coriolis effects in the strict sense apply to movements between different eccentricities in a rotating system and not combinations of rotations.

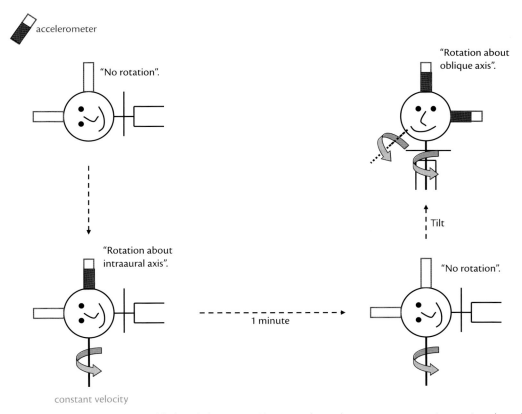

Fig. 2.20 Schema of a multiaxis rotation experiment. Simplified vestibular system with two angular accelerometers, one measuring rotations about the head-vertical axis, the other measuring rotations about the interaural axis. After the initial position (top left) the subject is continuously rotated about an earth-vertical axis. The multiaxis stimulus occurs when the subject is rotated upright (from bottom right to top right).

References

1. Lorente de Nó R (1933). Vestibulo-ocular reflex arc. *Arch Neurol Psychiatry*, 30, 245–91.

2. Aw ST, Haslwanter T, Halmagyi GM, Curthoys IS, Yavor RA, Todd MJ (1996). Three-dimensional vector analysis of the human vestibuloocular reflex in response to high-acceleration head rotations. I. Responses in normal subjects. *J Neurophysiol*, 76, 4009–20.

3. Collewijn H, Smeets JB (2000). Early components of the human vestibulo-ocular response to head rotation: latency and gain. *J Neurophysiol*, 84, 376–89.

4. Bockisch CJ, Straumann D, Haslwanter T (2005). Human 3-D aVOR with and without otolith stimulation. *Exp Brain Res*, 161, 358–67.

5. Weber KP, Aw ST, Todd MJ, McGarvie LA, Curthoys IS, Halmagyi GM (2008). Head impulse test in unilateral vestibular loss: vestibulo-ocular reflex and catch-up saccades. *Neurology*, 70, 454–63.

6. Van Valkenburg M (1984). In memoriam: Hendrik W. Bode (1905–1982). *Automatic Control, IEEE Trans Automat Contr*, 29, 193–4.

7. Bárány R (1907). *Physiologie und Pathologie (Funktions-Prufung) des Bogengang-Apparates beim Menschen*. Leipzig: F. Deuticke.

8. Dai M, Klein A, Cohen B, Raphan T (1999). Model-based study of the human cupular time constant. *J Vestib Res*, 9, 293–301.

9. Raphan T, Matsuo V, Cohen B (1979). Velocity storage in the vestibulo-ocular reflex arc (VOR). *Exp Brain Res*, 35, 229–48.

10. Robinson DA (1977). Vestibular and optokinetic symbiosis: an example of explaining by modelling. In Baker H, Berthoz A (Eds) *Control of gaze by brainstem neurons*, pp. 49–58. Amsterdam: Elsevier.

11. Fetter M, Zee DS (1988). Recovery from unilateral labyrinthectomy in rhesus monkey. *J Neurophysiol*, 59, 370–93.

12. Wade SW, Halmagyi GM, Black FO, McGarvie LA (1999). Time constant of nystagmus slow-phase velocity to yaw-axis rotation as a function of the severity of unilateral caloric paresis. *Am J Otol*, 20, 471–8.

13. Waespe W, Cohen B, Raphan T (1985). Dynamic modification of the vestibulo-ocular reflex by the nodulus and uvula. *Science*, 228, 199–202.

14. Goldberg JM, Fernandez C (1971). Physiology of peripheral neurons innervating semicircular canals of the squirrel monkey. I. Resting discharge and response to constant angular accelerations. *J Neurophysiol*, 34, 635–60.

15. Alexander G, Schlossmann A (Eds) (1912). Die Ohrenkrankheiten im Kindesalter, pp. 84–96. Leipzig: Verlag von F.C.W. Vogel.

16. Robinson DA, Zee DS, Hain TC, Holmes A, Rosenberg LF (1984). Alexander's law: its behavior and origin in the human vestibulo-ocular reflex. *Ann Neurol*, 16, 714–22.

17. Robinson DA (1964). The mechanics of human saccadic eye movements. *J Physiol*, 174, 245–64.

18. Robinson DA (1970). Oculomotor unit behavior in the monkey. *J Neurophysiol*, 33, 393–403.

19. Cannon SC, Robinson DA, Shamma S (1983). A proposed neural network for the integrator of the oculomotor system. *Biol Cybern*, 49, 127–36.

20. Cannon SC, Robinson DA (1987). Loss of the neural integrator of the oculomotor system from brain stem lesions in monkey. *J Neurophysiol*, 57, 1383–409.

21. Hess K (1983). Counterdrifting of the eyes following unilateral labyrinthine disorders. *Adv Otorhinolaryngol*, 30, 46–9.

22. Kattah JC, Talkad AV, Wang DZ, Hsieh YH, Newman-Toker DE (2009). HINTS to diagnose stroke in the acute vestibular syndrome: three-step bedside oculomotor examination more sensitive than early MRI diffusion-weighted imaging. *Stroke*, 40, 3504–10.

23. Straumann D, Zee DS, Solomon D (2000). Three-dimensional kinematics of ocular drift in humans with cerebellar atrophy. *J Neurophysiol*, 83, 1125–40.

24. Kalla R, Deutschlander A, Hufner K, *et al.* (2006). Detection of floccular hypometabolism in downbeat nystagmus by fMRI. *Neurology*, 66, 281–3.

25. Zee DS, Yamazaki A, Butler PH, Gücer G (1981). Effects of ablation of flocculus and paraflocculus of eye movements in primate. *J Neurophysiol*, 46, 878–99.

26. Marti S, Straumann D, Büttner U, Glasauer S (2008). A model-based theory on the origin of downbeat nystagmus. *Exp Brain Res*, 188, 613–31.

27. Glasauer S, Hoshi M, Kempermann U, Eggert T, Büttner U (2003). Three-dimensional eye position and slow phase velocity in humans with downbeat nystagmus. *J Neurophysiol*, 89, 338–54.

28. Pierrot-Deseilligny C, Milea D (2005). Vertical nystagmus: clinical facts and hypotheses. *Brain*, 128, 1237–46.

29. Szentagothai J (1950). The elementary vestibulo-ocular reflex arc. *J Neurophysiol*, 13, 395–407.

30. Ezure K, Graf W (1984). A quantitative analysis of the spatial organization of the vestibulo-ocular reflexes in lateral- and frontal-eyed animals—II. Neuronal networks underlying vestibulo-oculomotor coordination. *Neuroscience*, 12, 95–109.

31. Ewald JR (1892). *Physiologische Untersuchungen über das Endorgan des Nervus octavus*. Wiesbeden: J. F. Bergmann.

32. Baloh RW, Honrubia V, Konrad HR (1977). Ewald's second law re-evaluated. *Acta Otolaryngol*, 83, 475–9.

33. Lasker DM, Hullar TE, Minor LB (2000). Horizontal vestibuloocular reflex evoked by high-acceleration rotations in the squirrel monkey. III. Responses after labyrinthectomy. *J Neurophysiol*, 83, 2482–96.

34. Halmagyi GM, Curthoys IS (1988). A clinical sign of canal paresis. *Arch Neurol*, 45, 737–9.

35. Aw ST, Halmagyi GM, Haslwanter T, Curthoys IS, Yavor RA, Todd MJ (1996). Three-dimensional vector analysis of the human vestibuloocular reflex in response to high-acceleration head rotations. II. responses in subjects with unilateral vestibular loss and selective semicircular canal occlusion. *J Neurophysiol*, 76, 4021–30.

36. MacDougall HG, Weber KP, McGarvie LA, Halmagyi GM, Curthoys IS (2009). The video head impulse test: diagnostic accuracy in peripheral vestibulopathy. *Neurology*, 73, 1134–41.

37. Schwarz U, Busettini C, Miles FA (1989). Ocular responses to linear motion are inversely proportional to viewing distance. *Science*, 245, 1394–6.

38. Ramat S, Zee DS (2003). Ocular motor responses to abrupt interaural head translation in normal humans. *J Neurophysiol*, 90, 887–902.

39. Lichtenberg BK, Young LR, Arrott AP (1982). Human ocular counterrolling induced by varying linear accelerations. *Exp Brain Res*, 48, 127–36.

40. Nagel A (1896). Ueber das Vorkommen von wahren Rollungen des Auges um die Gesichtslinie. *Graefes Arch Clin Exp Ophthalmol*, 14, 228–46.

41. Einstein A (1907). Über das Relativitätsprinzip und die aus demselben gezogenen Folgerungen. *Jahrbuch der Radioaktivität und Elektronik*, 4, 411–62.

42. Angelaki DE, Shaikh AG, Green AM, Dickman JD (2004). Neurons compute internal models of the physical laws of motion. *Nature*, 430, 560–4.

43. Curthoys IS, Uzun-Coruhlu H, Wong CC, Jones AS, Bradshaw AP (2009). The configuration and attachment of the utricular and saccular maculae to the temporal bone. New evidence from microtomography-CT studies of the membranous labyrinth. *Ann N Y Acad Sci*, 1164, 13–8.

44. Ramat S, Zee DS, Minor LB (2001). Translational vestibulo-ocular reflex evoked by a 'head heave' stimulus. *Ann NY Acad Sci*, 942, 95–113.

45. Bronstein AM, Gresty MA (1988). Short latency compensatory eye movement responses to transient linear head acceleration: a specific function of the otolith-ocular reflex. *Exp Brain Res*, 71, 406–10.

46. Brown EL, Hecht H, Young LR (2002). Sensorimotor aspects of high-speed artificial gravity: I. Sensory conflict in vestibular adaptation. *J Vestib Res*, 12, 271–82.

47. Raphan T, Cohen B, Suzuki J, Henn V (1983). Nystagmus generated by sinusoidal pitch while rotating. *Brain Res*, 276, 165–72.

48. Bockisch CJ, Straumann D, Haslwanter T (2003). Eye movements during multi-axis whole-body rotations. *J Neurophysiol*, 89, 355–66.

CHAPTER 3

Eye Movements, Vision, and the Vestibulo-Ocular Reflexes

Alessandro Serra, Karim Salame,
Ke Liao, and R. John Leigh

Introduction: visual demands made of vestibular reflexes

The vestibulo-ocular reflexes (VORs) are essential for maintaining clear vision during locomotion. A striking demonstration of this fact is provided by the visual consequences of loss of the vestibular responses caused by aminoglycoside toxicity. These symptoms were originally reported by an anonymous physician, (1), who commented that 'during a walk, I found too much motion in my visual picture of the surroundings to permit recognition of fine detail. I learned that I must stand still in order to read the lettering on a sign'. The reason for such symptoms is that, during locomotion, head perturbations have a predominant frequency range of 0.5–5.0 Hz (2, 3), and visual processing is too slow (latency >70 ms) to stabilize gaze during such head movements. Conversely, the angular vestibulo-ocular reflex (aVOR) has a latency of less than 15 ms (4), and can generate eye rotations to hold the eye on target, and guarantee clear vision during locomotion.

Although the properties of aVOR in human subjects are well studied, head perturbations occurring during locomotion consist of both linear movements (translations) and rotations (3). The erect, straight-legged gait of humans induces substantial head translations in the vertical plane (referred to as heave or bob) (5), as well as side-to-side translations. The geometry of aVOR differs from that of linear or translational vestibulo-ocular reflex (tVOR), as is summarized in Figure 3.1 (discussed further later in the chapter), and dictates different properties of these two, distinct VORs. In this chapter, we approach properties and testing of aVOR and tVOR from the standpoint of how each reflex responds to visual demands by generating eye movements. Evaluation of each of the two VORs presents separate challenges. First, head-on-neck translations are more difficult to evoke at the bedside than rotations, as in the Halmagyi–Curthoys head impulse test (6). Second, although, the purpose and properties of aVOR are well defined, those of the human tVOR are still being clarified. Third, under natural condition, head rotations and translations normally occur together, when the properties of aVOR and tVOR may differ from when each reflex is separately tested. These issues are being addressed by rotating and translating subjects on moving platforms and measuring their head and eye movements with precision (7). Before describing these recent studies, we summarize the evaluation of vision during head movements at the bedside.

Clinical evaluation of VORs by testing vision

The clinical examination of the VORs is discussed in Chapter 12, but here we approach testing by considering their influence on vision. For aVOR and tVOR, the geometric rules are different: for aVOR, eye movements preserve clear vision of the environment (i.e. visual acuity), but tVOR seems more concerned with optimizing visual cues important for navigation.

Consider first aVOR. A standard test is to measure visual acuity with a test card of optotypes first with the patient's head stationary and then during small angular oscillations at about 1–2 Hz (which exceeds the range over which the visual system can respond). Normal subjects may show a slight degradation of visual acuity during such head rotations but patients who have vestibular insufficiency will report a substantial decline in visual acuity. A similar, objective, test is to view the patient's optic disc with an ophthalmoscope first with their head stationary, and then while they make small angular head oscillations at 1–2 Hz; the optic disc of the normal subject will remain stationary during head shaking, but the patients with an inadequate aVOR will show movements of the retina with each head rotation (8). Another objective demonstration is to perform the head impulse test and determine if aVOR holds the eye on target during a rapid head turn; for normal subjects the eye remains on target at the end of the head rotation but patients who have lost vestibular function must generate a corrective, visually-guided saccade.

Head translations (side-to-side) are more difficult to elicit at the bedside, but subjects can 'jog' up-and-down in place while they read a visual acuity card at about 15 cm; under these conditions, even in normal subjects, visual acuity declines compared with standing stationary. Using a moving platform and transient presentation of optotypes on a screen, it has been possible to confirm that visual acuity is substantially reduced during vertical translations compared with stationary visual acuity in normal subjects (9). Furthermore, if normal subjects' heads are abruptly translated in the interaural direction, then eye movements invariably fall short of those required to keep the line of sight pointing at a visual target (10). This behaviour suggests that tVOR is not normally concerned with generating eye movements to safeguard visual acuity during head translations. It also means that measurement of tVOR at the bedside using manual head perturbations may be less reliable than the angular head impulse test in distinguishing abnormal from normal behaviour, although asymmetries demonstrated in any one individual may be useful. Further insights into differences between aVOR and tVOR become apparent when normal subjects and patients with certain neurological disorders are tested using a moving platform and with precise measurements of eye movements. Such an approach allows application of pure rotations or translations, or combinations of head perturbations that approximate those occurring during locomotion. But first it is important to reconsider geometric factors that promoted the evolution of different properties of the two VORs.

How different visual geometry dictates different properties of aVOR and tVOR

Consider the geometry underlying aVOR and tVOR (Figure 3.1). On the one hand, aVOR acts to stabilize images across the whole visual field during head turns, and this can be achieved when viewing optical infinity. However, during viewing of a near target, eye rotations may be needed to rotate up to 30% more than the head rotations that induce them, because the rotational axis of the head lies posterior to that of the eyes (11). Therefore, under near-viewing conditions, there will be a small amount of relative motion between the image of a near target located on the retinal fovea, and images of the more distant background located on retinal periphery. On the other hand, tVOR is only really needed during near viewing (33); during far viewing, head translations do not induce retinal image slip, and tVOR is not necessary (Figure 3.1b). Geometry indicates that the eye rotations required to maintain foveal fixation of a target at 15 cm are over ten times greater than those required to fixate a target at 2 m. It follows that images of near and distant objects cannot be simultaneously held still on the retina during head translations. However, in older literature on tVOR, it is often assumed that the purpose of tVOR is to hold the image of a near target steady on the fovea. In fact, measurements of tVOR during head translation in humans do not substantiate this assumption. Thus, the *compensation gain* of tVOR (defined as eye rotational velocity/required eye rotational velocity to maintain foveal target fixation) is typically 0.6, or less (12, 13, 24–30). During combined head rotations and translations, a tVOR compensation gain of 0.6 is unlikely to be adequate to hold the eyes on a near target, and large amounts of retinal image slip (7–14 deg/sec) and oscillopsia—illusory motion of the near target—are reported as subjects walk on a treadmill (31, 32).

Quantitative comparisons of aVOR and tVOR in normal subjects and patients with neurological disorders

Here we summarize a series of our studies on aVOR and tVOR. Our initial goal was to study VORs as normal humans were subjected

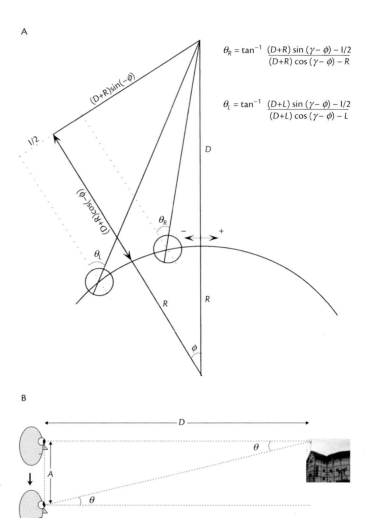

$$\theta_R = \tan^{-1} \frac{(D+R)\sin(\gamma-\phi) - I/2}{(D+R)\cos(\gamma-\phi) - R}$$

$$\theta_L = \tan^{-1} \frac{(D+L)\sin(\gamma-\phi) - I/2}{(D+L)\cos(\gamma-\phi) - L}$$

$$\theta = \tan^{-1} \frac{A}{D}$$

Fig. 3.1 (A) Geometry of the angular vestibulo-ocular reflex (aVOR), summarizing relationships between the angle of head rotation (ϕ), the radius of head rotation (R), the distance of the target from the centre of head rotation (R + D), interocular distance (I), target eccentricity (γ), and the rotation of the right eye (θ_R) required to maintain fixation of a stationary near target. Note that since the eyes do not lie at the centre of rotation of the head, the eyes must rotate more than the head during near viewing by as much as about 30%. (B) Geometry of the translational vestibulo-ocular reflex (tVOR). During vertical head translations (in the Z-axis, bob or heave), vertical eye rotations are required to hold the eyes on target. The magnitude (θ) of eye movements required to hold the foveal line of sight on the target is given by the equation at bottom, where D is the target distance, and A is the amplitude of the head translation. Note that during viewing a near target, larger eye rotations are required (by a factor of 10 or more). It follows that tVOR cannot generate eye rotations that hold images of far and near targets simultaneously still on the retina.

to combined translations and rotations in natural illumination, such as occur during locomotion, and to relate these properties to visual needs. We then studied VORs in patients with neurological

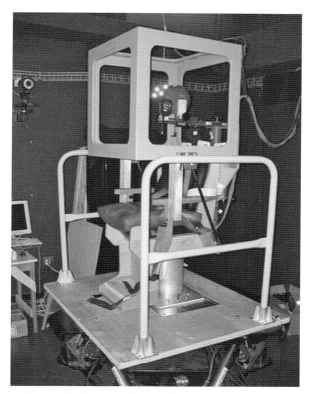

Fig. 3.2 Photograph of Moog platform used for testing. The attached cube held the field coils which allowed measurement of 3D eye rotations as subjects wore scleral search coils. The helmet served to stabilize the subject's head and reflective makers on it and the subject's face allowed measurement of head rotations and translations.

disorders that commonly lead to falls—progressive supranuclear palsy (PSP) and cerebellar ataxia.

The methodology of our approach to studying the VORs is described in detail elsewhere (7), and is briefly summarized here. Experiments were performed in ambient light, so that natural visual cues, such as motion parallax and relative size, were available. For safety reasons, one of the investigators monitored the subject on the platform, and could activate an emergency stop switch. Our subjects and patients sat in a chair on a Moog 6DOF2000E electric motion platform (Figure 3.2), which could move with six degrees of rotational and translational freedom through a range of +20° and +20 cm, with peak rotational acceleration of 400°/s², and peak linear acceleration of 5 m/s² (0.5 g). Belts secured the subject's torso and a snugly fitting skateboard helmet stabilized the subject's head. Head movements due to decoupling from chair or platform motion were measured.

Two main visual conditions were used to compare tVOR performance during heave versus combined heave-yaw under ambient illumination: 1) binocular viewing of a laser spot projected onto a wall at a distance of 2 m ('far target'), and 2) binocularly viewing of a 'near target' (a reflective ball, diameter 1 cm) suspended at a distance of about 17 cm in front of the left eye. All 20 normal subjects, including older individuals, were easily able to view these visual stimuli without refractive correction.

To determine the relative importance of vergence angle and viewing distance, subjects also viewed targets binocularly at 2 m, 40 cm, and 17 cm first directly and then with a 15- or 10-dioptre base-out

prism placed before the right eye; in this way, each stimulus was viewed binocularly at one distance with two different vergence angles. To determine whether tVOR behaviour in ambient lighting could be explained by the contribution of smooth visual tracking, subjects followed a moving visual stimulus, consisting of a grid subtending 25.6° horizontally and 18.6° vertically with a central dot, at a viewing distance of 110 cm. The stimulus moved sinusoidally, in the vertical plane through +5.6° at 2.0 Hz (peak velocity 70°/s), or through +2.8° at 2.0 Hz (peak velocity 35°/s).

Since prior studies indicate that tVOR does not keep the line of sight pointed at a stationary visual target, we estimated the ideal performance of the VORs by first applying three cycles of vertical translation at 0.2 Hz (typical amplitude +5.6 cm) followed, after a pause of seconds, by three cycles of horizontal rotation at 0.2 Hz (typical amplitude +6°). We assumed that our normal subjects could continuously fixate the visual target during these 0.2-Hz stimuli using smooth pursuit; thus their eye movements were those required to hold the line of sight on the object of regard.

Three-dimensional (3D) eye rotations were measured using the magnetic search coil technique (7). Linear and rotational movements of the chair frame and the subject's head were monitored by an infrared reflection system (Vicon Motion Systems, Los Angeles, CA). We measured gain of aVOR as eye-in-head rotational velocity/head rotational velocity. We measured tVOR performance in two ways. First, we calculated the responsivity of tVOR from eye rotational velocity/head translational acceleration (output/input). Note that while aVOR gain has no units, tVOR responsivity has units of degrees/second of eye rotation per metres/second² of head translation (stated as deg × s/m). We measured tVOR performance from the ratio: eye rotational velocity/required eye rotational velocity to maintain foveal fixation of the visual target (far or near), which we refer to as compensation gain (12, 13). Compensation gain allowed us to relate measured responses to the ideal response (1.0), assuming that the goal of tVOR is indeed to hold the line of sight on target. We similarly measured aVOR compensation gain. Thus, our studies tested the hypothesis that while aVOR compensation gain would be approximately equal to 1.0, tVOR compensation gain would not.

Studies of VORs in healthy subjects

We studied 20 healthy subjects, age range 27–72 years, median 55 years; eight were female (7). Representative responses are shown in Figure 3.3A, B, and results from all 20 subjects are summarized in Figure 3.4. As predicted by geometry (Figure 3.1B), tVOR responsivity (eye velocity/head acceleration) increased by a large amount (median increase was by a factor of 8.7) from far to near viewing (Figure 3.4A). Nonetheless, this was less than the calculated 'ideal' response to hold the foveal line of sight on the target. However, when we calculated compensation gain (Figure 3.4B), median values were 0.59 during viewing of the far target and 0.6 during viewing of the near target. These values were not substantially different from prior studies, even though we employed natural illumination, and we combined horizontal rotation with vertical translation. Thus, our subjects showed only a small increase in compensation gain during combined heave-yaw versus during simple heave (7). From these studies, we concluded that tVOR could not have evolved to hold the images of near objects steady on the fovea of the retina in humans. Before

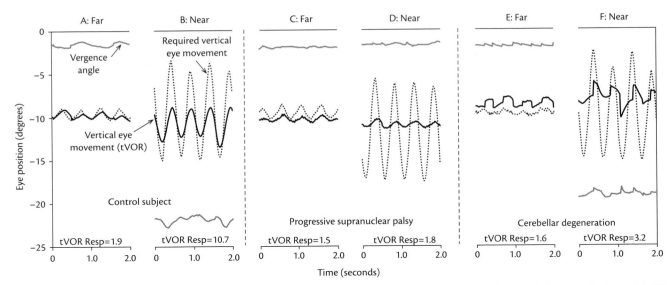

Fig. 3.3 Representative records from a normal subject (A, B), a patient with PSP (C, D), and a patient with cerebellar ataxia (E, F). At the bottom of each panel, tVOR responsivity (Resp) is stated in degrees × seconds/metre. Except for vergence (grey lines), individual traces have been offset in position to aid clarity of display. Positive values indicate downward and divergence movement. Note how tVOR (vertical eye rotation) increased during near viewing (17 cm) compared with far viewing (2 m) for the normal subject, but remained less than the eye movement required to keep the fovea (line of sight) pointed at the visual target (dotted lines). The PSP patient showed inability to converge at near, and tVOR did not increase. The patient with cerebellar ataxia was able to converge at near, but could not substantially increase tVOR responsivity. Required eye rotations were computed from measured head movements.

proposing an alternative hypothesis, we wanted to identify which visual factors determined tVOR behaviour. We first addressed the question of whether convergence angle or viewing distance was the more important determinant (7). Six subjects binocularly viewed targets at three distances either directly or with a base-out prism placed before one eye (to induce convergence). We found that viewing distance, not vergence angle, determined tVOR responses under conditions of ambient illumination. Next, we asked how much visual tracking, such as smooth pursuit, could be contributing to the overall response during head translation. We found, as expected, that smooth tracking of a large visual display moving vertically at 2.0 Hz had small gain and large phase shifts (typically 60°), which were three times greater than for tVOR (7).

Thus, although visual motion information seems important to determine the properties of tVOR, smooth tracking eye movements per se do not appear to contribute.

Based on this body of work, we proposed that tVOR evolved to optimize motion parallax during locomotion (7). It is possible for subjects to estimate the distance of objects in the visual environment while remaining stationary, using binocular cues (14). However, the ability to estimate relative distances of environmental objects is greatly increased when the observer's head translates along an axis perpendicular to the direction of motion through the environment. As noted in the introduction, vertical translations are prominent in human subjects because of their straight-legged bouncy gait (5). Side-to-side head translations also occur (3). It seems that these

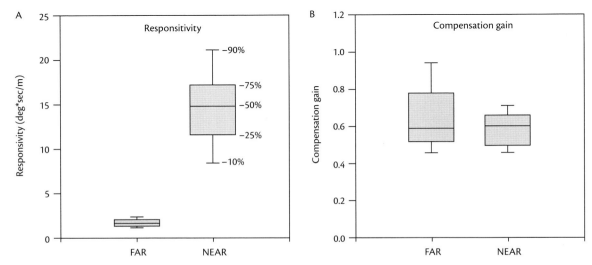

Fig. 3.4 Summary of tVOR responsivity (A) and tVOR compensation gain (B) for all 20 normal subjects during the three main viewing conditions (indicated at bottom). Data are illustrated as box plots with percentile values indicated. Note that although tVOR responsivity increases substantially from far to near viewing, compensation gain changes little.

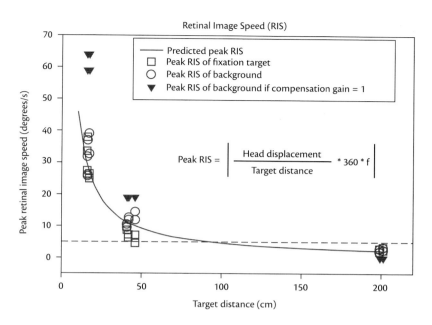

Fig. 3.5 Comparison of geometric prediction of peak retinal image speed (RIS) as a function of target distance for three subjects versus their measured peak retinal image speeds. The mean heave head displacement in these three subjects was +1.5 cm. Their mean compensation gain was 0.6, and the curve defined by the equation shown was accordingly scaled by a factor of 0.4. Squares indicate directly measured values of RIS of the fixation target at each of the target distances for three subjects for either pure heave or combined heave-yaw. There is generally good agreement, except that during viewing targets at 40 cm, peak RIS is lower than predicted due to greater compensation gain values. Circles indicate RIS of the background at 200 cm; although the direction of background image motion is opposite to that of the target image motion, the magnitude is similar. Inverted triangles indicate calculated RIS values of the background if tVOR compensation gain = 1.0; this is substantially increased during near viewing. The dashed horizontal line corresponds to a retinal image speed of 5°, above which visual acuity for high spatial frequencies will decline.

head translations provide potentially useful information on the distance of objects in the path of locomotion, provided the visual system can process their image motion. We assume that estimates of image speed will be optimized at lower image speed, because visual acuity is also optimized when image speed falls below about 5°/s (15). Thus, we proposed that it is in the brain's best interest to reduce image motion of *both* the near object of regard *and* the background, which may contain more distant objects lying near the path of locomotion.

From the measurements of head translations for our 20 normal subjects, it was possible to calculate the peak retinal image speed that will occur as subjects view targets over a range of target distances (16). We then scaled this curve by a factor of (1 − compensation gain) to estimate actual peak retinal image speed. For our group of normal subjects, compensation gain was close to 0.6, producing the curve shown in Figure 3.5 (7). To confirm our calculations, we measured directly the peak retinal image speed of fixation targets of three subjects, as they viewed targets located at 17 cm, 40 cm, or 200 cm; these data are plotted as squares in Figure 3.5. We also plotted in Figure 3.5 a dashed line corresponding to 5°/s, which is required for clear vision of objects with higher spatial frequencies (15, 17). Note that, for a compensation gain of 0.6, peak retinal image speed is less than 5°/s for target distances greater than 90 cm, corresponding to just one pace of a walk. Thus, only for very close viewing does retinal image speed increase to levels that degrade vision and cause oscillopsia. In Figure 3.5, we also plot the peak retinal image speed of the background lying at 200 cm for the three subjects (open circles); its speed was similar to that of the image of the fixation target (although opposite in direction). Finally, we estimated what motion of the background image would occur if tVOR did indeed perfectly compensate for head translations (compensation gain = 1.0) during view targets at the three distances; it is evident that, during near viewing, background image motion (inverted triangles,) would be expected to exceed 50°/s. These considerations led us to postulate that minimizing retinal

image motion of both near *and* distant objects might aid detection of motion parallax signals that are important for detecting relative distances of objects in the environment. If this is true, the human tVOR may have evolved to maintain compensation gain at a value of ~0.6 not to keep the eyes on target, but rather to optimize motion parallax estimates of the location of objects in the path of locomotion. This value also agrees with predictions of an optimization function that seeks to determine the best combination of image motion of a near target and distant background that will aid detection of relative motion of the two images so that their relative distances can be estimated (7). It also explains why the latency of tVOR (20–25 ms) is longer than that of aVOR (<15 ms); minimizing difference between two or more set of moving images (corresponding to several depth planes) is less likely to require tight regulation of responses than when aVOR minimizes motion of one set of images on the retina.

Abnormalities of VORs in neurological disorders leading to falls

After we had established the range of tVOR responses from normal subjects, we were able to study patients with neurological disorders. Our goal was to identify abnormal tVOR behaviour in patients who fall frequently. We selected patients with two disorders that commonly cause difficulty in walking: cerebellar ataxias and PSP.

It is known that the aVOR in cerebellar ataxias show inconsistent changes, and may sometimes be normal (18). One prior study of tVOR in cerebellar ataxia tested with transient translations along the interaural axis found that patients were unable to increase their responses during near viewing (19). We studied a group of eight patients with various cerebellar disorders and found similar results during sinusoidal heave stimulation (7). Representative records are shown in Figure 3.3E, F, and group results are summarized in Figure 3.6. Although patients could converge during viewing of a near target, they could only generate small increases in tVOR responses.

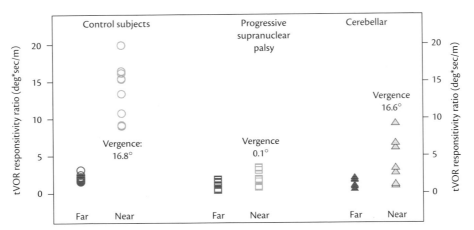

Fig. 3.6 Comparison of tVOR responsivity of nine older, healthy control subjects, nine patients with progressive supranuclear palsy (PSP), and eight patients with cerebellar ataxia during far (200 cm) and near (17 cm) viewing. Mean vergence angles are given during near viewing. Note how controls increase tVOR responsivity substantially from far to near, but PSP and cerebellar patients show no or small increases of responsivity at near. Vergence at near was similar for controls and cerebellar patients, but PSP patients were unable to converge.

PSP is a parkinsonian disorder characterized by frequent falls, vertical saccadic palsy, and dysphagia (18, 20, 21). Even in advanced stages of the disease, eye movements can still be elicited by turning the patient's head, indicating that aVOR is relatively preserved (22). Thus, there appears to be a paradox: PSP patients show substantial postural instability, suggesting early abnormalities of vestibulospinal reflexes, but some vestibulo-ocular reflexes continue to operate even in advanced disease. Convergence is impaired in PSP (18). We studied nine patients with PSP and compared their responses with nine age-matched healthy subjects (23). The PSP patients were unable to increase their tVOR responses at near. Representative responses are shown in Figure 3.3C, D and group data are summarized in Figure 3.6. Since they were also unable to converge their eyes, it could be argued that this was the cause of their inability to increase tVOR at near viewing. However, as our studies of normal subjects showed, convergence does not appear to be the key factor in setting tVOR responses at near viewing; the viewing distance seems more important. Rather, we argue that PSP patients are unable to direct their visual attention to a near stimulus, perhaps due to the midbrain involvement, and that this inability affects both tVOR and convergence. Studies of vestibular-evoked myogenic potentials (VEMPs) in PSP have shown reduced responses. Taken together with the reduced tVOR responses, this suggests that central otolithic mechanisms are impaired in patients with PSP, eventually causing falls. The combined defect of vertical saccades, convergence, and tVOR had led to a hypothesis that these defects in PSP reflect involvement of a newly evolved neural system concerned with coordination of gaze shifts in humans, who walk erect with their hands free.

Thus, on the one hand, our cerebellar patients could converge but could not increase tVOR responses during near viewing; on the other hand, our PSP patients could neither converge nor increase their tVOR responses during near viewing. Thus, different parts of the brainstem and cerebellum may contribute to setting tVOR appropriately for viewing distance. Thus, both patients with cerebellar ataxia and PSP may have impaired motion parallax, and this could cause difficulty in localizing objects in the path of locomotion and partly explain why these patients fall. Our studies employed only simple sinusoidal stimuli in one plane each for translation and rotation, with the goal of simulating locomotion. More systematic studies using a range of different frequencies and transient stimuli are likely to illuminate the role of the VORs during normal activities.

Summary

Clinicians routinely exam the aVOR and these tests rest on the assumption that the purpose of this reflex is to hold the eye on target during head rotations. In this way, motion of images on the retina is minimized and visual acuity is optimized. In contrast, clinicians seldom test tVOR, because this is more challenging at the bedside and its visual purpose is less well understood. We have summarized evidence to make the case that tVOR does not generate eye movements to hold the eye on target during linear head movements (translations). Rather the properties of tVOR are more suited to minimize image slip of near and distant objects so that visual cues of the locations of objects in the environment can be used to aid navigation. Abnormalities of aVOR and tVOR occur independently or in combination with peripheral or central vestibular disorders. New clinical tests of tVOR are needed.

Acknowledgements

Supported by NIH grant EY06717, the Office of Research and Development, Medical Research Service, Department of Veterans Affairs, NASA/NSBRI NA00208, and the Evenor Armington Fund.

References

1. (No authors listed) (1952). Living without a balancing mechanism. *N Eng J Med*, 246, 458–60.
2. Grossman GE, Leigh RJ, Abel LA, Lanska DJ, Thurston SE (1988). Frequency and velocity of rotational head perturbations during locomotion. *Exp Brain Res*, 70, 470–76.
3. Pozzo T, Berthoz A, Lefort L (1990). Head stabilization during various locomotor tasks in humans. I. Normal subjects. *Exp Brain Res*, 82, 97–106.
4. Maas EF, Huebner WP, Seidman SH, Leigh RJ (1989). Behavior of human horizontal vestibulo-ocular reflex in response to high-acceleration stimuli. *Brain Res*, 499, 153–6.

5. Massaad F, Lejeune TM, Detrembleur C (2007). The up and down bobbing of human walking: a compromise between muscle work and efficiency. *J Physiol*, 582, 789–99.

6. Halmagyi GM, Curthoys, IS (1988). A clinical sign of canal paresis. *Arch Neurol*, 45, 737–39.

7. Liao K, Walker MF, Joshi A, Reschke M, Leigh RJ (2008). Vestibulo-ocular responses to vertical translation in normal human subjects. *Exp Brain Res*, 185, 553–62.

8. Zee DS (1978). Ophthalmoscopy in examination of patients with vestibular disorders. *Ann Neurol*, 3, 373–4.

9. Cheng R, Walker MF (2011). Dynamic visual acuity during head translation. *Soc Neurosci Abstr*, 700.

10. Ramat S, Zee DS (2002). Translational VOR responses to abrupt interaural accelerations in normal humans. *Ann N Y Acad Sci*, 956, 551–4.

11. Viirre E, Tweed D, Milner, K, Vilis, T (1986). A reexamination of the gain of the vestibuloocular reflex. *J Neurophysiol*, 56, 439–50.

12. Ramat S, Zee, DS (2003). Ocular motor responses to abrupt interaural head translation in normal humans. *J Neurophysiol*, 90, 887–902.

13. Ramat S, Straumann D, Zee DS (2005). The interaural translational VOR: suppression, enhancement and cognitive control. *J Neurophysiol*, 94, 2391–402.

14. Howard IP, Rogers BJ (2002). Depth from motion parallax. In Howard IP, Rogers BJ (Eds) *Seeing in Depth, volume 2*, pp. 411–43. Toronto: I. Porteus.

15. Demer JL, Amjadi F (1993). Dynamic visual acuity of normal subjects during vertical optotype and head motion. *Invest Ophthalmol Vis Sci*, 34, 1894–1906.

16. Schwarz U, Miles FA (1991). Ocular responses to translation and their dependence on viewing distance. I. Motion of the observer. *J Neurophysiol*, 66, 851–64.

17. Carpenter RHS (1991). The visual origins of ocular motility. In Cronly-Dillon JR (Ed) *Vision and Visual Function. Vol 8. Eye Movements*, pp. 1–10. London: Macmillan Press.

18. Leigh RJ, Zee DS (2006). *The Neurology of Eye Movements (Book/DVD). Fourth Edition.* New York: Oxford University Press.

19. Wiest G, Tian JR, Baloh RW, Crane BT, Demer JL (2001). Otolith function in cerebellar ataxia due to mutations in the calcium channel gene CACNA1A. *Brain*, 124, 2407–16.

20. Steele JC, Richardson JC, Olszewski J (1964). Progressive supranuclear palsy. A heterogeneous degeneration involving the brain stem, basal ganglia and cerebellum with vertical gaze and pseudobulbar palsy, nuchal dystonia and dementia. *Arch Neurol*, 10, 333–59.

21. Litvan I (2005). Progressive supranuclear palsy. In Litvan I (Ed) *Atypical Parkinsonian Disorders. Clinical and Research Aspects*, pp. 287–308. Totowa, NJ: Humana Press.

22. Das VE, Leigh RJ (2000). Visual-vestibular interaction in progressive supranuclear palsy. *Vision Res*, 40, 2077–81.

23. Liao K, Wagner J, Joshi A, *et al.* (2008). Why do patients with PSP fall? Evidence for abnormal otolith responses. *Neurology*, 70, 802–9.

24. Bronstein AM, Gresty MA (1988). Short latency compensatory eye movement responses to transient linear head acceleration: a specific function of the otolith-ocular reflex. *Exp Brain Res*, 71, 406–10.

25. Israël I, Berthoz A (1989). Contribution of the otoliths to the calculation of linear displacement. *J Neurophysiol*, 62, 247–63.

26. Paige GD (1989). The influence of target distance on eye movement responses during vertical linear motion. *Exp Brain Res*, 77, 585–93.

27. Busettini C, Miles FA, Schwarz U, Carl JR (1994). Human ocular responses to translation of the observer and of the scene: dependence on viewing distance. *Exp Brain Res*, 100, 484–94.

28. Gianna CC, Gresty MA, Bronstein AM (2000). The human linear vestibulo-ocular reflex to transient accelerations: visual modulation of suppression and enhancement. *J Vestib. Res*, 10, 227–38.

29. Paige GD, Telford L, Seidman SH, Barnes GR (1998). Human vestibuloocular reflex and its interactions with vision and fixation distance during linear and angular head movement. *J Neurophysiol*, 80, 2391–404.

30. Tian JR, Mokuno E, Demer JL (2006). Vestibulo-ocular reflex to transient surge translation: complex geometric response ablated by normal aging. *J Neurophysiol*, 95, 2042–54.

31. Crane BT, Demer JL (1997). Human gaze stabilization during natural activities: translation, rotation, magnification, and target distance effects. *J Neurophysiol*, 78, 2129–44.

32. Moore ST, Hirasaki E, Cohen B, Raphan T (1999). Effect of viewing distance on the generation of vertical eye movements during locomotion. *Exp Brain Res*, 129, 347–61.

33. Angelaki DE (2004). Eyes on target: what neurons must do for the vestibuloocular reflex during linear motion. *J Neurophysiol*, 92, 20–35.

CHAPTER 4

Postural Control and the Vestibulospinal System

John H. J. Allum and Mark G. Carpenter

Introduction

Co-dependence of vestibular and proprioceptive inputs

It is quite well known in both animals and humans how leg proprioceptive inputs contribute to the recruitment of muscle responses via direct connections to lumbar motoneurons (1) from muscle stretch afferents. Very little is known about the corresponding processes for vestibular inputs. Although the vestibulospinal (VS) and reticulospinal tracts can excite motoneurons directly, they have more extensive connections to motoneurons via indirect pathways (2–4). How inputs from various semicircular canals and otoliths are distributed to these pathways and thence to spinal motoneurons is well established for the neck muscles (5), but not for muscles of the extremities (6). The information that is available is based on slow and rapid tilts of animals in roll and pitch planes (7, 8), vertical accelerations (9), and translations (10). While there is also some evidence of VS influence on human balance control, through the modulation of proximal and distal muscle activity (11–13), there are a number of analytical issues that must be overcome before the specific contribution of VS inputs to the recruitment of muscle responses maintaining human postural control can be identified. For example, unlike ocular reflexes, spinal motor control signals cannot be independently tested for the strength of the vestibular inputs. Other sensory influences, specifically proprioceptive inputs, have a far greater role in controlling the stability of the body than in the control of eye movements. Furthermore, these proprioceptive signals cannot be 'switched-off' like visual inputs (14, 15). When one source of proprioceptive input, for example, that from the ankle joints, is absent or deficient, others, at the knee or hip, become more influential (14, 15). Thus the study of balance control, with or without visual inputs, should always consider the relative roles, and co-dependence between vestibular and proprioceptive inputs.

Another issue that should be considered is that vestibulospinal reflexes (VSRs) originate from different first-order vestibular neurons and course along different brainstem pathways to spinal inter- and motoneurons, than those used by vestibulo-ocular reflexes

(VORs). Thus, it is to be expected that the contribution of the VS system to postural control during stance, gait, and recovery from perturbed balance will not be predictable from the amplitudes of VOR responses, nor have a similar time course of compensation for peripheral vestibular loss.

Methods of measuring balance control

Balance control can be divided into two types of tasks. Static balance control involves maintaining upright stance on a stable base of support while overcoming the downward forces of gravity. In contrast, dynamic postural control involves re-establishing upright equilibrium following a perturbation to stance caused by either external forces (i.e. movement of the support-surface, so-called dynamic posturography), or internal forces generated during voluntary movements (known as anticipatory postural adjustments). Note that a similar distinction applies to the control of balance during gait.

In the literature, generally two techniques for measuring static balance control have been described. One technique uses a forceplate to measure the forces generated at the feet to control sway of the centre of mass (CoM) within the base of support. From these forces estimates of the CoM sway can be made, assuming that the body moves as an inverted pendulum. Alternatively, body-mounted sensors can be used to quantify the actual displacement of the whole body CoM, or its individual segments, during postural sway. Body-mounted sensors have the added advantage that they can be used to measure balance during gait.

To measure balance recovery, a dynamic posturography system is used to perturb quiet stance in one direction or another. The influence of vestibular inputs on balance responses in different muscles can be tested using perturbations to stance induced by movements of the support surface. Such tests use instrumented moving support-surfaces to quantify balance control by recording the muscle reactions and body movements that follow the perturbation under different sensory conditions (16–18). These sensory manipulations can be used to emphasize contributions from a particular sensory system, for example, by having the subjects stand eyes-closed (removing visual inputs), moving the support surface in different directions, or servo-controlling it to reduce or enhance the efficacy of ankle proprioceptive inputs (11, 13, 16, 19).

In our work we have measured trunk sway with body-worn angular velocity transducers during both stance and gait tasks (20). The sensors are mounted near the body's CoM at lumbar segments L1–L3. These transducers have allowed us to quantify the effect of bilateral vestibular loss (BVL), track improvements in VS control following onset of a unilateral vestibular loss (UVL), and compare the rates of balance improvement following UVL between stance and gait tasks (21). The inclusion of both stance and gait tasks follows recommendations that a variety of such tasks should be used to quantify observations of gait deviations, loss of balance, and changes in postural stability when evaluating patients with vestibular deficits (22, 23).

As will become clear later in this chapter, body-mounted sensors provide a global, clinically oriented picture of the effect of vestibular loss on CoM stability during stance and gait, whereas dynamic posturography can be used to pinpoint the segment motion and muscles responses affected by vestibular loss. That is, how the VS system modulates muscle responses to achieve effective postural control.

Effect of vestibular loss on the control of stance and gait

How does bilateral vestibular loss and unilateral vestibular loss influence the control of stance and gait?

The difficulty with examining BVL patients in quiet stance (i.e. the Romberg test) is that these patients can adequately maintain their balance almost normally on a stable surface with their eyes open, and in some cases, with their eyes closed, given concentrated effort (24). To observe clearer differences in the balance control of BVL patients compared to those of healthy subjects it is better to have the patient stand on a foam support surface with eyes closed (see Figures 4.1 and 4.2). Typically, under this condition these patients fall slowly backwards often without realizing what is happening until they almost fall (see near falls marked in the traces of Figure 4.1C) because ankle proprioceptive inputs are not as effective in indicating body tilt on foam as on a firm surface, and particularly when vision is absent. As Weber and Cass (25) previously noted this task is a sensitive test for balance deficits of vestibular origin. Thus the results of Hegeman et al. (24) would also appear to indicate a direct influence of the vestibular system on CoM stability during quiet stance. However, the

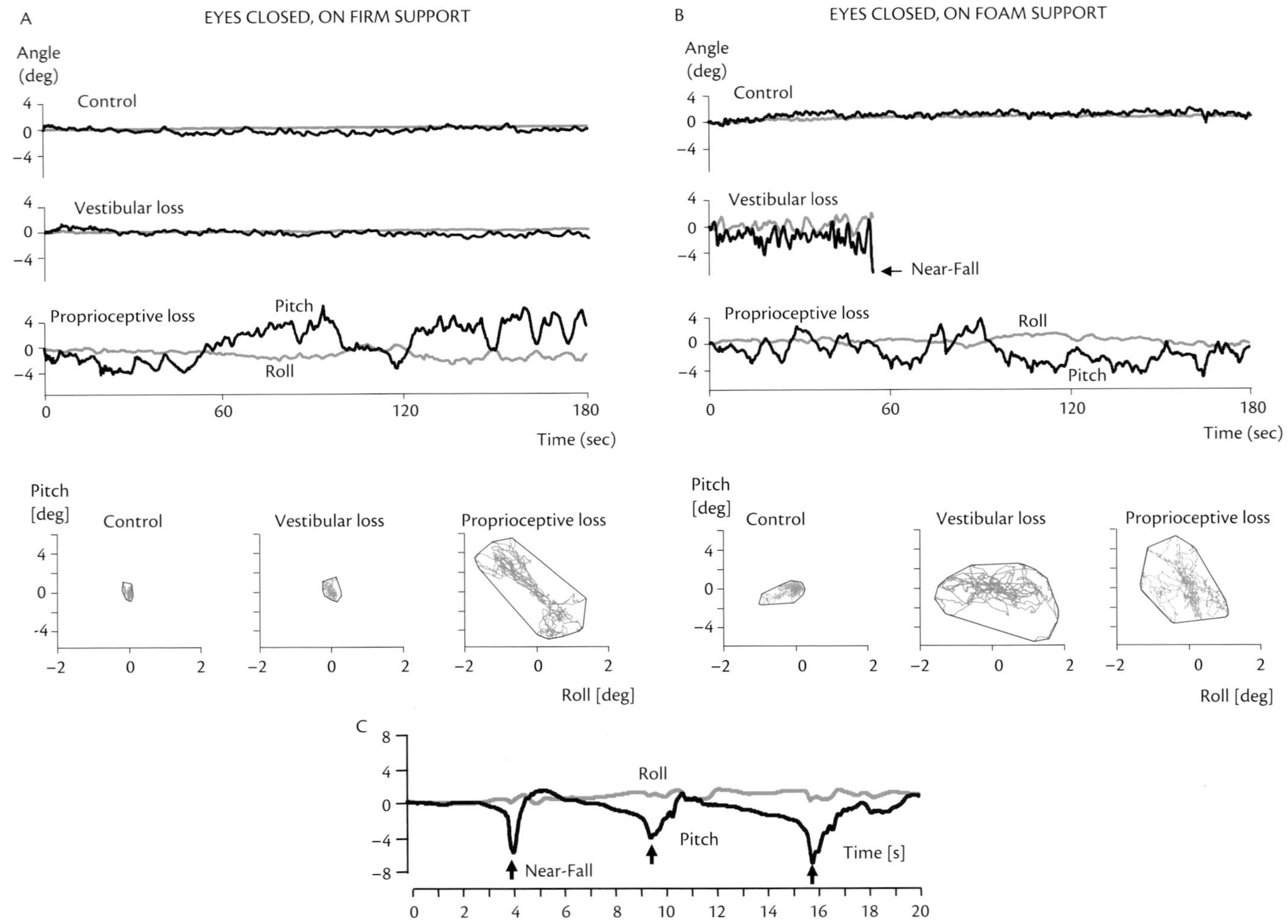

Fig. 4.1 Typical examples of pitch (dark green lines) and roll (light green lines) sway of the pelvis during standing with eyes closed on a normal firm floor (A) and on foam support surface (B) for a healthy control subject, a bilateral vestibular loss patient and a lower-leg proprioceptive loss patient. The lower three graphs of A and B are x–y plots showing roll (x-axis) versus pitch (y-axis) angle for the same subjects. Convex hulls have been drawn around the x–y plots. (C) shows a short segment with expanded time scale of the vestibular loss patient's traces eyes closed on foam. Data from Horlings et al. (26).

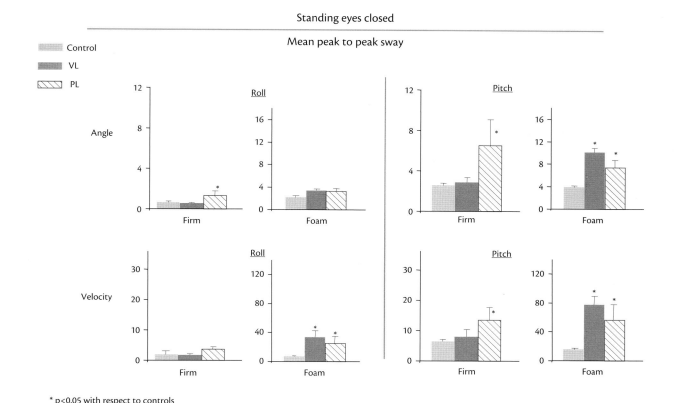

Fig. 4.2 Bar columns of group mean peak-to-peak pelvis sway angles and angular velocities in pitch and roll planes while standing with eyes closed on firm or foam support surface. Vertical bars indicate the standard error of the mean. Significant differences between the groups are indicated with: * p <0.05 for the six lower-leg proprioceptive loss patients versus the 26 age- and gender-matched controls, and for the six BVL patients versus controls. Data from Horlings et al. (26).

aforementioned instability on foam is not specific to bilateral or even unilateral vestibular loss (21) because a number of other diseases affecting the central nervous system (CNS) cause balance deficits which can be observed during this test (20). Among these diseases are those such as spinal cerebellar ataxia which affects the integration of proprioceptive and vestibular signals in the cerebellum (20). In addition, proprioceptive loss due to diabetes causes instability when standing eyes closed on foam. As an example, Figures 4.1 and 4.2 show that during this task both BVL and bilateral lower-leg proprioceptive loss (PL) patients have significantly increased CoM sway compared to controls. To establish test criteria specific for BVL it is necessary to distinguish the effects of other diseases from those of BVL, using additional tests. For example, abnormal sway behaviour in BVL subjects is restricted almost exclusively to the condition where proprioceptive inputs are unreliable and vision is absent (standing on foam with eyes closed), whereas PL subjects also have abnormal sway in roll and pitch directions when standing on a firm surface without vision (Figure 4.1A, B, and Figure 4.2), presumably because their ankle proprioceptive inputs are absent. When balance measures from these two stance conditions are taken into account, differentiating between vestibular loss (VL), PL patients, and controls is possible with a classification accuracy greater than 90% (26) with pitch angle and angular velocity for standing eyes closed on foam taking a prominent weighting in the separation of BVL patients from controls. This underlines the uniqueness of the BVL balance pathology and how well BVL subjects can compensate by using other inputs such as ankle proprioception and vision when these are available.

As will be described later in more detail for perturbations to stance using a rotating support surface, the backwards instability of BVL subjects during stance is to be expected (11, 19, 27). BVL subjects also show considerable instability to perturbed stance when the support surface is servo-referenced, thereby 'nulling' ankle angle inputs (11, 19). Thus, testing on a foam surface (a test which attempts to mimic servo-referencing) should reveal the dependence on the vestibular system for control of the CoM under these circumstances.

BVL subjects also suffer instabilities during gait tasks. When asked to walk 3 m eyes closed, pitch movements are larger than those of controls. During the get-up-and-go task (raising from a stool and walking 3 m) roll movements are greater than normal (24).

As documented in Figures 4.3–4.5, the instability suffered by UVL subjects at onset of their deficit is less than that of BVL subjects for stance tasks but greater for gait tasks (21). The stance tasks with eyes closed are, however, more unstable than for healthy controls. The gait tasks for which instability is greater are those either with simultaneous head movements (head rotations side-to-side or up and down) or walking eyes closed.

Recovery rates are different for stance and gait after unilateral vestibular loss

The compensation processes after BVL are difficult to follow because so few patients actually suffer an acute BVL. Usually the loss is first on one side then the other. Thus studying recovery from an acute UVL provides a clearer opportunity to monitor the compensation

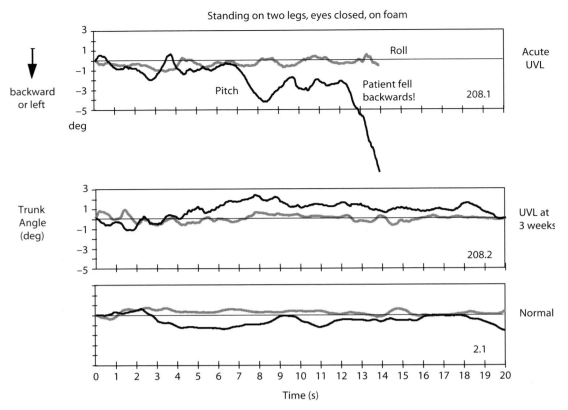

Fig. 4.3 Original traces of pitch and roll movements of the lower back (L1–3) recorded from a patient with a unilateral peripheral vestibular loss while standing eyes closed on a foam surface. The upper traces were recorded in the acute phase (within 5 days of loss onset), the middle traces 3 weeks later. These traces can be compared with those of a healthy subject of the same age and gender. Note the near fall backwards after 8 s until a final loss of balance control at 13 s in the upper traces. The recording duration of the other traces lasted the full 20 s. Data from Allum and Adkin (21).

processes involved. It is reasonable to test UVL patients who are presumably suffering from acute vestibular neuritis at three time points: at onset of the deficit and then 3 weeks and 3 months later (21). The 3-week interval can be justified based on reports that at this time point UVL patients recover normal control of stance (28–30), neurochemical changes associated with compensation are complete (31), and spontaneous nystagmus has subsided (32). The third test point at 3 months coincides with the time point when VOR responses to low acceleration (below 100°/s²) body rotations have achieved normal symmetry and gains (33, 34).

As Figures 4.3 and 4.4 show, UVL patients improve rapidly over 3 weeks for the two-legged stance task, standing eyes closed on foam. Slightly less rapid improvement can be noted for one-legged stance tasks. Specifically, stance time on one leg requires more than 3 months to reach normal durations (21). Trunk sway amplitudes, but not task durations, of simple gait tasks such as walking while turning the head, or walking eyes closed, reach normal values after 3 months (21). In contrast, trunk sway for more complex gait tasks such as walking tandem steps on foam or walking up and down stairs (see Figure 4.5) are not within normal limits at 3 months.

A number of conclusions can be drawn from results shown in Figures 4.3–4.5. Firstly, the lack of vestibular inputs from one ear is compensated more rapidly for stance compared to gait tasks. This signifies that using stance tasks alone to determine recovery from vestibular loss will provide a misleading underestimate of the patient's recovery. Secondly, it appears that for simple gait tasks,

patients aid their recovery by performing the task more slowly, presumably also stiffening their trunk control in order to reduce trunk sway. A similar mechanism of compensation has already been noted when gait tasks of the elderly were compared to those of the young (35, 36). Thirdly, for those tasks that inherently involve control of roll oscillations coupled with gaze control in planning future gait steps, such as walking tandem steps or up and down stairs, UVL subjects appear unable to control trunk roll oscillations within normal limits at 3 months. The difference for these complex gait tasks compared to the mainly pitch control of simple gait tasks suggests that trunk roll control has a different rate of compensation compared to trunk pitch control. This latter finding supports evidence that trunk roll and trunk pitch motion are controlled differently by the CNS (13, 37) due to differing trunk dynamics in these planes, especially with aging (38, 39).

The question arises whether the differing rates of recovery for stance and gait tasks parallel the rates of recovery observed with VOR function. VS and VOR neural pathways are no longer common beyond the vestibular nuclei, even if there may be functional relationships between the two. Thus, deficiencies in VS pathways during gaze fixation would need to be compensated for by enhanced VOR control and vice versa, suggesting that two simultaneous, but independent, compensation processes may well occur. For example, because both the level of spontaneous nystagmus (32, 40) and the stance instability on two legs (Figures 4.3 and 4.4) improves dramatically after 3 weeks it is tempting to believe that these two recovery processes are linked. The sway velocities recorded for

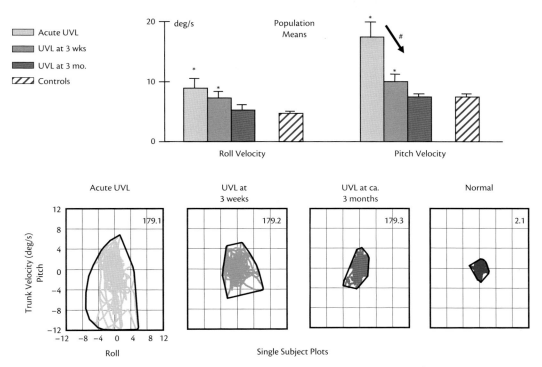

Fig. 4.4 Population means (and standard errors of the means) of peak-to-peak trunk angular velocities of subjects with an acute vestibular loss (UVL) and healthy controls while performing the task of standing on foam with eyes closed. The means were from 28 acute UVL subjects, 26 of these at 3 weeks, and 20 at 3 months. These subjects were compared with 100 age- and gender-matched controls. Significant differences to controls are marked with *, and significant changes over time with #. Note the velocities larger than controls for the first weeks after the acute onset of UVL. The lower part of the figure shows x–y plots of roll versus pitch velocity from typical subjects. Data from Allum and Adkin (21).

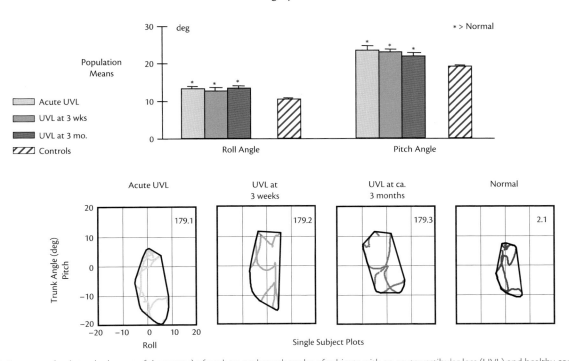

Fig. 4.5 Population means (and standard errors of the means) of peak-to-peak trunk angles of subjects with an acute vestibular loss (UVL) and healthy controls while performing the task of walking up and down a set of stairs consisting 2 steps up and down. For details of the figures see the legend to Figure 4.4. Note that the angle deviations remain larger than controls for the 3 months of follow-up after the acute onset of UVL. The lower part of the figure shows x-y plots of roll versus pitch angles from typical subjects (same subjects as in Figure 4.4). Data from Allum and Adkin 2003.

stance tasks even under difficult conditions (foam support surface and eyes closed) are less than 7°/s, that is of the order of the level of spontaneous nystagmus slow-phase velocity during the acute stage of the UVL. This level of spontaneous nystagmus presumably represents the bilateral static imbalance in afferent vestibular fibres caused by the UVL. Such an imbalance would make the detection of the small sway deviations involved with two-legged stance more difficult and lead to increased trunk sway.

Once the static imbalance due to UVL has been compensated for, the dynamic imbalance will still be prevalent in the VOR causing saturated responses for head and trunk movements towards the deficit side (34, 41). Linking these changes to the changes in gait stability observed in UVL patients is difficult for a number of reasons. Even though the rotating chair velocities observed for trunk sway of UVL patients are roughly equal to the velocities that have been used to test the VOR responses in such patients, the rates of compensation of VOR reflexes appear to be different in different planes with vertical canal VOR recovery being faster (33). Furthermore the more rapid improvement for gait tasks with horizontal head rotation compared to those with vertical head pitching (21) is counterintuitive to the differing rate of improvement for the VOR in these planes. If anything, the discrepancy between these findings indicates that compensation rates may be different for the VOR and the VS system.

One aspect that might be common between VOR and VS responses concerns the lack of compensation for high frequency (41, 42) compared to low-frequency VOR responses (33, 34). This would imply that gait tasks with larger and more rapid trunk (and head) movements (reaching 100°/s) when walking up and down stairs (see Figure 4.5), would more likely drive the remaining vestibular afferents into saturation and fail to provide adequate VS control. At 3 months after onset of a UVL, the results illustrated in Figure 4.5 indicate such a lack of compensation. Similarly, eye movement responses to rapid head turns do not acquire normal compensatory movements many months after an UVL imposed surgically (41). Therefore, tests after 3 months would be required to know if UVL patients eventually acquire normal control of the CoM for complex gait tasks compared to the VOR.

Summarizing, recovery rates for VS control of gait movements following vestibular afferent loss appear to be different for the pitch and roll planes, and considerably different from VOR response recovery rates.

Directional aspects of vestibular contributions to balance corrections

Characteristics of pitch and roll balance corrections after vestibular loss

Vestibular loss causes considerable instability when the CoM is perturbed backwards and/or into roll. As shown in Figures 4.6 and 4.7, during a pitch plane, toe-up, rotation of the support surface,

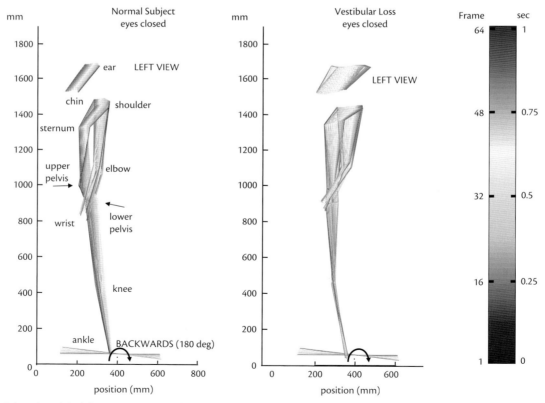

Fig. 4.6 (Also see Colour plate 1.) Stick figure representation of the movements of a normal and a bilateral vestibular loss (BVL) subject following a 7.5°, 60°/s backwards rotation of the support surface. Both subjects stood with eyes closed. Eighteen infrared Optotrak markers were placed on the body and 3 on the rotating support surface to track movements. The 64 time frames, recorded over 1 s, are indicated by the colour code. Blue frames mark the start of the recording, red the end. The platform rotation started at frame 6. To create the stick figure, marker movements in response to 8 identical stimuli were averaged, and then marker positions on a segment were joined. Note the backwards falling tendency in the vestibular loss subject and contrast this with the forward leaning of the normal subject. Data from Allum et al. (12).

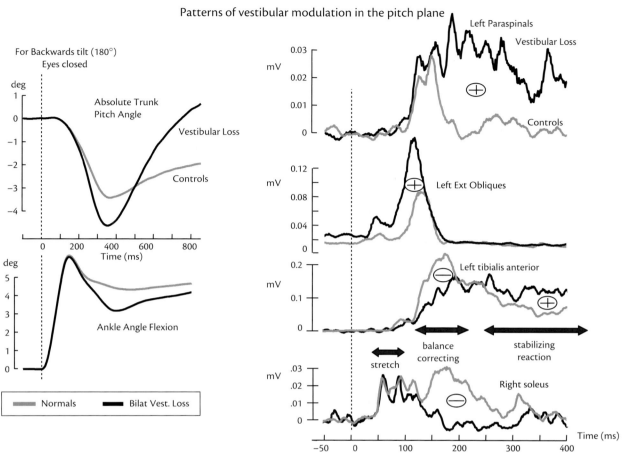

Fig. 4.7 Population pitch directed responses of 16 control and 6 bilateral vestibular loss subjects under eyes closed conditions for a toe up (180°) backward tilt of the support surface. Each subject response was repeated eight times. The vertical dotted line at 0 ms marks the onset of the stimulus (first deflection of platform angular velocity). On the left, plots are shown of trunk pitch angle and ankle dorsi-flexion angle over 800 ms. Note the correspondence with the stick figure of 7, with greater trunk movement and failure to brake backwards induced falling at the ankle joint. On the right, responses from a number of leg and trunk muscles are shown for the first 400 ms. Differences between the populations responses are marked. Note the reduced amplitudes in leg muscles and increased responses in trunk muscles with vestibular loss. Data from Allum et al. (12).

the body moves essentially as two links. The legs are initially rotated backwards by the platform rotation, while the trunk and pelvis, together are rotated slightly forward to counter the backward displacement of the COM. Compared to controls, VL subjects respond to the same backward support surface tilts with greater backward rotation of the leg, and increased forward pitch of the trunk followed by increased backward pitching of trunk (Figure 4.7). The final backwards tilt of the trunk causes a near fall. Underlying these biomechanical changes, VL subjects demonstrate decreased activity in the leg muscles, including tibialis anterior and quadriceps (11, 43) which is needed to counter the backward rotation of the legs induced by the platform. This is coupled with an initial increase in trunk flexor activity (i.e. abdominals), followed by increased late trunk extensors activity (i.e. paraspinals; Figure 4.7). There is little difference in the first 400ms of the responses with eyes open. Later stabilizing action driven by visual inputs prevents a fall when visual inputs are present (27, 44).

When the support surface is tilted laterally, the initial movement of the platform drives the uphill leg upwards, causing a roll of the pelvis toward the downhill side, while the trunk rotates in the opposite (uphill) direction due to joint coupling. The uphill knee

is rapidly flexed to stabilize the body with respect to the tilted platform, while the downhill leg is extended. Vestibular loss causes the trunk and CoM to rotate more downhill than is the case for healthy age-matched controls (Figures 4.8 and 4.9). As shown in Figures 4.8–4.10, there appears to be three underlying biomechanical causes for this instability. Firstly the uphill knee does not flex sufficiently, secondly the downhill knee has less extension (see Figure 4.10), and thirdly the uphill external oblique trunk muscles first over-react holding the trunk uphill and then a subsequent antagonist reaction in the downhill paraspinals moves the trunk into a roll downhill (see Figure 4.9). This reaction of the trunk muscles is very similar to that observed for pitch in BVL subjects—first excessive movement in the direction of motion initially induced by the stimulus, and then an instability in the opposite direction (see Figure 4.9). Lack of knee flexion may be a result of the excessive activation observed in the uphill quadriceps, thereby resisting normal flexion by knee flexors (see Figure 4.9). No reduction in knee flexion activity has been observed (unpublished observations, Grüneberg and Allum, 2005).

The available evidence suggests that the central control of responses to roll and pitch perturbations is separately organized in

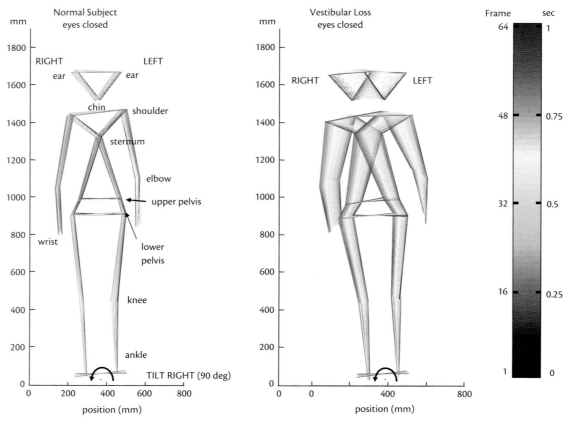

Fig. 4.8 (Also see Colour plate 2.) Stick figure representatives of body segment movements to right tilt of the support-surface in a typical VL and control subject under eyes closed conditions. For details of the figure refer to the legend of Figure 4.6. The views are from in front of the subjects. Note the similar arm and leg positions for the two subjects prior to tilt and tendency of the BVL subject to fall to the right. Data from Allum et al. (12).

man (13, 38). It is important to bear this information in mind when considering how vestibular and proprioceptive signals are combined to provide adequate balance corrections in pitch and roll. As a comparison of trunk angle traces in Figures 4.7 and 4.9 shows, an earlier stimulus-induced trunk roll compared to pitch is part of the biomechanical response of the body to the tilt perturbation on the support surface even when the stimulus is a combined roll and pitch tilt (38, 45, 46). As the stimulus-induced trunk roll motion occurs earlier than that of trunk pitch, one assumption is that the balance control centres located in the CNS require separate processing loops to generate balance corrections arresting unstable body motion in the roll and pitch planes (13). For example, provided that appropriate sensory information is available, it could be assumed that roll balance corrections would be generated first because roll motion occurs first. In fact, balance corrections of body motion in the pitch and roll planes begin simultaneously with onsets of 90–120 ms across many body segments (13, 38). Therefore it appears that balance command centres permit the roll instability of the trunk to continue well after the onset of roll movement in favour of generating roll and pitch balance correcting commands simultaneously across many segments. While this may be a factor underlying the greater roll than pitch plane instability in VL subjects, it is possible, as we will argue below that this instability occurs because the appropriate sensory signals required to generate balance corrections involve different types of processing in the roll and pitch directions.

Characteristics of vestibular sensory signals contributing to balance corrections

In order to focus on those signals that are most likely to contribute sensory inputs to balance corrections, the timing and amplitude of initial proprioceptive signals arising from muscles spanning ankle, knee, hip and lumbo-sacral joint needs to be examined along with head accelerations in pitch and roll planes which would be sensed by the vestibular system. Thereby, new insights into triggering and modulating aspects of proprioceptive and vestibular signals required for generating balance corrections in the roll and pitch planes can be obtained (12). It can be assumed that a significantly robust correlation between rotation velocity of a joint and short latency stretch reflex activity in a muscle spanning that joint would imply that central balance control centres would receive proprioceptive information from that joint at times dependent on transmission times of the fastest (Ia) afferents involved (14, 47). Examples of such responses are shown for ankle and trunk muscles in Figures 4.11 and 4.12, respectively. At the same time head accelerations can be measured, ideally with gyroscopes and linear accelerometers, thereby providing information on signals sensed by vestibular sensory systems as shown for vertical head linear and head roll angular acceleration traces in Figures 4.11 and 4.12 respectively. If the proprioceptive and vestibular sensory signals arrive sequentially and can be processed sequentially then replacement of an absent signal (here assumed to be a vestibular signal) may be easier than if parallel processing is

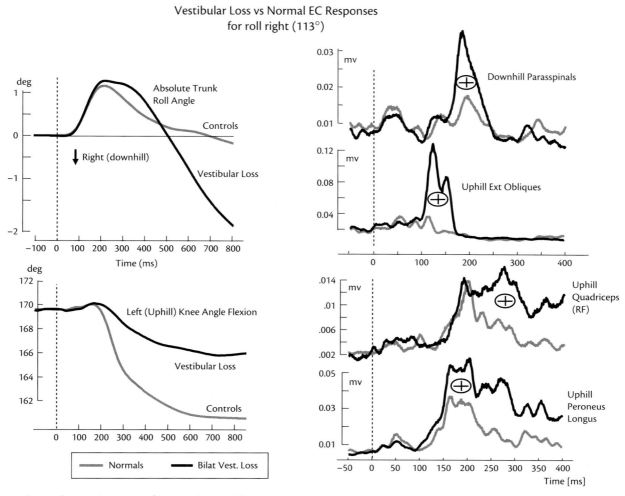

Fig. 4.9 Population roll-directed responses of 16 control and six bilateral vestibular loss subjects under eyes closed conditions for right (113°) tilt of the support surface. Each subject response was repeated eight times. The vertical dotted line at 0 ms marks the onset of the stimulus (first deflection of platform angular velocity). On the left, plots are shown of trunk roll angle and knee flexion angle over 800 ms. Note the correspondence with the stick figure of Figure 4.8, with greater trunk movement and failure to flex the uphill knee sufficiently. On the right, responses from a number of leg and trunk muscles are shown for the first 400 ms. Differences between the populations responses are marked. Note the increased amplitudes in leg muscles and increased responses in trunk muscles with vestibular loss. Previously unpublished data from Grüneberg and Allum, 2005.

required. Thus it could be expected that the direction with parallel processing would be the most unstable with vestibular loss.

Timing of sensory signals contributing to pitch and roll directed balance corrections

When a perturbation to upright stance occurs, the question arises as to when sensory signals elicited by the perturbation reach the CNS, and further, whether the times of arrival imply that these signals can be processed sequentially or simultaneously.

Pitch rotation of the support-surface is transmitted as a vertical linear acceleration to the head with a short delay of 10 ms (see Figure 4.12). Among the six head linear and angular accelerations present (12), the vertical linear acceleration provides the best vestibular sensory signal in terms of amplitude and polarity for pitch perturbations. In contrast, ankle proprioceptive inputs reach the CNS much later. Taking the onset of the stretch reflex in ankle muscles as the time to reach the CNS (assuming the time taken for the reflex response to travel back to the muscle from the spinal

cord is the same as that up to the CNS) this proprioceptive information will be present in the CNS at 46 ms. The proprioceptive information from the trunk will also be later than the head movement information as the trunk first starts to pitch forward or backward some 50 ms later. This difference in sensory transmission times suggest that processing these signals in the planning of an appropriate balance-correcting pitch response may occur sequentially.

Thus, we would argue that, in the pitch direction, proprioceptive and vestibular information is processed independently. This would allow VL subjects to use other proprioceptive information instead of vestibular information to successfully maintain balance in pitch. One such alternative signal might originate from load receptors in the spinal column registering the upward or downward thrust of the support-surface with pitch (48). The relative long delay, between the normally present vestibular input and proprioceptive input, suggests that alternative sources of vertical body acceleration signals could easily be integrated into the modulation of proprioceptive signals from the ankle joint, if vestibular signals were

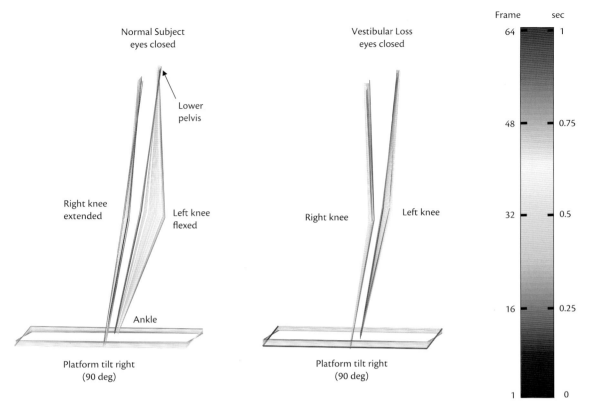

Fig. 4.10 (Also see Colour plate 3.) Stick figure representations of the knee flexion and extension movements following a right tilt of the support surface. On the left a normal subject and on the right a BVL subject, both standing with eyes closed. The views in the figures are from slightly in front (8°), slightly raised (4°) and from the right. Note the normal uphill knee flexion and downhill knee extension is reduced in the BVL subject. Same subjects as in Figure 4.9. For further details refer to the legend of Figure 4.6. Data from Allum et al. (12).

absent. Nonetheless, even if alternative proprioceptive inputs are used in the event of vestibular loss, responses from these patients are still deficient (Figure 4.7). Poor pitch balance control remains. We postulate that this arises because VL subjects tend to weight ankle inputs more heavily (49) but not heavily enough to replace the absent excitatory vestibular influences. There is also a need to reduce the weighting of trunk proprioceptive inputs in the absence of vestibular inhibitory influences, because otherwise the trunk motion is sensed as larger than it is and an overreaction occurs. The result for the legs and the trunk is a greater orientation of the body to the support surface tilt rather than to the vertical. That is the BVL subjects fall backwards like an inverted pendulum instead of flexing at the hips.

Proprioceptive roll information arrives at the CNS almost simultaneously with vestibular roll information. This is because roll plane perturbations elicit head movements later than pitch perturbations (compare traces in Figures 4.11 and 4.12), with roll accelerations of the head commencing around 31 ms (see Figure 4.11). This signal offers the best vestibular signal, in terms of amplitude and polarity for a roll perturbation (12). At the same time, the roll tilt is transmitted to the pelvis, with the legs acting as a parallelogram. Thereby, rotation of the pelvis with respect to the legs and trunk occurs, leading to stretch and unloading responses in gluteus medius and paraspinal muscles at 28 ms (see Figures 4.9 and 4.11). Later responses would arrive from the stretched peroneus muscles. Thus the time difference between the arrival of vestibular and proprioceptive roll

sensory inputs is much shorter (3 ms as shown in Figure 4.11) than that for pitch inputs. The small difference in the case of roll may lead to a restricted choice of alternative vestibular-like sensory signals for roll motion with vestibular loss, assuming that in roll the CNS would still parallel process sensory information in order to generate roll-directed balance corrections.

Based on this proposal, the roll sensory information can only be interpreted when the incoming sensory signals are combined. Given the distributed nature of the proprioceptive inputs best related to the pitch and roll stimuli (pitch at the ankle, roll at the hip and lumbo-sacral joints) and the timing of vestibular responses to pitch and roll head accelerations, one possible explanation for the later and larger roll instability than pitch plane instability observed in vestibular loss patients (12, 13) could be based on the different times when these sensory signals interact for perturbations in the roll and pitch directions. That is the types of processing balance control centres in the CNS use to form a perception of leg and trunk, roll and pitch may differ. If the head acceleration measurements we recorded represent the information transduced by the vestibular system to these centres, than it would appear from our results that stimulus-related pitch directional and amplitude information is received by the CNS via vestibular afferents within 13 ms of stimulus onset whereas roll information is received some 20 ms later (see Figures 4.1 and 4.3). Another explanation for the increased roll instability is, as mentioned previously, the simultaneous execution of balance

Head Roll Acceleration Responses

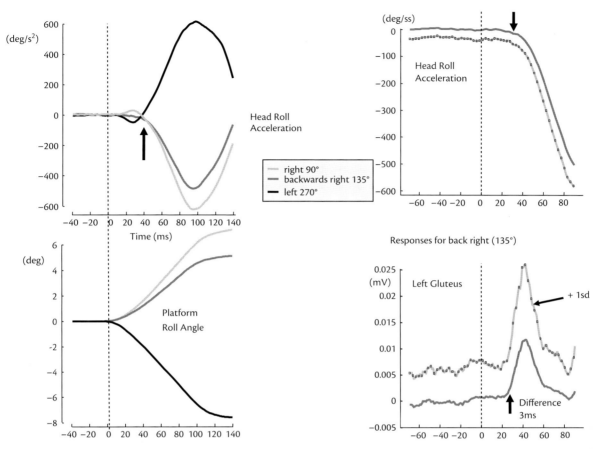

Fig. 4.11 Population roll directed responses of control subjects under eyes open conditions for a left (270°), right (90°), and combined pitch and roll directed (135° direction, backward right) tilt of the support surface. The vertical dotted line at 0 ms marks the onset of the stimulus (first deflection of platform angular velocity). On the right, plots are shown with the mean and standard deviation for the 135° direction for comparison with Figure 4.7. This direction produces the largest gluteus medius stretch reflex response. Gluteus medius responses are the largest stretch reflex responses to platform roll perturbations. The mean onsets (determined visually) of the head roll acceleration (recorded with an accelerometer) are marked on the traces. This acceleration response rises equally rapidly as head lateral linear acceleration and is equally well correlated with platform roll amplitude. Responses of vestibular loss subjects are within 1 SD of control subjects. Note that head roll acceleration rises less rapidly than the head vertical linear acceleration responses shown in Figure 4.7, leading to a lack of difference in arrival at the CNS of head roll directed acceleration and trunk proprioceptive information; difference of 3 ms. For further details of the figure refer to the legend of Figure 4.7. Data from Allum et al. (12).

corrections, despite the earlier trunk roll than pitch biomechanical response to the perturbation (38). Thus greater roll displacement will have occurred before it is corrected.

It should be noted that our conclusions on the perception of head accelerations by vestibular sensory systems are based on direct measurements of head accelerations recorded with precision sensors at high sample rates (1 kHz). Interpretations of head accelerations based on double differentiation of head position signals with low sampling rates (*c*.100 Hz) of position signals will be limited by both the low sampling rate and inherent noise following differentiation of position signals (see, e.g. (50, 51)). For this reason, early work on postural control in the pitch plane focussed more on proprioceptive rather than on vestibular sensory inputs contributing to balance corrections (17, 47) because the low sample rate recordings appeared to reveal a lack head motion. Direct measurements of head accelerations in the pitch plane such as those shown in Figures 4.11 and 4.12 provided a correction to this focus and more emphasis on vestibular inputs (12, 27, 52).

As illustrated in Figure 4.13, loss of vestibular information will lead to an overestimate of the required counter-tilt trunk lean in humans, and an underestimate of the required leg motion in the form of knee flexion. Correct interpretation of trunk lean is crucial for stability (45). A misinterpretation of the perturbation amplitude, as is shown in Figure 4.13, for the simple case in which the proprioceptive inputs are excitatory, and the vestibular inputs are excitatory for the legs, and inhibitory for the trunk, will lead to insufficient knee flexion (or insufficient ankle braking for pitch) to correct the response and movement of the trunk in the direction of tilt. It has been suggested that a similar misinterpretation process occurred in VL cats during voluntary horizontal head turns (53) or following support-surface tilt (51). Furthermore, spinal-cerebellar ataxia patients with normal vestibulo-ocular reflexes also provide insufficient knee flexion on roll tilt (54). This latter finding would support the viewpoint that a sensory integration deficit rather than loss of a sensory signal alone is the cause of balance instability in roll.

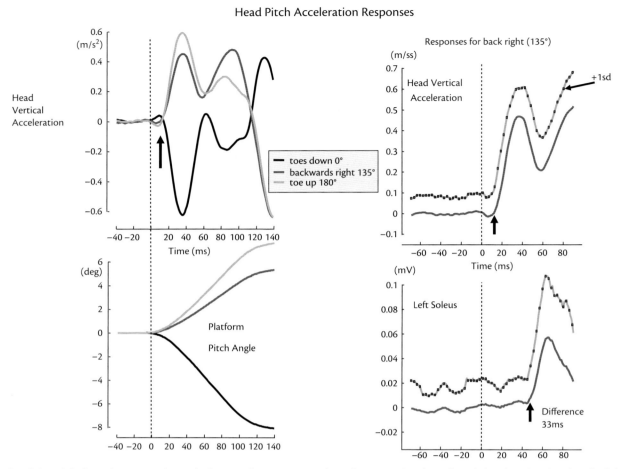

Fig. 4.12 Population pitch directed responses of control subjects under eyes open conditions for a toe up (180°), toe down (0°), and combined pitch and roll directed (135° direction, backward right) tilt of the support surface. The deviations of support surface tilt are indicated by different line types as indicated in the inserted legend. Each of the sets of responses on the left shows the mean in these directions for 12 control subjects. Each subject response was repeated eight times. The vertical dotted line at 0 ms marks the onset of the stimulus (first deflection of platform angular velocity). On the right, plots are shown with the mean and standard deviation for the 135° direction for comparison with Figure 4.11. This direction produces a slightly smaller soleus stretch reflex response than the 180°. Soleus responses are the largest stretch reflex responses to platform pitch perturbations. The traces were sampled directly as analogue signals at 1024 Hz. The sample times are shown in the right traces by open circles. The mean onsets (determined visually) of the head vertical linear acceleration (recorded with an accelerometer) are marked on the traces. This acceleration response rises more rapidly than that of pitch angular acceleration and is more strongly correlated with platform pitch amplitude. Responses of vestibular loss subjects are within 1 SD of control subjects for the first 80–140 ms shown here for both eyes open and eyes closed conditions. Note the much earlier arrival of head pitch directed acceleration than ankle proprioceptive information at the CNS; difference of 33 ms as indicated in the figure. Data from Allum et al. (12).

Comparisons with animal studies

Care needs to taken in applying balance corrections of cats to those of humans. In cats, due to the biomechanics of quadrupedal stance, both trunk and pelvis rotate in the direction of support-surface tilt (51). However, in young and middle aged humans the trunk and the pelvis move in opposite directions (46). Only with aging does the trunk stiffen, and move in concert with the pelvis toward the downhill side (38). Assuming, in the lack of evidence to the contrary, that head tilt also follows that of pelvis and trunk roll in quadrupeds, then the direction of roll acceleration perceived by cats and humans for the same direction of tilt must be of different polarity (see Figure 4.13). Nonetheless, the uphill leg flexion response and downhill leg extension responses (as shown for humans in Figure 4.10) are, however, functionally similar despite this opposite vestibulospinal polarity.

Numerous studies have examined the responses to roll tilts of the support surface in both normal and vestibular loss cats (4, 6–8, 55, 51). It is generally accepted that vestibular-spinal inputs contribute significantly to muscle responses flexing the uphill hind- and fore-limbs and extending the downhill limbs (7, 8, 56, 57). In these animal experiments, insufficient muscle activity following chronic loss of vestibular function was demonstrated (6, 7). More recently MacPherson et al. (51) have demonstrated that uphill leg muscle responses to tilt can be characterized by an overreaction not just a weaker response. Thus these authors have argued that the responses to tilt are dominated by an active extension of the uphill leg pushing the animal downhill. Despite the overreaction in knee extensor muscles as we have noted in Figure 4.9, the net reaction in humans is less flexion of the uphill leg and extension of downhill leg as shown in Figure 4.10. This would be an appropriate action if the perceived tilt was less than actual tilt. We would argue that the

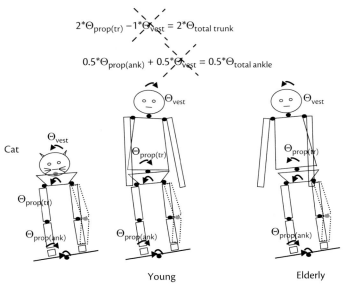

$$2*\Theta_{prop(tr)} - 1*\Theta_{vest} = 2*\Theta_{total\ trunk}$$

$$0.5*\Theta_{prop(ank)} + 0.5*\Theta_{vest} = 0.5*\Theta_{total\ ankle}$$

Fig. 4.13 Schematic illustrating the proposed misinterpretation of trunk and position in space after vestibular loss in humans. A combination of vestibular signals due to head roll and proprioceptive signals from trunk roll in the opposite direction to support surface tilt provide information on the tilt of the trunk. This is represented by the upper equation. For the leg it is assumed that the proprioceptive signals are combined in a different manner. With vestibular loss, the inhibitory signal is missing in the trunk and excitatory signal is missing for the legs. The remaining proprioceptive signal is misinterpreted as greater trunk roll than actually occurred and less ankle roll. A similar processing is assumed for pitch. In cats, the head is assumed to roll with the pelvis and trunk in the same direction as the support-surface tilt. Thus the vestibular and trunk proprioceptive signals have different polarities and the proprioceptive signals come from different muscles. With aging the trunk is stiffer, and rotates slightly downhill (as shown on the right) following a similar profile to that of cats.

clearer examples of overreaction are seen for the trunk muscles and movements in humans, as shown in Figures 4.7 and 4.9, rather than in the legs.

Summarizing, we have focused here on two aspects of VS control of human posture. First a global clinical picture of how vestibular loss affects stance and gait, and second we have attempted to pinpoint the contributions of vestibular inputs to muscle responses during recovery of balance following a perturbation in different directions. The picture we have painted of insufficient leg muscle and biomechanical responses for pitch, increased leg antagonist muscle responses leading to insufficient biomechanical responses for roll, and overreactions in the trunk muscles following vestibular loss, requires further investigation, possibly, with modelling studies in order to correlate muscle responses with the instability observed with motion analysis. Future work will need to consider the duality of these VS reactions in detail in order to develop rehabilitation programmes focusing on muscle responses which need to be retrained in order to compensate for falling tendencies in vestibular loss subjects.

Acknowledgements

This work was supported by National Swiss Research Fund grant number 32/117950 to J. H. J. Allum. Funding for M. G. Carpenter was provided by the Natural Sciences and Engineering Research Council of Canada.

References

1. Katz R, Pierrot-Deseilligny E (1999). Recurrent inhibition in humans. *Prog Neurobiol*, 57, 325–55.
2. Wilson VJ, Yoshida M (1969). Comparison of effects of stimulation of Dieters' nucleus and medial longitudinal fasciculus on neck, forelimb, and hindlimb motoneurons. *J Neurophysiol*, 32, 743–58.
3. Grillner S, Hongo T (1972). Vestibulo spinal effects on motoneurons and interneurons in the lumbosacral cord. *Prog Brain Res*, 37, 243–62.
4. Peterson BW, Fukushima K, Hirgi N, Schor RH, Wilson VJ (1980). Responses of vestibulospinal and recticulospinal neurons to sinusoidal vestibular stimulation. *J Neurophysiol*, 43, 1236–50.
5. Goldberg JM, Cullen KE (2011). Vestibular control of the head: possible functions of the vestibulocollic reflex. *Exp Brain Res*, 210, 331–45.
6. Wilson VJ, Schor RH (1999). The neural substrate of the vestibulo colic reflex. What needs to be learned. *Exp Brain Res*, 129, 483–93.
7. Pompeiano O (1984). Excitatory and inhibitory influences on the spinal cord during vestibular and neck reflexes. *Acta Otolaryngol (Stockh) Suppl* 406, 5–9.
8. Anderson JH, Soechting JF, Terzuolo CA (1977). Dynamic relations between natural vestibular inputs and activity of forelimb extensor muscles in the decerebrate cat. I. motor output during sinusoidal linear accelerations. *Brain Res*, 120, 1–15.
9. Lacour M, Xerri C, Hugen M (1979). Compensation of postural reactions to fall in the vestibular neurectomized monkey. Role of remaining labyrinthic afferences. *Exp Brain Res*, 37, 563–50.
10. Inglis JT, Macpherson JM (1995). Bilateral labyrinthectomy in the cat: effects on the postural response to translation. *J Neurophysiol*, 73, 1181–91.
11. Allum JHJ and Honegger F (1998). Interactions between vestibular and proprioceptive signals in triggering and modulating human balance-correcting responses differ across muscles. *Exp Brain Res*, 121, 478–94.
12. Allum JHJ, Oude Nijhuis LB, Carpenter MG (2008). Differences in coding provided by proprioceptive and vestibular sensory signals may contribute to alteral instability in vestibular loss subjects. *Exp Brain Res*, 184, 391–410.
13. Carpenter MG, Allum JHJ, Honegger F (2001). Vestibular influences on human postural control in combination of pitch and roll planes reveal differences in spatio temporal processing. *Exp Brain Res*, 140, 95–111.
14. Bloem BR, Allum JH, Carpenter MG, Honegger F (2000). Is lower leg proprioception essential for triggering human balance corrections? *Exp Brain Res*, 130, 375–91.
15. Bloem BR, Allum JHJ, Carpenter MG (2002). Triggering of balance corrections and compensatory strategies in a patient with total leg proprioceptive loss. *Exp Brain Res*, 142, 91–107.
16. Allum JHJ, Shepard N (1999). An overview of the clinical use of dynamic posturograhy in the differential diagnosis of balance disorders. *J Vest Res*, 9, 223–52.
17. Nashner LM, Black FO, Wall C III (1982). Adaptation to altered support and visual conditions during stance in patients with vestibular deficits. *J Neurosc*, 5, 536–44.
18. Nashner LM, Peters JF (1990). Dynamic posturography in the diagnosis and management of dizziness and balance disorders. *Neurol Clin*, 8, 331–49.
19. Allum JHJ, Bloem BR, Carpenter MG, Honegger F (2001). Differential diagnosis of proprioceptive and vestibular deficits using dynamic support-surface posturography. *Gait Posture*, 14, 217–26.
20. Allum JHJ, Carpenter MG (2005). A speedy solution for balance and gait analysis: angular velocity measured at the centre of mass. *Curr Opin Neurol*, 18, 15–21.
21. Allum JHJ, Adkin AL (2003). Improvements in trunk sway observed for stance and gait tasks during recovery from an acute unilateral peripheral vestibular deficit. *Audiol Neuro-Otol*, 8, 286–302.
22. Borello-France DF, Whitney SL, Herdman SJ, *et al.* (1994). Assessment of vestibular hypofunction. In Hardman SJ ed. *Vestibular* rehabilitation, pp. 247–86. Philadelphia, PA: FA Davis Co.

23. O'Neill DE, Gill-Body KM, Krebs DE (1998). Posturography changes do not predict functional performance changes. *Am J Otol*, 19, 797–803.

24. Hegeman J, Honegger F, Kupper M, Allum JHJ (2005). The balance control of bilateral vestibular loss subjects and its improvement with auditory prosthetic feedback. *J Vest Res*, 15, 1–9.

25. Weber PC, Cass SP (1993). Clinical assessment of postural stability. *Am J Otol*, 14(6), 566–9.

26. Horlings GC, Kueng UM, Honegger F, *et al.* (2008). Identifying deficits in balance control following vestibular or lower leg proprioceptive loss using posturographic analysis of stance tasks. *Clin Neurophysiol*, 119, 2338–346

27. Allum JHJ and Pfaltz CR (1985). Visual and vestibular contributions to pitch sway stabilization in the ankle muscles of normals and patients with bilateral peripheral vestibular deficits. *Exp Brain Res*, 58, 82–90.

28. Fetter M, Diener HC, Dichgans J (1991). Recovery of postural control after an acute unilateral vestibular lesion in humans. *J Vest Res*, 1, 373–83.

29. Lacour M, Barthemy J, Barel L, *et al.* (1997). Sensory strategies in human postural control before and after unilateral vestibular neurotomy. *Exp Brain Res*, 115, 301–10.

30. Strupp M, Arbusow V, Maag KP, Gall C, Brandt T (1998). Vestibular exercises improve central vestibulospinal compensation after vestibular neuritis. *Neurology*, 51, 838–44.

31. Li H, Godfrey DA, Rubin AM (1997). Quantitative autoradiography of 5-[^{3}]6-cyano-7-nitro-quinoxaline-2,3-dione and (+)-3-[^{3}H]dizocilpine maleate binding in rat vestibular nuclear complex after unilateral deafferentation, with comparison to cochlear nucleus. *Neuroscience*, 77, 473–84.

32. Ryu JH (1993). Vestibular neuritis: an overview using a classical case. *Acta Otolaryngol (Suppl)*, 503, 25–30.

33. Allum JHJ, Yamane M, Pfaltz CR (1988). Long-term modifications of vertical and horizontal vestibulo-ocular reflex dynamics in man. I. After acute unilateral peripheral vestibular paralysis. *Acta Otolaryngol (Stockh)*, 105, 328–37.

34. Allum JHJ, Ledin T (1999). Recovery of vestibulo-ocular function in subjects with acute peripheral vestibular loss. *J Vest Res*, 9, 135–44.

35. Gill J, Allum JHJ, Carpenter MG, Held-Ziolkowska M, Honegger F, Pierchala K (2001). Trunk sway measures of postural stability during clinical balance tests: effects of age. *J Gerontol*, 56A, M438–M447.

36. Goutier KTM, Janssen SL, Horlings CGC, Küng UM, Allum JHJ (2010). The influence of walking speed and gender on trunk sway for the healthy elderly and young. *Age Aging*, 39, 647–50.

37. Grüneberg C, Duysens J, Honegger F, Allum JHJ (2005). Spatio-temporal separation of roll and pitch balance correcting commands in man. *J Neurophysiol*, 94, 3143–58.

38. Allum JHJ, Carpenter MG, Bloem BR, Honegger F, Adkin AL (2002). Age-dependent variations in the directional sensitivity of balance corrections. *J Physiol (Lond)*, 542, 643–63.

39. Grüneberg C, Allum JHJ, Honegger F, Bloem BR (2004). The influence of artificially increased hip and trunk stiffness on balance control in the pitch and roll planes. *Exp Brain Res*, 157, 472–85.

40. Curthoys IS and Halmagyi GM (1995). Vestibular compensation: a review of the oculomotor, neural, and clinical consequences of unilateral vestibular loss. *J Vest Res*, 5, 67–107.

41. Halmagyi GM, Curthoys IS, Cremer PD, *et al.* (1990). The human horizontal vestibulo-ocular reflex in response to high acceleration stimuli before and after unilateral vestibular neurectomy. *Exp Brain Res*, 81, 479–90.

42. Aw ST, Halmagyi GM, Haslwanter T, Curthoys IS, Yavor RA, Todd MJ (1996). Three dimensional vector analysis of the human vestibulo ocular reflex in response to high-acceleration head rotations II Responses in subjects with unilateral vestibular loss and selective semicircular canal occlusion. *J Neurophysiol*, 76, 4021–90.

43. Allum JHJ, Honegger F, Schicks H (1993). Vestibular and proprioceptive modulation of postural synergies in normal subjects. *J Vest Res*, 3, 59–85.

44. Keshner EA, Allum JHJ and Pfaltz CR (1987). Postural coactivation and adaptation in the sway stabilizing responses of normals and patients with bilateral vestibular deficit. *Exp Brain Res*, 69, 77–92.

45. Carpenter MG, Allum JHJ, Honegger F (1999). Directional sensitivities of stretch reflexes and balance corrections for normal subjects in the roll and pitch planes. *Exp Brain Res*, 129, 93–113.

46. Allum JHJ, Carpenter MG, Honegger F (2003). Directional aspects of balance corrections in man. *IEEE Eng in Med Biol Mag*, 22, 37–47.

47. Diener HC, Horak FB, Nashner LM (1988). Influence of stimulus parameters on human postural responses. *J Neurophysiol*, 59, 1888–905.

48. Dietz V (1998). Evidence for a load receptor contribution to the control of posture and locomotion. *Neurosci Biobehav Rev*, 22, 495–9.

49. Peterka RJ, Loughlin PJ (2004). Dynamic regulation of sensorimotor integration in human postural control. *J Neurophysiol*, 91, 410–23.

50. Forssberg H, Hirschfeld H (1994). Postural adjustments in sitting humans following external perturbations. *Exp Brain Res*, 97, 515–27.

51. MacPherson JM, Everaert DG, Stapley PJ, Ting LH (2007). Bilateral vestibular loss in cats leads to active destabilization of balance during pitch and roll rotations of the support-surface. *J Neurophysiol*, 97, 4397–67.

52. Runge CF, Shepert CL, Horak FB, Zajac FE (1998). Role of vestibular information in initiation of rapid postural responses. *Exp Brain Res*, 122, 403–12.

53. Stapley PJ, Ting LH, Kuifu C, Everaert DG, MacPherson JM (2006). Bilateral vestibular loss leads to active destabilization of balance during voluntary head turns in the standing cat. *J Neurophysiol*, 95, 3783–97.

54. Bakker M, Allum JH, Visser JE, *et al.* (2006). Postural responses to multidirectional stance perturbations in cerebellar ataxia. *Exp Neurol*, 202(1), 21–35.

55. Lindsay KW, Roberts TD, Rosenberg JR (1976). Asymmetric tonic labyrinth reflexes in the decerebrate cat. *J Physiol*, 261, 583–601.

56. Krutki P, Jankowska E, Edgley SA (2003). Are crossed actions of reticulospinal and vestibulospinal neurons on feline motoneurons mediated by the same or separate commissural neurons? *J Neurosc*, 23, 8041–50.

57. Wilson VJ, Schor RH, Suzuki I, Parks BR (1986). Spatial organisation of neck and vestibular reflexes acting on the forelimbs of the decerebrate cat. *J Neurophysiol*, 55, 514–26.

CHAPTER 5

The Vestibulo-Autonomic System

Bill J. Yates, Ilan A. Kerman, Brian J. Jian, and Timothy D. Wilson

Many clinicians equate 'vestibulo-autonomic responses' with motion sickness. While motion sickness does include symptoms and signs such as pallor and cold sweating that result from the actions of the autonomic nervous system (1–3), research over the past 25 years has demonstrated the existence of vestibulo-autonomic responses that serve to maintain homeostasis during movement and changes in posture. Such homeostatic vestibulo-autonomic responses are the focus of this chapter, as they are not as widely recognized as motion sickness (Chapter 28), but dysfunction of the responses can have clinical manifestations. In particular, we will describe the role of the vestibular system in adjusting blood distribution in the body during postural alterations. The vestibular system also participates in altering the activity of respiratory muscles during movement to compensate for the effects of gravitational loading on the muscles and the flow of air into and out of the lungs. Although vestibulo-respiratory and vestibular-cardiovascular responses have similarities, the former have been the topic of several reviews (4–7), and will not be discussed here.

The physiological importance of vestibular influences on cardiovascular regulation relates to the prominent changes in blood distribution in the body that occur during some postural alterations. The top panel of Figure 5.1 illustrates the decline in venous return from the hindlimb that occurred in conscious cats during graded head-up tilts. A 60° head-up rotation resulted in an approximately 70% drop in blood flow in the femoral vein (relative to that when the animal was prone), which gradually dissipated to a 30% reduction in venous return as venoconstriction and skeletal muscle pumping occurred (8). Starling's law of the heart stipulates that cardiac output is proportional to venous return (9); the decline in venous return during some postural alterations demands that other physiological responses must occur rapidly to prevent hypotension. Besides cardiac output, the other major determinant of systemic arterial pressure is total peripheral resistance, or the resistance to blood flow provided by the vasculature (10, 11). Total peripheral resistance is adjusted by the sympathetic nervous system, which elicits constriction of smooth muscle in arterioles (10, 11). The middle panel of Figure 5.1 illustrates that within 10 s of the onset of

a 60° head-up tilt, blood flow to the hindlimb in the femoral artery declines proportionately to the reduction in blood flow from the hindlimb in the femoral vein. The bottom panel of Figure 5.1 shows that blood flow to and from the hindlimb are precisely matched, so that long-term blood accumulation in the limb does not occur (8).

A reduction in blood pressure causes the unloading of baroreceptors located in the aortic arch and carotid sinus, which elicits a baroreceptor reflex that increases heart rate, heart contractility, and total peripheral resistance (10, 11). However, this mechanism has two deficiencies. First, the baroreceptor reflex requires the presence of hypotension before it is engaged; it is practical to begin compensation for the effects of a postural alteration on the cardiovascular system before blood pressure changes substantially. Second, the baroreceptors cannot distinguish the aetiology of hypotension, and whether it is the result of postural changes, hypovolaemia, or other causes; they just reveal when blood pressure has changed. Integration of vestibular signals by the brainstem circuitry controlling sympathetic nervous system activity can provide for the onset of peripheral vasoconstriction before blood pressure changes substantially, as well as maximization of the vasoconstriction in the part of the body positioned below the heart, where venous pooling is maximal. A number of lines of evidence have demonstrated that the presence of vestibular inputs is necessary for appropriate cardiovascular adjustments to occur during postural alterations.

Cardiovascular responses elicited by vestibular stimulation in animal subjects

Electrical and caloric vestibular stimulation

As early as a century ago, it was recognized that stimulation of vestibular receptors in animals elicits changes in sympathetic nervous system activity and blood pressure (7). For example, caloric stimulation of the labyrinth in rabbits was reported to elicit a depression in blood pressure; placing lesions in the vestibular nuclei abolished this response, indicating that it was not due to stimulation of non-labyrinthine receptors (12, 13). A variety of laboratories

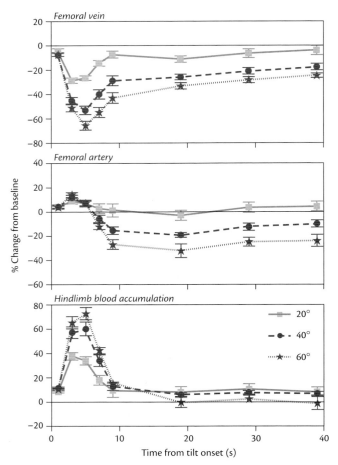

Fig. 5.1 Effects of head-up tilts of different amplitudes on mean blood flow to (*femoral artery flow, middle panel*) and from (*femoral vein flow, top panel*) the hindlimb of conscious cats. The bottom panel shows instantaneous blood accumulation in the hindlimb during the progression of the head-up tilt, which was determined by subtraction of percent difference from baseline in venous blood flow from per cent difference from baseline in arterial blood flow. At the onset of the head-up tilt, blood flow in the femoral vein plummeted due to the effects of gravity, but then rebounded as venoconstriction and skeletal muscle pumping occurred. Blood flow to the leg in the femoral artery was simultaneously reduced through vasoconstriction. This vasoconstriction was precisely matched to balance the decrease in venous return, such that after ~10 s there was no additional blood accumulation in the lower body. Data from (8).

also demonstrated that electrical stimulation of vestibular afferents produces changes in sympathetic nervous system activity, blood pressure, and peripheral blood flow (for reviews of this literature, see (14)). For example, Figure 5.2A shows the changes in activity of the superior mesenteric nerve and renal nerve that were elicited by delivery of a short train of electrical pulses to the vestibular nerve. The responses were compared when blood pressure was normal and elevated by the infusion of an alpha-receptor agonist, which produced peripheral vasoconstriction. When blood pressure was elevated, changes in sympathetic nervous system activity elicited by vestibular stimulation were attenuated or abolished (15). Stimulation of baroreceptors through increases in blood pressure selectively diminishes the excitability of sympathetic efferents that innervate vascular smooth muscle (16–18), but not those that regulate gastrointestinal activity and have other functions. This observation shows that electrical stimulation of vestibular afferents has its

strongest effects on sympathetic efferents involved in cardiovascular regulation.

Electrical stimulation of the vestibular nerve can have both excitatory and inhibitory effects on the activity of sympathetic efferents, although it always results in a decrease in blood pressure (19–22), as illustrated in Figure 5.2B. This could be partially explained by the observation that changes in blood flow elicited by electrical vestibular stimulation are patterned, and differ between the upper and lower body (23). Figure 5.2B shows that delivery of current pulses to the labyrinth results in an increase in hindlimb blood flow, while forelimb blood flow simultaneously decreases (23). The increase in lower body blood flow during electrical vestibular stimulation is due to a decrease in vascular resistance, whereas upper body vascular resistance increases. However, the magnitude of the decline in lower body vascular resistance was much greater than the increase in upper body vascular resistance, which explains the observation that blood pressure drops during vestibular stimulation (23).

Recordings of activity of individual sympathetic efferent fibres innervating skeletal muscle arterioles (muscle vasoconstrictor (MVC) fibres) in the face, forelimb and hindlimb confirmed that sympathetic nervous system responses to electrical vestibular stimulation differ between the upper and lower body. Most hindlimb MVC fibres were inhibited by electrical stimulation of vestibular afferents, whereas most forelimb and facial MVC fibres exhibited a response including early, powerful excitation (24). Such a response pattern of sympathetic efferents would evoke the increase in hindlimb blood flow (as vascular smooth muscle dilates) and decrease in forelimb blood flow (as vascular smooth muscle constricts) that is observed when current pulses are applied to the VIIIth nerve (23).

Selective natural vestibular stimulation

Delivery of electrical pulses to the vestibular nerve is a useful tool to determine whether labyrinthine inputs contribute to a particular physiological response, since vestibular afferents can be selectively activated. However, electrical vestibular stimulation is non-physiological, in that afferents signalling head movement in every direction are simultaneously stimulated. Another method to selectively activate vestibular afferents in decerebrate or anesthetized animals is to rotate the head on a fixed body following denervations to eliminate non-labyrinthine inputs that could be elicited by the stimulus, including bilateral transection of the upper cervical dorsal roots, vagus nerves, and aortic depressor nerves, ligation of the common carotid arteries, and denervation of the carotid sinus using blunt dissection and cauterization (25, 26). Figure 5.3 shows the effects of such natural vestibular stimulation on blood pressure (Figure 5.3A) and sympathetic nervous system activity (Figure 5.3B) in decerebrate cats. Fifty-degree nose-up trapezoidal (ramp-and hold) head tilts produced an increase in blood pressure of approximately 18 mmHg; ear-down tilt produced little change in blood pressure (26). The changes in blood pressure began approximately 1.4 s after the plateau of the stimulus. The responses to nose-up tilt were abolished following intracranial transections of the VIIIth cranial nerves, confirming that they were due to activation of labyrinthine afferents. These data suggest that vestibular inputs elicited by nose-up movements of the head act to rapidly increase blood pressure. However, it is noteworthy that the baroreceptors in the animals were denervated, which likely resulted in an exaggeration of the cardiovascular responses to head movements.

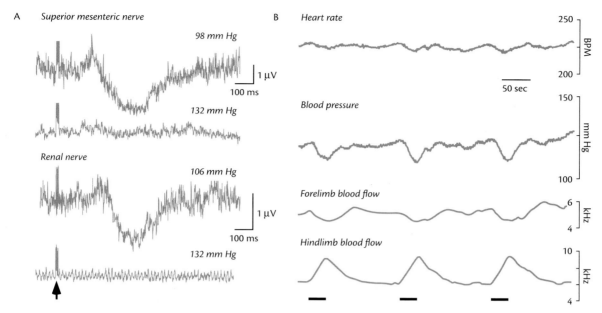

Fig. 5.2 Cardiovascular system responses to stimulation of electrical stimulation of vestibular afferents. (A) Effects of electrical stimulation of the vestibular nerve on sympathetic nerve activity in cats. A train of five shocks was delivered to the vestibular nerve at the time indicated by an arrow at the bottom of the panel. Averaged responses of the superior mesenteric nerve and renal nerve to the stimuli are illustrated; data were obtained when blood pressure was near normal, and when elevated by infusion of a peripherally-acting alpha receptor agonist. Vestibular-elicited sympathetic nerve responses were blunted when blood pressure was high. Adapted from (15). (B) Effects of delivery of a train of stimuli to the vestibular nerve on heart rate, blood pressure, and blood flow to the forelimb (brachial artery) and hindlimb (femoral artery). The stimulus produced depressor responses that were accompanied by small heart rate changes, increases in blood flow to the hindlimb, and decreases in flow to the forelimb. Adapted from (23).

Changes in sympathetic nervous system activity could be elicited by selective vestibular stimulation produced by relatively small (10–15°) head movements (25). Figure 5.3B illustrates the effects of combined roll and pitch head tilts on the activity of the splanchnic nerve, which innervates abdominal viscera. In the top panel, the head tilt rotated in the clockwise direction, and shifted from nose-down, to right-ear-down, to nose-up, to left-ear-down, and back to nose-down. In the bottom panel, the head tilt rotated in the counterclockwise direction. During both stimuli, the activity of the nerve was highest when the nose was tilted upwards, and lowest

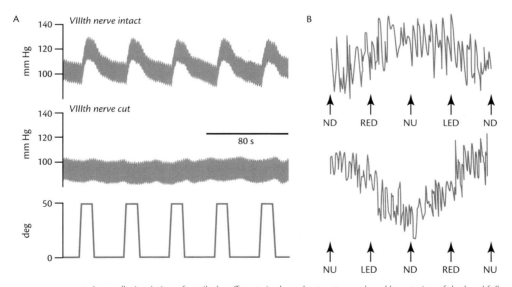

Fig. 5.3 Cardiovascular system responses to 'natural' stimulation of vestibular afferents in decerebrate cats, produced by rotation of the head following denervations to eliminate non-labyrinthine inputs that could be elicited by the movement (bilateral transection of the upper cervical dorsal roots, vagus nerves, and aortic depressor nerves, ligation of the common carotid arteries, and denervation of the carotid sinus using blunt dissection and cauterization). (A) Change in blood pressure elicited by 50° nose-up head tilt before and after transection of the VIIIth cranial nerves. Elimination of vestibular inputs abolished the approximately 30 mmHg increases in blood pressure elicited during nose-up head rotation. Adapted from (26). (B) Modulation of activity of a sympathetic nerve (splanchnic nerve) produced by 15° 'wobble' head rotations incorporating roll and pitch. In the top panel, clockwise wobble rotations were delivered, where the head was positioned nose down (ND), then right ear down (RED), nose up (NU), left ear down (LED). In the bottom panel, counterclockwise wobble stimulation was delivered. Splanchnic nerve activity was maximal when the head was tilted nose-up, and minimal when the head was tilted nose-down. Ear-down tilt had little impact on sympathetic nerve activity. Adapted from (25).

when the head was positioned downwards. Ear-down tilt had little effect on splanchnic nerve activity (25). The gains of the responses remained relatively constant when rotations were delivered at different frequencies, and the responses were in phase with the position of the head, as opposed to stimulus velocity (25). These response dynamics are similar to those of otolith afferents (27). As such, the properties of vestibulosympathetic responses recorded from the splanchnic nerve support the hypothesis that the vestibular system participates in compensating for cardiovascular challenges elicited by head-up rotations of the body.

Deficiencies in adjusting blood distribution in the body during postural alterations subsequent to vestibular system lesions.

Another approach that has been used to determine whether the vestibular system contributes to cardiovascular regulation is to compare the effects of postural alterations on blood pressure and blood distribution in the body before and after the removal of vestibular inputs. This approach was first employed in the 1970s by Doba and Reis (28), who compared blood pressure during head-up tilts of anesthetized cats before and after the transection of the VIIIth cranial nerves. It was reported that blood pressure remained stable in vestibular-intact cats during 60° head-up rotations, but dropped approximately 50 mmHg during the movements after the removal of labyrinthine inputs (28). This experiment was subsequently repeated in conscious cats that were instrumented for telemetric recordings of blood pressure (29). In agreement with the findings of Doba and Reis, blood pressure remained stable during head-up rotations in conscious, vestibular-intact animals. Following the removal of labyrinthine inputs, blood pressure was labile, and either increased or decreased appreciably at the onset of head-up tilts (29). This posturally-related lability in blood pressure resolved after approximately 1 week. The presence of lability in blood pressure during orthostatic challenges following bilateral peripheral vestibular lesions has been verified in conscious rats, in experiments where gravitational stress on the cardiovascular system was induced by head-up tilts (30), linear acceleration (31), free fall (32), and centrifugation (33).

Studies in conscious animals have also examined the effects of postural changes and vestibular lesions on blood flow to a variety of vascular beds. Following a bilateral labyrinthectomy, basal blood flow to the head increased ~40% (34), whereas basal levels of blood flow to the forelimb and hindlimb were relatively unchanged (35). As noted earlier, hindlimb blood flow ordinarily decreases markedly during head-up tilts (>20% reduction during 60° rotations), due to an increase in hindlimb vascular resistance. This increase in vascular resistance was blunted following a bilateral labyrinthectomy (35), as illustrated in Figure 5.4 by comparing solid lines of different colours. However, the changes in forelimb blood flow and vascular resistance during head-up rotations were unaffected by removal of vestibular inputs, as shown in Figure 5.4 by dashed lines of different colours (35). Similarly, bilateral peripheral vestibular lesions did not affect the adjustments in head blood flow that occur during postural alterations, despite the fact that basal blood flow to the head, measured when the animal was in the prone position, increased dramatically (34). These data show that vestibular inputs have distinct effects on the regulation of blood flow to different

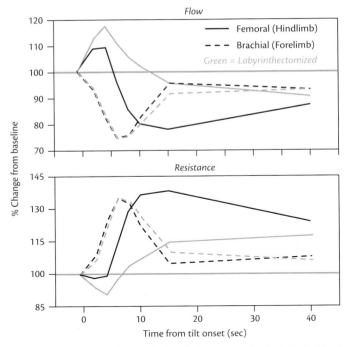

Fig. 5.4 Effects of bilateral removal of vestibular inputs on forelimb (*dashed lines*) and hindlimb (*solid lines*) blood flow (*top panel*) and vascular resistance (*bottom panel*) during 60° head-up tilts of conscious cats. Black lines indicate responses when vestibular inputs were intact, whereas grey lines designate responses during the first week after bilateral transection of the VIIIth cranial nerves. Removal of labyrinthine inputs attenuated the increase in hindlimb vascular resistance and decline in hindlimb blood flow that ordinarily occurs during large head-up tilts. However, forelimb vascular responses to head-up tilts were unaffected by vestibular lesions. Data from (35).

parts of the body, and support the notion arising from experiments involving electrical vestibular stimulation (23, 24) that vestibulosympathetic responses differ between body regions.

Neural pathways crucial for producing vestibulosympathetic responses

Vestibular nuclei

The vestibular nucleus complex is large in mammals, and extends from the level of the caudal medulla to the middle region of the pons (36). Ablation studies have explored whether a specific region of the vestibular nucleus complex mediates vestibulosympathetic responses. Chemical or electrical lesions confined to the caudal aspect of the medial and inferior vestibular nuclei abolish changes in sympathetic nervous system activity produced by electrical stimulation of the vestibular nerve (15, 22, 37). Furthermore, anatomical studies in rats, rabbits, and cats demonstrated that the caudal region of the vestibular nuclei makes connections with areas of the brainstem that participate in controlling autonomic functions, including nucleus tractus solitarius (NTS; 38–40), the rostral ventrolateral medulla (RVLM; 41, 42), and lateral regions of the caudal medullary reticular formation that provide inputs to the RVLM (41, 43, 44). Neurons in the caudal vestibular nuclei also contain imidazoleacetic acid-ribotide, a putative neurotransmitter involved in blood pressure regulation (45). In combination, these findings

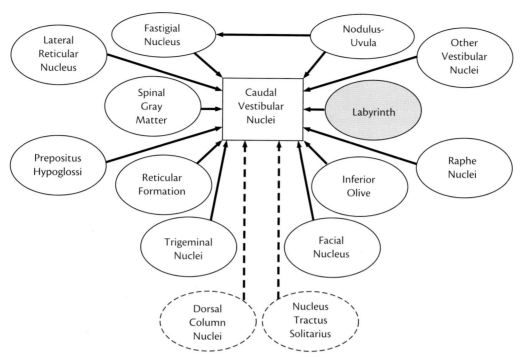

Fig. 5.5 Regions of the brainstem and cerebellum providing inputs to the caudal aspects of the medial and inferior vestibular nuclei (caudal vestibular nuclei). Solid ovals and lines designate direct inputs that were established by injecting a retrogradely-transported tracer (the beta subunit of cholera toxin) into the caudal vestibular nuclei of ferrets. Dashed ovals and lines indicate additional indirect inputs that were revealed by injecting a transneuronal tracer (pseudorabies virus) into the same area. The brainstem regions providing inputs to the caudal vestibular nuclei process labyrinthine, somatosensory, and visual inputs, such that this area receives a variety of sensory signals that reflect body position in space.

demonstrate that the caudal aspect of the vestibular nucleus complex participates in the regulation of sympathetic outflow.

The caudal region of the vestibular nucleus complex receives substantial inputs from otolith organs, as well as semicircular canals (46–48). The activity of a majority of caudal vestibular nucleus neurons is also modulated by stimulation of muscle and cutaneous afferents in forelimb and hindlimb nerves, as well as by the stimulation of visceral nerves (47). The injection of retrogradely-transported tracers into the caudal vestibular nuclei showed that this region receives direct inputs from several areas of the nervous system that process non-labyrinthine inputs, including the spinal grey matter, prepositus hypoglossi, pontomedullary reticular formation, inferior olivary nucleus, lateral reticular nucleus, medullary raphe nuclei, the spinal and principal trigeminal nuclei, and the facial nucleus (49). Injections of transneuronally-transported viral tracers revealed that the caudal vestibular nuclei additionally receive multisynaptic inputs from nucleus tractus solitarius and the gracile and cuneate nuclei (49). Other studies demonstrated that the posterior cerebellar cortex (lobules IX–X) and cerebellar fastigial nucleus project to the caudal vestibular nuclei (50). The inputs to the caudal vestibular nuclei are summarized in Figure 5.5. These data suggest that the responses of caudal vestibular nucleus neurons to changes in body position in space likely reflect an integration of inputs from vestibular, proprioceptive, cutaneous, and visceral afferents (51).

Rostral ventrolateral medulla

The RVLM, a longitudinal column of bulbospinal neurons located near the ventrolateral surface of the rostral medulla, plays a

predominant role in controlling blood pressure (52–54). Stimulation of the RVLM produces large increases in blood pressure (52, 55), and the activity of RVLM neurons is powerfully inhibited by activation of baroreceptors (56–61). Furthermore, bilateral destruction or inhibition of this region produces a profound drop in blood pressure similar to that observed after transecting the cervical spinal cord (62–64), and also eliminates baroreceptor reflexes (65–67).

The RVLM plays a critical role in generating vestibulosympathetic responses. Bilateral chemical lesions of the RVLM abolished changes in sympathetic nervous system activity elicited by stimulation of vestibular afferents (68). In addition, the activity of about half of RVLM neurons is modulated by moderate-amplitude (≤10°) rotations in vertical planes (69, 70). The dynamic properties of the responses of RVLM neurons to rotations in vertical planes are similar to those of sympathetic nerves (25), as well as otolith afferents (69, 70). The direction of tilt that elicited maximal modulation of RVLM neuronal activity was highly variable from cell to cell, with some units being activated by ear-down tilts and others responding to head-up rotations (69, 70). In contrast, sympathetic nerve activity is selectively modulated by rotations in the sagittal (pitch) plane (25). These findings show that the responses of sympathetic preganglionic neurons to changes in body position in space are not a simple reflection of the activity of RVLM neurons. Instead, spinal cord neurons regulating sympathetic outflow likely receive convergent inputs from multiple cells in the RVLM, and perhaps other brainstem regions that contribute to controlling vasomotor activity; integration of these signals generates sympathetic nerve responses to tilts with properties that deviate from those of individual bulbospinal neurons.

Sympathetic efferents innervating blood vessels in the lower body are inhibited by electrical stimulation of the vestibular nerve, which results in a regional increase in blood flow, as illustrated in Figure 5.2B (23, 24). In contrast, the response to electrical vestibular stimulation of sympathetic efferents innervating blood vessels in the upper body includes prominent excitation, which induces a reduction in upper body blood flow (23, 24). It thus seemed likely that the responses of RVLM neurons to vestibular stimulation would differ depending on whether the cell projected to upper thoracic spinal cord segments providing sympathetic nervous system influences on the upper body, or more caudally to lower thoracic spinal segments containing lower body sympathetic preganglionic neurons. Contrary to this expectation, the majority of RVLM neurons were excited by vestibular stimulation, despite their level of projection in the spinal cord (71). These results suggest that the RVLM is not solely responsible for establishing the patterning of vestibular-sympathetic responses. This patterning apparently requires the integration by spinal circuitry of labyrinthine signals transmitted from brainstem regions in addition to the RVLM, perhaps from the medullary raphe nuclei. Anatomical studies have demonstrated that the caudal medullary raphe nuclei provide inputs to sympathetic preganglionic neurons that regulate blood flow (72, 73). In the cat, the RVLM and caudal medullary raphe nuclei are the only areas containing bulbospinal neurons that have been demonstrated to be essential for shaping

the discharges of sympathetic efferents that participate in cardiovascular regulation (74–76). In addition, many caudal medullary raphe neurons, including those with projections to the thoracic spinal cord, respond robustly to vestibular stimulation (77, 78). Further experiments will be needed to establish the relative roles of the RVLM and caudal medullary raphe nuclei in shaping the patterning of vestibulosympathetic responses.

Brainstem interneurons

Direct projections exist from the caudal aspect of the vestibular nucleus complex to the RVLM (41, 42), which likely mediate the short-latency responses of a subset of RVLM neurons to electrical stimulation of vestibular afferents (71, 79). However, the latencies of the responses of most RVLM neurons to vestibular nerve stimulation are over 10 ms, suggesting that multisynaptic connections also are present between the vestibular nuclei and RVLM (71, 79). Two regions of the caudal medullary reticular formation, the lateral tegmental field (44) and caudal ventrolateral medulla (80), contain neurons that can be antidromically activated by stimulation within the RVLM and respond to vestibular nerve stimulation at shorter latency than RVLM units. Ablation of these areas of the brainstem also abolish or attenuate the effects of vestibular stimulation on sympathetic nervous system activity, suggesting that they participate in generating vestibulosympathetic responses (81). However, it is unclear how labyrinthine signals are integrated with non-labyrinthine inputs

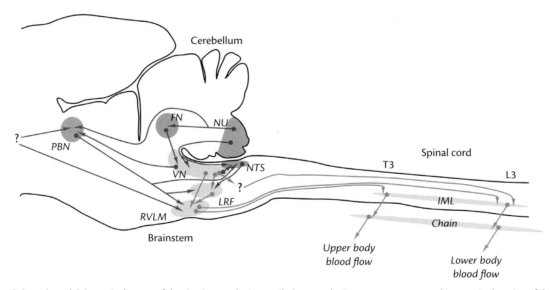

Fig. 5.6 (Also see Colour plate 4.) Schematic diagram of the circuitry producing vestibulosympathetic responses, transposed on a sagittal section of the cat brainstem and spinal cord. Areas and connections that play a primary role in generating these responses are indicated in red, and those that modulate the responses are indicated in blue. Vestibulosympathetic responses are mediated by the caudal regions of the medial and inferior vestibular nuclei (*VN*), which provide direct inputs to bulbospinal neurons in the rostral ventrolateral medulla (*RVLM*) as well as indirect inputs conveyed through the lateral portions of the caudal medullary reticular formation (*LRF*). The RVLM plays a critical role in relaying vestibular signals to sympathetic preganglionic neurons in the intermediolateral cell column (*IML*), which spans from the third thoracic (*T3*) to the third lumbar (*L3*) spinal cord segments. In turn, sympathetic preganglionic neurons provide inputs to sympathetic postganglionic cells positioned in the sympathetic chain (*chain*). Vestibulosympathetic responses are patterned, as indicated by the observation that vestibular stimulation produces opposite changes in forelimb and hindlimb blood flow. Since RVLM neurons respond similarly to vestibular stimulation despite their level of projection in the spinal cord, it is likely that additional areas of the brainstem that are presently unidentified also participate in relaying vestibular signals to sympathetic preganglionic neurons. The responses of RVLM neurons to vestibular stimulation are blunted in conscious animals, suggesting that the responses are modulated by higher brain regions that are currently unidentified. Descending influences of forebrain neurons on cardiovascular regulation may also be mediated through the parabrachial nucleus (*PBN*). Vestibulosympathetic responses are also altered by damage of the nodulus-uvula (*NU*) region of the caudal cerebellar vermis, which influences the activity of neurons in the caudal VN both directly and indirectly through connections in the cerebellar fastigial nucleus (*FN*). It has been proposed that NU indirectly influences the activity of neurons in nucleus tractus solitarius, presumably through relays in PBN or the caudal VN. These connections may participate in adjusting the gain of the baroreceptor reflex in accordance with body position in space or behavioural context.

and modified as they are passed through lateral regions of the caudal medullary reticular formation to the RVLM.

Summary

The most direct central nervous system pathways through which labyrinthine inputs contribute to the regulation of blood pressure are indicated in red in Figure 5.6. This minimal pathway includes connections from the caudal aspect of the vestibular nucleus complex to the RVLM, which are both direct and indirect via interneurons in the lateral portion of the caudal medullary reticular formation. Bulbospinal neurons in the RVLM in turn modulate the activity of sympathetic preganglionic neurons in the thoracic and upper lumbar spinal cord in accordance with body position in space. Brainstem regions in addition to the RVLM, including the caudal medullary raphe nuclei, may also participate in generating vestibulosympathetic responses; these additional pathways are indicated by a question mark in Figure 5.6, since they are speculative.

Modulation of vestibulosympathetic responses

Higher brain centres

A recent study compared RVLM neuronal responses to whole-body rotations in vertical planes in conscious and decerebrate cats (70). As noted earlier, approximately 50% of RVLM neurons responded to moderate-amplitude vertical tilts of decerebrate cats. In contrast, the firing of less than 1% of RVLM units was modulated by whole-body rotations in conscious animals (70). These data suggest that RVLM neurons are highly sensitive to changes in body position in space, but that their responses to vestibular inputs are ordinarily suppressed by higher brain centres when the nervous system is intact. Such response suppression is physiologically appropriate, since the vestibular system responds robustly during movements that are too small to affect fluid distribution in the body. For example, a less than 5° deviation in head position would degrade visual acuity unless the vestibulo-ocular reflex produced a compensatory eye movement (82, 83). In contrast, movements less than 20° do not affect blood distribution in the body and blood pressure, and thus don't require adjustments in sympathetic nerve activity (8, 35). Nevertheless, 15° head-up rotations in decerebrate cats elicit robust increases in the activity of sympathetic efferents, indicating that vestibular system influences on sympathetic nervous system activity are exaggerated in this preparation. Further studies are required to determine the identity of the nervous system regions that suppress RVLM neuronal responses to vestibular stimulation, although higher centres of the brain are likely involved. The parabrachial nucleus of the pons may also participate in modulating the gain of vestibulo-sympathetic responses, since some parabrachial neurons relay signals from the forebrain to brainstem regions that regulate blood pressure (84–86). The parabrachial nucleus additionally receives vestibular inputs (41, 87), raising the possibility that the integration of forebrain and labyrinthine signals by this region provides complex modulatory influences on the activity of RVLM neurons.

Posterior cerebellar cortex

Regions of the posterior cerebellar cortex, particularly the nodulus-uvula (lobules IX–X), participate in regulating blood pressure. Stimulation of the nodulus-uvula produces changes in blood pressure, typically a depressor response (88–90). Furthermore, the firing rate of RVLM neurons is modified by stimulation of these cerebellar regions (91). Lesions of the posterior cerebellar cortex in anesthetized, baroreceptor-denervated cats alter the rhythmic properties of sympathetic nerve discharges and result in an increase in blood pressure (92). Nodulus-uvula lesions have also been reported to affect the acquisition of conditioned cardiovascular responses (93).

Purkinje cells in the nodulus-uvula project to the regions of the caudal medial and inferior vestibular nuclei that mediate autonomic responses (50, 94). Cardiovascular responses elicited by stimulation of the uvula may also be elicited through direct connections of this region with the parabrachial nucleus in the pons, or indirectly via the fastigial nucleus (50). Nonetheless, because of the extensive connections between the uvula/nodulus and areas of the vestibular nuclei that participate in cardiovascular regulation, it seems likely that the 'autonomic region' of the cerebellum modulates vestibulo-sympathetic reflexes.

As of yet, the role of the caudal cerebellar vermis in cardiovascular regulation is not clear. However, insights may be gained by considering other responses affected by this cerebellar region. Lesions of the nodulus and uvula alter the characteristics of vestibulo-ocular reflexes (95–100). In general, the vestibulocerebellum, which is comprised of the flocculus, nodulus, and uvula, is believed to be critically involved in adaptive changes in vestibulo-ocular responses (99, 101–104). These findings raise the possibility that the nodulus/uvula may also participate in adaptive plasticity in cardiovascular responses elicited through the vestibular system.

As noted earlier, a bilateral labyrinthectomy results in lability in blood pressure during postural alterations, which dissipates after about a week (29). It has been postulated that the recovery of compensatory cardiovascular responses to postural alterations following vestibular lesions is at least partly related to the capacity of the central nervous system to substitute non-labyrinthine signals for vestibular inputs in the neural pathways that mediate vestibulosympathetic responses (51). As indicated in Figure 5.5, neurons in the caudal portions of the medial and inferior vestibular nuclei integrate a variety of non-labyrinthine inputs that signal body position in space. For example, proprioceptive inputs related to the stretching of muscles, visceral inputs elicited by the shifting of internal organs, and somatosensory signals produced by contact of particular regions of skin on surfaces provide cues that indicate body orientation in space. Several lines of evidence suggest that caudal vestibular nucleus neurons substitute non-labyrinthine signals for vestibular inputs following damage to the inner ear. Some neurons positioned in the caudal aspect of the vestibular nucleus complex regain the capacity to respond to particular alterations in body position in space after a bilateral labyrinthectomy (46, 105). Caudal vestibular nucleus neurons also become more sensitive to somatosensory and visceral stimulation subsequent to a bilateral labyrinthectomy, suggesting that their postural-related responses after removal of vestibular inputs are due to these inputs (47). Furthermore, spinalization eliminates vestibular nucleus neuronal responses to tilts in animals with a bilateral labyrinthectomy (106). In addition, bilateral lesions placed in the caudal portions of the vestibular nuclei resulted in deficits in regulating blood pressure during postural alterations that persisted longer than those occurring after a bilateral labyrinthectomy (107). Cumulatively, these data show that plastic changes in the caudal vestibular nuclei following the removal of labyrinthine inputs permit the substitution of non-labyrinthine for vestibular inputs in this region, which is at least partially responsible for recovery of the ability to adjust blood pressure during postural alterations.

Ablation of the posterior cerebellar cortex also attenuated the adjustments in heart rate and blood pressure that ordinarily occur during postural changes in conscious cats (108). Furthermore, animals with posterior cerebellar lesions experienced more severe orthostatic hypotension following the subsequent removal of vestibular inputs than in cerebellum-intact animals with bilateral labyrinthectomies (108). These deficits were only noted when the lesions included both the dorsal and ventral areas of the cerebellar uvula; lesions of the adjacent cerebellar nodulus had no discernable effect on cardiovascular regulation. The consequences of posterior cerebellar lesions on cardiovascular regulation are consistent with the notion that the cerebellum facilitates substitution of non-labyrinthine for vestibular inputs in the neural pathways that mediate vestibulosympathetic responses following damage to the inner ear (51). However, in addition to projecting to the vestibular nuclei, the posterior cerebellar vermis makes connections with the parabrachial nucleus in the pons (50, 109), which in turn provides inputs to brainstem regions regulating blood pressure including NTS (110–112). It has been postulated that a cerebellar–parabrachial–NTS pathway modulates the gain of the baroreceptor reflex (110). A recent study also suggested that recovery of the capacity to adjust blood pressure following vestibular lesions is partly due to increased sensitivity of RVLM neurons to baroreceptor inputs that are elicited during changes in posture (113). Further experiments are needed to examine this possibility, as well as the role of the posterior cerebellar cortex in adjusting the gain of the baroreceptor reflex following the loss of labyrinthine inputs.

Nucleus tractus solitarius

The NTS receives inputs from baroreceptor afferents and other visceral inputs, and plays a critical role in generating baroreceptor reflexes (114–116). The NTS additionally receives projections from the caudal portions of the medial and inferior vestibular nuclei (38–40), suggesting that labyrinthine inputs affect the processing of signals by this region. Only 20% of NTS neurons with discharges synchronized to fluctuations in blood pressure during the cardiac cycle responded to electrical stimulation of the vestibular nerve in anesthetized animals, leading to the conclusion that the vestibular nucleus to NTS projections did not play an appreciable role in cardiovascular regulation (40). A problem with this study is that it did not consider NTS neurons with weaker baroreceptor inputs, whose activity was not modulated by the modest cardiac-related changes in blood pressure. One possibility is that the vestibular system increases the excitability of these cells during changes in posture that may affect blood pressure, so that their sensitivity to baroreceptor inputs increases. As noted earlier, NTS neurons appear to receive signals from the vestibulocerebellum that are relayed through the parabrachial nucleus (110); this circuit may be well-suited to provide for posturally-related adaptive plasticity in baroreceptor responses. Further experiments are thus required to determine the physiological relevance of connections from the caudal vestibular nuclei and vestibulocerebellum to NTS.

Additional regions

Recent work employing retrograde trans-synaptic tract-tracing using attenuated pseudorabies virus recombinants has revealed the existence of central somatomotor-sympathetic circuits. These brain pathways are composed of neurons, which have been called somatomotor-sympathetic neurons (SMSNs), which polysynaptically regulate the activity of both somatic motoneurons and sympathetic efferents (117–121). SMSNs have the potential to coordinate activation, or inhibition, of the somatic motor and sympathetic nervous system, and are thus ideally positioned to be engaged during postural changes. Interestingly, several brain regions that are enriched in their content of SMSNs have been implicated in a variety of responses that require integrated motor and autonomic responses. These include the lateral hypothalamus, dorsal medial hypothalamus, and the paraventricular nucleus of the hypothalamus, which have all been implicated in fight-or-flight type of responses (117–119, 121–124). Other prominent nodes in this circuitry include the ventromedial medulla, a complex integrative region that mediates motor and autonomic responses to pain and thermal stimuli, and the ventrolateral periaqueductal grey, which mediates passive coping behaviours in response to acute threats that are characterized by freezing and tachycardia (117–119, 125, 126). Other regions that contain considerable numbers of SMSNs include locus coeruleus, Kölliker-Fuse nucleus, and RVLM all of which have been shown to interact with the vestibular system (120). These regions may also contribute to shaping vestibularly-elicited responses in a variety of situations.

Summary

The indirect central nervous system connections through which labyrinthine inputs modulate the regulation of blood pressure are indicated in blue in Figure 5.6. Physiological studies have shown that neurons located rostral to the brainstem regulate the sensitivity of RVLM neurons to labyrinthine inputs. These influences could be direct or indirect, perhaps being relayed through the parabrachial nucleus in the pons. In addition, portions of the vestibulocerebellum participate in cardiovascular control, possibly by enhancing the effects of non-labyrinthine inputs on the regulation of blood pressure following damage to the inner ear. NTS receives indirect inputs from the vestibulocerebellum, relayed through the parabrachial nucleus, which may participate in adjusting the sensitivity of the baroreceptor reflex in accordance with body position in space and perhaps behavioural context.

Effects of vestibular stimulation on sympathetic nervous system activity and blood flow in human subjects

Considerable experimental evidence shows that the vestibular system participates in the adjustment of blood pressure during postural alterations of humans. During these experiments, a variety of approaches were used to stimulate the vestibular system, which generated changes in heart rate, blood pressure, and the activity of sympathetic efferent fibres innervating blood vessels in muscle (muscle sympathetic nerve activity, MSNA). Some of the studies employed electrical stimulation to activate vestibular afferents. Sinusoidal galvanic vestibular stimulation was demonstrated to alter MSNA, which became partially entrained to the frequency of the stimulus (127–130). Application of current pulses to the inner ear also elicited a transient increase in MSNA (131). Galvanic vestibular stimulation has also been shown to alter the cardiovascular

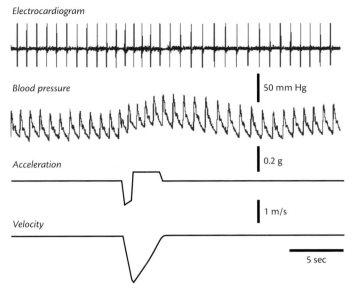

Fig. 5.7 Changes in heart rate and blood pressure during forward linear acceleration with the head restrained in the upright position. The bottom two traces respectively show stimulus acceleration and stimulus velocity. The acceleration evoked a transient increase in heart rate and blood pressure. Adapted from (143).

system responses during conditions that challenge the maintenance of stable blood pressure (132, 133).

A variety of different natural (movement) stimuli that activate the otolith organs also have been shown to affect the regulation of blood pressure. Unfortunately, unlike in studies in animals, it is difficult to perform controls in humans that demonstrate that the effects of movement stimuli are selectively due to activation of the vestibular system. Essandoh (134) introduced a manoeuvre, termed head-down neck flexion (HDNF), where a prone subject allows their neck to extend over the end of table, which is flexed downwards to stimulate the otolith organs. This manoeuvre has been used very frequently in studies of vestibulosympathetic responses, since it is very simple to deliver and has robust effects. Shortt and Ray (135) provided evidence that HDNF increased vascular resistance in the calf musculature in association with augmented MSNA. When subjects that were positioned supine or on their side were subjected to the same head movement, no alterations in MSNA occurred (136, 137). Horizontal head rotation also failed to modulate MSNA (137). These observations were used to bolster the claim that changes in sympathetic nerve activity elicited by HDNF were due to activation of the otolith organs. In addition, aging attenuates the sympathetic nervous system response to HDNF, as hair cells are lost in the inner ear and vestibular hypofunction ensues (138, 139).

The findings from studies involving HDNF are supported by the demonstration that otolith organ stimulation during off-vertical axis rotation (OVAR) also modulated sympathetic nervous system activity in humans (140). In addition, linear acceleration of the head produced by oscillating a subject in a linear sled (141–143) or dropping the head for a short distance (144, 145) modified MSNA, heart rate and blood pressure. For example, Figure 5.7 illustrates the changes in heart rate and blood pressure during forward linear acceleration in a sled. Some of the experiments involving linear acceleration included labyrinthine-defective subjects (143, 145),

which did not exhibit the same cardiovascular system responses to accelerations as normal subjects. These data further confirm that inputs from otolith organs participate in the regulation of blood pressure in humans.

There is some evidence from experiments in human subjects that vestibulosympathetic responses are patterned, as documented in animals and described previously (23, 24, 34, 35, 146). One study (147) incorporated central blood volume challenges using moderate (−40 mmHg) lower body negative pressure and stimulation of vestibular receptors using HDNF and head-down neck extension (HDNE, downward tilt of the head in supine subjects). HDNF in this experiment elicited peripheral vasoconstriction coupled with a compensatory cerebral artery relaxation, while HDNE did not affect peripheral sympathetic outflow but augmented cerebral constriction. A recent study in women also indicated that forelimb and hindlimb MSNA responses to head-down flexion diverge in certain phases of the menstrual cycle (148); hormonal changes have not been shown to affect patterning of responses to other stimuli in humans.

Vestibulo-autonomic system: relevance for clinicians

Vestibular system dysfunction can occur as a result of damage to the inner ear, VIIIth cranial nerve, or structures within the central nervous system that process labyrinthine signals. Vascular and immunological insults of the vestibular system can occur (149) but truly isolated vascular lesions to the central nervous system, bilateral immunological attack of the labyrinths, VIIIth nerves, or vestibular nuclei are rare. Neurosurgical problems such as vestibular schwannoma are not generally associated with the hallmark symptom of vestibular disorders: dizziness (150). The rarity of dizziness in the patient with vestibular schwannoma is likely due to the slow indolent growth pattern of the tumour, and resulting central nervous system compensation. Common neurological pathologies affecting the vestibular system, such as benign paroxysmal positional vertigo, Ménière's disease, and vestibular labyrinthitis often present acutely, but undergo a slow chronic pathologic transformation (151–153). The symptoms are often at their greatest at the onset of the disease, and diminish over the course of the disease's lifetime. It is thus not surprising that patients with vestibular disorders do not ordinarily report overt signs or symptoms related to the regulation of blood pressure, such as orthostatic intolerance, since their problems are typically unilateral and/or they develop slowly enough for compensation to occur. For example, in a retrospective study of 56 patients with known peripheral vestibular nerve dysfunction, which was unilateral and chronic in most of the individuals, an incidence of 10.7% of neurocardiogenic dysfunction was noted although no significant association was observed between cardiovascular response abnormalities and tilt-table testing (154). The conclusion from this study was that there is no difference in the rate of orthostatic intolerance between patients with poor or normal caloric function. These findings are in accordance with data collected during studies on animals. As noted above, studies in animals showed that fluctuations in blood pressure during postural alterations are only prevalent within the first week after bilateral removal of vestibular inputs (29).

Non-physiological activation of vestibular afferents can elicit a pattern of autonomic responses that is physiologically maladaptive.

For example, caloric stimulation, visual-vestibular mismatch, as well as electrical and galvanic stimuli of vestibular afferents can lead to nausea, vomiting, hypotension, skin vasoconstriction, or sweating (23, 24, 127, 155, 156). In contrast to the physiologically-salient head-up tilts, which trigger a vestibularly-elicited decrease in blood pooling within the lower extremity and maintain the cardiac output, such autonomic responses do not have a clear adaptive role and their persistent activation is likely to be interpreted as stressful by the central nervous system. Extensive literature points to a strong bidirectional relationship between autonomic hyperactivity as well as aberrant, and stressful autonomic responses and anxiety (157). This relationship is thought to be due to the persistent activation of the fight-or-flight response, which serves an important adaptive role in the times of immediate danger, but has a deleterious effect when it is chronically activated. The resultant hypervigilance and sympathetic overactivity leads to the development of anxiety and phobias that often generalize to non-specific triggers (158–160). Stressful interoceptive cues triggered by sympathetic hyperactivation play a powerful role in the emergence of anxious and phobic responses, and interoceptive exposure via hyperventilation, spinning, or breathing through a straw can elicit panic reactions, anxiety, and re-experience of traumatic memories in susceptible individuals (161). It is likely that in the decompensated state following vestibular damage persistent non-physiological activation of vestibular afferents triggers autonomic responses that act as interoceptive stressors and potentiate emergence of anxiety. Indeed, agoraphobia and related anxiety disorders have been strongly linked with vestibular dysfunction, especially in panic disorder with agoraphobia (162). This relationship is likely bidirectional since hyperventilation, a common physical manifestation of panic, can negatively impact vestibular function (163), while anxiety patients often manifest abnormalities on vestibular function tests and patients with known balance disorders are more likely to develop anxiety (164, 165). Anxiety patients most frequently exhibit vestibulospinal, vestibulo-ocular, or peripheral vestibular dysfunction (162). In addition, anxiety is strongly associated with migraines, and is comorbid with dizziness (165, 166), suggesting that migraine anxiety dizziness (MARD) may represent a distinct disorder rather a random association (165). While the pathophysiology of MARD is unknown, Furman et al. have suggested that caudal medial and inferior vestibular nuclei play key roles in mediating its manifestations (165). Because these same areas mediate vestibulosympathetic interactions (see earlier), it seems feasible that vestibulosympathetic dysfunction may contribute to the aetiology of MARD. Interestingly, MARD patients exhibit visual dependence, presumably as part of a compensatory response to vestibular dysfunction (165), and because removal of visual cues worsens blood pressure lability in vestibularly-lesioned animals (29), this clinical observation suggests that MARD patients rely on the visual cues to maintain their cardiovascular and autonomic functions to prevent development of migraines and anxiety along with maintaining their postural stability.

Given this complexity, patients with vestibular dysfunction can present with a variety of symptoms, and with chief complaints focusing on cardiovascular, headache, or balance issues. These individuals are often evaluated by diverse healthcare practitioners, including primary care physicians, cardiologists, otolaryngologists, neurologists, and psychiatrists (165). Awareness of the underlying physiology of these systems and the potential consequences of vestibular dysfunction coupled with autonomic changes and mood alterations by these healthcare professionals is essential for effective treatment of these disorders.

Acknowledgements

This authors' research related to information presented in this chapter is supported by National Institutes of Health grants R01–DC00693 and R01–DC03732 (to B.J.Y.), R00–MH081927 (to I.A.K.), and a Brain and Behavior Research Foundation (NARSAD) Young Investigator Award (to I.A.K.).

References

1. Lackner JR, Dizio P (2006). Space motion sickness. *Exp Brain Res*, 175, 377–99.
2. Money KE (1970). Motion sickness. *Physiol Rev*, 50, 1–39.
3. Yates BJ (2009). Motion Sickness. In Binder MD, Hirokawa N, Windhorst U (Eds) *Encyclopedia of Neuroscience*, pp. 2410–3. Heidelberg: Springer.
4. Yates BJ, Wilson TD (2009). Vestibulo-autonomic responses. In Squire LR (Ed) *Encyclopedia of Neuroscience*, pp. 133–8. Oxford: Academic Press.
5. Yates BJ, Bronstein AM (2005). The effects of vestibular system lesions on autonomic regulation: observations, mechanisms, and clinical implications. *J Vestib Res*, 15, 119–29.
6. Yates BJ, Billig I, Cotter LA, Mori RL, Card JP (2002). Role of the vestibular system in regulating respiratory muscle activity during movement. *Clin Exp Pharmacol Physiol*, 29, 112–17.
7. Balaban CD, Yates BJ (2004). Vestibulo-autonomic interactions: a teleologic perspective. In Highstein SM, Fay RR, Popper AN (Eds) *Anatomy and Physiology of the Central and Peripheral Vestibular System*, pp. 286–342. Heidelberg: Springer.
8. Yavorcik KJ, Reighard DA, Misra SP, *et al.* (2009). Effects of postural changes and removal of vestibular inputs on blood flow to and from the hindlimb of conscious felines. *Am J Physiol Regul Integr Comp Physiol*, 297, R1777–84.
9. Starling EH (1918). *The Linacre Lecture on the Law of the Heart*. London: Longmans, Green.
10. Hall JE (2011). *Guyton and Hall Textbook of Medical Physiology* (12th ed). Philadelphia, PA: Saunders.
11. Rushmer RF (1976). *Cardiovascular Dynamics* (4th ed). Philadelphia, PA: Saunders.
12. Spiegel EA (1946). Effect of labyrinthine reflexes on the vegetative nervous system. *Arch Otolaryngol*, 44, 61–72.
13. Spiegel EA, Démétriades TD (1922). Der Einfluss des Vestibular-apparates auf das Gefässsystem. *Pflügers Arch ges Physiol*, 196, 185–8.
14. Yates BJ (1992). Vestibular influences on the sympathetic nervous system. *Brain Res Rev*, 17, 51–9.
15. Kerman IA, Yates BJ (1998). Regional and functional differences in the distribution of vestibulosympathetic reflexes. *Am J Physiol Regul Integr Comp Physiol*, 275, R824–R35.
16. Bahr R, Bartel B, Blumberg H, Janig W (1986). Functional characterization of preganglionic neurons projecting in the lumbar splanchnic nerves: vasoconstrictor neurons. *J Autonom Nerv Syst*, 15, 131–40.
17. Bahr R, Blumberg H, Janig W (198). Do dichotomizing afferent fibers exist which supply visceral organs as well as somatic structures? A contribution to the problem or referred pain. *Neurosci Lett*, 24, 25–8.
18. Janig W, McLachlan EM (1992). Characteristics of function-specific pathways in the sympathetic nervous system. *Trends Neurosci*, 15, 475–81.
19. Ishikawa T, Miyazawa T (1980). Sympathetic responses evoked by vestibular stimulation and their interactions with somato-sympathetic reflexes. *J Autonom Nerv Syst*, 1, 243–54.
20. Ishikawa T, Miyazawa T, Shimizu I, Tomita H (1979). Similarity between vestibulo-sympathetic response and supraspinal sympathetic reflex. *Nihon Univ J Med*, 21, 201–10.

21. Tang PC, Gernandt BE (1969). Autonomic responses to vestibular stimulation. *Exp Neurol*, 24, 558–78.

22. Uchino Y, Kudo N, Tsuda K, Iwamura Y (1970). Vestibular inhibition of sympathetic nerve activities. *Brain Res*, 22, 195–206.

23. Kerman IA, Emanuel BA, Yates BJ (2000). Vestibular stimulation leads to distinct hemodynamic patterning. *Am J Physiol Regul Integr Comp Physiol*, 279, R118–25.

24. Kerman IA, Yates BJ, McAllen RM (2000). Anatomic patterning in the expression of vestibulosympathetic reflexes. *Am J Physiol Regul Integr Comp Physiol*, 279, R109–17.

25. Yates BJ, Miller AD (1994). Properties of sympathetic reflexes elicited by natural vestibular stimulation: implications for cardiovascular control. *J Neurophysiol*, 71, 2087–92.

26. Woodring SF, Rossiter CD, Yates BJ (1997). Pressor response elicited by nose-up vestibular stimulation in cats. *Exp Brain Res*, 113, 165–8.

27. Fernandez C, Goldberg JM (1976). Physiology of peripheral neurons innervating otolith organs of the squirrel monkey. III. Response dynamics. *J Neurophysiol*, 39, 996–1008.

28. Doba N, Reis DJ (1974). Role of the cerebellum and vestibular apparatus in regulation of orthostatic reflexes in the cat. *Circ Res*, 34, 9–18.

29. Jian BJ, Cotter LA, Emanuel BA, Cass SP, Yates BJ (1999). Effects of bilateral vestibular lesions on orthostatic tolerance in awake cats. *J Appl Physiol*, 86, 1552–60.

30. Raffai G, Cseko C, Nadasy G, Monos E (2010). Vestibular control of intermediate- and long-term cardiovascular responses to experimental orthostasis. *Physiol Res*, 59, 43–51.

31. Zhu H, Jordan JR, Hardy SP, et al. (2007). Linear acceleration-evoked cardiovascular responses in awake rats. *J Appl Physiol*, 103, 646–54.

32. Abe C, Tanaka K, Awazu C, Morita H (2008). The vestibular system is integral in regulating plastic alterations in the pressor response to free drop mediated by the nonvestibular system. *Neurosci Lett*, 445, 149–52.

33. Abe C, Tanaka K, Awazu C, Chen H, Morita H (2007). Plastic alteration of vestibulo-cardiovascular reflex induced by 2 weeks of 3–G load in conscious rats. *Exp Brain Res*, 181, 639–46.

34. Wilson TD, Cotter LA, Draper JA, et al. (2006). Effects of postural changes and removal of vestibular inputs on blood flow to the head of conscious felines. *J Appl Physiol*, 100, 1475–82.

35. Wilson TD, Cotter LA, Draper JA, et al. (2006). Vestibular inputs elicit patterned changes in limb blood flow in conscious cats. *J Physiol*, 575, 671–84.

36. Goldberg JM, Fernández C (1984). The vestibular system. In Darian-Smith I (Ed) *Handbook of Physiology Section I: The Nervous System Volume III, Sensory Processes, Part 2*, pp. 977–1022. Bethesda, MD: American Physiological Society.

37. Yates BJ, Jakus J, Miller AD (1993). Vestibular effects on respiratory outflow in the decerebrate cat. *Brain Res*, 629, 209–17.

38. Balaban CD, Beryozkin G (1994). Vestibular nucleus projections to nucleus tractus solitarius and the dorsal motor nucleus of the vagus nerve: potential substrates for vestibulo-autonomic interactions. *Exp Brain Res*, 98, 200–12.

39. Ruggiero DA, Mtui EP, Otake K, Anwar M (1996). Vestibular afferents to the dorsal vagal complex: substrate for vestibular-autonomic interactions in the rat. *Brain Res*, 743, 294–302.

40. Yates BJ, Grelot L, Kerman IA, Balaban CD, Jakus J, Miller AD (1994). Organization of vestibular inputs to nucleus tractus solitarius and adjacent structures in cat brain stem. *Am J Physiol*, 267, R974–83.

41. Porter JD, Balaban CD (1997). Connections between the vestibular nuclei and brain stem regions that mediate autonomic function in the rat. *J Vestib Res*, 7, 63–76.

42. Holstein GR, Friedrich VL, Jr, Kang T, Kukielka E, Martinelli GP (2011). Direct projections from the caudal vestibular nuclei to the ventrolateral medulla in the rat. *Neuroscience*, 175, 104–17.

43. Stocker SD, Steinbacher BC, Balaban CD, Yates BJ (1997). Connections of the caudal ventrolateral medullary reticular formation in the cat brainstem. *Exp Brain Res*, 116, 270–82.

44. Yates BJ, Balaban CD, Miller AD, Endo K, Yamaguchi Y (1995). Vestibular inputs to the lateral tegmental field of the cat: potential role in autonomic control. *Brain Res*, 689, 197–206.

45. Martinelli GP, Friedrich VL, Jr, Prell GD, Holstein GR (2007). Vestibular neurons in the rat contain imidazoleacetic acid-ribotide, a putative neurotransmitter involved in blood pressure regulation. *J Comp Neurol*, 501, 568–81.

46. Miller DM, Cotter LA, Gandhi NJ, et al. (2008). Responses of caudal vestibular nucleus neurons of conscious cats to rotations in vertical planes, before and after a bilateral vestibular neurectomy. *Exp Brain Res*, 188, 175–86.

47. Jian BJ, Shintani T, Emanuel BA, Yates BJ (2002). Convergence of limb, visceral, and vertical semicircular canal or otolith inputs onto vestibular nucleus neurons. *Exp Brain Res*, 144, 247–57.

48. Endo K, Thomson DB, Wilson VJ, Yamaguchi T, Yates BJ (1995). Vertical vestibular input to and projections from the caudal parts of the vestibular nuclei of the decerebrate cat. *J Neurophysiol*, 74, 428–36.

49. Jian BJ, Acernese AW, Lorenzo J, Card JP, Yates BJ (2005). Afferent pathways to the region of the vestibular nuclei that participates in cardiovascular and respiratory control. *Brain Res*, 1044, 241–50.

50. Paton JF, La Noce A, Sykes RM, et al. (1991). Efferent connections of lobule IX of the posterior cerebellar cortex in the rabbit—some functional considerations. *J Auton Nerv Syst*, 36, 209–24.

51. Yates BJ, Miller DM (2009). Integration of nonlabyrinthine inputs by the vestibular system: role in compensation following bilateral damage to the inner ear. *J Vestib Res*, 19, 183–9.

52. Dampney RA, Goodchild AK, McAllen RM (1987). Vasomotor control by subretrofacial neurones in the rostral ventrolateral medulla. *Can J Physiol Pharmacol*, 65, 1572–9.

53. Dampney RAL (1990). The subretrofacial nucleus: its pivotal role in cardiovascular regulation. *News Physiol Sci*, 5, 63–7.

54. Dampney RAL (1994). The subretrofacial vasomotor nucleus – anatomical, chemical and pharmacological properties and role in cardiovascular regulation. *Prog Neurobiol*, 42, 197–227.

55. Dampney RA, Goodchild AK, Robertson LG, Montgomery W (1982). Role of ventrolateral medulla in vasomotor regulation: a correlative anatomical and physiological study. *Brain Res*, 249, 223–35.

56. Barman SM, Gebber GL (1985). Axonal projection patterns of ventrolateral medullospinal sympathoexcitatory neurons. *J Neurophysiol*, 53, 1551–66.

57. Dembowsky K, McAllen RM (1990). Baroreceptor inhibition of subretrofacial neurons: evidence from intracellular recordings in the cat. *Neurosci Lett*, 111, 139–43.

58. McAllen RM (1986). Identification and properties of sub-retrofacial bulbospinal neurones: a descending cardiovascular pathway in the cat. *J Auton Nerv Syst*, 17, 151–64.

59. McAllen RM, Habler HJ, Michaelis M, Peters O, Janig W (1994). Monosynaptic excitation of preganglionic vasomotor neurons by subretrofacial neurons of the rostral ventrolateral medulla. *Brain Res*, 634, 227–34.

60. McAllen RM, May CN, Campos RR (1997). The supply of vasomotor drive to individual classes of sympathetic neuron. *Clin Exp Hypertension*, 19, 607–18.

61. McAllen RM, Trevaks D, Allen AM (2001). Analysis of firing correlations between sympathetic premotor neuron pairs in anesthetized cats. *J Neurophysiol*, 85, 1697–708.

62. Dean C, Coote JH (1986). A ventromedullary relay involved in the hypothalamic and chemoreceptor activation of sympathetic postganglionic neurones to skeletal muscle, kidney and splanchnic area. *Brain Res*, 377, 279–85.

63. Feldberg W, Guertzenstein PG (1976). Vasopressor effects obtained by drugs acting on the ventral surface of the brain stem. *J Physiol*, 258, 337–55.

64. Stein RD, Weaver LC, Yardley CP (1989). Ventrolateral medullary neurones: effects on magnitude and rhythm of discharge of mesenteric and renal nerves in cats. *J Physiol*, 408, 571–86.

65. Dampney RA (1981). Brain stem mechanisms in the control of arterial pressure. *Clin Exp Hypertens*, 3, 379–91.

66. Reis DJ, Ross CA, Ruggiero DA, Granata AR, Joh TH (1984). Role of adrenaline neurons of ventrolateral medulla (the C1 group) in the tonic and phasic control of arterial pressure. *Clin Exp Hypertens A*, 6, 221–41.

67. Granata AR, Ruggiero DA, Park DH, Joh TH, Reis DJ (1985). Brain stem area with C1 epinephrine neurons mediates baroreflex vasodepressor responses. *Am J Physiol*, 248, H547–H67.

68. Yates BJ, Siniaia MS, Miller AD (1995). Descending pathways necessary for vestibular influences on sympathetic and inspiratory outflow. *Am J Physiol Regul Integr Comp Physiol*, 37, R1381–R5.

69. Yates BJ, Goto T, Bolton PS (1993). Responses of neurons in the rostral ventrolateral medulla of the cat to natural vestibular stimulation. *Brain Res*, 601, 255–64.

70. Destefino VJ, Reighard DA, Sugiyama Y, et al. (2011). Responses of neurons in the rostral ventrolateral medulla (RVLM) to whole-body rotations: comparisons in decerebrate and conscious cats. *J Appl Physiol*, 110, 1699–707.

71. Sugiyama Y, Suzuki T, Yates BJ (2011). Role of the rostral ventrolateral medulla (RVLM) in the patterning of vestibular system influences on sympathetic nervous system outflow to the upper and lower body. *Exp Brain Res*, 210, 515–27.

72. Schramm LP, Strack AM, Platt KB, Loewy AD (1993). Peripheral and central pathways regulating the kidney – a study using pseudorabies virus. *Brain Res*, 616, 251–62.

73. Lee TK, Lois JH, Troupe JH, Wilson TD, Yates BJ (2007). Transneuronal tracing of neural pathways that regulate hindlimb muscle blood flow. *Am J Physiol Regul Integr Comp Physiol*, 292, R1532–41.

74. Barman SM, Gebber GL (1992). Rostral ventrolateral medullary and caudal medullary raphe neurons with activity correlated to the 10–Hz rhythm in sympathetic nerve discharge. *J Neurophysiol*, 68, 1535–47.

75. Zhong S, Barman SM, Gebber GL (1992). Effects of brain stem lesions on 10-Hz and 2- to 6-Hz rhythms in sympathetic nerve discharge. *Am J Physiol*, 262, R1015–24.

76. Zhong S, Huang ZS, Gebber GL, Barman SM (1993). The 10–Hz sympathetic rhythm is dependent on raphe and rostral ventrolateral medullary neurons. *Am J Physiol*, 264, R857–R66.

77. Yates BJ, Goto T, Bolton PS (1992). Responses of neurons in the caudal medullary raphe nuclei of the cat to stimulation of the vestibular nerve. *Exp Brain Res*, 89, 323–32.

78. Yates BJ, Goto T, Kerman I, Bolton PS (1993). Responses of caudal medullary raphe neurons to natural vestibular stimulation. *J Neurophysiol*, 70, 938–46.

79. Yates BJ, Yamagata Y, Bolton PS (1991). The ventrolateral medulla of the cat mediates vestibulosympathetic reflexes. *Brain Res*, 552, 265–72.

80. Steinbacher BC, Yates BJ (1996). Processing of vestibular and other inputs by the caudal ventrolateral medullary reticular formation. *Am J Physiol Regul Integr Comp Physiol*, 271, R1070–R7.

81. Steinbacher BC, Yates BJ (1996). Brainstem interneurons necessary for vestibular influences on sympathetic outflow. *Brain Res*, 720, 204–10.

82. Demer JL, Honrubia V, Baloh RW (1994). Dynamic visual acuity: a test for oscillopsia and vestibulo-ocular reflex function. *Am J Otol*, 15, 340–7.

83. Tian JR, Shubayev I, Demer JL (2002). Dynamic visual acuity during passive and self-generated transient head rotation in normal and unilaterally vestibulopathic humans. *Exp Brain Res*, 142, 486–95.

84. Hayward LF (2007). Midbrain modulation of the cardiac baroreflex involves excitation of lateral parabrachial neurons in the rat. *Brain Res*, 1145, 117–27.

85. Allen GV, Cechetto DF (1992). Functional and anatomical organization of cardiovascular pressor and depressor sites in the lateral hypothalamic area: I. Descending projections. *J Comp Neurol*, 315, 313–32.

86. Cechetto DF, Calaresu FR (1983). Parabrachial units responding to stimulation of buffer nerves and forebrain in the cat. *Am J Physiol*, 245, R811–R9.

87. Balaban CD (1996). Vestibular nucleus projections to the parabrachial nucleus in rabbits: implications for vestibular influences on the autonomic nervous system. *Exp Brain Res*, 108, 367–81.

88. Bradley DJ, Ghelarducci B, Paton JF, Spyer KM (1987). The cardiovascular responses elicited from the posterior cerebellar cortex in the anaesthetized and decerebrate rabbit. *J Physiol*, 383, 537–50.

89. Bradley DJ, Pascoe JP, Paton JF, Spyer KM (1987). Cardiovascular and respiratory responses evoked from the posterior cerebellar cortex and fastigial nucleus in the cat. *J Physiol*, 393, 107–21.

90. Henry RT, Connor JD, Balaban CD (1989). Nodulus-uvula depressor response: central GABA-mediated inhibition of alpha-adrenergic outflow. *Am J Physiol*, 256, H1601–H8.

91. Silva-Carvalho L, Paton JF, Goldsmith GE, Spyer KM(1991). The effects of electrical stimulation of lobule IXb of the posterior cerebellar vermis on neurones within the rostral ventrolateral medulla in the anaesthetised cat. *J Autonom Nerv Syst*, 36, 97–106.

92. Barman SM, Gebber GL (2009). The posterior vermis of the cerebellum selectively inhibits 10-Hz sympathetic nerve discharge in anesthetized cats. *Am J Physiol Regul Integr Comp Physiol*, 297, R210–7.

93. Sebastiani L, La Noce A, Paton JF, Ghelarducci B (1992). Influence of the cerebellar posterior vermis on the acquisition of the classically conditioned bradycardic response in the rabbit. *Exp Brain Res*, 88, 193–8.

94. Shojaku H, Sato Y, Ikarashi K, Kawasaki T (1987). Topographical distribution of Purkinje cells in the uvula and the nodulus projecting to the vestibular nuclei in cats. *Brain Res*, 416, 100–12.

95. Angelaki DE, Hess BJ (1994). The cerebellar nodulus and ventral uvula control the torsional vestibulo-ocular reflex. *J Neurophysiol*, 72, 1443–7.

96. Angelaki DE, Hess BJM (1995). Inertial representation of angular motion in the vestibular system of rhesus monkeys. 2. otolith-controlled transformation that depends on an intact cerebellar nodulus. *J Neurophysiol*, 73, 1729–51.

97. Angelaki DE, Hess BJ (1995). Lesion of the nodulus and ventral uvula abolish steady-state off-vertical axis otolith response. *J Neurophysiol*, 73, 1716–20.

98. Solomon D, Cohen B (1994). Stimulation of the nodulus and uvula discharges velocity storage in the vestibulo-ocular reflex. *Exp Brain Res*, 102, 57–68.

99. Wearne S, Raphan T, Waespe W, Cohen B (1997). Control of the three-dimensional dynamic characteristics of the angular vestibulo-ocular reflex by the nodulus and uvula. In Dezeeuw CI, Strata P, Voogd J (Eds) *Cerebellum: from Structure to Control*, pp. 321–34. Amsterdam: Elsevier.

100. Wiest G, Deecke L, Trattnig S, Mueller C (1999). Abolished tilt suppression of the vestibulo-ocular reflex caused by a selective uvulo-nodular lesion. *Neurology*, 52, 417–9.

101. Dulac S, Raymond JL, Sejnowski TJ, Lisberger SG (1995). Learning and memory in the vestibulo-ocular reflex. *Annu Rev Neurosci*, 18, 409–41.

102. Lisberger SG (1988). The neural basis for learning of simple motor skills. *Science*, 242, 728–35.

103. Miles FA, Lisberger SG (1981). Plasticity in the vestibulo-ocular reflex: a new hypothesis. *Ann Rev Neurosci*, 4, 273–99.

104. Nagao S, Yoshioka N, Hensch T, et al. (1991). The role of cerebellar flocculus in adaptive gain control of ocular reflexes. *Acta Oto-Laryngol Suppl*, 481, 234–6.

105. Yates BJ, Jian BJ, Cotter LA, Cass SP (2000). Responses of vestibular nucleus neurons to tilt following chronic bilateral removal of vestibular inputs. *Exp Brain Res*, 130, 151–8.

106. Cotter LA, Arendt HE, Cass SP, et al. (2004). Effects of postural changes and vestibular lesions on genioglossal muscle activity in conscious cats. *J Appl Physiol*, 96, 923–30.

107. Mori RL, Cotter LA, Arendt HE, Olsheski CJ, Yates BJ (2005). Effects of bilateral vestibular nucleus lesions on cardiovascular regulation in conscious cats. *J Appl Physiol*, 98, 526–33.

108. Holmes MJ, Cotter LA, Arendt HE, Cass SP, Yates BJ (2002). Effects of lesions of the caudal cerebellar vermis on cardiovascular regulation in awake cats. *Brain Res*, 938, 62–72.

109. Sadakane K, Kondo M, Nisimaru N (2000). Direct projection from the cardiovascular control region of the cerebellar cortex, the lateral nodulus-uvula, to the brainstem in rabbits. *Neurosci Res*, 36, 15–26.

110. Paton JFR, Silva-Carvalho L, Thompson CS, Spyer KM (1990). Nucleus tractus solitarius as mediator of evoked parabrachial cardiovascular responses in the decerebrate rabbit. *J Physiol*, 428, 693–705.

111. Smith JC, Morrison DE, Ellenberger HH, Otto MR, Feldman JL (1989). Brainstem projections to the major respiratory neuron populations in the medulla of the cat. *J Comp Neurol*, 281, 69–96.

112. Fulwiler CE, Saper CB (1984). Subnuclear organization of the efferent connections of the parabrachial nucleus in the rat. *Brain Res*, 319, 229–59.

113. Barman SM, Suzuki T, Sugiyama Y, *et al.* (2011). Cardiac-related and other rhythmic activity of neurons in the rostral ventrolateral medulla (RVLM) of conscious cats: effects of vestibular lesions. *FASEB J*, 25, 1027.4.

114. Lawrence AJ, Jarrott B (1996). Neurochemical modulation of cardiovascular control in the nucleus tractus solitarius. *Prog Neurobiol*, 48, 21–53.

115. Loewy AD (1981). Descending pathways to sympathetic and parasympathetic preganglionic neurons. *J Autonom Nerv Syst*, 3, 265–75.

116. Pilowsky PM, Goodchild AK (2002). Baroreceptor reflex pathways and neurotransmitters: 10 years on. *J Hypertens*, 20, 1675–88.

117. Kerman IA (2008). Organization of brain somatomotor-sympathetic circuits. *Exp Brain Res*, 187, 1–16.

118. Kerman IA, Akil H, Watson SJ (2006). Rostral elements of sympatho-motor circuitry: a virally mediated transsynaptic tracing study. *J Neurosci*, 26, 3423–33.

119. Kerman IA, Bernard R, Rosenthal D, Beals J, Akil H, Watson SJ (2007). Distinct populations of presympathetic-premotor neurons express orexin or melanin-concentrating hormone in the rat lateral hypothalamus. *J Comp Neurol*, 505, 586–601.

120. Kerman IA, Enquist LW, Watson SJ, Yates BJ (2003). Brainstem substrates of sympatho-motor circuitry identified using trans-synaptic tracing with pseudorabies virus recombinants. *J Neurosci*, 23, 4657–66.

121. Krout KE, Mettenleiter TC, Loewy AD (2003). Single CNS neurons link both central motor and cardiosympathetic systems: a double-virus tracing study. *Neuroscience*, 118, 853–66.

122. Zhang Y, Kerman IA, Laque A, *et al.* (2011). Leptin-receptor-expressing neurons in the dorsomedial hypothalamus and median preoptic area regulate sympathetic brown adipose tissue circuits. *J Neurosci*, 31, 1873–84.

123. Sonmez K, Zaveri NT, Kerman IA, *et al.* (2009). Evolutionary sequence modeling for discovery of peptide hormones. *PLoS Comp Biol*, 5, e1000258.

124. Zhang W, Shimoyama M, Fukuda Y, Kuwaki T (2006). Multiple components of the defense response depend on orexin: evidence from orexin knockout mice and orexin neuron-ablated mice. *Autonom Neurosci*, 126–127, 139–45.

125. Mason P (2005). Ventromedial medulla: pain modulation and beyond. *J Comp Neurol*, 493, 2–8.

126. Johnson PL, Lightman SL, Lowry CA (2004). A functional subset of serotonergic neurons in the rat ventrolateral periaqueductal gray implicated in the inhibition of sympathoexcitation and panic. *Ann N Y Acad Sci*, 1018, 58–64.

127. Bent LR, Bolton PS, Macefield VG (2006). Modulation of muscle sympathetic bursts by sinusoidal galvanic vestibular stimulation in human subjects. *Exp Brain Res*, 174, 701–11.

128. Grewal T, James C, Macefield VG (2009). Frequency-dependent modulation of muscle sympathetic nerve activity by sinusoidal galvanic vestibular stimulation in human subjects. *Exp Brain Res*, 197, 379–86.

129. James C, Macefield VG (2010). Competitive interactions between vestibular and cardiac rhythms in the modulation of muscle sympathetic nerve activity. *Autonom Neurosci*, 158, 127–31.

130. James C, Stathis A, Macefield VG (2010). Vestibular and pulse-related modulation of skin sympathetic nerve activity during sinusoidal galvanic vestibular stimulation in human subjects. *Exp Brain Res*, 202, 291–8.

131. Voustianiouk A, Kaufmann H, Diedrich A, *et al.* (2006). Electrical activation of the human vestibulo-sympathetic reflex. *Exp Brain Res*, 171, 251–61.

132. Iwata C, Abe C, Tanaka K, Morita H (2011). Role of the vestibular system in the arterial pressure response to parabolic-flight-induced gravitational changes in human subjects. *Neurosci Lett*, 495, 121–5.

133. Tanaka K, Abe C, Awazu C, Morita H (2009). Vestibular system plays a significant role in arterial pressure control during head-up tilt in young subjects. *Auton Neurosci*, 148, 90–6.

134. Essandoh LK, Duprez DA, Shepherd JT (1988). Reflex constriction of human resistance vessels to head-down neck flexion. *Am J Physiol*, 64, 767–70.

135. Shortt TL, Ray CA (1997). Sympathetic and vascular responses to head-down neck flexion in humans. *Am J Physiol*, 272, H1780–4.

136. Hume KM, Ray CA (1999). Sympathetic responses to head-down rotations in humans. *J Appl Physiol*, 86, 1971–6.

137. Ray CA, Hume KM, Steele SL (1998). Sympathetic nerve activity during natural stimulation of horizontal semicircular canals in humans. *Am J Physiol*, 275, R1274–8.

138. Ray CA, Monahan KD (2002). Aging attenuates the vestibulosympathetic reflex in humans. *Circulation*, 105, 956–61.

139. Monahan KD, Ray CA (2002). Vestibulosympathetic reflex during orthostatic challenge in aging humans. *Am J Physiol Regul Integr Comp Physiol*, 283, R1027–32.

140. Kaufmann H, Biaggioni I, Voustianiouk A, *et al.* (2002). Vestibular control of sympathetic activity. An otolith-sympathetic reflex in humans. *Exp Brain Res*, 143, 463–9.

141. Cui J, Iwase S, Mano T, Katayama N, Mori S (2001). Muscle sympathetic outflow during horizontal linear acceleration in humans. *Am J Physiol Regul Integr Comp Physiol*, 281, R625–34.

142. Cui JA, Iwase S, Mano T, Katayama N, Mori S (1999). Muscle sympathetic nerve response to vestibular stimulation by sinusoidal linear acceleration in humans. *Neurosci Lett*, 267, 181–4.

143. Yates BJ, Aoki M, Burchill P, Bronstein AM, Gresty MA (1999). Cardiovascular responses elicited by linear acceleration in humans. *Exp Brain Res*, 125, 476–84.

144. Radtke A, Popov K, Bronstein AM, Gresty MA (2000). Evidence for a vestibulo-cardiac reflex in man. *Lancet*, 356, 736–7.

145. Radtke A, Popov K, Bronstein AM, Gresty MA (2003). Vestibulo-autonomic control in man: Short- and long-latency vestibular effects on cardiovascular function. *J Vestib Res*, 13, 25–37.

146. Kerman IA, McAllen RM, Yates BJ (2000). Patterning of sympathetic nerve activity in response to vestibular stimulation. *Brain Res Bul*, 53, 11–6.

147. Wilson TD, Serrador JM, Shoemaker JK (2003). Head position modifies cerebrovascular response to orthostatic stress. *Brain Res*, 961, 261–8.

148. Lawrence JE, Klein JC, Carter JR (2010). Menstrual cycle elicits divergent forearm vascular responses to vestibular activation in humans. *Auton Neurosci*, 154, 89–93.

149. Karatas M (2008). Central vertigo and dizziness: epidemiology, differential diagnosis, and common causes. *Neurologist*, 14, 355–64.

150. Kentala E, Pyykko I (2001). Clinical picture of vestibular schwannoma. *Auris, Nasus, Larynx*, 28, 15–22.

151. Furman JM, Cass SP (1999). Benign paroxysmal positional vertigo. *New Engl J Med*, 341, 1590–6.

152. Charles J, Fahridin S, Britt H (2008). Vertiginous syndrome. *Austr Fam Phys*, 37, 299.

153. Weber PC (1998). Vertigo: strategies for evaluating/treating the patient with dizziness or vertigo. *J S Carolina Med Assoc*, 94, 526–9.

154. Heidenreich KD, Weisend S, Fouad-Tarazi FM, White JA (2009). The incidence of coexistent autonomic and vestibular dysfunction in patients with postural dizziness. *Am J Otolaryngol*, 30, 225–9.

155. Bolton PS, Wardman DL, Macefield VG (2004). Absence of short-term vestibular modulation of muscle sympathetic outflow, assessed by brief galvanic vestibular stimulation in awake human subjects. *Exp Brain Res*, 154, 39–43.

156. Yates BJ, Holmes MJ, Jian BJ, Kerman IA (2003). Vestibular influences on cardiovascular control during movement. In Luxon LM (Ed) *Textbook of Audiological Medicine*, pp. 691–700. London: Taylor and Francis.

157. Dugas MJ, Gagnon F, Ladouceur R, Freeston MH (1998). Generalized anxiety disorder: a preliminary test of a conceptual model. *Behav Res Ther*, 36, 215–26.

158. Jovanovic T, Ressler KJ (2010). How the neurocircuitry and genetics of fear inhibition may inform our understanding of PTSD. *Am J Psych*, 167, 648–62.

159. Ressler KJ (2010). Amygdala activity, fear, and anxiety: modulation by stress. *Biol Psych*, 67, 1117–9.

160. Martin EI, Ressler KJ, Binder E, Nemeroff CB (2010). The neurobiology of anxiety disorders: brain imaging, genetics, and psychoneuroendocrinology. *Clin Lab Med*, 30, 865–91.

161. Wald J, Taylor S (2008). Responses to interoceptive exposure in people with posttraumatic stress disorder (PTSD): a preliminary analysis of induced anxiety reactions and trauma memories and their relationship to anxiety sensitivity and PTSD symptom severity. *Cog Behav Ther*, 37, 90–100.

162. Jacob RG, Redfern MS, Furman JM (2009). Space and motion discomfort and abnormal balance control in patients with anxiety disorders. *J Neurol Neurosurg Psych*, 80, 74–8.

163. Park HJ, Shin JE, Lee YJ, Park MS, Kim JM, Na BR (2010). Hyperventilation-induced nystagmus in patients with vestibular neuritis in the acute and follow-up stages. *Audiol Neuro-Otol*, 16, 248–53.

164. Jacob G, Biaggioni I (1999). Idiopathic orthostatic intolerance and postural tachycardia syndromes. *Am J Med Sci*, 317, 88–101.

165. Furman JM, Balaban CD, Jacob RG, Marcus DA (2005). Migraine-anxiety related dizziness (MARD): a new disorder? *J Neurol Neurosurg Psych*, 76, 1–8.

166. Staab JP (2006). Chronic dizziness: the interface between psychiatry and neuro-otology. *Cur Opin Neurol*, 19, 41–8.

CHAPTER 6

Multisensory Interaction and Vestibular Compensation

Ian S. Curthoys and G. Michael Halmagyi

Introduction

This chapter aims to provide a perspective for understanding the huge literature on vestibular compensation. At 28 September 2012 The Web of Science listed 1069 papers on this topic. Why is it so enormous? Because it is so important and because vestibular sensory input is such a fundamental and far-reaching sense that directly or indirectly impinges on so many other systems—not just motor systems but even cognitive systems since vestibular information projects to the hippocampus and is now being implicated in memory and spatial navigation. In this chapter we aim to give a coherent picture, rather than a wiki-like recitation of every fact known about vestibular compensation but there are many papers which provide these facts (1, 2, 3, 4, 5, 6, 7, 8, 9, 10).

Immediately after unilateral loss of vestibular function there are very dramatic symptoms—rapid eye movements (nystagmus), vertigo, nausea, falling to the affected side, ataxia—and the patient is incapacitated. We will use the term uVD syndrome (for unilateral vestibular deafferentation) to refer to these symptoms. These symptoms usually diminish within days or weeks and, almost miraculously after such a devastating loss, most patients return to their normal lifestyle. That term used to describe that overall recovery is 'vestibular compensation'. The recovery appears to be a simple general improvement but closer examination shows a different picture.

Loss of one eye or one ear's hearing leads to sensory losses but nothing as devastating as the loss of one vestibular system. Why does a uVD cause these symptoms? Why aren't these symptoms permanent? How do these patients recover? The answers to those questions are not straightforward. On the one hand, the pragmatist can simply point out that normal function effectively returns—the patient recovers even without any intervention—so why worry? The analyst wants to know the reasons—what neural changes are taking place? What synapses are directly involved? What transmitters are involved? Is this really a good model of neural plasticity? Can the recovery process be speeded up? Does rehabilitation help? And most importantly, why do some patients *not* recover?

To start to put this huge field into perspective consider the schematic diagram (Figure 6.1). It shows that the two vestibular nuclei in the brainstem are hubs for multisensory integration—they receive direct and indirect neural input from many different systems: neural input from the vestibular sensory regions in the inner ear, from proprioceptors in neck muscles, from distant levels of the spinal cord, indirect input from the visual system, from nuclei concerned with autonomic function, as well as from the reticular formation and from the cerebellum (1). The output of these vestibular nuclei, these hubs of multimodal integration, are almost as diverse—to control eye movements and posture and to generate sensations. Most importantly the two vestibular nuclei 'talk to each other'—there are functionally inhibitory connections called commissural connections between the two vestibular nuclei.

The vestibular system may seem like an input–output system. Far from it! The operation of this system is totally different depending on *how* the vestibular sensory input was generated. If the vestibular input is caused by 'passive', involuntary head movements then many reflexes are initiated. If *exactly the same* vestibular sensory input is generated by the subject *actively* generating the same movements then many of the reflexes are suppressed. So a skater or an acrobat during an active spin completely suppresses the same compensatory responses which would have been triggered to prevent falling if it had been a passively received stimulus. Clearly this is not just some simple transmission system.

Animal studies

The labyrinth has a similar structure and function across all mammals and the vestibular control of eye movements and posture are very similar across mammals. Recovery after vestibular loss in animals has a similar sequence to that in humans. The major difference being the time course—slower in humans (days and weeks), faster in guinea pigs (days), very fast in goldfish (hours). Given this similarity in structure and function across species it is assumed that similar neural processes underlie the recovery in these different species. So results from experimental studies on animals are used to understand human vestibular compensation and its neural basis (2, 11, 12).

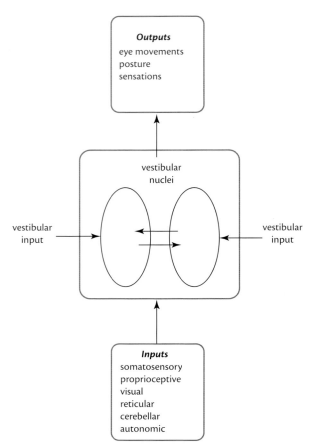

Fig. 6.1 A very simple schematic representation of the neural basis of the multimodal interaction underlying vestibular compensation. There are functionally inhibitory interconnections between the two vestibular nuclei. These nuclei receive input from a wide variety of sources and their output projects to systems concerned with movement and sensation.

The normal system and its disruption

Even from the simple schematic diagram (Figure 6.1) it is easy to see that many factors can influence the normal processing of vestibular information and of course these factors also affect the recovery after uVD. But we must elaborate a bit more. Patients with uVD are a very heterogeneous group, because they vary so much in the causes of their dysfunction. Experimental work has focussed on complete unilateral surgical vestibular loss of sensory input from all five vestibular sense organs in the one labyrinth at the one moment in a young healthy animal, while the remaining labyrinth remains healthy. This is a very atypical example for the clinic—most patients tend to be middle aged and have had a chronic progressive disease of one labyrinth which has been ongoing for months or years with the other labyrinth affected to an unknown extent. So one needs to be cautious about simple extrapolations from results in animals to human patients. It is rare for a normal healthy person to suddenly lose all vestibular function in one labyrinth. Much more common is the progressive loss of function on one side accompanied by less severe loss of the sensory input from the other 'healthy' side. Vestibular loss in patients ranges from partial unilateral loss, e.g. from loss of

just the utricular macula, to complete unilateral vestibular loss to complete *bilateral* vestibular loss. In these cases the functional status of the other side—the 'healthy' vestibular labyrinth—is of crucial importance in determining the final outcome. So the cause of the vestibular loss and the pre-existing conditions are important considerations in understanding vestibular compensation in the clinic (1, 5).

Someone who has had a slowly growing acoustic schwannoma on one vestibular nerve—and then had that entire vestibular nerve removed at surgery—may exhibit virtually none of the symptoms of a uVD. So by the time the surgery takes place, the patient has no effective vestibular function in the affected ear and so there is no uVD syndrome and so no vestibular compensation takes place after surgery—none is necessary, it has all happened before the surgery. Without knowing the preoperative level of vestibular function and having an understanding of the mechanism of vestibular compensation, these totally different uVD syndromes would be inexplicable.

Causes of loss of vestibular input

There are many possible causes of loss of peripheral vestibular function, including disease, such as vestibular neuritis (13), trauma, surgery (e.g. for removal of an acoustic schwannoma), and therapeutic intratympanic injection of gentamicin for the treatment of peripheral vestibular disorders.

Not surprisingly these different procedures have very different outcomes—some procedures totally remove all vestibular afferent input, some remove all input from some sensory regions, while others preserve the resting neural activity from all sensory regions but remove the modulation of that resting activity by vestibular stimulation.

One procedure now very widely used to treat unilateral peripheral vestibular dysfunction, largely because of its safety, is injection of a solution of the ototoxic antibiotic gentamicin via a fine needle inserted through the eardrum into the middle ear. The gentamicin is taken up through the round and oval windows of the cochlea into the inner ear and selectively attacks vestibular hair cell receptors in preference to cochlear receptors, even though both auditory and vestibular receptors are hair cells.

The intratympanic gentamicin injection procedure is now so successful that surgical uVD procedures are becoming less common. However, in patients after intratympanic gentamicin the final level of vestibular function is unknown. After the same intratympanic gentamicin injection procedure some patients may lose almost all vestibular function, others may lose much less.

At low doses gentamicin destroys the cilia of vestibular hair-cells disabling their response to natural vestibular stimuli, but with little effect on cochlear receptors so hearing is minimally affected. During the course of the gentamicin treatment, the cell bodies of the vestibular receptors may be preserved and the cilia on these vestibular receptor cells may re-grow following the procedure, so that vestibular function (and possibly vestibular symptoms) may reappear following gentamicin treatment. So what may appear as compensation is in fact the actual return of peripheral vestibular function. A similar situation applies in some cases of vestibular neuritis where the affected peripheral vestibular afferent neurons recover and start to function again (14). These are not examples of vestibular compensation but vestibular restoration. So one needs to be careful in using data from patients with vestibular neuritis to understand vestibular compensation.

The unilateral vestibular deafferentation syndrome

What are the symptoms after uVD? Humans have intense disequilibrium which has both sensory and motor components. In turn these can be categorized into static or dynamic symptoms. Static symptoms are present continuously, even when the person is totally stationary. Dynamic symptoms occur during changing stimulation, i.e. during movement (1, 5).

Static symptoms

Spontaneous nystagmus

Immediately after uVD there is a spontaneous, mainly horizontal, nystagmus. The eyes appear to be beating away from the affected (lesioned) side. Recordings of eye position show there are slow eye deviations (called slow phases) towards the affected side, followed by rapid eye movements (called quick phases) away from the affected side. It is the quick phases which the observer sees—so to the observer both eyes of the patient appear to be *beating away from the affected ear*. Spontaneous nystagmus due to peripheral vestibular loss can be reduced or entirely suppressed by visual stimuli, whereas nystagmus due to central causes (such as congenital nystagmus) is present with vision. Tested in darkness the spontaneous nystagmus declines over days or weeks after the uVD but for some patients there is always a very small spontaneous nystagmus present in darkness.

Vertigo

Immediately after uVD, patients have the strong sensation that they are turning—a sensation called vertigo. Vertigo is totally subjective and it can be difficult for patients to describe. In darkness or with eyes closed the patient feels that they are turning towards the side of the uVD (i.e. ipsilesional rotation). However if visual stimuli are present, then they report typically that they feel like they are stationary but the world is rotating around them (but now in the opposite direction—towards their intact side). Nausea usually accompanies this vertigo.

Otolithic symptoms

In addition to spontaneous nystagmus and vertigo there are symptoms which appear to be primarily otolithic:

- There is a skew deviation of vertical eye position: the ipsilesional eye is positioned lower in its orbit relative to the position of the contralesional eye in its orbit.
- Conjugate ocular torsion to the lesioned side. Both eyes adopt a rolled position in the orbit with the upper pole of both eyes rolled toward the lesioned ear. This maintained ocular torsional position can be up to 15° of roll away from the usual torsional position. Corresponding to this ocular torsion there is a change in the patient's judgement of the subjective visual horizontal (or vertical) in an otherwise darkened room. This judgement of the visual horizontal in the absence of other visual cues depends heavily on the exact position of the retina in the orbit (15).

Postural symptoms

As well as the oculomotor symptoms there are postural symptoms. In darkness the patient has a small roll-tilt of the head towards the lesioned side. On standing or trying to walk there is a tendency to fall towards the lesioned side. Most patients report that the floor feels unstable, like a rocking boat.

Why does the unilateral vestibular deafferentation syndrome occur and how does compensation take place?

Static symptoms

These symptoms can be best understood by considering what happens in the vestibular nuclei of a healthy person at rest and during a horizontal head rotation. When a healthy subject has their head still, the neural activity in the two vestibular nuclei is approximately equal, i.e. 'balanced.' If the subject receives a horizontal angular acceleration in one direction, e.g. a head turn to the person's *left*, then it causes an imbalance in neural activity: many neurons in the ipsilateral (left) vestibular nucleus increase their rate of firing of action potentials, whilst many neurons in the right vestibular nucleus simultaneously decrease their firing and the result is an imbalance in neural activity between the two nuclei (1, 5). The imbalance is enhanced by the functionally inhibitory interactions between the two vestibular nuclei. That neural imbalance causes corrective responses (vestibulo-ocular and vestibulospinal reflexes) and changes in perception.

Measures of neural activity in animals after a uVD show that the uVD causes massive changes in neural activity in the two vestibular nuclei in the brainstem (1, 4, 5). The uVD causes a total loss of vestibular afferent input to the vestibular nucleus on the affected side (the *ipsilesional* vestibular nucleus) so there is a great reduction in neural activity of that nucleus. Simultaneously there is an increase in the activity of neurons in the vestibular nucleus on the healthy side (the *contralesional* vestibular nucleus). Again the inhibitory connections between the two nuclei act to enhance that imbalance even further. This very large imbalance in neural activity is what would occur if the person received a very large angular acceleration towards their healthy ear, and the sensations and responses correspond to such a stimulus. Within a short space of time (about 24–48 h in the guinea pig) neural activity starts to return to the ipsilesional vestibular nucleus—the silenced neurons in the ipsilesional vestibular nucleus start to fire again and the very active cells in the contralesional vestibular nucleus start to decrease their activity (1, 4, 6, 7, 10). As the imbalance between the two vestibular nuclei starts to be reduced the major symptoms of the uVD correspondingly decrease, the spontaneous nystagmus decreases, the ocular torsion decreases.

So the uVD generates a very similar imbalance in neural activity to that produced by a natural head turn, but in a totally different way—by silencing the input from one labyrinth. In both cases, the acceleration and the uVD, the responses and the sensations are similar—the person perceives themselves as *rotating*, there is nystagmus, and there are corrective postural responses. Most real-life acceleration stimuli are usually of fairly short duration and at the end of the acceleration the vestibular nuclei return to their balanced state. But after uVD the imbalance in neural activity persists for hours or days.

This evidence for the initial imbalance and the rebalancing of activity between the two vestibular nuclei has been demonstrated by single-neuron recording studies in the vestibular nuclei on both sides in healthy and compensating cats and guinea pigs (1, 16). Studies of cells in brain slice preparations from animals at various stages after a uVD allow one to examine mechanisms. How could the balance be restored? Adaptation is one possibility—that the firing rate of the more active neurons reduces over time so they exert less inhibition onto neurons on the ipsilesional side. Another is that the neurotransmitter receptors in the ipsilesional neurons become less sensitive to the inhibitory transmitter released by the overactive inhibitory neurons driven from the intact side. Most interest has focused on the neurotransmitter gamma-aminobyric acid (GABA). A reduction in the efficacy of the neurotransmitter receptor for GABA would allow for greater activity by ipsilesional neurons. This idea is referred to as 'down regulation of GABA sensitivity' and it is likely at least partly responsible for the restoration of balanced activity in the two vestibular nuclei (7, 17).

There are changes in the intrinsic membrane potential of central vestibular neurons together with reorganization of synaptic connections with stronger input from neck proprioceptors and spinal input (2, 4). Kitahara has shown that neurons in the flocculus of the cerebellum play an important role in the early stages of vestibular compensation for static symptoms. He has proposed that neurons in the flocculus may inhibit the hyperactive neurons in the contralesional vestibular nucleus and so act to relieve the inhibition on the ipsilesional neurons (18, 19) and so restore the balance. Human patients with cerebellar lesions do show slow compensation (20).

These and many other possibilities are not mutually exclusive—many of these processes probably occur concurrently.

Dynamic symptoms

The vestibulo-ocular reflex

One major function of the semicircular canals is to generate eye movements to correct for head movement, so that during the head movement the image on the retina remains stable. This is the vestibulo-ocular reflex (VOR) and it is an important function of the semicircular canals. The gain of the VOR is an indicator of dynamic semicircular canal function and is defined as the ratio of the eye velocity response to the head velocity stimulus. If the VOR gain is not 1, the eye movement does not compensate for head movement then the image of the world is smeared across the retina and patients report their visual world is blurred, bouncing, and nauseating. Measuring the eye movement response during the head movement yields an index of how well the semicircular canals are operating. Ideally the eye velocity should exactly cancel head velocity (and so the VOR gain should be 1).

Passive stimulation

For practical reasons, low-frequency (less than 1Hz), low-acceleration, horizontal sinusoidal rotation has been used extensively to test dynamic semicircular canal function. Unfortunately the results of such tests are indefinite because at low frequencies and low accelerations the eye movement response to the acceleration can be controlled not just by vestibular activation but by a variety of different sensory systems apart from the vestibular system. We found that a patient with bilateral surgical loss of vestibular function could generate slow eye movements to 0.2-Hz horizontal rotations, probably because of predictive pursuit cued by somatosensory input. Unless these extraneous sources of oculomotor control are excluded there may appear to be recovery of dynamic vestibular function, whereas when careful measures with specific vestibular tests are made the clear answer

is that there is no such recovery. Very low sinusoidal test frequencies are not common in real life—when did you last turn your head back and forth at a rate of 1 turn per 10 seconds?—most natural head movements are very brief, high-acceleration, high-frequency stimuli. The head accelerations during walking or running, which post-uVD patients complain about, have high acceleration (2,000–3,000, up to 8,000°/s²) and high frequencies (5–12 Hz). When these stimuli are used—passive, unpredictable, high-acceleration head rotations—the head impulse test—it is clear that there is very little if any recovery of dynamic semicircular canal function after uVD (21).

Active stimulation

If one asks a patient with a uVD to maintain gaze on a spot on the wall while they actively turn their head abruptly to left or right, most patients can quickly learn to do so. However, detailed high-speed measures show that uVD patients produce a small saccade to correct their inadequate VOR during this active head movement. This is an important observation since it shows that during *active* head movements there can be a *substitution* of a saccade for the deficient vestibular slow phase (22). This saccade acts to minimize the effect of the uVD on the patients' permanent dynamic VOR deficit: the saccade minimizes retinal smear. More recently we have shown that some uVD patients can generate this saccade even during *passive* unpredictable, high-acceleration head turns (23, 24, 25). These are called covert saccades.

Manipulations which affect the recovery

Given the many and varied inputs to the vestibular nuclei one can understand how it is that many different sensory manipulations can influence uVD and the rate of recovery.

Deprivation of all visual input after uVD retards the compensation of dynamic VOR and the recovery of the static roll head tilt. But visual deprivation seems to have little effect on the reduction of spontaneous nystagmus after uVD (1, 5, 11). Visual inputs do augment the diminished motor responses to linear acceleration and the deficient righting reflexes that occur after uVD. Visual motion deprivation delays recovery of locomotor equilibrium (1).

Stimulation of proprioceptive sensory input appears to facilitate the recovery of dynamic postural equilibrium and conversely deprivation of such input appears to retard the recovery of postural equilibrium. Cervical proprioceptive input could be important in static compensation since head restraint retards resolution of head tilt and spontaneous nystagmus. Somatosensory proprioceptive deprivation appears to retard static compensation.

Even within the vestibular nuclei, the networks concerned with different functions have different substrates and the process of their recovery is different; the recovery of oculomotor and postural symptoms are clearly different. This has recently been shown in cats: procedures which prevent the usual neurogenesis in the vestibular nuclei of cats after uVD have dramatic delaying effects on recovery of postural stability, but have no effect on the disappearance of nystagmus. These differential effects clearly demonstrate the different recovery processes of vestibulo-ocular and vestibulospinal symptoms (26).

Learning, substitution, and rehabilitation

During compensation there are probably many new strategies being learned but there is one simple example which illustrates how valuable even a very simple learned response can be. The example is the saccade during passive, unpredictable, high-acceleration head turns ('head impulses'). Some uVD patients can produce these 'covert saccades' even during unpredictable passive head rotations to their affected side. Why is this saccade so useful? It is eliminating the smeared retinal image which would have occurred during the head turn because of the inadequate VOR and also by virtue of saccadic suppression—the suppression of vision during saccades (27). So that saccade and saccadic suppression yields a visual stimulus, and a visual percept, free of the retinal smear which otherwise would have occurred.

If people can be so good at learning such a saccade during a passive unpredictable head rotation, how much better will they be during an active, completely predictable head rotation? There are probably a host of behavioural strategies which patients can learn to minimize the challenge of their vestibular loss, apart from any neural changes. For example, to blink, to restrict their head movements, to insert a corrective saccade even during the head movement.

Taking such patients into a laboratory and trying to assess the mechanism of their recovery based on a few classical measures of oculomotor performance may not reveal the subtle but effective compensatory strategies which people use in real life. It was only by using high-speed, high-resolution measures of eye movement that we detected the very small covert saccades during the passive high acceleration head movements (23, 24, 25).

Rehabilitation

Many years ago Cawthorne and Cooksey suggested a number of exercises to assist in the rehabilitation of patients with vestibular disorders. Those exercises are similar to those in use today. If there is little or no change in purely vestibular function how can these exercises benefit patients? How can patients improve? As we have shown, substitution of other responses can effectively conceal the vestibular deficit and so protect the patient from receiving smeared retinal images during head movements. We suggest that the Cawthorne Cooksey exercises and other such exercises are acting to teach patients how to substitute these other responses to conceal and thus overcome their vestibular loss.

We suggest that the process of vestibular rehabilitation should be thought of as an opportunity for other non-vestibular sensory inputs and cognitive behavioural strategies to increase their role in controlling the patient's equilibrium, rather than thinking of rehabilitation as a means of restoring the lost vestibular sensory input. It is essentially a substitution rather than a restoration. Dealing with vestibular loss is more analogous to the rehabilitation procedures after an amputated limb, rather than the rehabilitation procedures after a broken limb.

The problem: poor compensation

Most human patients recover well after uVD and have an apparently normal lifestyle with good quality of life. But some patients with apparently similar vestibular losses do not.

Detailed comparison of the vestibular performance of such patients has not been able to identify any clear differences post-uVD between well- and poorly-compensated patients. Why should this poor compensation occur? In some cases it seems that events such as postoperative complications within the first few days after a surgical uVD procedure may be important for determining the success or otherwise of the eventual recovery. In other words, that there may be a sensitive period, a critical period, for the establishment of vestibular compensation. Certainly there is neural and behavioural evidence from animal studies which underpins this distinction

between the initiation and maintenance of vestibular compensation (4, 5).

Some of these poorly-compensated patients may have had inadequate vestibular function or even central (e.g. cerebellar) deficits before the uVD procedure. Thus the uVD procedure is potentially dangerous and that is why careful preprocedural testing is needed to ensure there is an adequate level of function of the remaining labyrinth and an absence of central deficits before the procedure is undertaken. Unless such care is taken the patient may suffer postural disequilibrium and gait ataxia virtually for the rest of their lives. 'Recovery' has a large subjective component and it is probable that some of these patients had expected a much better outcome.

The final question—are they happy?

What is the final outcome? Most patients return to a lifestyle similar to what they had before the uVD. It seems as if one labyrinth was as good as two—that the vestibular system could function just as well on 'one cylinder as on two'. But we have shown that this is not correct in detail—when the correct tests are done the deficits are revealed.

Summary

The vestibular system is a very fundamental system whose activity impinges on so many other motor systems so that the ramifications of disruption of its function are indeed far-reaching. Some symptoms do recover, in the sense that vestibular-dependent performance resumes, some do not. Over time the patient resumes their lifestyle because of this patchwork recovery and because they learn a variety of new behaviours to allow normal function. However, if the appropriate tests are carried out, probing vestibular function and preventing some of the other 'tricks', then the permanent loss of vestibular function is very clear.

Although vestibular compensation appears to be a simple recovery of function there is overwhelming evidence that there are many different processes taking place during vestibular compensation and that the various processes recover at different rates, or, in some cases, do not recover at all, while new behaviours are being learned to substitute for the lost vestibular function.

Acknowledgements

This chapter is supported by the Australian National Health and Medical Research Council grant 632746 and the Garnett Passe and Rodney Williams Foundation. We thank Ann Burgess for her meticulous proofreading of this manuscript.

References

1. Curthoys IS, Halmagyi GM (1995). Vestibular compensation: a review of the oculomotor, neural, and clinical consequences of unilateral vestibular loss *J Vestib Res*, 5, 67–107.
2. Dieringer N (1995). 'Vestibular compensation': neural plasticity and its relations to functional recovery after labyrinthine lesions in frogs and other vertebrates. *ProgNeurobiol*, 46, 97–129.
3. Brandt T, Strupp M, Arbusow V, Dieringer N (1997). Plasticity of the vestibular system: central compensation and sensory substitution for vestibular deficits. *AdvNeurol*, 73, 297–309.
4. Vidal PP, de Waele C, Vibert N, Muhlethaler M (1998). Vestibular compensation revisited. *Otolaryngol Head Neck Surg*, 119, 34–42.

5. Curthoys IS, Halmagyi GM (1999). Vestibular compensation. *Adv Otorhinolaryngol*, 55, 82–110.

6. Peusner K, Vidal PP, Minor L, *et al.* (2009). Vestibular compensation: new clinical and basic science perspectives. *J Vestib Res*, 19, 143–6.

7. Dutia MB (2010). Mechanisms of vestibular compensation: recent advances. *CurrOpinOtolaryngol Head Neck Surg*, 18, 420–4.

8. Horak FB (2010). Postural compensation for vestibular loss and implications for rehabilitation. *RestorNeurolNeurosci*, 28, 57–68.

9. Allum JH (2012). Recovery of vestibular ocular reflex function and balance control after a unilateral peripheral vestibular deficit. *Front Neurol*, 3, 83.

10. Peusner KD, Shao M, Reddaway R, Hirsch JC (2012) Basic concepts in understanding recovery of function in vestibular reflex networks during vestibular compensation. *Front Neurol*, 3, 17.

11. Curthoys IS, Smith PF, Darlington CL (1988). Postural compensation in the guinea pig following unilateral labyrinthectomy. *Prog Brain Res*, 76, 375–84.

12. Fetter M, Zee DS (1988). Recovery from unilateral labyrinthectomy in rhesus monkey. *J Neurophysiol*, 59, 370–93.

13. Strupp M, Brandt T (2009). Vestibular neuritis. *Semin Neurol*, 29, 509–19.

14. Manzari L, Burgess AM, MacDougall HG, Curthoys IS (2011). Objective verification of full recovery of dynamic vestibular function after superior vestibular neuritis. *Laryngoscope*, 121, 2496–500.

15. Curthoys IS, Dai MJ, Halmagyi GM (1991). Human ocular torsional position before and after unilateral vestibular neurectomy. *Exp Brain Res*, 85, 218–25.

16. Precht W, Shimazu H, Markham CH (1966). A mechanism of central compensation of vestibular function following hemilabyrinthectomy. *J Neurophysiol*, 29, 996–1010.

17. Bergquist F, Ludwig M, Dutia MB (2008). Role of the commissural inhibitory system in vestibular compensation in the rat. *J Physiol*, 586, 4441–52.

18. Kitahara T, Takeda N, Saika T, Kubo T, Kiyama H (1997). Role of the flocculus in the development of vestibular compensation: immunohistochemical studies with retrograde tracing and flocculectomy using Fos expression as a marker in the rat brainstem. *Neuroscience*, 76, 571–80.

19. Beraneck M, McKee JL, Aleisa M, Cullen KE (2008). Asymmetric recovery in cerebellar-deficient mice following unilateral labyrinthectomy. *J Neurophysiol*, 100, 945–58.

20. Furman JM, Balaban CD, Pollack IF (1997). Vestibular compensation in a patient with a cerebellar infarction. *Neurology*, 48, 916–20.

21. Halmagyi GM, Curthoys IS, Cremer PD, *et al.* (1990). The human horizontal vestibulo-ocular reflex in response to high-acceleration stimulation before and after unilateral vestibular neurectomy. *Exp Brain Res*, 81, 479–90.

22. Berthoz A (1988). The role of gaze in compensation of vestibular disfunction: the gaze substitution hypothesis. *Prog Brain Res*, 76, 411–20.

23. Weber KP, Aw ST, Todd MJ, McGarvie LA, Curthoys IS, Halmagyi GM (2008). Head impulse test in unilateral vestibular loss: vestibulo-ocular reflex and catch-up saccades. *Neurology*, 70, 454–63.

24. MacDougall HG, Weber KP, McGarvie LA, Halmagyi GM, Curthoys IS (2009). The video head impulse test: diagnostic accuracy in peripheral vestibulopathy. *Neurology*, 73, 1134–41.

25. Macdougall HG, Curthoys IS (2012). Plasticity during Vestibular Compensation: The Role of Saccades. *Front Neurol*, 3, 21.

26. Dutheil S, Brezun JM, Leonard J, Lacour M, Tighilet B (2009). Neurogenesis and astrogenesis contribution to recovery of vestibular functions in the adult cat following unilateral vestibular neurectomy: cellular and behavioral evidence. *Neuroscience*, 164, 1444–56.

27. Matin E (1974). Saccadic suppression: a review and an analysis. *Psychol Bull*, 81, 899–917.

Further Reading

Allum JH (2012). Recovery of vestibular ocular reflex function and balance control after a unilateral peripheral vestibular deficit. *Front Neurol*, 3 (83), 1–7.

Dutia MB (2010). Mechanisms of vestibular compensation: recent advances. *CurrOpinOtolaryngol Head Neck Surg*, 18, 420–24.

Halmagyi GM, Weber KP, Curthoys IS (2010). Vestibular function after acute vestibular neuritis. *RestorNeurolNeurosci*, 28, 37–46.

Horak FB (2010). Postural compensation for vestibular loss and implications for rehabilitation. *RestorNeurolNeurosci*, 28, 57–68.

Lacour M, Tighilet B (2010). Plastic events in the vestibular nuclei during vestibular compensation: the brain orchestration of a "deafferentation" code. *RestorNeurolNeurosci*, 28, 19–35.

Macdougall HG, Curthoys IS (2012). Plasticity during vestibular compensation: the role of saccades. *Front Neurol*, 3 (21), 1–9.

Sadeghi SG, Minor LB, Cullen KE (2011). Multimodal integration after unilateral labyrinthine lesion: single vestibular nuclei neuron responses and implications for postural compensation. *J Neurophysiol*, 105, 661–73.

Saman Y, Bamiou DE, Gleeson M, Dutia MB (2012). Interactions between stress and vestibular compensation—A Review. *Front Neurol* 3 (116), 1–8.

CHAPTER 7

Functional Imaging of the Vestibular System

Marianne Dieterich and Thomas Brandt

Introduction

In-depth knowledge of the vestibular structures in humans has been gained from several sources. Caloric irrigation and galvanic currents, for example, have been used to stimulate experimentally the intact vestibular system and thus acquire insights into its structure and functions. Nowadays, positron emission tomography (PET) and functional magnetic resonance imaging (fMRI) are used in brain activation studies to image the central connectivity and interactions of the vestibular system with other sensory systems. While these methods are quite reliable for determining cortical and subcortical as well as cerebellar activation patterns, they are still limited when it comes to brainstem structures. When combined with vestibular stimulation in normal subjects, however, they reveal the existence of a specific cortical pattern of activations and deactivations in the sensory systems. Patients with lesions of peripheral and central vestibular structures exhibit certain modifications of these patterns.

The following review summarizes findings that have elucidated the interconnections of vestibular structures, their activations and interactions with other sensory modalities, the correlations of perceptual and motor functions in normal humans, and the changes that result from strategic unilateral peripheral and central vestibular lesions. First the typical cortical activation pattern of unilateral vestibular stimulation in normal subjects is described. Then the alterations of this pattern are addressed, e.g. in patients with acute unilateral and chronic bilateral peripheral vestibular failure, and in those with lesions within the central vestibular system (e.g. acute lesions of the vestibular nuclei, Wallenberg syndrome, and the vestibular posterolateral thalamus) (for review see (1, 2)).

The intact vestibular system

The existence of several separate and distinct cortical areas was first confirmed by tracer and electrophysiological studies in animals, especially in monkeys. The most robust cortical structures involved were the parieto-insular vestibular cortex (PIVC), the visual temporal sylvian area (VTS) in the retroinsular cortex, the superior temporal gyrus (STG), the inferior parietal lobule (IPL), the anterior cingulum, the hippocampus, and area 6a. All belong to a multisensory (vestibular) cortical circuit. In monkeys the PIVC seems to be the dominant multimodal vestibular cortex area which is closely connected to the other areas and to the opposite hemisphere; it is considered the 'core region' within this network (3) (Figure 7.1). Otolith input to this region was only recently characterized in detail (4). The roles of the ventral-intraparietal area (VIP) and periarcuate cortex in the frontal lobes in the cortical vestibular circuit have been further defined (5–7). During the last 10 years functional imaging studies using vestibular, somatosensory, and visual optokinetic stimulation have suggested that such multisensory vestibular cortical areas are located and connected in similar sites in humans.

Activations during vestibular stimulation

A complex network of areas has been found mainly in the temporo-insular and temporo-parietal cortex in both hemispheres of healthy subjects during caloric irrigation of the horizontal semicircular canals (8–14) as well as during galvanic stimulation of the vestibular nerve (15–20), and even during stimulation of the sacculus otolith (sound induced; 21–23). These activated areas in humans

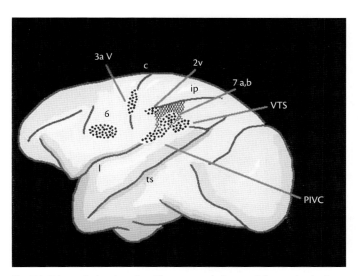

Fig. 7.1 Schematic drawing of multisensory cortical areas of the monkey brain the neurons of which respond to vestibular stimulation.

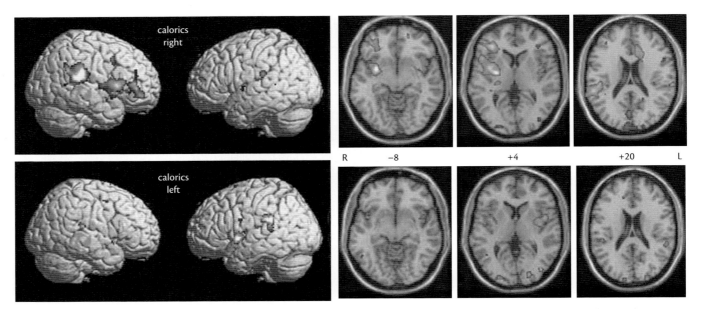

Fig. 7.2 (Also see Colour plate 5.) Illustration of the normal activation–deactivation pattern during unilateral vestibular stimulation in healthy volunteers (activations in yellow-red, deactivations in blue). For comparison, a schematic drawing is given of a monkey brain with the neurophysiologically determined multisensory vestibular areas 6, 3aV, 2v, 7a,b, PIVC and VTS (Figure 7.1). Note that the locations of the activated areas during galvanic stimulation of the vestibular nerve in humans (fMRI; top left) are similar to those in monkey. During caloric irrigation of the right ear in healthy right-handers, activations ($H_2^{15}O$-PET) occur in the temporo-parieto-insular areas of both hemispheres, but there is a dominance of the non-dominant right hemisphere (left: surface view of the right and left hemispheres; right: transverse sections Z = −10, +10, +20 mm). Deactivations are located in areas of the visual cortex bilaterally. Modified after (13).

are located in the posterior insula (first and second long insular gyri) and retroinsular regions (which correspond to the PIVC and the posterior adjacent VTS (3) in the monkey), the STG, parts of the IPL, deep within the intraparietal sulcus representing monkey area VIP, the postcentral and precentral gyrus, the anterior insula and adjacent inferior frontal gyrus, the anterior cingulate gyrus, the precuneus, and the hippocampus (Figure 7.2). Interestingly, this cortical network is not activated symmetrically in the two hemispheres. Instead, the pattern is determined by three factors, which were defined in a study of healthy right- and left-handers during caloric irrigation in PET (13) (Figure 7.2). These are: 1) the subject's handedness, 2) the side of the stimulated ear, and 3) the direction of the induced vestibular nystagmus. Activation was found to be stronger in the non-dominant hemisphere (right hemisphere in right-handers, left hemisphere in left-handers), in the hemisphere ipsilateral to the stimulated ear, and in the hemisphere ipsilateral to the slow phase of vestibular caloric nystagmus (12, 13, 24, 25).

Deactivations during vestibular stimulation

At the same time that activations occur in areas within the visual and somatosensory systems of both hemispheres there are also deactivations (12, 17, 26). The activation–deactivation patterns are opposite to each other. Originally the patterns were found during visually-induced self-motion perception, for example, activations of occipital and parietal visual areas co-occurred with deactivations of the multisensory vestibular cortex, e.g. the PIVC (13, 27) (Figure 7.3). These findings led to the assumption that there is a reciprocal inhibitory cortical interaction between the visual and the vestibular systems (27). The interaction shifts the dominant sensorial weight from one modality to the other, and so resolves conflicts between incongruent sensory inputs. It was subsequently hypothesized that reciprocal inhibitory interactions between the sensory systems

are likely to be a fundamental mechanism of the central nervous system (28). Such interactions also occur between other sensory modalities, e.g. the somatosensory and nociceptive, the nociceptive and the vestibular, the tactile sensory and visual, and the visual and auditory systems (17, 29–31). The psychophysical consequences of these interactions were revealed in a study investigating

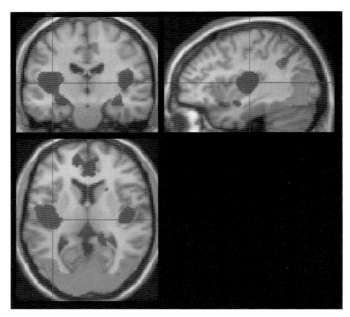

Fig. 7.3 (Also see Colour plate 6.) Activated areas during visual optokinetic stimulation in 7 healthy volunteers. While activations are located in the visual cortex bilaterally, areas with BOLD signal decreases are found in the temporal, insular and parietal cortex areas and the anterior cingulate cortex (p for activations: ≤0.001, p for deactivations: ≤0.0001).

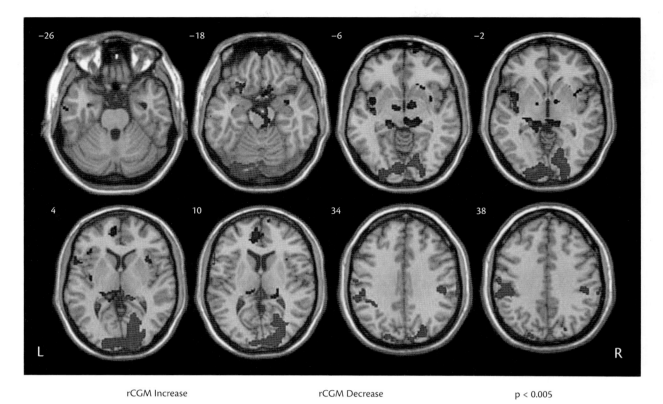

rCGM Increase   rCGM Decrease   p < 0.005

Fig. 7.4 (Also see Colour plate 7.) Statistical group analysis of five patients with vestibular neuritis of the right ear versus the control condition 3 months later (eyes closed, without stimulation). A significant increase (red) of regional cerebral glucose metabolism (rCGM) is seen in the contralateral left vestibular cortex, left superior temporal gyrus, hippocampus, thalamus bilaterally; it is also pronounced in the anterior cingulate gyrus. Simultaneously rCGM decreases (blue) are located in the visual and somatosensory cortex bilaterally. For illustrative purposes, voxels above a threshold of p ≤0.005, uncorrected, are shown.

high-resolution visual mental imagery and mental rotation tasks, which were significantly impaired during vestibular caloric stimulation in healthy subjects (32).

The psychophysical and functional imaging data of an inhibitory interaction within the visual system (33, 34) support the interpretation that the deactivation of neural activity in the visual system (measured by fMRI and PET) may be associated with a functional decrement in sensitivity needed to perceive motion and orientation. This might reflect transcallosal attentional shifts between the two hemispheres, i.e. so-called 'cross-talk' between the two cerebral hemispheres to resolve sensory conflicts. Indeed, negative fMRI responses correlated with decreases in neural activity in the monkey visual area V1 (35). Taken together the deactivations found in normal subjects in PET and fMRI studies seem to represent decreases of function at the neural level.

The non-intact vestibular system

During an acute unilateral lesion of the vestibular nerve

Does the acute lesion-induced vestibular tonus imbalance between the two labyrinths, e.g. in vestibular neuritis, lead to a modulation of neural activity within the thalamo-cortical vestibular system? If it does, is this activation pattern asymmetrical and thus reflects the perceptual correlate of the tonus imbalance at the cortical level? To answer these questions the cortical activation patterns in patients with unilateral lesions were compared to the functional imaging data

of healthy volunteers during unilateral caloric (10–13) or galvanic (16, 17, 19) stimulation. Unilateral vestibular stimulation, on the one hand, and unilateral failure of the vestibular end organ, on the other, should create a vestibular tonus imbalance. However, each occurs at different levels of activity of the vestibular system. A unilateral lesion reduces the resting discharge input, whereas a unilateral stimulation increases the resting discharge input from an end organ.

Activations and deactivations

During the acute stage of vestibular neuritis (mean: 6.6 days after symptom onset) it was indeed possible to demonstrate that the central vestibular system exhibited a visual-vestibular activation–deactivation pattern similar to that described earlier in healthy volunteers during unilateral vestibular stimulation. Right-handed patients with a right-sided vestibular neuritis were examined with fluorodeoxyglucose (FDG)-PET in the acute stage and 3 months later after central vestibular compensation when the patients were symptom-free (36). The regional cerebral glucose metabolism was significantly increased during the acute stage in multisensory vestibular cortical and subcortical areas such as the PIVC in the posterior insula, posterolateral thalamus, anterior cingulate gyrus, ponto-mesencephalic brainstem, and hippocampus (Figure 7.4). Thus, FDG-PET could image a cortical activation pattern of the vestibular system, which was induced by unilateral peripheral vestibular loss and may reflect the tonus imbalance. Simultaneously, there was a significant decrease of regional cerebral glucose metabolism in the visual and somatosensory cortex as well as in parts of the auditory cortex (transverse temporal gyrus) (36). These decreases were very similar to those in the visual and somatosensory systems during vestibular stimulation in healthy subjects (12, 17, 20). This pattern probably reflects a non-specific inhibition of other sensory areas in response to vestibular activation.

The details, however, also revealed certain differences from the activation–deactivation pattern during experimental vestibular stimulation in healthy volunteers. In the patients, the activation of the vestibular cortex in the posterior insula (PIVC) was not bilateral with a dominance of the right side, but unilateral and contralateral (left) to the right labyrinthine failure. This asymmetry of activations within the PIVC can be explained by assuming that the more dominant ipsilateral right-sided ascending projections to the right insular cortex were depressed by the right vestibular neuritis, because the tonic end-organ input was absent (resting discharge). Another explanation might be that the vestibular tonus imbalance at the vestibular nuclei level mimics a left-sided vestibular excitation due to a higher resting discharge rate of the unaffected left vestibular nuclei complex. This would be compatible with the activation-deactivation pattern in healthy subjects, i.e. activation of the pontine and ponto-mesencephalic brainstem and left temporo-insular vestibular cortex areas (dominance of ipsilateral pathways) as well as the concurrent deactivation of the visual and somatosensory cortex areas.

These suggestions are in line with recent animal data on vestibular neuronal excitability and molecular mechanisms of neural and synaptic plasticity in the vestibular nuclei during the vestibular compensation following deafferentation of one rat labyrinth (37–39). Rapid compensatory changes in gamma-aminobutyric acid (GABA) receptor efficacy in medial vestibular nucleus neurons lead to a downregulation in the ipsilesional and a simultaneous upregulation in contralesional neurons. Furthermore, examinations of the histaminergic and glycinergic modulation of GABA release in the medial vestibular nuclei of normal and labyrinthectomized rats showed a profoundly downregulated GABA release on both sides for at least 3 weeks after unilateral labyrinthectomy. Stimulation of the histamine H(3) receptors restored normality but only on the contralateral side.

Correlation analyses in patients with vestibular neuritis have, furthermore, shown that some of the other multisensory vestibular cortex areas such as the STG, IPL, and precuneus seem to be involved in special aspects of vestibular function or dysfunction (36). First, the amount of spontaneous nystagmus during the acute stage of vestibular neuritis positively correlated with the increase of glucose metabolism in the area of the superior temporal gyrus bilaterally (Brodmann area (BA) 22) as well as with that of an ocular motor area in the right inferior medial frontal gyrus (BA 9/44) that includes the frontal eye field. Second, a measure of the index of vestibular failure is the caloric asymmetry between the affected and unaffected ears. It positively correlated with an area in the left IPL (BA 40) known to represent a multisensory (vestibular) cortex area that is also involved in the modulation of gain and time constants of the vestibulo-ocular reflex (VOR) (40).

During chronic bilateral vestibular failure

Bilateral vestibular failure (BVF) is a rare chronic disorder of the labyrinth or the VIIIth cranial nerve with various aetiologies (see Chapter 26). Its key symptoms are unsteadiness of gait, particularly in the dark and on unlevel ground, and blurred vision due to oscillopsia. Oscillopsia, the illusory motion of the visual scene, is caused by involuntary retinal slip due to an insufficient VOR. BVF patients do not usually have a vestibular tonus imbalance like patients with

vestibular neuritis, and their signs and symptoms can only be elicited by locomotion and head movements.

Activations and deactivations

The differential effects of caloric irrigation in right-handed patients with complete and incomplete BVF are of special interest. These patients exhibit no caloric vestibular nystagmus and do not perceive any illusory self-motion or have vegetative sensations due to caloric irrigation. Their activation-deactivation patterns during vestibular caloric stimulation are generally decreased ($H_2^{15}O$-PET; 41). In particular, there is only a small area of activation in the PIVC contralateral to the irrigated ear and no significant activation on the side of the irrigated ear. In contrast healthy right-handers have bilateral activation and the activation on the ipsilateral right side is stronger. BVF patients largely lack bilateral deactivation of the visual cortex. This general absence suggests that bilaterality depends on a 'normal' activation of the vestibular cortex. There is also no evidence of common non-vestibular (e.g. auditory, somatosensory) responses in other cortex areas. Since vestibular input is reduced in these patients, causing them to have reduced or absent vestibular nystagmus and concurrent oscillopsia, there is perhaps no need for a 'protective' reduction of visual cortex functions. On the one hand, BVF might cause the sensorial weight to be permanently shifted to the visual system, because no valid vestibular information can be generated. On the other, there is obviously no shift of the sensorial weight to the somatosensory or auditory modalities, since no signal changes in other sensory cortex areas were found during vestibular stimulation.

A functional imaging study on visual optokinetic stimulation in BVF patients provides first evidence of visual substitution for vestibular loss (42). Visual optokinetic stimulation in these patients induced a significantly stronger activation and larger activation clusters of the primary visual cortex bilaterally (inferior and middle occipital gyri, BA 17, 18, 19), the motion-sensitive areas V5 in the middle and inferior temporal gyri (BA 37), and the frontal eye field (BA 8), the right paracentral and superior parietal lobule, and the right fusiform and parahippocampal gyri compared to that of age-matched healthy controls (Figure 7.5). Functionally, the enhanced activations were independent of optokinetic performance, since the mean slow-phase velocity of optokinetic nystagmus in the patients did not differ from that in normals. Furthermore, small areas of blood oxygen-level-dependent (BOLD) signal decreases (deactivations), located primarily in the right posterior insula containing the PIVC, were similar to those in healthy controls. These enhanced activations within the visual and ocular motor systems of BVF patients suggest that they might be correlated with an upregulation of visual sensitivity during tracking of visual motion patterns. Functional brain imaging techniques have now complemented the psychophysical and neurophysiological tests showing how sensory loss in one modality leads to a substitutional increase of functional sensitivity in other modalities (e.g. 43–45).

During an acute unilateral lesion of the vestibular nucleus (infarction of the posterolateral medulla)

Vestibular nucleus lesions due to an acute infarction of the posterolateral medulla (Wallenberg syndrome) affect the medial and/or superior vestibular subnuclei, causing a central vestibular disorder. This central vestibular syndrome is characterized by static vestibular signs such as ipsiversive cyclorotation of one or both eyes (82%), skew deviation with the ipsilateral eye lowermost (44%), complete ocular

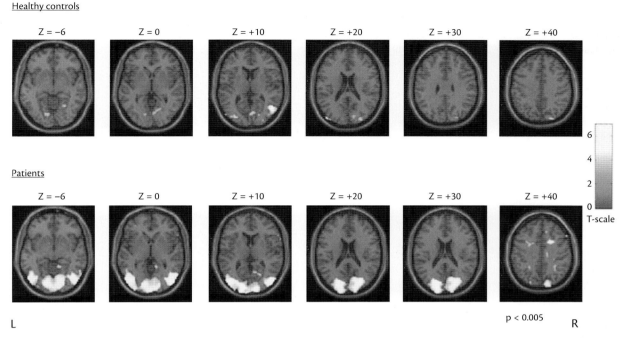

Fig. 7.5 (Also see Colour plate 8.) Head-to-head display of the activation in the t-contrast optokinetic nystagmus (OPK) vs. stationary visual stimulus (SVS) condition in fMRI for BVF patients (bottom) and the age-matched healthy control group (top). For illustrative purposes, voxels above a threshold of p < 0.005, uncorrected, are shown. Modified after Dieterich et al. (42).

tilt reaction (33%), tilts of the perceived vertical in most patients (94%), dynamic vestibular signs such as ipsilateral lateropulsion of eyes and body (46, 47), torsional nystagmus, as well as dysmetria of saccades and limbs (48, 49). Additionally, a normal head impulse test most often differentiates the acute stroke from peripheral vestibular lesions (50). Vestibular signs are combined with other neurological deficits such as Horner's syndrome, impairment of facial pain and temperature sensation, paralysis of the pharynx and larynx with dysphagia and dysphonia, and contralateral impairment of pain and temperature sensation over the trunk and limbs.

Activations and deactivations

Caloric irrigation of the ears in patients with Wallenberg syndrome elicits asymmetrical activations at the cortical level as it does in patients with vestibular neuritis. These patients show typical signs of acute unilateral vestibular dysfunction (i.e. transient rotatory vertigo with vomiting at the onset, ipsiversive body and ocular lateropulsion, and a complete ocular tilt reaction with tilts of the subjective visual vertical). When examined during warm water caloric vestibular stimulation ($H_2{}^{15}O$-PET; 51), their activation pattern was typically different from that of healthy volunteers. During caloric irrigation of the ear ipsilateral to the side of the lesion, there was either no activation or significantly reduced activation in the contralateral hemisphere, whereas the activation pattern in the ipsilateral hemisphere appeared 'normal'. These results agree with the existence of bilaterally ascending vestibular pathways from the vestibular nuclei (especially the medial vestibular subnucleus) to vestibular cortex areas, in which only the contralateral tract is affected. The novel finding was that the activation patterns support the assumption that only the fibres crossing from the medial vestibular subnucleus to the contralateral

medial longitudinal fasciculus are lesioned, whereas the ipsilateral vestibular thalamo-cortical projections via the superior vestibular subnucleus are spared.

Additional findings comparable to those in patients with vestibular neuritis were recently reported for right-handed patients with an acute unilateral medullary infarction (six right, six left) (FDG-PET: 52). The patients were examined twice without any stimulation: 1) in the acute phase on day 7 as a mean after symptom onset when they showed vestibular signs and 2) again 6 months later after recovery (Figure 7.6). There were widespread *decreases* of regional glucose metabolism not only in the visual cortex (BA 17–19) bilaterally, including the motion-sensitive areas MT/V5 and merging into the secondary visual areas in the upper occipital cortex (BA 19/37), but also in the multisensory temporo-parietal areas of the medial and superior temporal gyrus and the IPL. Interestingly, no relevant activations were seen at the cortical level, in contrast to patients with vestibular neuritis. However, the findings for deactivations in visual cortex areas parallel the data for vestibular neuritis. This means that the concept of a reciprocally inhibitory interaction between the vestibular and visual systems is modified by the type of central vestibular lesion: areas become deactivated (GTS, IPL) which are normally activated during vestibular stimulation conditions in healthy subjects.

In general, Wallenberg patients showed signal increases in the acute phase of disease. These were located mainly in the medulla and cerebellar peduncle contralateral to the infarction, but also in the vermis and extensively in both cerebellar hemispheres (52). The signal increases seem to represent an essential circuit for the central compensation in unilateral central vestibular lesions (Wallenberg syndrome), since such relevant cerebellar activations were not observed in the patients with unilateral or bilateral peripheral vestibular lesions.

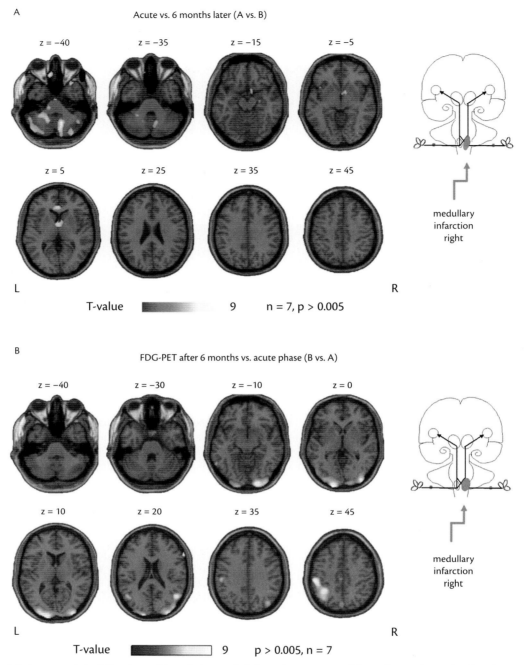

Fig. 7.6 FDG-PET statistical group analysis of 12 patients with vestibular tone imbalance due to acute medullary infarction (situated in the right brainstem) versus the control scan 6 months later at recovery (contrast A vs. B), and the inverse contrast (B vs. A). The contrast A versus B mainly showed cerebellar signal differences, whereas the inverse contrast (PET B vs. A) revealed widespread bilateral signal changes in the visual cortex (BA 17–19), including the motion-sensitive area MT/V5 (BA 19/37) and merging into secondary visual areas in the upper occipital cortex (BA 19/39) as well as in temporo-parietal areas (GTm/s, LPi, BA 39/40).

During acute unilateral lesions of the vestibular thalamic nuclei (infarction of the posterolateral thalamus)

Unilateral lesions of the posterolateral thalamus and—at the cortical level—the superior temporal and the insular cortex (including the PIVC) cause vestibular tonus imbalance without ocular motor signs. These patients, however, have perceptual deficits (e.g. deviations of the perceived visual vertical) as well as postural deficits, i.e.

an imbalance of stance and gait with lateral falls (51, 53, 54). This type of vestibular imbalance is probably identical to the earlier term 'thalamic astasia', a condition of irresistible falls without paresis or sensory or cerebellar signs (55).

Vestibular stimulation investigations in animal experiments in the 1970s (56–58) showed that the posterolateral thalamus—including the subnuclei ventrocaudalis externus, ventro-oralis intermedius (Vim), dorsocaudalis, ventrocaudalis internus, and ventroposterior lateralis (VPLo)—is the afferent relay station for multiple multisensory vestibular cortex areas. In animals vestibular information reaches several separate and distinct cortex areas via the subnuclei of this relay station: for example, the PIVC in the posterior insula, adjacent retroinsular areas and the granular insular region (3, 59, 60), the VTS area posterior to PIVC (3), parts of area 7 in the IPL (BA 40) (40, 61, 62), the VIP in the fundus of the intraparietal sulcus (5, 63, 64), area 3aV in the central sulcus (65, 66), and probably area 2v at the tip of the intraparietal sulcus (65, 67). In patients with three different types of acute unilateral thalamic infarctions only posterolateral lesions cause transient vestibular signs and symptoms like perceptual deficits with ipsi- or contralateral tilts of the subjective visual vertical, corresponding deviations of stance and gait, but no ocular motor deficits (53).

These signs of thalamic lesions agree with earlier findings in electrical stimulation studies of the thalamic subnucleus Vim in humans. Such stimulation elicited a corresponding rotation or spinning of the body, head, or eyes in either a counterclockwise (more often) or clockwise direction (68, 69). Vestibular thalamic deficits found in humans (53) also agreed with findings of electrophysiological studies on the posterolateral thalamus in non-human primates (56–58).

Activations and deactivations

In view of the vestibular thalamo-cortical network in both hemispheres, the question arose as to the consequences of a unilateral lesion of the 'vestibular relay station' in the posterolateral thalamus. Therefore, the differential effects of unilateral caloric vestibular stimulation (right or left ear irrigation with warm water) on the cortical and subcortical activation pattern of both hemispheres were

analysed in right-handed patients who had had an acute unilateral stroke of the posterolateral thalamus (H_2^{15}O-PET: 24) (Figure 7.7). It was found that: 1) activation of the multisensory vestibular cortex was significantly reduced in the ipsilateral hemisphere, when the ear ipsilateral to the thalamic lesion was stimulated; 2) activation of multisensory vestibular cortex areas of the hemisphere contralateral to the irrigated ear was also diminished, but to a lesser extent; 3) the right hemispheric dominance in right-handers was preserved in patients with right and left thalamic lesions. Thus, these data demonstrated the functional importance of the posterolateral thalamus as a gatekeeper, of the dominance of ipsilateral ascending pathways, and of the right hemisphere in right handedness.

This asymmetrical pattern of cortical activation during calorics was neither associated with directional asymmetry of caloric nystagmus nor with motion perception for the entire group (24). The caloric nystagmus tended to be stronger during stimulation of the ear contralateral to the lesion and the contrast between significant hemispheric differences in the mediation of vestibular input (activations) and minimal vestibular signs and symptoms of the patients was striking. The finding that the caloric nystagmus was not significantly influenced by the vestibular thalamic lesion is not trivial: there are cortical areas (e.g. the suprasylvian cortex in cats and monkeys, particularly area 7, corresponding to an area at the occipito-temporo-parietal junction in humans) which influence VOR symmetry in terms of directional preponderance of VOR gain and VOR time constant and nystagmus frequency (40, 61, 62, 70). Since activation of the multisensory vestibular cortex ensemble was significantly reduced in the ipsilateral hemisphere during stimulation of the ear ipsilateral to the thalamic lesion, the diminished

Patient BS: thalamus infarction left

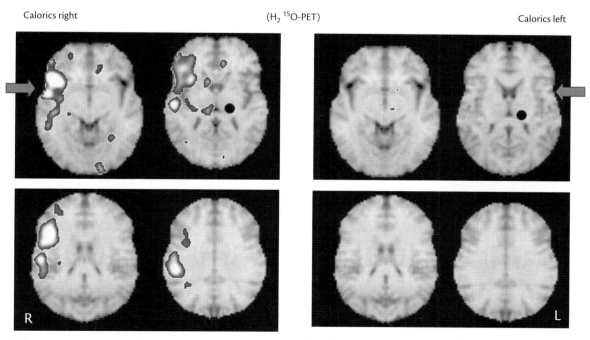

Calorics right   (H_2 ^{15}O-PET)   Calorics left

Fig. 7.7 Activated areas during caloric stimulation of the right or left ear in a patient with a left-sided posterolateral thalamic infarction (p <0.001). Left: activations for the left-sided lesions during right calorics (non-affected side) occur as large clusters in the posterior and anterior insula, inferior frontal gyrus, superior temporal gyrus, inferior parietal lobule, and superior parts of the parietal lobule, hippocampus, paramedian thalamus, and midbrain, nucleus ruber, putamen, medial and superior frontal gyrus, and cerebellar vermis of the right hemisphere. Activations of the left hemisphere are found in only the anterior cingulate gyrus, and diagonal frontal gyrus. Right: caloric irrigation of the affected left side shows no significant activations.

activation of the occipito-temporo-parietal region could have modulated the VOR symmetry and thereby reduced the caloric nystagmus.

Vestibular stimulation in healthy volunteers not only activates vestibular cortex areas but at the same time deactivates visual cortex areas bilaterally (17, 20, 26). Patients with posterolateral thalamic infarctions generally showed deactivations of the visual cortex areas in only one hemisphere, namely in the hemisphere contralateral to the stimulated ear and contralateral to activated vestibular cortex areas (24). This suggests a crossed inhibition, i.e. the normal interaction between the vestibular and the visual systems (described earlier as a reciprocal inhibitory interaction in both hemispheres in Brandt et al. (27)) is disturbed in these patients: their ipsilateral hemisphere was 'functionally disconnected.'

Conclusions

Advances have been made in identifying the cortical areas involved in the processing of vestibular, ocular motor, and visual information and the cortical interaction between these systems in healthy subjects. These areas appear in fMRI and PET as activations or deactivations. The typical cortical activation–deactivation pattern during vestibular stimulation of normal subjects is modified in patients. These alterations have revealed the following:

1) In patients with acute unilateral peripheral vestibular lesions the modified pattern is most likely due to adaptive substitution or compensation within the central vestibular system of the unaffected side.

2) The reciprocal inhibitory interaction between the vestibular and visual systems appears to be preserved in BVF patients but at a significantly lower level during vestibular stimulation (i.e. there are less activations and less deactivations). However, it is enhanced during visual stimulation within the visual cortex; this is probably a visual substitution for vestibular loss.

3) Central compensatory processes of vestibular imbalance during the acute phase after medullary infarctions take place mainly in brainstem–cerebellar loops (upregulation). The visual cortical system—primary visual areas as well as secondary visual cortex areas and even multisensory (vestibular) areas—are deactivated (probably downregulated) at the cortical level (decreases of glucose metabolism) in the acute phase.

4) The functional relevance of deactivations at neural levels is still not known, since adequate psychophysical tests for the visual system are rare.

5) Calorically-induced vestibular nystagmus appears to be mainly mediated by a subthalamic brainstem VOR circuitry and the vestibular cerebellum rather than by thalamo-cortical structures. Patients with acute and subacute lesions of the vestibular thalamus lack spontaneous vestibular nystagmus and rotational vertigo. Moreover, their ipsilateral hemisphere does not show activations, nor does the contralateral hemisphere show deactivations. Thus, the inhibitory interaction between the visual and the vestibular systems may be organized by pathways that cross the hemispheres.

Although we have also learned how certain vestibular and ocular motor disorders modify visuo-vestibular interaction by changing the 'normal' cortical activation–deactivation pattern, it is still early days for functional imaging studies that aim to determine the neural basis of the underlying disorders. Several vestibular, ocular motor, and cerebellar disorders still await investigation with fMRI and PET. These studies promise to provide further insights into the complex neural networks of the human cortex and the changes occurring during compensatory processes after strategic lesions.

References

1. Dieterich M, Brandt T (2008). Functional imaging of peripheral and central vestibular disorders. *Brain*, 131, 2538–52.
2. Dieterich M, Brandt T (2010).Imaging cortical activity after vestibular lesions. *Restor Neurol Neurosci*, 28(1), 47–56.
3. Guldin WO, Grüsser OJ (1996). The anatomy of the vestibular cortices of primates. In Collard M, Jeannerod M, Christen Y (Eds) *Le cortex vestibulaire. Editions IRVINN*, pp. 17–26. Paris: Ipsen.
4. Chen A, DeAngelis GC, Angelaki DE (2010) Macaque parieto-insular vestibular cortex: responses to self-motion and optic flow. *J Neurosci*, 30, 3022–42.
5. Bremmer F, Klam F, Duhamel J-R, Hamed SB, Graf W (2002). Visual-vestibular interactive responses in the macaque ventral intraparietal area (VIP). *Eur J Neurosci*, 16, 1569–86.
6. Ebata S, Sugiuchi Y, Izawa Y, Shinomiya K, Shinoda Y (2004). Vestibular projection to the periarcuate cortex in the monkey. *Neurosci Res*, 49, 55–68.
7. Schlack A, Sterbing-D'Angelo SJ, Hartung K, Hoffmann KP, Bremmer F (2005). Multisensory space representations in the macaque ventral intraparietal area. *J Neurosci*, 25, 4616–25.
8. Bottini G, Sterzi R, Paulesu E, *et al.* (1994). Identification of the central vestibular projections in man: a positron emission tomography activation study. *Exp Brain Res*, 99, 164–9.
9. Bottini G, Karnath HO, Vallar G, *et al.* (2001). Cerebral representations for egocentric space: functional-anatomical evidence from caloric vestibular stimulation and neck vibration. *Brain*, 124, 1182–96.
10. Suzuki M, Kitano H, Ito R, *et al.* (2001). Cortical and subcortical vestibular response to caloric stimulation detected by functional magnetic resonance imaging. *Brain Res Cogn Brain Res*, 12, 441–9.
11. Fasold O, von Brevern M, Kuhberg M, *et al.* (2002). Human vestibular cortex as identified with caloric stimulation in functional magnetic resonance imaging. *NeuroImage*, 17, 1384–93.
12. Naito Y, Tateya I, Hirano S, *et al.* (2003). Cortical correlates of vestibulo-ocular refelx modulation: a PET study. *Brain*, 126, 1562–78.
13. Dieterich M, Bense S, Lutz S, *et al.* (2003). Dominance for vestibular cortical function in the non-dominant hemisphere. *Cerebral Cortex*, 13, 994–1007.
14. Emri M, Kisely M, Lengyel Z, *et al.* (2003). Cortical projection of peripheral vestibular signaling. *J Neurophysiol*, 89, 2639–46.
15. Bucher SF, Dieterich M, Wiesmann M, *et al.* (1998). Cerebral functional MRI of vestibular, auditory, and nociceptive areas during galvanic stimulation. *Ann Neurol*, 44, 120–5.
16. Lobel E, Kleine JF, Le Bihan D, Leroy-Willig A, Berthoz A (1998). Functional MRI of galvanic vestibular stimulation. *J Neurophysiol*, 80, 2699–709.
17. Bense S, Stephan T, Yousry TA, Brandt T, Dieterich M (2001). Multisensory cortical signal increases and decreases during vestibular galvanic stimulation (fMRI). *J Neurophysiol*, 85, 886–99.
18. Bremmer F, Schlack A, Duhamel J-R, Graf W, Fink GR (2001). Space coding in primate posterior parietal cortex. *NeuroImage*, 14, 46–51.
19. Fink GR, Marshall JC, Weiss PH, *et al.* (2003). Performing allocentric visuospatial judgements with induced distortion of the egocentric reference frame: an fMRI study with clinical implications. *NeuroImage*, 20, 1505–17.
20. Stephan T, Deutschländer A, Nolte A, *et al.* (2005). Functional MRI of galvanic vestibular stimulation with alternating currents at different frequencies. *NeuroImage*, 26, 721–32.

21. Miyamato T, Fukushima K, Takada T, de Waele C, Vidal PP (2007). Saccular stimulation of the human cortex: a functional magnetic resonance imaging study. *Neurosci Lett*, 423(1), 68–72.

22. Janzen J, Schlindwein P, Bense S, *et al.* (2008). Neural correlates of hemispheric dominance and ipsilaterality within the vestibular system. *NeuroImage*, 42(2), 1508–18

23. Schlindwein P, Mueller M, Bauermann T, Brandt T, Stoeter P, Dieterich M (2008). Cortical representation of saccular vestibular stimulation: VEMPs in fMRI. *NeuroImage*, 39(1), 19–31

24. Dieterich M, Bartenstein P, Spiegel S, Bense S, Schwaiger M, Brandt T (2005). Thalamic infarctions cause side-specific suppression of vestibular cortex activations. *Brain*, 128, 2052–67.

25. Bense S, Bartenstein P, Lutz S, *et al.* (2003). Three determinants of vestibular hemispheric dominance during caloric stimulation. *Ann N Y Acad Sci*, 1004, 440–5.

26. Wenzel R, Bartenstein P, Dieterich M, *et al.* (1996). Deactivation of human visual cortex during involuntary ocular oscillations. A PET activation study. *Brain*, 119, 101–10.

27. Brandt T, Bartenstein P, Janek A, Dieterich M (1998). Reciprocal inhibitory visual-vestibular interaction: visual motion stimulation deactivates the parieto-insular vestibular cortex. *Brain*, 121, 1749–58.

28. Brandt T, Dieterich M (1999). The vestibular cortex. Its locations, functions, and disorders. *Ann N Y Acad Sci*, 871, 293–312.

29. Laurienti PJ, Burdette JH, Wallace MT, Yen YF, Field AS, Stein BE (2002). Deactivation of sensory-specific cortex by cross-modal stimuli. *J Cogn Neurosci*, 14, 420–9.

30. Maihöfner C, Handwerker HO, Birklein F (2006). Functional imaging of allodynia in complex regional pain syndrome. *Neurology*, 66(5), 711–17.

31. Merabet LB, Swisher JD, McMains SA, *et al.* (2007). Combined activation and deactivation of visual cortex during tactile sensory processing. *J Neurophysiol*, 97, 1633–41.

32. Mast FW, Merfeld DM, Kosslyn SM (2006). Visual mental imagery during caloric vestibular stimulation. *Neuropsychologia*, 44 (1), 101–9.

33. Brandt T, Stephan T, Bense S, Yousry TA, Dieterich M (2000). Hemifield visual motion stimulation: an example of interhemispheric crosstalk. *NeuroReport*, 11, 2803–9.

34. Brandt T, Marx E, Stephan T, Bense S Dieterich M (2003). Inhibitory interhemispheric visuovisual interaction in motion perception. *Ann NY Acad Sci*, 1004, 283–8.

35. Shmuel A, Augath M, Oeltermann A, Logothetis NK (2006). Negative functional MRI response correlates with decreases in neuronal activity in monkey visual area V1. *Nat Neurosci*, 9, 569–77.

36. Bense S, Bartenstein P, Lochmann M, Schlindwein P, Brandt T, Dieterich M (2004). Metabolic changes in vestibular and visual cortices in acute vestibular neuritis. *Ann Neurol*, 56, 624–30.

37. Yamanaka T, Him A, Cameron SA, Dutia MB (2000). Rapid compensatory changes in GABA receptor efficacy in rat vestibular neurons after unilateral labyrinthectomy. *J Physiol*, 523, 413–24.

38. Guilding C, Dutia MB (2005). Early and late changes in vestibular neuronal excitability after deafferentation. *Neuroreport*, 16, 1415–18.

39. Bergquist F, Ruthven A, Ludwig M, Dutia MB (2006). Histaminergic and glycinergic modulation of GABA release in the vestibular nuclei of normal and labyrinthectomised rats. *J Physiol*, 577, 857–68.

40. Ventre-Dominey J, Nighoghossian N, Denise P (2003). Evidence for interacting cortical control of vestibular function and spatial representation in man. *Neuropsychologia*, 41, 1884–98.

41. Bense S, Deutschländer A, Stephan T, Bartenstein P, Schwaiger M, Brandt T, Dieterich M (2004). Preserved visual-vestibular interaction in patients with bilateral vestibular failure. *Neurology*, 63, 122–8.

42. Dieterich M, Bauermann T, Best C, Stoeter P, Schlindwein P (2007). Evidence for cortical visual substitution of chronic bilateral vestibular failure (an fMRI study). *Brain*, 130(Pt 8), 2108–16.

43. Bles W, Klören T, Büchele W, Brandt T (1983). Somatosensory nystagmus: Physiological and clinical aspects. *Adv Oto-Rhino-Laryngol*, 30, 30–3.

44. Bles W, de Jong JM, de Wit G (1984). Somatosensory compensation for loss of labyrinthine function. *Acta Otolaryngol (Stockh)*, 97, 213–21.

45. Curthoys IS, Halmagyi GM (1994). Vestibular compensation: a review of the oculomotor, neural, and clinical consequences of unilateral vestibular loss. *J Vest Res*, 5, 67–107.

46. Dieterich M, Brandt T (1992). Wallenberg's syndrome: Lateropulsion, cyclorotation, and subjective visual vertical in thirty-six patients. *Ann Neurol*, 31, 399–408.

47. Dieterich M, Brandt T (1993). Ocular torsion and tilt of subjective visual vertical are sensitive brainstem signs. *Ann Neurol*, 33, 292–9.

48. Kommerell G, Hoyt WF (1973). Lateropulsion of saccadic eye movements: electro-oculographic studies in a patient with Wallenberg's syndrome. *Arch Neurol*, 28, 313–18.

49. Morrow MJ, Sharpe A (1988). Torsional nystagmus in the lateral medullary syndrome. *Ann Neurol*, 24, 390–8.

50. Newman-Toker DE, Kattah JC, Alvernia JE, Wang DZ (2008). Normal head impulse test differentiates acute cerebellar strokes from vestibular neuritis. *Neurology*, 70, 2378–85.

51. Dieterich M, Bense S, Stephan T, Schwaiger M, Bartenstein P, Brandt TH (2005). Medial vestibular nucleus lesions in Wallenberg's syndrome cause decreased activity of the contralateral vestibular cortex. *Ann N Y Acad Sci*, 1039, 1–16.

52. Bense S, Buchholz H-G, Best C, Schlindwein P, *et al.* (2006). Compensation for central vestibular dysfunction in patients with acute medullary infarction (FDG-PET study). *J Neurol*, 253(S2), 33.

53. Dieterich M, Brandt T (1993). Thalamic infarctions: Differential effects on vestibular function in the roll plane (35 patients). *Neurology*, 43, 1732–40.

54. Brandt T, Dieterich M (1994). Vestibular syndromes in the roll plane: topographic diagnosis from brainstem to cortex. *Ann Neurol*, 36, 337–47.

55. Masdeu JC, Gorelick PB (1988). Thalamic astasia: Inability to stand after unilateral thalamic lesions. *Ann Neurol*, 23, 596–602.

56. Sans A, Raymond J, Marty R (1970). Response thalamiques et corticales a la stimulation electrique du nerf vestibulaire chez le chat. *Exp Brain Res*, 10, 265–75.

57. Deecke L, Schwarz DWF, Fredrickson JM (1974). Nucleus ventroposterior inferior (VPI) as the thalamic relay in the rhesus monkey. I. Field potential investigation. *Exp Brain Res*, 20, 88–100.

58. Büttner U, Henn V (1976). Thalamic unit activity in the alert monkey during natural vestibular stimulation. *Brain Res*, 103, 127–32.

59. Grüsser OJ, Pause M, Schreiter U (1990). Localization and responses of neurons in the parieto-insular cortex of awake monkeys (Macaca fascicularis). *J Physiol (Lond)*, 430, 537–57.

60. Grüsser OJ, Pause M, Schreiter U (1990). Vestibular neurones in the parieto-insular cortex of monkeys (Macaca fascicularis): visual and neck receptor responses. *J Physiol (Lond)*, 430, 559–83.

61. Ventre J (1985). Cortical control of oculomotor function. II. Vestibulo-ocular reflex and visual-vestibular interaction. *Behav Brain Res*, 17, 221–34.

62. Faugier-Grimaud S, Ventre J (1989). Anatomic connections of inferior parietal cortex (Area 7) with subcortical structures related to vestibulo-ocular function in a monkey (Macaca fascicularis). *J Compar Neurol*, 280, 1–14.

63. Klam F, Graf W (2003). Vestibular response kinematics in posterior parietal cortex neurons of macaque monkeys. *Eur J Neurosci*, 18, 995–1010.

64. Klam F, Graf W (2003). Vestibular signals of posterior parietal cortex neurons during active and passive head movements in macaque monkeys. *Ann N Y Acad Sci*, 1004, 271–82.

65. Schwarz DWF, Fredrickson JM (1971). Rhesus monkey vestibular cortex: a bimodal primary projection field. *Science*, 172, 280–1.

66. Ödkvist LM, Schwarz DWF, Fredrickson JM, Hassler R (1974). Projection of the vestibular nerve to the area 3a arm field in the squirrel monkey (Saimiri sciureus). *Exp Brain Res*, 21, 97–105.

67. Büttner U, Buettner UW (1978). Parietal cortex area 2 V neuronal activity in the alert monkey during natural vestibular and optokinetic stimulation. *Brain Res*, 153, 392–7.

68. Hassler R (1959). Anatomy of the thalamus. In Schaltenbrand G, Bailey P (Eds) *Introduction to stereotaxis with an atlas of the human brain*, vol. 1, pp. 230–90. Stuttgart: Thieme.

69. Tasker RR, Organ LW, Hawrylyshyn PA (1982). *The thalamus and midbrain of man. A physiological atlas using electrical stimulation*. Springfield, IL: Charles C Thomas.

70. Tusa RJ, Demer JL, Herdman SJ (1989). Cortical areas involved in OKN and VOR in cats: cortical lesions. *J Neurosci*, 9, 1163–78.

CHAPTER 8

Clinical Anatomy and Physiology of the Vestibular System

G. Michael Halmagyi and Ian S. Curthoys

Some knowledge of the basic structure and function of the vestibular system, all the way from the labyrinth of inner ears, to the vestibular ganglia and nerves, to the brainstem vestibular nuclei and the extraocular muscles, to the cortex, to the spinal cord, then axial and limb muscles, is needed if the clinician is to diagnose and manage patients with vertigo and imbalance from principles as well as from pattern recognition. For a recent monograph on vestibular physiology see Goldberg et al. (1).

Why have labyrinths?

The vestibular system exists to sense motion of the head and the orientation of the head with respect to gravity. It does this by the inertial bending of exquisitely sensitive cilia on hair cells in the labyrinth—on the cristae of the three semicircular canals and the maculae of the two otoliths, in each inner ear (Figures 8.1 and 8.2). The cristae and maculae are situated within the inner chamber of

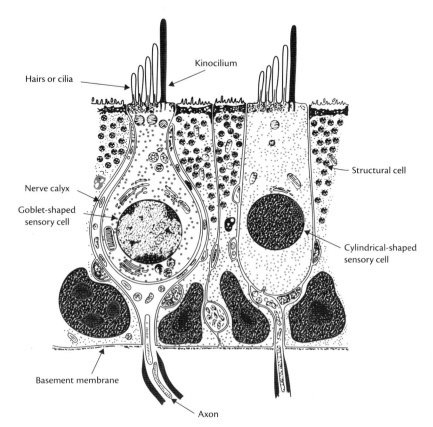

Fig. 8.1 Vestibular hair cells. Schematic representation of the two types of receptor hair cells in the mammalian vestibular system. The large goblet-shaped receptor cells are called type I cells and the afferent nerve ending forms a chalice (or calyx) around most of the receptor cell. In contrast the type II cells are cylindrical in shape and the afferent endings make bouton terminations on the cell-body. These two types are found in each vestibular sense organ—the type I cells are clustered at the striola and the peak of the cristae, whereas the type II cells are spread throughout the sense region. From Engstrom et al. (21).

Hairs or cilia

Kinocilium

Nerve calyx

Goblet-shaped sensory cell

Structural cell

Cylindrical-shaped sensory cell

Basement membrane

Axon

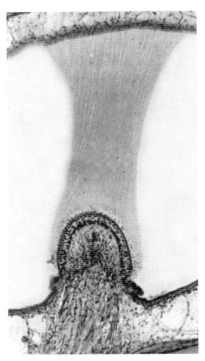

Fig. 8.2 The cupula. The cupula stretches from the top of the crista to the roof of the ampulla of the semicircular canal. The cilia of the receptor hair cells lie within the cupula. Each crista is covered by receptor hair cells with the kinocilia of every cell oriented in the same direction. Angular acceleration causes fluid flow within the semicircular canal and so results in small deflections of the cupula so that all the embedded hair cells are deflected and, depending on the direction of the deflection, are all excited or all inhibited. From Igarashi & Alford (22).

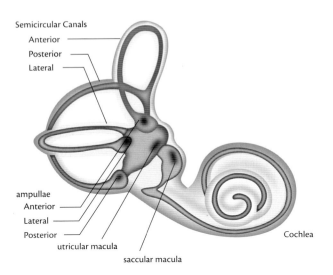

Fig. 8.3 Schematic of membranous labyrinth. Schematic representation of the membranous labyrinth showing the relative locations of the sensory regions—for each semicircular canal at the ampulla and for the otoliths at the utricular macula and saccular macula. The cochlea is also part of the membranous labyrinth but it is spatially separated as shown.

the inner ear—the membranous labyrinth (Figure 8.3) which contains endolymph, a fluid with a high potassium content in contrast to the outer compartment of the inner ear which contains perilymph, a fluid which is high in sodium content and in continuity with cerebrospinal fluid via the cochlear aqueduct, a channel in the temporal bone.

Since force equals mass times acceleration the cilia of vestibular hairs cells can be bent (i.e. displaced) only by acceleration and not by velocity. Each semicircular canal (SCC) is structurally specialized to

transduce angular acceleration (i.e. head rotation) whereas each otolith is structurally specialized to sense linear acceleration, which can be produced by head movement (translation from side-to-side, up-and-down, or back-and-forward) or head tilt (change of orientation). The structure and geometry of each SCC makes its hair cells sense rotation rather than translation of the head, whereas the presence of otoconia allows the macular hair cells to sense tilt and translation. Vestibular hair cells have one kinocilium and 40–70 stereocilia; when these stereocilia are bent towards the kinocilium the cell depolarizes and this increases the neural firing of its ganglion cell; when these are bent away from the kinocilium the hair cell hyperpolarizes and this reduces the resting neural activity of its ganglion cell (Figure 8.4). The three SCCs in each ear are angled at about 90° to each other so that the vestibular system has information about angular acceleration in three dimensions (Figures 8.5 and 8.6).

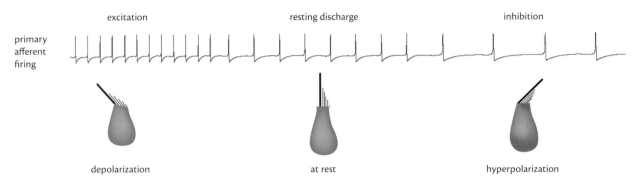

Fig. 8.4 Schematic of hair cell activation. A representation of how the deflection of hair cells results in changes in primary vestibular afferent firing. At rest the cilia are upright and there is a resting discharge. When the cilia are deflected towards the kinocilium (the longest cilium) the cell is depolarized and the resting discharge rate increases (excitation). When the cilia are deflected away from the kinocilium the receptor is hyperpolarized and there is a decrease in resting discharge rate. This kind of excitation–inhibition is exemplified for both afferents from cells in semicircular canals (corresponding to the two directions of angular acceleration) and also for otolithic afferents (corresponding to the two opposing directions of linear acceleration).

The two otoliths in each ear are also angled at about 90° to each other—the utricular macula (Figure 8.7) close to horizontal while the saccular macula is close to vertical (Figure 8.8), so that the vestibular system has information about linear acceleration in three dimensions. Signals from the labyrinth are conveyed to the vestibular nuclei by the axons of Scarpa's ganglion cells in the vestibular nerves: the superior and lateral SCCs and the utricle are innervated by the superior vestibular nerve, the posterior SCC and the saccule by the inferior vestibular nerve (Figure 8.9). Normal people are, of course, constantly aware of the function of their cochlear hair cells; in contrast they are totally unaware of the function of their vestibular hair cells until something goes wrong.

How you can tell that your patient doesn't have a functioning labyrinth

The symptoms and signs of bilateral loss of vestibular function are unmistakable: imbalance and jiggling vision (oscillopsia), both only while walking (see Chapters 13 and 26). There are no symptoms while the patient sits or lies down. The imbalance is due to impaired vestibulospinal reflexes and is worse if vision and proprioception—the two other sensory modalities used to help humans stay upright—are disrupted. Walking on a soft surface in the dark (e.g. a beach or field at night) is particularly challenging. The imbalance can be easily shown doing a Romberg test, first on the firm floor—possible, and then on a thick (10 cm) foam mat—impossible (2). The oscillopsia is due to impaired vestibulo-ocular reflexes (VORs; Figure 8.10) and it can be easily demonstrated by showing that the patient's vision will drop to 6/36 or less during rapid (>1 Hz) vertical head-shaking (dynamic visual acuity test) (3, 4). If the patient tries to stare at any fixed target while the examiner rapidly turns her head to one side, the patient will make easily visible delayed compensatory rapid eye movements (saccades) rather the immediate smooth eye movements (VOR); this is the head impulse test (Figure 8.11). Gentamicin ototoxicity is a frequent reason for patients to have no labyrinthine function (5, 6).

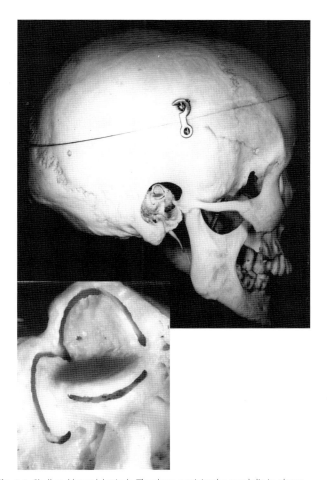

Fig. 8.5 Skull and bony labyrinth. The three semicircular canals lie in planes approximately perpendicular to one another. The ampullae of the horizontal and anterior canals are at the anterior end of the canals, whereas the ampulla of the posterior canal is ventral and well below the horizontal canal. This figure shows the orientation of the canals in the skull and that they are located about 2.5 cm in from the surface of the skull.

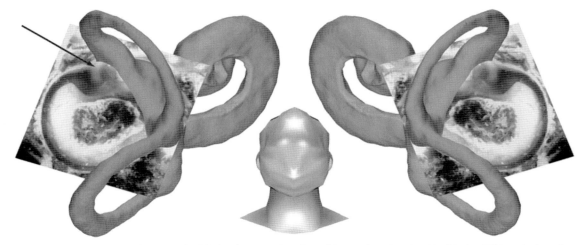

Fig. 8.6 CT bony labyrinth. The semicircular canals on one side of the head are approximately parallel to canals on the other side of the head. This semi-schematic representation shows reconstructions from CT scans (courtesy Andrew Bradshaw). The labyrinths have been enlarged and translated to be close to one another but the spatial relationships of the canals have not been changed. Superimposed on the horizontal canals is a photo (to scale) of the membranous horizontal duct and ampullae from a dissected human specimen. The arrow points to the crista of the canal which is approximately in the median plane of the head. The point of view of the head is as shown on the Oscar style head. As the head is turned to the left the cupula on the left is deflected in an excitatory direction and simultaneously the cupula on the right side is deflected in an inhibitory direction. The neural circuitry at the brainstem level uses that symmetrical and opposite change in neural afferent input to enhance the sensitivity of the system (see Figure 8.16). From Curthoys et al. (25).

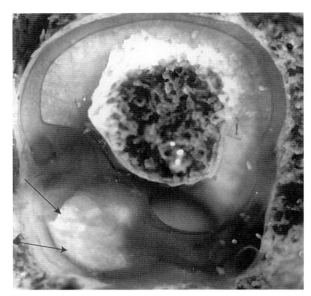

Fig. 8.7 The macula. View directly perpendicularly down onto an exposed human horizontal semicircular canal, ampulla, and utricle. The membranous wall of the utricle has been opened to expose the otoconia on the surface of the utricular macula (arrows). The bulk of the utricular macula lies close to the plane of the horizontal canal.

How you can tell that your patient has only one functioning labyrinth

Unlike other paired sensory organs, such as the eyes or the cochleas, the two labyrinths work as a push–pull system; neural

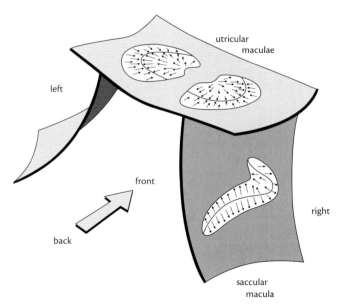

Fig. 8.8 Otolithic planes. Schematic representation of the approximate orientation of the utricular and saccular maculae in the head. Each macula is covered by a sheet of receptor hair cells, each one with a preferred orientation as shown by the small arrows on the maculae. A linear acceleration in the preferred direction stimulates that receptor optimally. The utricular macula is approximately in the plane of the horizontal semicircular canal (see Figure 8.7) and the long arm (the 'shank') of the saccular macula is roughly parallel to the plane of the horizontal canal. From Curthoys & Betts (26).

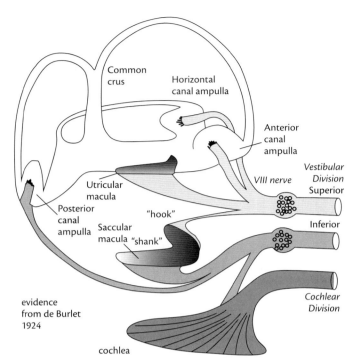

Fig. 8.9 Innervation of the inner ear. Schematic representation of the divisions of the VIIIth nerve and the sensory regions innervated (evidence from de Burlet (23)). The superior division of the vestibular nerve contains afferents from the horizontal and anterior canals, the utricular macula and from the rostral part (the 'hook' of the saccular macula). The inferior division contains the afferents from the posterior canal and the bulk of the saccular macula (the 'shank'). Afferents from the cochlea also travel in the VIIIth nerve. The cell bodies of Scarpa's ganglion are shown as the dots within the vestibular nerve.

excitation of one side is invariably accompanied by neural inhibition (strictly, disfacilitation) of the other. In order to have disfacilitation there has to be resting neural activity; in axons of vestibular ganglion cells originating in the lateral SCC of the monkey this is about 40 action potentials (spikes) per second. Rapid angular acceleration (say $10,000°/s^2$) in the excitatory direction will drive this neural activity to a maximum of say 800 spikes/s, an increase of 760 spikes/s. The same acceleration in the opposite (inhibitory) direction can of course drive the neural activity to 0 spikes/s—it will silence the neuron, a decrease of 40 spikes/s, which gives rising to an inherent ('hard-wired') asymmetry in the bidirectional responses of the SCC (Figures 8.12 and 8.13).

So it should be, and it is, possible to show this inhibitory saturation during rapid angular accelerations away from the one functioning lateral SCC in the patient who has only one. This is the head impulse test which relies on the examiner recognizing the tell-tale catch-up saccade in response to rapid passive head rotations away from the normal SSC, towards the defective SCC (Figure 8.14) (7, 8). Labyrinthitis and vestibular schwannoma surgery are common reasons for patients to have only one functioning labyrinth.

But having only one labyrinth is rarely as good as having two: many patients who have only one will notice the same symptoms as those who don't have even one: imbalance and oscillopsia with a positive foam Romberg test and decreased dynamic visual acuity (9, 10). Vestibular rehabilitation might have something to offer them (Chapter 17).

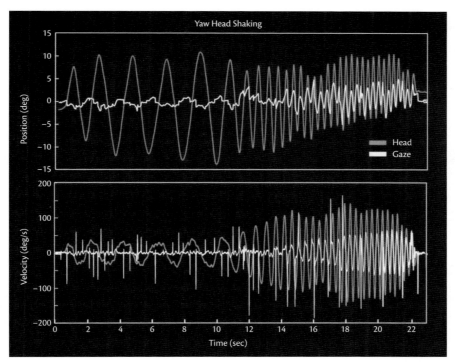

Fig. 8.10 Mechanism of oscillopsia. Horizontal and head and gaze position (top panel) and head and gaze velocity (bottom panel) in a patient with bilateral vestibular loss due to gentamicin toxicity. Gaze is eye position/velocity relative to space. The patient is actively shaking her head from side-to-side increasing in frequency from about 0.5 Hz to about 3 Hz and in peak velocity from 30°/s to about 130°/s. At 0.5-Hz gaze is stable (velocity close to 0°/s) so that there is no oscillopsia. At 3.0 Hz, gaze velocity reaches 70°/s (equivalent to the VOR gain of only 0.3) and the patient experiences extreme horizontal oscillopsia with a visual acuity of 6/60. In a normal subject, VOR gain at 3.0 Hz would be close to 1.0, gaze velocity would be close to 0, visual acuity would be close to 6/6 and there would be no oscillopsia—as in this patient at 0.5 Hz.

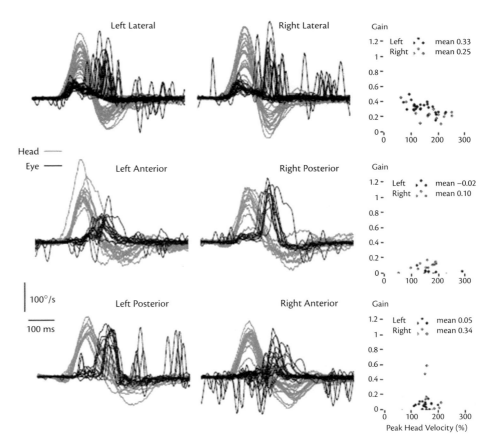

Fig. 8.11 Head impulse test with bilateral vestibular loss. Bilateral vestibulopathy shown on horizontal and vertical impulsive testing using the GN Otometrics video-oculography system in a patient with bilateral vestibular loss. The head rotation stimulus is shown in grey (up to a peak angular velocity of 250°/s and an angular acceleration of 2000°/s²); eye movement response is shown in black. With horizontal impulses the maximum gain of the VOR is less than 0.4 (normal >0.95) in each direction. There are overt catch-up saccades. With vertical head impulses in the plane of individual vertical semicircular canals the peak VOR gain is less than 0.2 (normal > 0.8) and there are again overt catch-up saccades. For details of the method see MacDougall et al. (15).

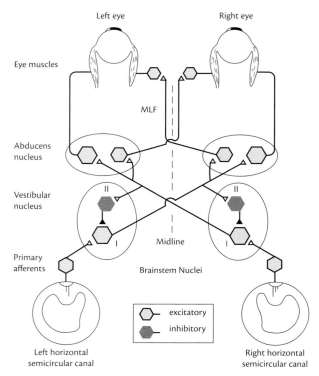

Fig. 8.12 Neurons of the VOR. Schematic representation of the basic projections from the horizontal semicircular canal to the eye muscles. The primary afferents project to vestibular nucleus and synapse on an excitatory neuron which projects to contralateral abducens motoneurons and excites them. So a head rotation to the left will increase the firing of these afferents and so result in increased activity of the contralateral abducens neurons and so the lateral rectus will be activated and the eye will rotate to the right to counteract the leftwards rotation. Importantly the excitatory neuron from the vestibular nucleus also excites an inhibitory neuron (II) which acts to inhibit neurons in the contralateral vestibular nucleus and so inhibit the abducens neurons on the left side, allowing for a smooth synergistic response—activation of right lateral rectus and inhibition of the left lateral rectus. The abducens internuclear neurons project to the medial rectus in the medial longitudinal fasciculus (MLF). All the connections shown here have been established by physiological experiments.

How you can tell that your patient has just lost one labyrinth

If it happens slowly, then not much. One day the patient might notice (you guessed it) imbalance and oscillopsia—see earlier section. In contrast if it happens quickly, then all hell breaks loose: terrible, relentless, wild spinning with nausea, retching, sweating, vomiting (see Chapter 13). Some patients are terrified about dying; others about not. Some patients will have the full acute unilateral vestibular loss syndrome (present and almost identical in all vertebrates): third-degree nystagmus with slow phases towards the lost side and an ocular tilt reaction (head tilt, skew deviation and conjugate ocular torsion—Figure 8.15), also towards the lost side. The head impulse test will be positive to the lost side (Figure 8.14). The acute vestibular syndrome is of course due to loss of resting neural activity from the affected side, which then results in a decrease in resting neural activity in vestibular nucleus neurons on the affected side (Figure 8.16). While vestibular nucleus resting activity is relatively higher on the normal side than on the affected side, your patient cannot help but feel that she is spinning

towards her normal side. But through the magic of vestibular compensation (see Chapter 6) a miracle always occurs—although the labyrinth does not recover, the resting vestibular nucleus activity on the two sides gradually equalizes, the acute vestibular syndrome resolves, the spinning stops and the patient is cured usually within a week (2 days in guinea pigs). The most frequent cause of acute unilateral vestibular loss is vestibular neuritis/labyrinthitis/neuro-labyrinthitis (Chapter 19) but can also occur from traumatic or surgical injuries of the inner ear (11).

How you can tell that your patient has just lost the other labyrinth

It depends when—there are three possibilities. 1) If the other labyrinth is lost at exactly the same time as the first (simultaneous loss) then there will be no vestibular asymmetry, no acute vestibular syndrome, no vertigo, no nystagmus, no ocular tilt, just sudden onset of imbalance and oscillopsia—i.e. sudden bilateral labyrinthine loss. 2) If the other labyrinth is lost soon after the first (close sequential loss) then the asymmetry is abolished so the acute vestibular syndrome stops in its tracks, but imbalance and oscillopsia take over. 3) If the other labyrinth is lost after the acute vestibular syndrome, the vertigo, the nystagmus, the ocular tilt has resolved (remote sequential loss) then a second acute vestibular syndrome occurs, opposite in direction to the first, and eventually that also resolves spontaneously, also by compensation and again imbalance and oscillopsia due to absent labyrinthine function take over (12). All this was described and explained over 100 years ago by Vladimir Bechterev, the great Russian neurologist (and discoverer of ankylosing spondylitis).

Where and how the brain uses all this vestibular information

Neural impulses from the labyrinths are turned into information about the position and motion of the head at the level of the vestibular nuclei. Although the SCCs respond only to angular acceleration and not to velocity, much of the neural code in the axons of the vestibular ganglion cells equates to head velocity not acceleration, indicating that some form of neural-mathematical integration takes place in the inner ear itself (Figure 8.13). This signal is then relayed to vestibular nuclei on both sides—as an excitatory signal to the ipsilateral vestibular nucleus and as a crossed inhibitory signal to the contralateral vestibular nucleus (Figure 8.12). From vestibular nuclei the signal goes to cerebral cortex via the thalamus, to spinal cord via the vestibulospinal tracts and to the brainstem ocular motor nuclei mainly via the medial longitudinal fasciculus. Abnormal vestibulocortical signals about illusions of motion are the vestibular patient's chief complaint; they cause illusions of rotating (vertigo), tilting (13), rocking up and down (mal-de debarquement) (14)—these are impossible to measure. Abnormal vestibulospinal signals cause the common complaints of imbalance and disequilibrium. It is possible to measure standing and walking for clinical purposes, but the results can be non-specific as the measurements are subject to many variables apart from vestibular inputs (see Chapters 4 and 26). Abnormal vestibular signals to brainstem autonomic nuclei are perhaps the greatest source of distress for patients—with spinning some might be willing to put up but with throwing up, they won't. Autonomic responses are also non-specific and cannot be accurately measured in a clinical setting (see Chapter 5).

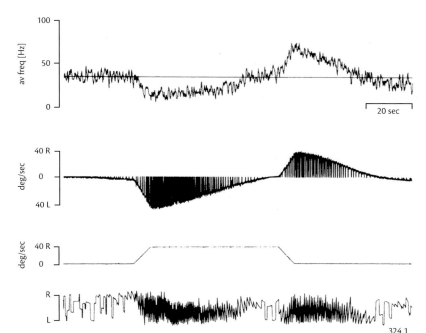

Fig. 8.13 Monkey VOR with vestibular nucleus neural response in response to constant angular acceleration. Eye velocity in the dark (2nd trace) closely follows vestibular nucleus neuron firing rate (top trace) during and after a step of acceleration at 6°/s² to a constant velocity of 40°/s. Eye velocity and neural firing rate together decay exponentially once constant velocity is reached since the semicircular canals respond only to angular acceleration. The neural responses to the acceleration are about the same—a change of 20 impulses/s in both the inhibitory and the excitatory directions. In response to higher accelerations the inhibitory response would have saturated at zero impulses/s whereas the firing rate in the excitatory direction could have increased to over 100/s. This inhibitory saturation is the basis of the head impulse test. Rotating chair (=head) velocity is 3rd trace, eye position showing saw-tooth nystagmus pattern is bottom trace. From Waespe and Henn (24).

Abnormal vestibular signals to the ocular motor nuclei produce only one symptom, oscillopsia, but can be measured with unique precision. The normal VOR response to rapid head rotation is a precisely equal and opposite eye rotation (Figure 8.14)—sometimes still referred to by the quaint old term the 'doll's head' or the 'doll's eye' reflex (it's time to move on) (7, 15).

Why eye movements matter for the diagnosis of vestibular disorders

Patients coming to a Balance Disorders Clinic might say: 'Doctor, I have come to see you about my balance—I am spinning and wobbling all over the place, but all you do is look at my eyes; do you really know what you are doing?' One might reply: 'Yes I do—what you need to know is that the eyes are the speedometers of the ears; from looking at how your eyes spin I can tell how your ears work.' This message is reinforced by using video Frenzel goggles and recording the examination to show the partner as well as the patient.

There are four totally different eye movement systems: vestibular, visual (pursuit/optokinetic), vergence, and saccadic (see Chapter 3). It is only through the nature of the stimulus eliciting the eye movement and the dynamic properties of the eye movement response itself that it is possible to distinguish these from each other. The differences between the latency, peak velocity, and frequency of an eye movement will distinguish saccadic and pursuit movements from vestibular. There are important interactions between visual

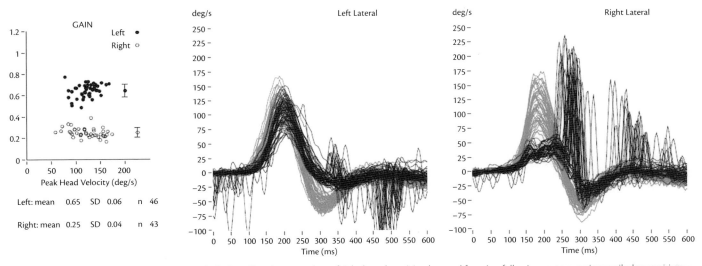

Fig. 8.14 Head impulse test with unilateral vestibular loss. Showing severe loss of right lateral semicircular canal function following acute superior vestibular neuritis. Head velocity in grey, eye (in-head) velocity in black. In response to head impulses in increasing peak velocity to the left, eye velocity closely approximates head velocity—the gain is about 0.6. With impulses to the right, the eye velocity saturates at about 30°/s producing a gain of only 0.25 and a stereotyped overt catch-up saccade starting just as the head stops moving. Recording and measurement with a GN Otometrics video-oculographic system.

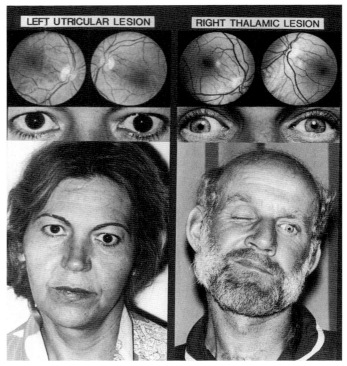

Fig. 8.15 Ocular tilt reaction (OTR). OTR is a triad comprising head tilt, conjugate ocular torsion, and hypotropia due to skew deviation, all to one side. An OTR indicates an ipsilateral lesion of the otolith (utricle), vestibular nerve, or vestibular nucleus, or a contralateral lesion of the medial longitudinal fasciculus or interstitial nucleus (in the subthalamus). With lesions in the cerebellum it can be ipsilateral or contralateral. From Halmagyi *et al.* (27).

and vestibular eye movements—both additive and subtractive. Additive interaction of visual and vestibular eye movements occurs in everyday life as a subject views fixed or moving targets—the so called 'visual VOR'. Subtractive interaction occurs in the special case when a subject views a head-fixed target so that visual and vestibular signals are actually in the opposite direction—this is called VOR suppression. Critical to understanding these interactions are the differences in the latency and peak velocity and frequency of smooth pursuit (about 140 ms, 80°/s, 0.8 Hz) versus the vestibulo-ocular reflex (about 7 ms, 800°/s, 8 Hz). These differences explain why smooth pursuit can only interact with the VOR at low head accelerations, not at the high accelerations used in the head impulse test (Figures 8.11 and 8.14) (15) (see Chapter 2)—which in the clinical setting relies on being able to identify the tell-tale catch-up saccades that indicate an inadequate VOR.

Saccadic eye movements have an amplitude–velocity–duration relationship that allows them to be distinguished from visual or vestibular eye movements. Although voluntary saccades are planned and triggered from the cortex, especially in the frontal eye fields, they are finally generated in the brainstem: horizontal saccades in the pons and vertical saccades in the midbrain.

How vestibular nystagmus is made and why it matters for diagnosis

Clinical examination of the vestibular system requires accurate evaluation of the patient for any spontaneous nystagmus and also

for abnormal provoked nystagmus. For the clinician it is important not just to recognize the patterns but also to understand the mechanisms of the various types of peripheral vestibular nystagmus—spontaneous and provoked—and their differentiation from various types of central vestibular disorders.

Quick phases of vestibular nystagmus are saccades triggered in the brainstem from vestibular stimulation. For example, consider a seated patient being passively rotated from side-to-side in the dark at about 0.5 Hz with a peak velocity of 50°/s (Figure 8.17). (Note the same result would be obtained if the patient actively turned his own head at the same frequency and peak velocity.) This stimulus produces a pattern of horizontal eye movements comprising slow components away from the direction of rotation at about the same speed as the rotation, and quick components in the direction of rotation of about 10° magnitude and 3000°/s peak velocity. These are saccades serving as the quick phases of vestibular nystagmus. Note that if the patient had stared at an earth fixed target there would have been slow but no quick components in the vestibular response—vision would have been adding to the VOR producing the visual-VOR. If, on the other hand, the patient had stared at a head/chair fixed target there would have been no eye movements at all as VOR suppression is normally complete at that stimulus magnitude. These are typical examples of additive and subtractive visual–vestibular interaction.

A constant acceleration stimulus can also produce vestibular nystagmus (Figures 8.13 and 8.18). Irrigating the ear canal with water below or above body temperature will do just that by setting up a convection current in the endolymph of the lateral semicircular canal if the canal is in a vertical position—as it is when the patient is supine with the head elevated about 30° from the horizontal. This, of course, is the time-honoured caloric test in which the slow phase component velocity of the horizontal nystagmus is taken as a measure of lateral SCC function (see Chapter 14).

Much is now known about the neural circuitry producing this horizontal vestibular nystagmus, too much for the busy clinician but of interest to those who can still admire the precision of the central nervous system.

The slow or compensatory component of peripheral vestibular nystagmus is generated in the vestibular and the ocular motor nuclei (Figure 8.16). Consider a patient being rotated to the left at a constant acceleration producing left-beating nystagmus, rightward slow phases, and then leftward quick phases. The leftward acceleration produces rightward displacement of stereocilia on hair cells in the cristae of the both lateral SCCs (see Figure 8.4). Because of the orientation of the hair cells a rightward displacement of stereocilia in the left lateral SCC is towards the kinocilium, and this produces an increase in the resting discharge rate of the hair cell and of its ganglion cell and of type 1 (excitatory) neurons in the left medial vestibular nucleus and then in the right abducens nucleus in the pons and via abducens interneurons and the medial longitudinal fasciculus in the medial rectus portion of the left oculomotor nucleus in the midbrain. From this activation arises the rightward slow phase of vestibular nystagmus. This, however, is not the whole story. The rightward displacement of stereocilia in hair cells of the right lateral SCC crista is away from the kinocilium and is therefore inhibitory, which will reduce the neural discharge rate of ganglion cells in the right vestibular nerve and of type 1 neurons in the right medial vestibular nucleus. These right medial vestibular nucleus type 1 neurons send axons to the left medial vestibular nucleus where they synapse with inhibitory (type 2) neurons, which in their turn synapse with adjacent excitatory

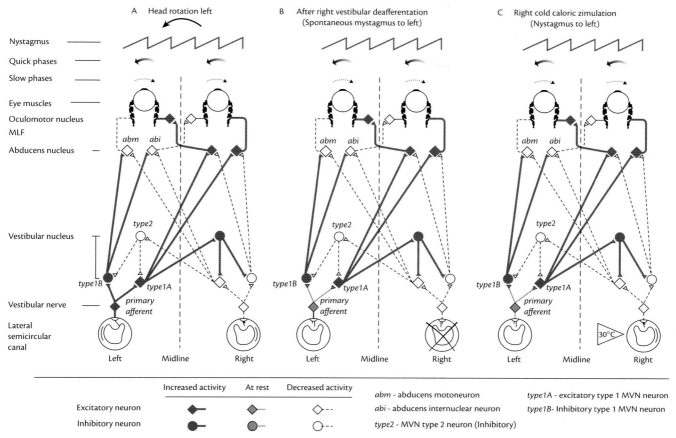

Fig. 8.16 Activity of vestibular neurons during unilateral vestibular loss and caloric stimulation. Schematic representation of brainstem neurons responsible for the direct, disynaptic VOR. The activity of the neurons is shown during (A) head rotation to the left, (B) after right vestibular deafferentation, and (C) during right ear cold caloric stimulation. In all three situations there is left-beating nystagmus which is generated by the same pattern of neural activation and inactivation in the two vestibular nuclei.

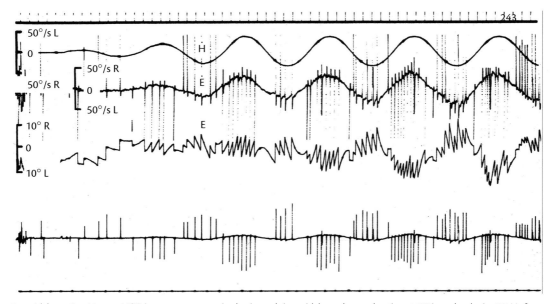

Fig. 8.17 VOR to sinusoidal rotation. Human VOR in response to passive horizontal sinusoidal angular acceleration at 50°/s peak velocity, 0.1 Hz frequency in a rotating chair. The 2nd trace is head (= chair) velocity, inverted to facilitate comparison with eye velocity in the 3rd tracing. The 4th trace is eye position showing the typical saw-tooth nystagmus pattern of slow-phase eye movements away from the direction of head movement and quick-phase eye movements in the direction of head movement. The bottom trace is eye velocity displayed at lower gain to show that quick-phases increase in frequency with increasing head velocity. Since quick-phases are what is obvious to a clinical observer the direction of nystagmus is traditionally reported as the direction in which the quick phases beat. Time in seconds is shown in the top trace.

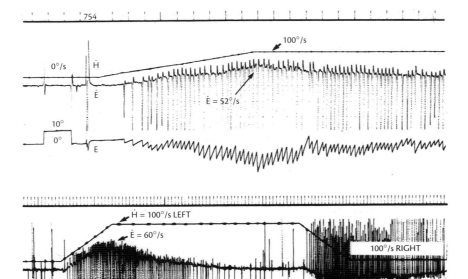

Fig. 8.18 Eye position and velocity in the dark during and after constant angular acceleration to 100°/s at 10°/s² (top trace). The typical saw-tooth pattern of vestibular nystagmus is seen in eye position (3rd trace). Peak slow-phase eye velocity (2nd trace) reaches only 52°/s, since the gain of the VOR is less than 1.0 at low stimulus (i.e. angular acceleration) magnitudes. Contrast this with gain of nearly 1.0 at high stimulus magnitude with head impulse testing. Bottom two traces show the same response on lower gain with compressed time. The nystagmus response decays exponentially since the semicircular canals respond only to angular acceleration; the time constant of this decay has both a peripheral component reflecting the elasticity of the cupula and a central component reflecting the neural process of 'velocity storage'. Time is shown in 1-s intervals.

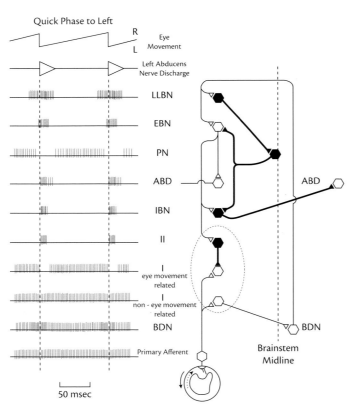

Fig. 8.19 Schematic of quick phase generation. To show how the quick phase of vestibular nystagmus may be generated by the network of excitatory and inhibitory neurons in the brainstem. During ipsilateral accelerations, primary afferents increase firing and a burster driver neuron (BDN) also increases firing. This neuron projects to inhibitory neurons (LLBN) which inhibit pause neurons. That cessation of PN inhibition triggers a burst of firing in excitatory burst neurons which project to ipsilateral abducens and so generate a quick phase. The synapses shown in this circuit have been demonstrated by physiological studies (see Curthoys (20) for details).

(type 1) neurons—neurons which are already receiving excitatory input from the left lateral SCC cupula. The reduced activation of the left medial vestibular nucleus inhibitory (type 2 neurons) therefore act as contralateral disinhibition (the pull) to ipsilateral excitation (the push) in order to produce the horizontal VOR.

The fast or anticompensatory component of peripheral vestibular nystagmus is produced by a series of neurons in the pons (Figure 8.19). The final burst neurons that produce the leftward fast phases in response to leftward rotation are all located rostral to the left vestibular nucleus, near the abducens nucleus in the left pontine reticular formation. They themselves are driven by driver neurons in the right prepositus hypoglossi nucleus. Excitatory burst neurons in the left pons also synapse with inhibitory (type 2) left vestibular nucleus neurons which then send a burst on inhibition to left excitatory (type 1) vestibular nucleus neurons so that they are silenced during the leftward quick phases of the nystagmus.

Before considering the types of peripheral vestibular nystagmus one might encounter in a patient with vertigo it is important to review two useful rules about peripheral vestibular nystagmus: 1) peripheral vestibular nystagmus, especially horizontal nystagmus, is suppressed by vision so that if the clinician has no way of examining the eyes in the absence of visual fixation (best with video Frenzel goggles—the neuro-otologist's tendon hammer) she or he is guaranteed of missing important clinical signs every day; 2) the rotation axis of peripheral vestibular nystagmus is orthogonal (at 90°) to the plane of the stimulated SCCs.

Some common types of peripheral vestibular nystagmus are now considered. The patient with acute left labyrinthitis/vestibular neuritis will have a right-beating, mainly horizontal nystagmus with a subtle torsional component (indicating vertical—usually only superior SCC involvement) (11). The nystagmus will be faster in right gaze, slower in left gaze (Alexander's law) and may only be obvious with Frenzel goggles—that is, absent on direct inspection. Within a week the nystagmus is much less; within a month it's gone, except that it can be made to reappear briefly after vigorous horizontal head-shaking or during neck vibration especially on the affected side. In the

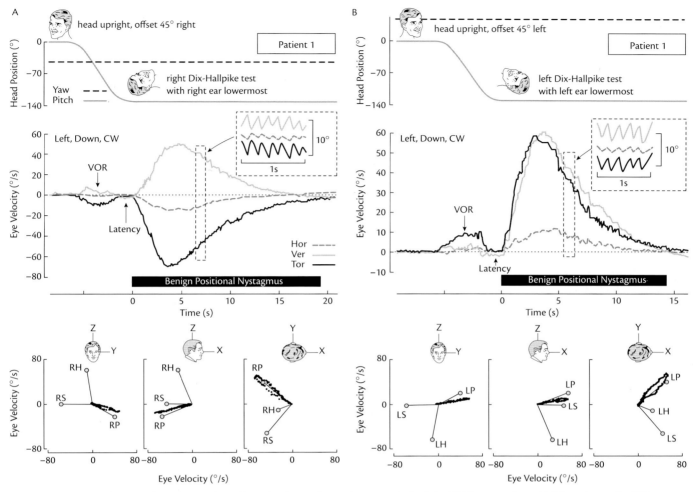

Fig. 8.20 Posterior canal positional nystagmus. Three-dimensional recording and vector analysis of the BPN from a patient with bilateral posterior SCC BPV in response to Dix–Hallpike tests in the two-axis whole-body rotator. (A) A right Dix–Hallpike test elicited a VOR and then after a latency of 1.4 s the BPN began. When the head was stationary, the BPN was paroxysmal in onset, peaked in magnitude after 3.5 s and decayed after 19 s. The BPN was upbeat geotropic-torsional towards the lowermost right ear (inset). Peak eye velocity of the BPN comprised large counterclockwise-torsional (−69°/s) with downward (48°/s) and small rightward (−15°/s) components. This BPN rotation axis displayed in roll, pitch and yaw plane views was directed along the right posterior SCC axis indicating right posterior SCC BPV. (B) A left Dix–Hallpike test elicited a VOR followed by a latency of 1.2 s. The BPN was again paroxysmal in onset, upbeat geotropic-torsional (inset) towards the lowermost left ear and decayed after 14 s. Peak eye velocity of this BPN comprised large clockwise-torsional (61°/s) with downward (55°/s) and small leftward (11°/s) components. The BPN rotation axis was directed along the left posterior SCC axis, indicating left posterior SCC BPV. Right horizontal (RH), right superior (RS), right posterior (RP), left horizontal (LH), left superior (LS), left posterior (LP) semicircular canal axis. From Aw et al. (16).

patient with left posterior SCC benign positional vertigo the left Dix–Hallpike test (Chapter 20) will provoke a positional nystagmus that is upbeating left-beating torsional, that is, it has a rotation axis that is orthogonal to the plane of the stimulated left posterior SCC (Figure 8.20) (16). In the patient with a left superior SCC dehiscence, sound and pressure stimulation produces nystagmus that is down-beating and leftward torsional, that is, it has a rotation axis that is orthogonal to the plane of the stimulated superior SCC (Figure 8.21) (17).

Summary

Clinical examination of the vestibular system is physiologically based. Abnormalities that can be demonstrated on each of the 10 standard clinical tests (listed here) have a basis in pathophysiology. Interpretation of the clinical signs and of vestibular test abnormalities requires some understanding of vestibular anatomy and physiology (18).

1) Spontaneous nystagmus with and without fixation (i.e. with Frenzel goggles)

2) Gaze-evoked nystagmus

3) Head-shaking nystagmus

4) Sound/pressure/vibration/hyperventilation-induced nystagmus.

5) Positional nystagmus

6) Head impulse test

7) Visual suppression of vestibular nystagmus

8) Smooth pursuit

9) Standing; Romberg test (on firm and then on foam surface)

10) Marching; Unterberger/Fukuda test.

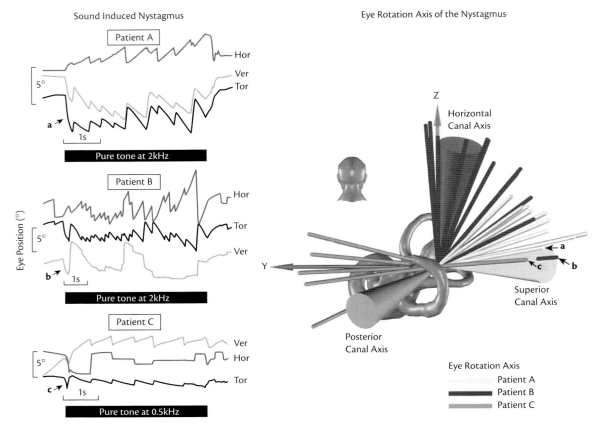

Fig. 8.21 The nystagmus of superior (anterior) semicircular canal dehiscence. Three-dimensional sound-induced nystagmus with horizontal (Hor), vertical (Ver), and torsional (Tor) eye movements for three unilateral superior canal dehiscence patients confirmed by high-resolution temporal bone computed tomography imaging. The patients were hypersensitive when stimulated by pure tone sound at either 0.5 or 2 kHz. The eye rotation axis for each slow-phase beat of the sound-induced nystagmus was computed and compared to the horizontal, superior, and posterior canal axes. The initial slow-phase beat of the nystagmus from each patient was notated as a, b, c. These examples show that the eye rotation axes from sound-induced nystagmus can be variable and align with any of three semicircular canals, which can be hypersensitive in superior canal dehiscence. From Aw et al. (19).

References

1. Goldberg JM, Wilson VJ, Cullen KE, Angelaki DE (2011). *The Vestibular System: A Sixth Sense*. New York: Oxford University Press.
2. Fujimoto C, Murofushi T, Chihara Y, *et al.* (2009). Assessment of diagnostic accuracy of foam posturography for peripheral vestibular disorders: analysis of parameters related to visual and somatosensory dependence. *Clin Neurophysiol*, 120, 1408–14.
3. Vital D, Hegemann SC, Straumann D, *et al.* (2010). A new dynamic visual acuity test to assess peripheral vestibular function. *Arch Otolaryngol Head Neck Surg*, 136, 686–91.
4. Badaracco C, Labini FS, Meli A, Tufarelli D (2010). Oscillopsia in labyrinthine defective patients: comparison of objective and subjective measures. *Am J Otolaryngol*, 31, 399–403.
5. Halmagyi GM, Fattore CM, Curthoys IS, Wade S (1994). Gentamicin vestibulotoxicity. *Otolaryngol Head Neck Surg*, 111, 571–4.
6. Weber KP, Aw ST, Todd MJ, McGarvie LA, Curthoys IS, Halmagyi GM (2009). Horizontal head impulse test detects gentamicin vestibulotoxicity. *Neurology*, 72, 1417–24.
7. Halmagyi GM, Curthoys IS (1988). A clinical sign of canal paresis. *Arch Neurol*, 45, 737–9.
8. Weber KP, Aw ST, Todd MJ, McGarvie LA, Curthoys IS, Halmagyi GM (2008). Head impulse test in unilateral vestibular loss: vestibulo-ocular reflex and catch-up saccades. *Neurology*, 70(6), 454–63.
9. Reid C, Eisenberg R, Fagan PA, *et al.* (1996). The outcome of vestibular neurectomy – the patient's point of view. *Laryngoscope*, 106, 1553–6.
10. Tufarelli D, Meli A, Labini FS, *et al.* (2007). Balance impairment after acoustic neuroma surgery. *Otol Neurotol*, 28(6), 814–21.
11. Halmagyi GM, Weber KP, Curthoys IS (2010). Vestibular function after acute vestibular neuritis. *Restor Neurol Neurosci*, 28(1), 37–46.
12. Zee DS, Preziosi TJ, Proctor LR (1982). Bechterew's phenomenon in a human patient. *Ann Neurol*, 12, 495–6.
13. Malis DD, Guyot JP (2003). Room tilt illusion as a manifestation of peripheral vestibular disorders. *Ann Otol Rhinol Laryngol*, 112(7), 600–5.
14. Clark BC, Quick A (2011). Exploring the pathophysiology of Mal de Debarquement. *J Neurol*, 258, 1166–8.
15. MacDougall HG, Weber KP, McGarvie LA, Halmagyi GM, Curthoys IS (2009). The video head impulse test: diagnostic accuracy in peripheral vestibulopathy. *Neurology*, 73(14), 1134–41.
16. Aw ST, Todd MJ, Aw GE, McGarvie LA, Halmagyi GM (2005) Benign positional nystagmus: a study of its three-dimensional spatio-temporal characteristics. *Neurology*, 64, 1897–905.
17. Minor LB (2005) Clinical manifestations of superior semicircular canal dehiscence. *Laryngoscope*, 115, 1717–27.
18. Halmagyi GM, Curthoys IS, Aw ST, Jenn JC (2004). Clinical applications of basic vestibular research. In Highstein SM, Fay RR, Popper AN (Eds) *The Vestibular System*, pp. 496–546. New York: Springer.

19. Aw ST, Todd MJ, Curthoys IS, Halmagyi GM (2009). Vestibular responses to sound and electrical stimulation. In Eggers SD, Zee, DS (Eds) *Vertigo and Imbalance. Clinical neurophysiology of the vestibular system*. Amsterdam: Elsevier.

20. Curthoys IS (2002). Generation of the quick phase of horizontal vestibular nystagmus. *Exp Brain Res*, 143(4), 397–405.

21. Engström H (1967). The morphology of the normal sensory cells. *Acta Otolaryngol*, 63(2, Suppl), 5–19.

22. Igarashi M, Alford BR (1969). Cupula, cupular zone of otolithic membrane, and tectorial membrane in the squirrel monkey. *Acta Otolaryngol*, 68, 420–6.

23. De Burlet HM (1924). Zur Innervation der Macula sacculi bei Säugetieren. *Anat Anzeig*, 58, 26–32.

24. Waespe W, Henn V (1979). The velocity response of vestibular nucleus neurons during vestibular, visual, and combined angular acceleration. *Exp Brain Res*, 37, 337–47.

25. Curthoys IS, Uzun-Coruhlu H, Wong CC, Jones AS, Bradshaw AP (2009). The configuration and attachment of the utricular and saccular maculae to the temporal bone. New evidence from micro-CT studies of the membranous labyrinth. *Ann N Y Acad Sci*, 1164, 13–8.

26. Curthoys IS, Betts GA (1997). The role of utricular stimulation in determining perceived postural roll-tilt. *Aust J Psych*, 49(3), 134–8.

27. Halmagyi GM, Curthoys IS, Brandt T, Dieterich M (1991). Ocular tilt reaction: clinical sign of vestibular lesion. *Acta Otolaryngol Suppl* 481, 47–50.

CHAPTER 9

I am an Otologist, What Neurology do I Need to Know?

Thomas Lempert

Introduction

Vertigo and dizziness are not exclusively related to inner ear disease but span several medical specialities—a fact that troubles patients and doctors alike. Thus, dizziness experts need to acquire skills and knowledge from neighbouring areas to serve their patients adequately. But also non-experts who see dizzy patients should have a basic understanding of the relevant disorders outside their field of specialization. This chapter deals with common neurological problems in the world of dizziness.

Acute persistent vertigo—how to recognize strokes

Missing a posterior fossa stroke in a patient with acute vertigo is a worst case scenario for the otologist in the emergency room. Most vestibular stroke syndromes result from occlusion of the posterior inferior cerebellar artery (PICA) or the anterior inferior cerebellar artery (AICA) and are easy to recognize when presenting with the full spectrum of signs and symptoms (1). Partial manifestations are sometimes tricky but can still be diagnosed clinically as we will see later in this section.

Infarction of the posterior inferior cerebellar artery territory

The PICA supplies the lateral medulla including the vestibular nuclei and most of the caudal cerebellum. Infarction of the PICA territory, usually caused by dissection or occlusion of the vertebral artery, presents with diverse nystagmus patterns, most commonly a horizontal-torsional spontaneous nystagmus beating towards the intact side and gaze-evoked nystagmus towards the affected side. Ipsilesional and alternating spontaneous nystagmus may also occur. A skew deviation with the ipsilateral eye deviated downward occurs in about half of the patients. Skew deviation designates a vertical misalignment of the eyes of central origin. In contrast to squints resulting from paresis of extraocular muscles, skew deviations show a fairly stable squint in all directions of gaze. It is best searched for by covering the eyes in an alternating fashion, which results in vertical corrections of the eye position for refixation (2).

Associated neurological findings on the side of PICA stroke include falls to the affected side, lateropulsion of saccades, broken pursuit, limb ataxia, trigeminal sensory loss to pain and temperature, facial paralysis, decreased gag reflex, hoarseness due to vocal chord paralysis, dysphagia, Horner's syndrome, and decreased sweating. On the contralesional side, there is hemisensory loss to pain and temperature (3, 4). Incomplete PICA syndromes are common due to individual variations of the vascular territory and isolated occlusion of the brainstem or cerebellar branches. These patients often present with isolated vertigo and spontaneous horizontal nystagmus, thus mimicking acute vestibular neuritis (Figure 9.1). Spontaneous nystagmus results from increased activity of the ipsilateral vestibular nucleus which is normally inhibited by the caudal cerebellum, resulting in asymmetric firing of central vestibular neurons. A normal head impulse test is regarded as the most reliable sign for a cerebellar lesion as it indicates an intact peripheral vestibular system (5).

Infarction of the anterior inferior cerebellar artery territory

The AICA supplies three arterial territories all of which are part of the vestibular system:

1. The labyrinth and VIIIth nerve.

2. The lateral brainstem at pontine level including the root entry zone of the VIIIth nerve.

3. The anterior and caudal cerebellum including parts of the vestibulo-cerebellum.

Therefore, complete infarction of the AICA territory produces a variety of symptoms (6) including a mixed peripheral and central pattern of vestibular dysfunction:

1. Horizontal-torsional spontaneous nystagmus to the healthy side, an abnormal head impulse test, and hearing loss, which often precedes other symptoms (labyrinth and VIIIth nerve) (7, 8).

2. Horner's syndrome, facial paralysis, trigeminal sensory loss to pain and temperature and crossed hemisensory loss to pain and temperature. Variable involvement of parts of the vestibular nucleus may modify the labyrinthine spontaneous nystagmus (lateral pons).

3. Gait and limb ataxia and gaze-evoked nystagmus when looking to the affected side (cerebellum).

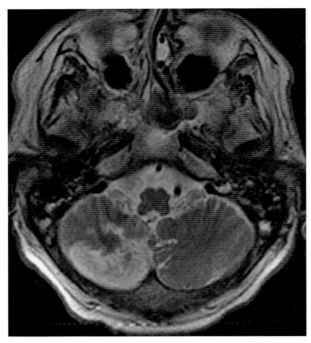

Fig. 9.1 Cerebellar stroke presenting with an acute vertigo. Magnetic resonance imaging of a partial PICA infarction involving the caudal and medial cerebellum, but sparing the lateral brainstem.

Branch occlusion may lead to partial infarction of the AICA territory with limited clinical symptoms only. Isolated infarction of the root entry zone of the VIIIth nerve, resulting in an abnormal head impulse test, may falsely suggest a peripheral lesion. Sometimes, acute bilateral deafness is the first symptom in the course of acute basilar artery thrombosis (9, 10). When large portions of the cerebellum are supplied by the AICA, extended infarcts may develop with cerebellar swelling and subsequent brainstem herniation. Therefore, rapid imaging is critical for appropriate management (11).

Recognizing small PICA or AICA strokes in patients with isolated vertigo

Patients presenting with a first episode of acute prolonged vertigo should be thoroughly examined for eye movement abnormalities, cranial nerve dysfunction, cerebellar ataxia, and long tract signs. One or more of the following features should lead to neurological referral and cerebral imaging:

- Age above 65 years.
- Pre-existing vascular disease.
- History of vascular risk factors (smoking, hypertension, diabetes, elevated cholesterol).
- A normal head impulse test (12).
- Any neurological finding which would not be explained by acute vestibular neuritis (which presents with abnormal head-thrust test and veering towards the affected side, horizontal-torsional spontaneous nystagmus to the healthy side (13)).

A recent study identified three ocular motor signs which proved particularly useful: a normal impulse test, gaze-evoked nystagmus beating in the opposite direction of the spontaneous nystagmus, and skew deviation. The presence of one or more of these signs

was 100% sensitive and 96% specific for identification of stroke in a series of 101 elderly patients with an acute vestibular syndrome and at least one vascular risk factor. In contrast, the initial diffusion-weighted magnetic resonance image (MRI) missed 12% of the strokes (14). The authors coined the acronymic mnemonic HINTS for: Head Impulse, Nystagmus, Test-of-Skew.

Key points: strokes causing vertigo

- The posterior and anterior cerebellar arteries (PICA and AICA) irrigate the vestibular system.
- Associated neurological symptoms characterize PICA and AICA strokes.
- Small PICA and AICA infarcts may cause isolated vertigo.
- Recognition is possible by head impulse testing and by searching for gaze-evoked nystagmus and skew deviation.

Recurrent vertigo—when to consider vertebrobasilar transient ischaemic attacks?

Vertebrobasilar transient ischaemic attacks (TIAs; or 'vertebrobasilar insufficiency' in outdated terminology) were once regarded as a frequent cause of recurrent vertigo, but account for only about 1% of diagnoses in our dizziness clinic (unpublished observation).

The typical patient with vertigo due to vertebrobasilar TIA is above 55 years of age and burdened with vascular risk factors such as smoking, hypertension, diabetes, or hyperlipidaemia. Embolic heart disease is not a usual risk factor as repeated embolization to the labyrinth or to the vestibular nuclei is quite unlikely. Attacks usually present with associated symptoms from the posterior circulation territory, such as diplopia, field defects, drop attacks, unsteadiness, incoordination, extremity weakness, confusion, headache, or hearing loss (15). About 10–20% of patients have attacks with isolated vertigo (16, 17), but most patients with isolated vertigo have other paroxysmal symptoms from the vertebrobasilar territory on other occasions. Therefore, when a patient presents with recurrent isolated vertigo over an extended period (say, 6 months), the diagnosis of vertebrobasilar TIA is unconvincing.

Vertigo due to vertebrobasilar TIA occurs spontaneously and starts abruptly. The duration of TIAs has been arbitrarily limited to 24 hours, the majority, however, last in the order of minutes or 1–2 hours. Ischaemic vertigo can be (rarely) provoked by turning or extending the neck, thus compressing the ipsilateral vertebral artery (18). But most neck movement-related vertigo is in fact *head* movement-related, reflecting vestibular disease such as benign positional vertigo or poorly compensated unilateral vestibular loss.

Audiometry and vestibular testing is useful in these patients to document permanent damage to the labyrinth or, occasionally, to central pathways. Doppler ultrasound studies can identify narrowing or occlusion of large extra- and intracranial vessels, whereas magnetic resonance angiography can also visualize medium-sized vessels.

When it comes to treatment, both doctors and patients should do their best for correcting vascular risk factors. In a patient with vertebrobasilar TIA the annual rate of cerebral infarction is around 20% and the risk can be reduced by antiplatelet drugs such as aspirin or clopidogrel. Oral anticoagulation is not indicated in patients with TIAs due to atherosclerosis. Angioplasty of the vertebral and basilar arteries is employed in selected high-risk patients (19).

Key points: vertebrobasilar TIAs

- TIAs rarely cause isolated recurrent vertigo.
- Affected individuals are mostly old and have vascular risk factors.
- Most of them have associated symptoms from the posterior circulation.
- Attacks usually last less than an hour.

Dizziness during standing and walking—the neurological gait disorders

You may have met these elderly patients who enter your office saying 'I am always dizzy, doctor'. When questioned, they often admit that they feel perfectly good while sitting or lying and that problems start only after getting up and walking around. They describe a sensation of permanent unsteadiness rather than spinning vertigo. The diagnosis is usually clarified by a simple neurological examination focusing on cerebellar, sensory, and motor functions. Common conditions include polyneuropathy, myelopathy, cerebellar disorders, normal pressure hydrocephalus, cerebral small-vessel disease, and Parkinson's disease. Combinations of these disorders are quite common, particularly in the elderly. Patients with only transient dizziness after getting up may have orthostatic hypotension and are discussed in the next section.

Polyneuropathy

Usually, the first symptom of polyneuropathy is tingling or numbness in the feet. Some patients, however, present with a primary complaint of unsteadiness which worsens in the dark and distal sensory loss may become evident only on clinical examination. The most sensitive sign of peripheral neuropathy is diminished vibration sense on the toes and ankles using a 128- or 256-Hz tuning fork (20). Similarly common, but less specific, is a positive Romberg with increased swaying after eye closure. Diminished sensation to touch and pin prick or a decreased joint position sense is usually noted later in the course of the disease. Weakness may also develop, often beginning in the toes. Decreased motor and sensory conduction velocities on electrophysiological testing will usually confirm the diagnosis, but may be negative in the early stages of the disorder (21). An aetiology can be found in about 70% of patients with diabetes and alcohol abuse accounting for at least half of them. Other causes include hereditary neuropathies, vitamin deficiency (e.g. B1, B6, B12), autoimmune disorders (vasculitis, rheumatological diseases, paraproteinaemia, Guillain–Barré syndrome, chronic inflammatory demyelinating polyneuropathy), renal failure, chronic liver disease, paraneoplastic disorders (particularly with small-cell carcinoma of the lung), toxins (e.g. organic solvents) and medications (e.g. vincristin, cisplatin, tacrin). An initial work-up should include fasting blood glucose, HbA1c, renal and liver function tests, blood count, erythrocyte sedimentation rate, antinuclear antibodies, immune electrophoresis, and B12. For patients with subacute neuropathy developing within weeks a search for occult malignancy including antineuronal antibodies is advisable (22). Once the cause of neuropathy is known, specific treatment (or elimination of toxins) may lead to remission of the neuropathy or at least retard its progression.

Myelopathy

While acute disorders of the spinal cord usually present with flaccid paraparesis and a sensory level, chronic myelopathy is often characterized by progressive spasticity before weakness and sensory dysfunction become evident. Consequently, patients complain about gait problems with stiffness in their legs and it takes a neurological examination to detect extensor plantar responses, increased tendon reflexes, spasticity and (sometimes subtle) sensory dysfunction in the legs. In the absence of a sensory level the lesion may be difficult to localize and MRI both of the cervical and thoracic cord may be required. However, involvement of the hands, e.g. wasting of hand muscles or numb fingers, clearly points to the cervical cord. Common causes of myelopathy include cervical spondylotic compression of the spinal cord, B12 deficiency, tumours such as meningioma or low-grade glioma, and primary progressive multiple sclerosis which often manifests itself with a pure spinal syndrome. In populations with dizziness and unsteadiness as presenting symptoms, cervical spondylotic myelopathy is by far the leading spinal cord disease. The archetypical patient would be about 70 years old and complain about gait problems and numb, clumsy hands. MRI visualizes narrowing of the cervical spine, most often at the C5/C6 level. T2 hyperintensities within the cord at the level of compression indicate secondary ischaemic damage which is usually permanent. Patients with mild symptoms can be monitored, while surgery is commonly advised when symptoms are moderate to severe and progressive (23).

Cerebellar disorders

The symptoms of cerebellar disease can be attributed to the three subsections of the cerebellum: ataxia of the extremities reflects dysfunction of the cerebellar hemispheres; gait and truncal ataxia results from involvement of midline structures (cerebellar vermis); while ocular motor signs such as saccadic pursuit, gaze-evoked nystagmus, impaired vestibulo-ocular reflex (VOR) suppression, and downbeat nystagmus point to the caudal cerebellum (flocculus and paraflocculus). Neurological disorders commonly affect various parts of the cerebellum so that a mixture of symptoms is found in most patients. The differential diagnosis of a chronic cerebellar syndrome includes hereditary degeneration, sporadic degenerations such as the cerebellar type of multiple system atrophy, Arnold–Chiari malformation, multiple sclerosis, tumours such as haemangioblastoma or meningioma, alcohol abuse, hypothyroidism, and paraneoplastic cerebellar degeneration. MRI is required to detect cerebellar lesions or atrophy and to search for associated findings such as brainstem atrophy in multiple systems atrophy or periventricular demyelination in multiple sclerosis. Extensive genetic testing for identification of one of the almost 30 subtypes of autosomal dominant spinocerebellar degeneration is useful only when the risk for relatives and offspring needs to be assessed. Most cerebellar disorders are not amenable to medical treatment. Similarly, physiotherapy has little effect on ataxia but can be employed as a supportive measure (24).

Downbeat nystagmus syndrome

Downbeat nystagmus syndrome deserves special consideration as it is easily missed in the chronically dizzy and unsteady patient. Patients complain of slight unsteadiness and sometimes vertical oscillopsia (25). Detection of downbeat nystagmus in primary position requires close inspection and sometimes magnification by fundoscopy (remember that you will see the eye jerking up through the ophthalmoscope as you are looking at the back of the eye). Downbeat nystagmus increases on lateral gaze sometimes adding up with a horizontal gaze-evoked nystagmus to an oblique pattern. Saccadic pursuit and defective VOR suppression are commonly associated. On Romberg testing, patients tend to sway backwards. Other cerebellar signs are often lacking, but some patients develop bilateral vestibular loss and/or polyneuropathy concomitantly, which aggravates their balance problem (26). Downbeat nystagmus is thought to result from disinhibition of the anterior canal VOR as the caudal cerebellum inhibits signals from the anterior canal signals more than those from the antagonistic posterior canal. As a rule of thumb, cerebellar degeneration, idiopathic variants, Arnold–Chiari malformation, and miscellaneous causes account for a quarter of the cases each. Treatment is rarely effective, but 4-aminopyridine, clonazepam, baclofen, and memantine have all been successfully tried in individual patients bothered by oscillopsia (27).

Normal pressure hydrocephalus

Normal pressure hydrocephalus is actually a misnomer because the ventricular enlargement in this condition is the consequence of brief and moderate increases in cerebrospinal fluid (CSF) pressure. Clinically, these elderly patients present with a triad of gait disorder, urinary urge incontinence, and slight dementia. Abnormal gait is the earliest and most prominent symptom and is characterized by a hesitant, non-fluent cadence, often with some stiffness and a moderately widened base as well as imbalance on turning around. As the disease progresses it becomes increasingly small-stepped and may lead to falls, eventually immobilizing the patient. Cerebral imaging shows enlarged ventricles while external CSF spaces are normal or even narrowed over the vertex. In addition, there are white matter alterations around the anterior and posterior extensions of the lateral ventricles (hypodense on computed tomography or T2 hyperintense on MRI), which result from CSF pressed into the adjacent white matter. The diagnosis is confirmed when spinal tapping with removal of 50 ml CSF produces a substantial gait improvement within a day or two. This can be measured by the time needed to walk a defined distance, say 20 metres, before and after puncture. Long-term treatment may include repeated lumbar punctures or CSF drainage through a ventriculo-peritoneal or lumbo-peritoneal shunt and will improve also cognitive and bladder symptoms (28).

Cerebral small-vessel disease

Small-vessel disease affecting the cerebral white matter may cause imbalance when multiple periventricular lesions affect sensory and motor fibres connecting the cortical gait and leg areas with the thalamus, basal ganglia, cerebellum, and spinal chord. The typical patient presents with a small-stepped gait with a somewhat widened base and imbalance, particularly when turning. Severely affected patients have additional features such as incontinence and subcortical dementia (note that clinical features are quite similar to normal pressure hydrocephalus). Most patients have longstanding hypertension. The neurological examination may reveal focal signs such as hemiparesis, spasticity, or extensor plantar responses. MRI shows enlarged perivascular spaces in the basal ganglia and cerebral white matter, lacunar infarctions, and patchy or confluent, T2 hyperintense white matter lesions resulting from vascular demyelination (29). The severity of white matter changes is significantly associated with a history of falls (30). As these changes reflect permanent ischaemic damage to the brain, treatment options are limited. Antiplatelet agents such as aspirin and clopidogrel are often prescribed, but have no proven effect on the progression of cerebral small-vessel disease. Hypertension should be strictly controlled, but one should be careful to avoid orthostatic hypotension on an already hypoperfused brain. Physiotherapy with gait and balance exercises may enhance the patient's residual function.

Parkinson's disease

In its early stages Parkinson's disease is difficult to diagnose. Unilateral resting tremor, the most distinctive feature of Parkinson's disease, is lacking in more than half of the patients at this time and sometimes for the entire course of the disease. Instead, patients may complain about unsteadiness, loss of dexterity, hoarseness, stiffness, and muscle aches. On examination, one can search for hypokinesia by asking the patient to perform rapidly alternating hand movements, to get up from a chair, or to turn 360° on the spot which should take no more than six steps. Unilateral loss of arm swing is another early sign whereas the characteristic slow, small stepped and shuffling gait develops only later on. Rigidity is best noted when the patient performs gripping hand movements on one side while the contralateral arms is passively moved by the examiner. Improvement of symptoms after a single dose of 125 or 250 mg L-dopa (after premedication with domperidone to prevent nausea) is another diagnostic criterion for Parkinson's disease. There are other (less treatable) Parkinsonian syndromes, which can usually be diagnosed by the presence of additional symptoms and signs. Slow saccades and early falls point to progressive supranuclear palsy, autonomic symptoms such as orthostatic hypotension, and erectile dysfunction to multiple system atrophy while dementia and urge incontinence are typical for normal pressure hydrocephalus and cerebral small-vessel disease. A diagnosis of Parkinson's disease should not be missed because anti-Parkinson drugs such as L-dopa and dopamine agonists can relieve symptoms by about 70%, even if doses need to be increased in later stages of the disease (31).

Fear of falling and cautious gait

Fear of falling develops in fallers, in patients who sustained a vestibular disorder, but also in elderly patients who have never fallen and look otherwise normal. This can be associated to a 'cautious gait' with reduced stride length and speed or even sliding the feet on the floor as if 'walking on ice'. The arms are outstretched and seeking support (32). Sometimes a cautious gait complicates or even predates an organic gait disorder. It would seem that the patients react to a perceived unsteadiness before it is apparent to an observer.

Key points: neurological gait disorders

- A neurological examination will usually localize the lesion.
- MRI, electrophysiological studies, and laboratory investigations may help to establish the final diagnosis.
- Be prepared to search for multiple causes of imbalance in the elderly.
- Make friends with a neurologist (for discussions and the occasional referral).

Transient dizziness immediately after standing up—orthostatic hypotension

Clinical features

Dizziness after standing up due to orthostatic hypotension is probably the most common type of dizziness with a lifetime prevalence of 12.5%. It may have severe consequences, causing syncope in 19 % and traumatic injury in 5% of affected individuals (33). Symptomatic orthostatic hypotension manifests itself shortly after standing up with light-headedness, inability to concentrate, blackening or fading out of vision, ringing of the ears or bilateral hearing loss, and eventually syncope. Pallor and sweating may be associated. The whole sequence can evolve within a few seconds or may take 1 or 2 minutes. All symptoms can be quickly reversed by sitting or lying down. When syncope occurs, the circulatory origin of the preceding dizziness is obvious but many patients experience only the presyncopal stage of orthostatic hypotension.

Clinically significant orthostatic hypotension becomes more prevalent with advancing age (33). Apart from age-related degeneration of the autonomic system there are specific neurological disorders of the elderly compromising autonomic function such as pure autonomic failure, multiple system atrophy, Parkinson's disease, and diabetic neuropathy (34). Orthostatic hypotension is aggravated by several factors which may cause orthostatic symptoms even in the absence of autonomic failure such as bed rest, fever, salt and volume depletion, heat, and anaemia. Orthostatic tolerance may be further impaired by various drugs including diuretics, vasodilators, antihypertensives, antiparkinsonians, and tricyclic antidepressants (35).

Pathophysiology

Maintenance of cerebral perfusion during upright stance depends critically on peripheral vasoconstriction mediated by sympathetic nerve fibres and cerebral autoregulation. The efficacy of both of these mechanisms declines with advancing age. Dizziness due to orthostatic hypotension is not related to ischaemia of the labyrinth but rather to widespread cortical hypoperfusion. This results in impaired processing of sensory signals for spatial orientation, diminished attention and cognition, and eventually loss of consciousness.

Investigations

Measurement of blood pressure supine and then repeatedly after standing up for 3 minutes should be a routine investigation in elderly dizzy patients and in anyone complaining of orthostatic dizziness or syncope (36). A fall of 20 mmHg or more in systolic blood pressure or 10 mmHg or more in diastolic pressure is regarded as relevant, particularly when typical symptoms are provoked. Orthostatic hypotension can go unrecognized when measurements are made at times that do not correspond to the patient's usual symptomatic periods, which are often in the morning or after meals. Hypertensive blood pressure measurements at rest do not argue against a diagnosis of orthostatic hypotension, on the contrary: orthostatic hypotension is quite common in elderly patients treated for hypertension (37). Moreover, patients with autonomic failure often suffer from supine hypertension (38). Quite unexpectedly, these *hyper*tensive patients return with a diagnosis of orthostatic *hypo*tension after referral to a dizziness clinic. Observation of the heart rate during orthostatic

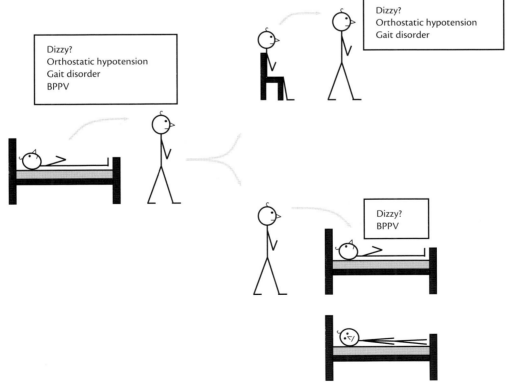

Fig. 9.2 Dizziness after getting up can imply orthostatic hypotension, a gait disorder or BPPV. If the dizziness is provoked by standing up from sitting (top right), orthostatic hypotension or a gait disorder is more likely than BPPV because head orientation remains unchanged with respect to gravity in this situation. In contrast, dizziness after lying down or turning over in bed (bottom right) usually indicates BPPV. Adapted from Bronstein and Lempert (1).

testing provides further clues with a fixed frequency pointing to an underlying disorder of the autonomic nervous system. Extended autonomic testing is only rarely required.

Differential diagnosis

Orthostatic dizziness can be readily identified from the patient's history. It should be easily distinguished from positional vertigo which depends on head position with respect to gravity and not on body posture. Thus, positional vertigo may appear after sitting up from lying but not after standing up from sitting with the head kept upright. Also, positional vertigo is usually provoked in supine positions whereas orthostatic hypotension is relieved by lying down (Figure 9.2). Orthostatic symptoms with normal orthostatic blood pressure may occur with hyperventilation and with the postural tachycardia syndrome.

Treatment

The first step is reduction or replacement of drugs that interfere with orthostatic tolerance. An equally important measure is increase of salt (extra 3–6 g) and fluid intake (3 L per day) (39), unless the patient is hypertensive or suffers from heart failure. Sleeping with the head and trunk elevated by 30–40°, e.g. by placing telephone directory books under the bed legs at the head end, prevents supine hypertension and nocturnal pressure-natriuresis, thus preserving plasma volume. Drinking 400–500 ml water from the night table immediately after awakening induces a sympathetic response which improves orthostatic tolerance during the following hours (40). Isometric leg exercises improve muscle tone and thereby support venous return to the heart. Hot baths should be avoided. Hypertensive patients with concurrent orthostatic hypotension should stay upright during the day and take antihypertensives at night. When postprandial hypotension is a problem, frequent small meals with coffee are helpful. Patient education includes simple advice on how to get up from bed: Sit up, wait a minute, stand up and go.

Pharmacological intervention is necessary only when behavioural measures fail (41). The alpha 1 adrenergic agonist midodrine (10 mg two or three times a day, starting with 2.5 mg, avoid bedtime dose) and fludocortisone (0.1 mg/day starting dose, followed by slow increases) are both effective.

Key points: orthostatic hypotension

- Orthostatic hypotension causes non-spinning dizziness after standing up.
- Syncope, falls, and trauma are common sequelae.
- Measure supine and orthostatic blood pressure in these patients (nobody else will do it!).
- Treat with behavioural measures and removal of offending drugs.

References

1. Bronstein A, Lempert T (2007). *Dizziness. A practical approach to diagnosis and management*. Cambridge: Cambridge University Press.
2. Brandt T, Dieterich M (1991). Different types of skew deviation. *J Neurol Neurosurg Psychiat*, 54, 549–50.
3. Duncan GW, Parker SW, Fisher CM (1975). Acute cerebellar infarction in the PICA territory. *Arch Neurol*, 32, 364–8.
4. Dieterich M, Brandt T (1992). Wallenberg's syndrome: lateropulsion, cyclorotation, and subjective visual vertical in thirty-six patients. *Ann Neurol*, 31(4), 399–408.
5. Lee H (2009). Neuro-otological aspects of cerebellar stroke syndrome. *J Clin Neurol*, 5, 65–73.
6. Amarenco P, Hauww JJ (1990). Cerebellar infarction in the territory of the anterior inferior cerebellar artery. A clinicopathological study of 20 cases. *Brain*, 113, 139–55.
7. Lee H, Kim JS, Chung EJ, et al. (2009). Infarction in the territory of anterior inferior cerebellar artery: spectrum of audiovestibular loss. *Stroke*, 40, 3745–51.
8. Lee H, Cho YW (2003). Auditory disturbance as a prodrome of anterior inferior cerebellar artery infarction. *J Neurol Neurosurg Psychiatry*, 74, 1644–8.
9. Bovo R, Ortore R, Ciorba A, Berto A, Martini A (2007). Bilateral sudden profound hearing loss and vertigo as a unique manifestation of bilateral symmetric inferior pontine infarctions. *Ann Otol Rhinol Laryngol*, 116(6), 407–10
10. Toyoda K, Hirano T, Kumai Y, Fujii K, Kiritoshi S, Ibayashi S (2002). Bilateral deafness as a prodromal symptom of basilar artery occlusion. *J Neurol Sci*, 193(2), 147–50.
11. Koh MG, Phan TG, Atkinson JL, Wijdicks EF (2000). Neuroimaging in deteriorating patients with cerebellar infarcts and mass effect. *Stroke*, 31, 2062–7.
12. Halmagyi GM, Cuthoys IS (1988). A clinical sign of canal paresis. *Arch Neurol*, 45, 737–9.
13. Baloh RW (2003). Clinical practice. Vestibular neuritis. *N Engl J Med*, 348, 1027–32.
14. Kattah JC, Talkad AV, Wang DZ, et al. (2009). HINTS to diagnose stroke in acute vestibular syndrome: three step bedside oculomotor examination more sensitive than early MRI diffusion-weighted imaging. *Stroke*, 40, 3504–10.
15. Grad A, Baloh RW (1989). Vertigo of vascular origin: clinical and electronystagmographic features in 84 cases. *Arch Neurol*, 46, 281–4.
16. Ferbert A, Brückmann H, Drummen R (1990). Clinical features of proven basilar artery occlusion. *Stroke*, 21(8), 1135–42.
17. Gomez CR, Cruz-Flores S, Malkoff MD, Sauer CM, Burch CM (1996). Isolated vertigo as a manifestation of vertebrobasilar ischemia. *Neurology*, 47(1), 94–7.
18. Bulsara KR, Velez DA, Villavicencio A (2006). Rotational vertebral artery insufficiency resulting from cervical spondylosis: case report and review of the literature. *Surg Neurol*, 65(6), 625–7.
19. Kerber KA, Rasmussen PA, Masaryk TJ, Baloh RW (2005). Recurrent vertigo attacks cured by stenting a basilar artery stenosis. *Neurology*, 65(6), 962.
20. Overell-JR (2011). Peripheral neuropathy: pattern recognition for the pragmatist. *Pract Neurol*, 11(2), 62–70.
21. Rosenberg NR, Slotema CW, Hoogendijk JE, Vermeulen M (2005). Follow-up of patients with signs and symptoms of polyneuropathy not confirmed by electrophysiological studies. *J Neurol Neurosurg Psychiatry*, 76(6), 879–81.
22. England JD, Gronseth GS, Franklin G, et al. (2009). Practice parameter: evaluation of distal symmetric polyneuropathy: role of laboratory and genetic testing (an evidence-based review). *Neurology*, 72(2), 185–92.
23. Tracy JA, Bartleson JD (2010). Cervical spondylotic myelopathy. *Neurologist*, 16(3), 176–87.
24. Manto M, Marmolino D (2009). Cerebellar ataxias. *Curr Opin Neurol*, 22(4), 419–29.
25. Bronstein AM (2004). Vision and vertigo. *J Neurol Neurosurg Psychiatry*, 251(4), 381–7.
26. Wagner JN, Glaser M, Brandt T, Strupp M. (2008). Downbeat nystagmus: aetiology and comorbidity in 117 patients. *J Neurol Neurosurg Psychiatry*, 79(6), 672–7.
27. Huppert D, Strupp M, Mückter H, Brandt T (2011). Which medication do I need to manage dizzy patients? *Acta Otolaryngol*, 131(3), 228–41.

28. Finney GR (2009). Normal pressure hydrocephalus. *Int Rev Neurobiol*, 84, 263–81.

29. Pantoni L (2010). Cerebral small vessel disease: from pathogenesis and clinical characteristics to therapeutic challenges. *Lancet Neurol*, 9(7), 689–701.

30. Blahak C, Baezner H, Pantoni L, *et al.* (2009). Deep frontal and periventricular age related white matter changes but not basal ganglia and infratentorial hyperintensities are associated with falls: cross sectional results from the LADIS study. LADIS Study Group. *J Neurol Neurosurg Psychiat*, 80, 608–13.

31. Lees AJ, Hardy J, Revesz T (2009) Parkinson's disease. *Lancet*, 373(9680), 2055–66.

32. Lempert T, Brandt T, Dieterich M, Huppert D (1991). How to identify psychogenic disorders of stance and gait. A video study in 37 patients. *J Neurol*, 238(3), 140–6.

33. Radtke A, Lempert T, von Brevern M, Feldmann M, Lezius F, Neuhauser H (2011). Prevalence and complications of orthostatic dizziness in the general population. *Clin Auton Res*, 21, 161–8.

34. Goldstein DS, Sharabi Y (2009). Neurogenic orthostatic hypotension: a pathophysiological approach. *Circulation*, 119(1), 139–46.

35. Kamaruzzaman S, Watt H, Carson C, Ebrahim S (2010). The association between orthostatic hypotension and medication use in the British Women's Heart and Health Study. *Age Ageing*, 39(1), 51–6.

36. Moya A, Sutton R, Ammirati F, *et al.*, Task Force for the Diagnosis and Management of Syncope(2009). Guidelines for the diagnosis and management of syncope (version 2009). *Eur Heart J*, 30(21), 2631–71.

37. Lee T, Donegan C, Moore A (2005). Combined hypertension and orthostatic hypotension in older patients: a treatment dilemma for clinicians. *Expert Rev Cardiovasc Ther*, 3(3), 433–40.

38. Goldstein DS, Pechnik S, Holmes C, Eldadah B, Sharabi Y (2003). Association between supine hypertension and orthostatic hypotension in autonomic failure. *Hypertension*, 42(2), 136–42.

39. Low PA, Singer W (2008). Management of neurogenic orthostatic hypotension: an update. *Lancet Neurol*, 7(5), 451–8.

40. May M, Jordan J (2011). The osmopressor response to water drinking. *Am J Physiol Regul Integr Comp Physiol*, 300(1), R40–6.

41. Figueroa JJ, Basford JR, Low PA (2010). Preventing and treating orthostatic hypotension: As easy as A, B, C. *Cleve Clin J Med*, 77(5), 298–306.

CHAPTER 10

I am a Neurologist, What Otology do I Need to Know?

Rosalyn A. Davies and Louisa J. Murdin

The natural inclination of the neurologist is to perceive the ear as an end organ transmitting vital sensory information about hearing and balance via a cranial nerve to the brain. The clinician may only be challenged to think from an otological perspective when the patient describes hearing loss or tinnitus or is confronted with a discharging ear. However, because the end organs of hearing and balance are paired in the labyrinth and the peripheral auditory and vestibular pathways travel together proximally in the VIIIth cranial nerve, a comprehensive assessment of the dizzy patient should include examination of the ear and an assessment of hearing. Otological assessment is best made using both otological and audiological information because of the complex inter-relationship between structure and function in the auditory system.

Hearing impairment is classified according to the site of the lesion along the auditory pathway: e.g. from the external and middle ear (*conductive*), through the cochlea of the inner ear (*cochlear*), along the VIIIth cranial nerve and within the brainstem (*retrocochlear*), and thence to the higher auditory centres (*central auditory processing disorder*). This classification is of great value to the practising clinician since the clinical presentation, the pattern of abnormalities on the auditory test battery, and likely aetiology all vary according to this anatomically-based system (Figure 10.1).

The first part of the chapter describes the examination of the ear, and the second part itemizes disorders of hearing and the site-specific evaluation of hearing.

Clinical examination of the ear

Examination includes careful inspection of the pinna and the external auditory meatus (EAM). Otoscopy allows examination of the tympanic membrane (TM) which offers a window into the middle-ear cleft and is affected by most of the changes that can take place in the middle ear. Two common problems which can be encountered on initial otoscopic inspection need attention before further evaluation as they may cause a spurious hearing loss: a collapsing external auditory canal, and presence of obstruction due to wax (cerumen). The audiologist needs to be alerted to the former as a device can be used to open up the meatus for audiometric testing. Excessive amounts of wax should be removed either by direct vision or by syringing as impaction can not only cause pain but also a conductive hearing loss.

The external ear and external auditory meatus

The pinna (auricle) and post-aural area are examined for signs of inflammation or trauma, as well as for congenital deformities. Most developmental anomalies are fairly obvious but must be carefully identified because of the likely association with middle and inner ear abnormalities and possible associated vestibular dysplasias. Atresia of the EAM is likely to be an indication of a congenital abnormality and requires further evaluation with audiological assessment.

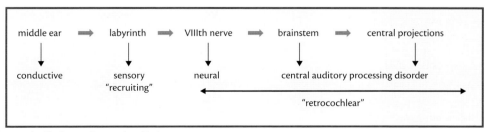

Fig. 10.1 Hearing impairment classified according to site of lesion.

Tympanic membrane and middle ear

Inspection of the ear can be carried out with the use of an otoscope, or with a head–worn light source so the hands are free to remove wax or discharge, or alternatively with a binocular microscope. The microscope is used with the patient lying on the couch or sitting close to horizontal. The largest speculum comfortable is inserted into the ear canal with the pinna held between the thumb and fore-finger and gently pulled backwards to straighten out the curve in the collagenous meatus. The little finger should be placed against the cheek to steady the otoscope and prevent the speculum penetrating too deeply into the outer ear canal.

The standard landmarks of the TM include the central portion and the handle of the malleus; the distinction between the pars tensa and the pars flaccida of the drum; and identification of the long process of the incus and stapedius tendon which may be visible with transparent TMs. The speculum should be directed so as to examine the entire rim of the TM and the attic portion of the pars flaccida. The normal TM has the appearance of mother of pearl and the light reflex should be seen anteroinferiorly, and is due to reflection of the examining light. Congenital abnormalities of the middle ear include stapes fixation, absent stapedius tendons and uncovered or aberrant VIIth nerves.

Perforations are classified as marginal or central according to location and whether the rim of the TM forms part of the circumference of the perforation. A large perforation is generally associated with a greater loss of sound pressure and more marked conductive hearing loss. A defect of the attic is described as an attic perforation and should be characterized as small or large and may be associated with cholesteatoma when keratin debris is seen in the pars flaccida.

The fistula sign is a particularly important part of the assessment of the dizzy patient, especially where there is a history of balance symptoms triggered by sound. It is elicited when there is transmission of air pressure changes from the external meatus via the middle ear through a fistula into the labyrinth causing endolymph movement and resulting in nystagmus. The pressure in the EAM may be raised by finger pressure on the tragus, but more accurately by tympanometry (see Box 10.4). Raised pressure causes a conjugate deviation of the eyes towards the opposite ear, and with maintenance of pressure, a corrective fast phase will be introduced and nystagmus will beat towards the affected ear. If the fistula is through to the horizontal semicircular canal, the nystagmus will be horizontal. Hennebert's sign is a positive fistula test in the presence of an intact TM.

Assessment of hearing and hearing disorders

This begins with an accurate history of difficulties hearing and the effect of the hearing loss on the patient, their social situation, and any past attempts at rehabilitation (Box 10.1).

Hearing impairment is classified according to the site of the lesion along the auditory pathway as described in Figure 10.1. Hearing disorders will be described here according to their likely site of lesion, e.g. conductive, cochlear, retrocochlear, or central auditory processing disorders. Site of lesion testing is described.

Conductive hearing loss

Disorders affecting the external and middle ear that cause significant impediment to sound transmission cause a conductive hearing loss. This is frequently unilateral, but may be bilateral. Since the deficit is caused purely by a failure to amplify sound in the middle ear, the patient complains that sounds are not loud enough, but distortion of sound is not a predominant feature. The loss needs to be characterized according to hearing thresholds measured with both air and bone conduction using pure tone audiometry (see Box 10.2), and with tympanometry (see Box 10.3). The maximum threshold of conductive hearing loss is 60 Db HL (decibels hearing level), meaning that conductive loss per se cannot cause a severe, profound, or total hearing loss. A conductive hearing loss is relevant not only in identifying a potential cause for vertigo, but is also relevant for the interpretation of some neuro-otological tests such as vestibular-evoked myogenic potentials and auditory evoked brainstem responses.

Box 10.1 Anamnesis

Hearing loss
- Date of onset
- Gradual or sudden
- Progressive, stable, or fluctuating
- Unilateral or bilateral
- Any difficulties localizing sound.

Associated symptoms
- Fullness, discharge, pain, vertigo, autophony
- Tinnitus (pitch, pulsatile, or clicking)
- Diplacusis (difference in pitch perception between the two ears), hyperacusis, distortion of sound.

Past medical history
- Noise exposure, trauma, ototoxic medications, otological surgery, infection, cardiovascular risk factors
- Birth and neonatal history
- Family history including pedigree of any syndromal/non-syndromal hearing loss.

Box 10.2 Pure tone audiometry

Pure tone audiometry (PTA) is a psychoacoustic test of hearing sensitivity that requires cooperation from the subject, and is thus a *subjective* estimate of hearing threshold. A quiet test environment is required and audiometric test booths are specifically designed to minimize external noise, particularly at low sound levels. PTA has two main purposes: to determine the sensitivity of an individual's hearing across a range of specified frequencies; and to distinguish conductive hearing loss from other kinds of hearing loss.

Procedure
Pure tones are presented at frequencies ranging from 250 Hz to 8 kHz, incorporating the speech frequency range according to a standardized procedure (e.g. British Society of Audiology (BSA) protocol; 1) designed to maximize reliability of results. The *threshold of hearing* is defined as the lowest level of the tone which can still be heard on at least 50% of occasions. This level is influenced by the manner in which the intensity of tones is presented, i.e. using 5-dB steps the apparent threshold is lower if approached from

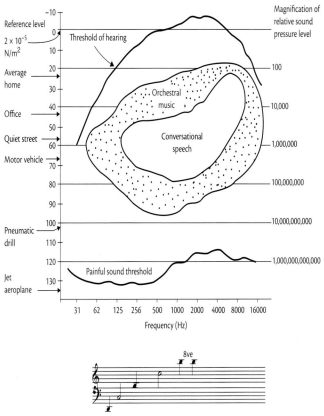

Fig. 10.2 This figure indicates the relative loudness of different intensities of sound in terms of everyday sounds and as magnitudes of amplification of sound pressure levels.

above (descending threshold). The reference intensity level which is designated 0 dB at each frequency is the mean value of the minimal audible intensity of pure tones in a group of healthy, young, male adults with normal hearing and corresponds to sound pressure levels set by the International Standards Organization (Figure 10.2).

Left and right ears are tested separately. Any hearing loss identified is classified in degree, as in the BSA system, as mild (21–40 dB HL), moderate (41–70 dB HL), severe (71–95 dB HL), or profound (≥ 96 dB HL) (1). Any level of hearing loss can cause symptoms, but those with a moderate or more severe loss are likely to have some degree of functional impairment, especially if the hearing loss is more recent or suddenly acquired.

Site of lesion
During testing, tones can be presented via air conduction (AC) through headphones or ear inserts, or by bone conduction (BC) using a vibrator placed on the mastoid. AC stimuli are sensed predominantly by the ipsilateral cochlea once the sound has travelled through the external and middle ear on that side. BC stimuli are transmitted via the bones of the skull to be heard by either cochlea, bypassing the external and middle ear systems. BC thresholds therefore correspond to the hearing threshold in the better hearing cochlea. During audiometry, white noise can be presented to the non-test ear, in order to prevent the phenomenon of cross-hearing, whereby sounds presented to one side are picked up by the contralateral cochlea. This procedure is known as *masking* and narrow bands of noise (⅓ to ½ octave wide) centred on the frequency of

the test tone are most effective. The need for masking is indicated by the degree of difference between AC thresholds on the two sides and the unmasked BC thresholds, e.g. 40 dB or more difference between the unmasked AC thresholds of the two ears. This means that a pure tone audiogram can be carried out to provide AC and BC thresholds, masked as necessary, for both ears.

If hearing sensitivity is normal, then the masked BC threshold is equal to or marginally better than the AC threshold. If there is a difference between the AC and BC thresholds of more than 15 dB, this is known as an *air–bone gap*. An air–bone gap is an indication of a conductive hearing loss, and localizes the auditory lesion to the external or middle ear.

Caveats
Pure tone audiometry is a behavioural test involving cooperation from the subject. It cannot therefore be used in unconscious individuals or those unwilling or unable to understand or follow the instructions. Testers also need to be alert to the possibility of non-organic hearing loss, where the apparent thresholds on audiometry do not correspond to the true threshold of hearing. It is essential that the need for any masking of AC or BC stimuli is identified, and, if required, the masking is carried out appropriately, since otherwise unilateral hearing losses can be missed. These caveats mean that audiometry should always be carried out by trained individuals in a suitably sound-proofed environment. Where the thresholds obtained are unreliable, further objective audiometry should be undertaken measuring acoustic reflex thresholds (see Box 10.3) and/or otoacoustic emissions (OAEs; see Box 10.4).

Table 10.1 Interpretation of tuning fork tests

	Rinne	Weber
Normal hearing	Positive bilaterally	No lateralization
Unilateral conductive hearing loss	Negative on the side of the pathology	Sound lateralizes to pathological ear
Unilateral sensorineural hearing loss	Positive bilaterally	Sound lateralizes to non-pathological ear

Conductive hearing loss: assessment

Tuning fork tests

Unilateral conductive hearing loss is traditionally identified using a 256-Hz tuning fork. Tuning fork tests rely on two general principles: 1) that the inner ear is more sensitive to sound conducted by air than bone; and 2) in a pure conductive hearing loss, the affected ear is subject to less environmental noise and is more sensitive to bone conducted sound. *Rinne's test* assesses whether sound is perceived more loudly by air or bone conduction, and is *negative* when the sound heard in front of the ear (by air conduction) is quieter than the sound heard via the mastoid (by bone conduction). It indicates a conductive hearing loss where the air–bone gap is 15 dB or more. *Weber's test* identifies where the sound from a tuning fork placed on the middle of the vertex is perceived and *lateralizes to the side of any asymmetric conductive loss, or to the better hearing ear in a pure sensorineural hearing loss.* These findings are summarized in Table 10.1. Dysacusis is present if the sound is described as being distorted or rough, and diplacusis is documented when the sound in the two ears is perceived as being of different pitch. Tuning fork tests in experienced hands are useful bedside tests but their sensitivity is limited, and formal audiometry is always indicated where patients complain of hearing disturbance even in the presence of normal tuning fork tests. They are not useful in the diagnosis of mild to moderate symmetric sensorineural hearing losses.

Box 10.3 Acoustic impedance measurements

Acoustic impedance measurements assess the amount of sound transmitted or reflected through the middle ear and give information about the state of the middle ear as a function of ear canal pressure.

Tympanometry

A probe assembly is inserted into the outer ear to make an air-tight seal. The probe not only delivers a tone, usually 226 Hz, but also measures the reflected sound in the outer ear canal as the pressure is varied from −400 to +300 daPa. The amount of transmitted sound is greatest when external ear pressure is equal to middle ear pressure, resulting in a peak at this point. The graph produced may take a variety of shapes: if the middle ear system is stiff, as in otosclerosis, then the magnitude of the peak is reduced (Type A_S). The peak can be raised by a floppy middle ear system (Type A_D), for example ossicular discontinuity due to trauma. A flat tracing, with no peak (Type B) is obtained when the middle ear is filled with fluid, so that the external ear pressure cannot be matched with middle ear pressure. If the peak occurs at a very negative value (Type C), i.e. more than −50 daPa, it suggests Eustachian tube dysfunction with failure of adequate ventilation of the middle ear and development of negative middle ear pressure.

Acoustic reflex thresholds (ARTs)

Ipsilateral and contralateral acoustic reflexes can be assessed using acoustic impedance measurements. The reflex pathway travels cranially via the VIIIth nerve, passes through the cochlear nuclei in the brainstem and thence to the effector organ via the VIIth nerve both ipsi- or contralaterally. The effector organ is the stapedius muscle which, when it contracts, results in TM displacement and a sudden shift in acoustic impedance. ARTs are documented as the lowest sound intensity for a given frequency that elicits measurable and reproducible displacement of the TM. The sound stimulus can be presented ipsi- or contralaterally to the recorded side. Acoustic reflex responses are usually *absent* on the side of sound presentation with significant hearing loss, and absent on the side of sound recording with significant middle ear pathology. *Recruitment* (see 'Cochlear hearing loss') can sometimes be seen with normal ARTs despite raised air conduction thresholds and is suggestive of a cochlear hearing loss.

Conductive hearing loss: aetiologies

Wax impaction

The commonest cause of conductive hearing loss is wax impaction in the external ear. Although small amounts of wax generally cause no bother, in some situations wax can become impacted resulting in impaired hearing. This is usually caused by the patient attempting to clean the ear with cotton buds or similar-shaped instruments and pushing the wax further down the EAM, but can occur where there is a plug in the external ear, such as an ear mould from a hearing aid. The effects of wax impaction and its removal on a moderate high-frequency sensorineural hearing loss are illustrated in Figure 10.3. Wax impaction can also impede sound transmission in vestibular tests such as vestibular-evoked myogenic potentials, or heat energy transmission in caloric testing, potentially resulting in spurious test results.

Otitis media

Otitis media refers to inflammation within the middle ear. When there is fluid in the middle ear that impedes sound transmission, as occurs in otitis media with effusion, this can be seen as a characteristic trace on tympanometry (Type B) with absence of the normal peaked response (see Box 10.3). Otitis media can be acute or chronic. Chronic suppurative otitis media can be divided into tubotympanic or attico-antral disease. Tubo-tympanic disease essentially comprises a central perforation of the TM and hearing loss and otorrhoea are the principal features. It is unlikely to be associated with vertigo or VIIth nerve symptoms. Treatment aims to secure a dry ear free from recurrent infections and optimize hearing. Attico-antral disease involves the rim of the TM (Figure 10.4). It is often associated with progressive destruction of middle ear cleft structures including VIIth nerve. It predisposes to cholesteatoma, and needs to be treated actively with a combination of aural toilet, local, and systemic antibiotics. Surgery may be required.

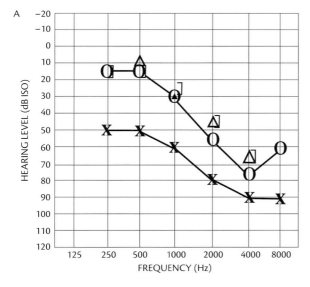

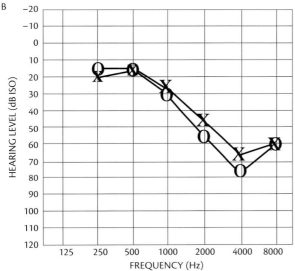

Fig. 10.3 (A) Impacted wax can result in an air-bone gap on the audiogram. (O and X represent right and left ear air conduction thresholds respectively, Δ is unmasked bone conduction and [is right masked bone conduction); (B) shows resolution of the air–bone gap after removal of the wax. From Davies (2).

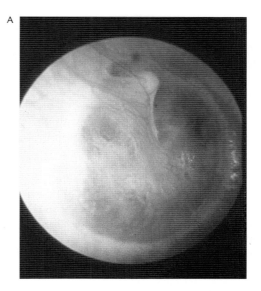

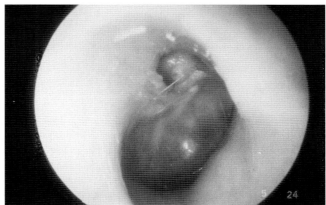

Fig. 10.4 (A) The otoscopic appearance of the normal left tympanic membrane. (B) Attico-antral disease with cholesteatoma.

Cholesteatoma

Cholesteatoma is a cyst lined with squamous epithelium which can arise in ears undergoing long periods of negative middle ear pressure and infection. It is associated with a history of perforation and foul-smelling discharge. It tends to begin in the attic of the ear and extend into the middle ear antrum. It can lead to intracranial complications by eroding through the dura of the middle or posterior fossa or into the lateral sinus, resulting in meningitis or cerebral abscess. It can also erode into the horizontal semicircular canal producing a fistula and causing vertigo (see discussion of fistula sign in earlier 'Tympanic membrane and middle ear' section). The eardrum will usually appear abnormal on otoscopy with keratin debris in the pars flaccida. Because of the progressive and destructive nature of cholesteatoma, surgical removal is indicated.

Bone and joint disorders

Otosclerosis is a disorder of bone within the ear in which mature lamellar bone is gradually replaced by immature woven bone. It can affect the ossicular chain, causing fixation of the stapes footplate, as well as involving other parts of the bony labyrinth with the potential for associated vestibular symptoms. It is a genetic disorder, following an autosomal dominant inheritance pattern with incomplete penetrance. It is often exacerbated during pregnancy. It can be addressed with surgery by stapedectomy with prosthesis insertion at the stapes footplate. Paget's disease of bone can also cause a conductive hearing loss, and this can resolve with treatment of the underlying disorder. The joints within the ossicular chain are true synovial joints, and can become involved in inflammatory arthritides such as rheumatoid arthritis.

Temporal bone skull fractures

Typically, trauma causing a longitudinal temporal bone fracture is associated with haemo-tympanum, TM perforation with haemorrhagic otorrhoea, or ossicular discontinuity. Each of these may be associated with a conductive hearing loss. This is by contrast with transverse temporal bone fractures which can cause a complete sensorineural hearing loss as well as vestibular deficits (see below).

Anterior canal dehiscence—Minor's syndrome (see Chapter 15)

Autophony, pulsatile tinnitus, and noise-induced vertigo (the Tullio phenomenon) are characteristic symptoms of a dehiscence of the anterior semicircular canal due to incomplete bony covering of the roof of this canal. This syndrome is included here because of the air–bone gap elicited on the side of the dehiscence on pure tone audiometric testing. Frequently the audiometric thresholds are normal (though in some with disease progression, a low-frequency sensorineural hearing loss is found) and the bone conduction thresholds are supranormal. It is considered that there is a 'gain' in bone conduction thresholds as a result of the dehiscence acting as a third labyrinthine window. Thus, despite the air–bone gap, this is not a true conductive hearing loss and the stapedius reflex thresholds are normal. The diagnosis is made by first screening with vestibular-evoked myogenic potentials, which show an abnormally low threshold, and by coronal computed tomography scanning with fine cuts through the petrous temporal bone.

Glomus tumour

A glomus tympanicum tumour may be identified as a vascular mass behind the TM (the 'setting sun' sign) and the patient may describe pulsatile tinnitus. This can often be correlated with a pulsatile movement on tympanometry.

Cochlear hearing loss

In the physiological process of hearing, the next stage after mechanical sound transmission through the external and middle ear is the transduction of sound energy into electrical nerve activity within the cochlea. Hearing loss caused by failure of this energy transduction process causes a distinctive pattern of symptoms and results in test abnormalities identifiable as cochlear hearing loss. Because of the embryological anatomical, physiological, and neurological relationship of the labyrinth and cochlea, neuro-otological disorders are commonly associated with cochlear hearing loss, and presence of cochlear hearing loss can therefore provide valuable diagnostic information.

Cochlear hearing loss can be of any severity from mild to profound. Since signal transduction is affected, patients may also complain of distortion of sound perception as well as sounds being of inadequate volume, although this distortion is less pronounced than occurs with retrocochlear hearing losses. Classically, cochlear hearing loss is also associated with loudness recruitment. This is an abnormal, large growth of loudness with increased stimulus intensity. Patients with cochlear recruitment may describe a reduced range of sound intensities between 'too quiet, can't hear' and 'too loud, don't shout'.

Cochlear hearing loss: assessment

Pure tone audiometry shows a sensorineural hearing loss. A pure cochlear hearing loss shows no air–bone gap. Loudness recruitment can be seen on acoustic (stapedius) reflex threshold measurements, where the difference between the reflex threshold and the audiometric threshold is less than 60 dB. Loudness discomfort levels can also be measured, although these are more subjective than ARTs and are less useful for localizing pathology. In addition, OAEs are lost in cochlear forms of hearing loss if hearing thresholds are 40 dB HL or worse (see Box 10.4).

Box 10.4 Otoacoustic emissions

Transient-evoked otoacoustic emissions (TEOAEs) were first reported in 1978 (3). OAEs are a by-product of outer hair-cell activity. In the transduction process, some sound energy escapes back through the middle and outer ear, and this can be picked up by a probe microphone placed just inside the ear canal. Computer processing is able to distinguish these sound emissions from background noise. The test requires reasonably quiet recording conditions and the ear canal to be clean and free of debris, so cannot be performed on restless or active individuals, but is otherwise not dependent on subject cooperation. The presence of OAEs indicates healthy outer hair cells. Since most forms of cochlear hearing loss appear to involve the outer hair cells primarily, loss of OAEs is characteristic of cochlear hearing loss (Figure 10.5). However, absence of OAEs can also occur in other circumstances, such as conductive hearing loss, or hearing loss from any cause where the threshold is greater than 40 dB HL for a prolonged period. Cochlear hearing loss can be distinguished from auditory neuropathy/desynchrony (see later) using OAEs, since in auditory neuropathy OAEs can be preserved despite moderate or more severe audiometric thresholds.

Cochlear hearing loss: aetiologies

Genetic

Genetic disorders can underlie conductive, cochlear, and retrocochlear causes of hearing loss. However, most congenital genetic sensorineural hearing loss is due to cochlear outer hair-cell dysfunction resulting in a cochlear-type hearing loss. This observation underlies the rationale behind the use of OAEs as a screening tool for the neonatal hearing screening programmes in the UK and other countries.

Genetic cochlear hearing loss is considered as either syndromic or non-syndromic. The number of genes identified as causing both is rapidly increasing (4). The commonest cause of non-syndromic hereditary hearing loss in the UK population, accounting for 30–60% of such cases, is a mutation in the gene (*GJB2*) for connexin 26, a protein involved in cellular gap junctions and inherited in an autosomal recessive fashion. Connexin 26 hearing loss is usually associated with normal vestibular function. There are many causes of syndromic hearing loss, and some, such as Usher syndrome type I, are associated with significant vestibular dysfunction.

There are documented pedigrees of adult-onset hearing loss inherited in an autosomal dominant manner, associated with mutations in the *COCH* gene, and causing a presentation similar to that of endolymphatic hydrops (Ménière's disease) with fluctuating or progressive hearing loss and episodic vertigo. Diseases with mitochondrial inheritance can also be associated with hearing loss, including: myoclonic epilepsy with red ragged fibres (MERRF), mitochondrially inherited diabetes and deafness (MIDD), and diabetes insipidus, diabetes mellitus, optic atrophy and deafness (DIDMOAD). Inherited metabolic disorders such as the mucopolysaccharidoses are also associated with hearing loss. When seen, this hearing loss can be associated with central and retrocochlear components in addition to the cochlear deficit.

Infective

Mumps, polio, adeno, parainfluenza, and measles viruses can be all associated with hearing loss. Reductions in vaccination rates and subsequent epidemics of mumps and measles have resulted in a corresponding increase in the complications from these diseases, including cochlear hearing loss. Bacterial meningitis can cause cochlear hearing

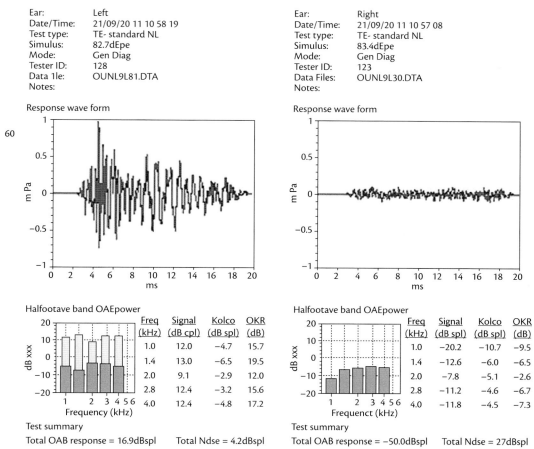

Ear:	Left
Date/Time:	21/09/20 11 10 58 19
Test type:	TE- standard NL
Simulus:	82.7dEpe
Mode:	Gen Diag
Tester ID:	128
Data 1le:	OUNL9L81.DTA
Notes:	

Ear:	Right
Date/Time:	21/09/20 11 10 57 08
Test type:	TE- standard NL
Simulus:	83.4dEpe
Mode:	Gen Diag
Tester ID:	123
Data Files:	OUNL9L30.DTA
Notes:	

Halfootave band OAEpower (Left)

Freq (kHz)	Signal (dB cpl)	Kolco (dB spl)	OKR (dB)
1.0	12.0	−4.7	15.7
1.4	13.0	−6.5	19.5
2.0	9.1	−2.9	12.0
2.8	12.4	−3.2	15.6
4.0	12.4	−4.8	17.2

Test summary: Total OAB response = 16.9dBspl   Total Ndse = 4.2dBspl

Halfootave band OAEpower (Right)

Freq (kHz)	Signal (dB spl)	Kolco (dB spl)	OKR (dB)
1.0	−20.2	−10.7	−9.5
1.4	−12.6	−6.0	−6.5
2.0	−7.8	−5.1	−2.6
2.8	−11.2	−4.6	−6.7
4.0	−11.8	−4.5	−7.3

Test summary: Total OAB response = −50.0dBspl   Total Ndse = 27dBspl

Fig. 10.5 Otoacoustic emissions: the bar chart shows the presence of any OAE signal (upper bars on left) above the noise floor (lower bars). Response intensity is shown on the y-axis across the frequency range on the x axis. Note therefore that in this example, no response is recorded on the right ear, but the response from the left ear is robust, in keeping with the clinical presentation of sudden right sided unilateral hearing loss.

loss of a profound degree that can require cochlear implantation. It is particularly important that audiological assessment is carried out swiftly in individuals who have had bacterial meningitis. Meningitis can be followed by labyrinthitis ossificans, whereby the whole of the labyrinth ossifies over a period of weeks or months, rendering subsequent cochlear implantation less successful or even impossible. Less commonly seen is cochlear hearing loss due to syphilitic otitis.

Ménière's disease (see Chapter 22)

Ménière's disease has been included here as it is an important cause of cochlear hearing loss. It is conventionally attributed to endolymphatic hydrops, and is an inner ear disorder characterized by fluctuating hearing loss, tinnitus and aural fullness associated with prolonged attacks of vertigo. Ménière's disease is usually idiopathic but can be acquired, e.g. after an inflammatory or traumatic insult to the labyrinth when it is sometimes known as delayed endolymphatic hydrops. It occurs in about 21/100,000 of the population, presenting between 40–60 years of age. To make a definite diagnosis American Academy of Otolaryngology 1995 criteria are commonly used (5), although it is important to keep a watching brief on those patients whose initial symptoms do not initially match the full criteria as the full picture may only develop with time. The mechanism underlying the disorder is thought to be an over accumulation of endolymph leading to distortion of the membranous labyrinth and eventually rupture of Reissner's membrane (Figure 10.6).

Typically the major loss of hearing occurs in the first few years. In the early stages the hearing loss tends to be reversible, affecting the low frequencies only, but with advancing cochlear involvement, a peaked audiogram can be seen (best threshold at 2000 Hz) and

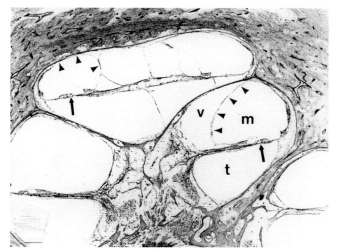

Fig. 10.6 Temporal bone preparation in a 79-year-old man with Ménière's disease: endolymphatic hydrops with ballooning of the membranous labyrinth (arrow-heads) and a dilated scala media (m) displacing much of the scala vestibuli (v). The organ of Corti (arrows) and the scala tympani (t) are seen. From Andrews and Honrubia (6).

eventually a flat loss is found in a majority of patients. The hearing loss is typically recruiting as identified by acoustic reflex thresholds (Box 10.3). In general, the longer the patients are followed, the greater the percentage of those who develop bilateral disease: 15% have bilateral disease by 2 years, and by 20 years, 30–60% are bilaterally affected. At autopsy, 30% of the temporal bones in patients with Ménière's disease have bilateral involvement.

Immune mediated

Cochlear hearing loss and associated peripheral vestibular deficits are a feature of a number of systemic autoimmune disorders (7; Table 10.2). These vary in terms of epidemiology, neuro-otological presentation, associated autoantibodies, and other systemic involvement. In Cogan syndrome, young adults and older children experience Ménière-like attacks, in association with eye inflammation and systemic vasculitis. Wegener's granulomatosis affects the middle ear more than the inner ear, although sensorineural hearing loss is reported. It is also associated with rhinorrhoea, sinusitis, pulmonary and renal manifestations. Systemic lupus erythematosus, sarcoid, Behçet's disease, rheumatoid arthritis, and Sjögren's syndrome are all associated with sensorineural hearing loss which can be subacute or even subclinical, detectable only as the absence of OAEs in an otherwise apparently healthy ear. In polyarteritis nodosa, cochlear hearing loss can be rapidly progressive.

Table 10.2 Autoimmune causes of hearing loss

Condition	Neuro-otologic syndrome	Associated findings	Epidemiology	Laboratory markers/diagnostic tests
Cogan syndrome	Ménière's-like attacks	Eye inflammation (keratitis, scleritis, conjunctivitis, uveitis, retinal vasculitis) Systemic vasculitis in 10%	Young adults and older children (median 25 years)	Neutrophilia, raised ESR/CRP MRI enhancement of vestibulocochlear structures
Vogt–Koyanagi–Harada syndrome	4 phases: 1. prodromal 2. uveitis (tinnitus) 3. convalescent 4. chronic recurrent	Meningo-encephalitis, bilateral uveitis, vitiligo, alopecia and poliosis	More common in Japan; presents in children or young adults	CSF pleocytosis in first phase .
Susac syndrome	SNHL, tinnitus, and vertigo	Encephalopathy and retinopathy: retinal branch occlusion and sectoral blindness	Female > male adults	MRI: multiple lesions in corpus callosum, cerebellum, and elsewhere; retinal fluorescein angiography; biopsy of CNS lesions or muscle; CSF pleocytosis and raised protein
Sarcoid	Acute, fluctuating, or progressive hearing loss which may be conductive, cochlear or VIIIth nerve Basal meningitis	Systemic auto-immune disorder with protean manifestations including lung, skin, ocular and CNS presentations	Commonest in young adults, females commoner than males	Chest X-ray: hilar lymphadenopathy; bronchoscopy; serum angiotensin-converting enzyme; biopsy may show non-caseating granulomatous change
Behçet's disease	Bilateral cochlear hearing impairment; peripheral vestibular dysfunction	Oral and genital ulceration; pustular rash; eye inflammation	Common in the Middle East and Asia	Pathergy reaction; HLA B51
Wegener's granulomatosis	Usually conductive hearing loss often have otitis media; SNHL reported	Rhinorrhoea and sinusitis pulmonary, renal, joint manifestations peripheral nervous system involvement	40–50 years males and females equally affected	Raised ESR/CRP raised c-ANCA (proteinase 3) Granulomatous infiltration on MRI Biopsy
Polyarteritis nodosa	Rapid SNHL	Systemic vasculitis (kidney, gut, skin) constitutional symptoms; mononeuritis multiplex	Male > female older age of onset	Leucocytosis, raised ESR, p-ANCA, visceral angiography, organ/nerve/muscle biopsy
Systemic lupus erythematosus	Subacute SNHL, uni- or bilateral vestibular failure	Dermatologic, joint, renal, neuropsychiatric; constitutional symptoms	Female > male (5:1) age 15–40 years	Raised ESR, ANA, dsDNA antibodies, antiphospholipid Ab, complement consumption
Sjögren's syndrome	Often subclinical	Dry eyes, dry mouth, Raynauds, joint, neuropathies (axonal, sensory ataxic, trigeminal)	Female > male	ANA, Ro, La Schirmer test, lip biopsy
Rheumatoid arthritis	Gradual, bilateral cochlear hearing loss Rarely synovial middle ear pathology	Symmetrical deforming polyarthropathy, multiple systemic involvement	Female>male adults	Plain film imaging, rheumatoid factor; anti-citrullinated protein antibodies; raised inflammatory markers

Adapted from Overell et al. (7).

It is also thought that immune-mediated hearing loss can be specific to the inner ear. Over 30 years ago it was hypothesized that autoantibodies against inner ear antigens could cause rapidly progressive or sudden sensorineural hearing loss (8). No specific or sensitive markers for autoimmune inner ear disease have been identified to date. Many patients in whom there is a sudden onset of hearing loss will be assessed to exclude autoimmune inner ear disease and require a full blood count, erythrocyte sedimentation rate, C-reactive protein, antinuclear antibodies, anticardiolipin antibodies, lupus anticoagulant, rheumatoid factor, antineutrophil cytoplasmic antibodies, clotting factors, and syphilis serology. Many clinicians treat such patients with oral steroids, although the evidence supporting such treatment is weak (9).

Trauma

Head injury can be associated with cochlear hearing loss and peripheral vestibular deficits through direct trauma to the labyrinth, i.e. as seen in transverse temporal bone fractures (Figure 10.7).

Hazardous noise exposure is a major cause of hearing loss, especially via occupational exposure in industrialized countries so that it is important to enquire in detail about occupational history, including work in industrial and military settings but also leisure industries such as music, in patients with unexplained cochlear hearing loss. Although health and safety regulations now require protective equipment to be worn at work by individuals exposed to hazardous levels of noise, it is relatively recent that provision and use of such equipment has become common practice. The audiogram in noise exposure classically has the worst threshold at 4 kHz, but other configurations including sloping high frequency loss are also seen.

Endocrine, metabolic, and toxic

Diabetes mellitus, hyperthyroidism, hypothyroidism, and chronic renal failure are among the commoner endocrine and metabolic disorders associated with cochlear hearing loss both with and without vestibular dysfunction. There are some drugs in common usage known to be toxic to the ear, via their action on the outer hair cells of the cochlea and similarly on vestibular hair cells. Some have generally reversible effects, such as salicylates, whereas others, such as platinum-based chemotherapy agents and aminoglycoside antibiotics, can cause permanent damage.

Vascular

Labyrinthine or 'ear' strokes can cause sudden unilateral hearing loss and peripheral vestibular failure. The anterior inferior cerebellar artery (AICA) supplies the inner ear through the internal auditory artery (IAA) in a majority of cases, and IAA occlusion will give varying degrees of hearing loss and/or peripheral vestibular deficits according to the vascular territory distal to the occlusion. Central vestibular dysfunction can also be found in patients with more extensive AICA occlusive disease giving rise to brainstem and cerebellar symptoms and signs.

Retrocochlear hearing loss

The term 'retrocochlear hearing loss' has been used for many decades to classify hearing loss caused by lesions more proximal to the brain than the cochlea, i.e. in the VIIIth nerve (first-order cochlear neurons), brainstem (second-order cochlear neurons) or the central auditory projections upwards from the brainstem. More recently however, the term *auditory neuropathy/dys-synchrony spectrum disorder* (AN/AD) has been coined to describe hearing disorders with VIIIth nerve hearing loss, in which the principal histopathological correlate is a lesion of the primary cochlear neuron. Recent developments in site-of-lesion testing, e.g. recording of TEOAEs and their suppression with contralateral noise (see Box 10.5) have allowed us to distinguish these VIIIth nerve lesions from preneural hearing loss. From an electrophysiological perspective the cochlear inner hair cell functions as part of the cochleovestibular nerve.

Retrocochlear hearing loss: clinical features

The common clinical feature of patients with auditory neuropathy is that their hearing difficulties are worse with speech than with simple environmental sound, and using the telephone causes particular difficulty. Patients complain that they can hear loudness, but they cannot understand words. Their difficulties are always more

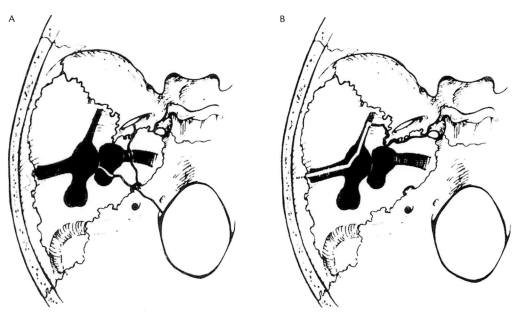

Fig. 10.7 Temporal bone fractures; (A) transverse fracture; (B) longitudinal fracture. From Hilger et al. (10).

Box 10.5 Retrocochlear hearing loss: test battery

Baseline audiometric tests
- Pure tone audiogram (thresholds can be normal or significantly impaired)
- Tympanogram (normal)
- Stapedius reflex thresholds (typically absent when ipsi- and contralaterally recorded).
- Electrophysiological tests
- Auditory brainstem-evoked responses (abnormal or absent)
- Cochlear microphonics (present)
- TEOAEs (typically present early on but lost with duration of disease)
- TEOAEs with contralateral suppression (suppression may be lost)
- Distortion product OAEs (typically present)
- Middle latency responses (may be absent).

Behavioural auditory tests
- Speech recognition tests (disproportionately impaired for pure tone threshold)
- Other central auditory tests to exclude CAPD e.g.:
  - Frequency pattern tests
  - Temporal gap detection.

marked in noisy environments when there are competing signals. The effect of an auditory neuropathy can be thought of as causing a 'time-smear' of sound. The severity of the hearing impairment may be variable and can range from transient, intermittent, to stable and deteriorating.

Retrocochlear hearing loss: assessment

Typically, the patient with AN/AD has relatively well-preserved pure tone audiometric thresholds, but markedly impaired speech thresholds and the synchronization of acoustic signals is not adequate to evoke an ABR, or to elicit the stapedius reflex, or to suppress contralateral OAEs.

Retrocochlear hearing loss: aetiologies

There are many causes of retrocochlear hearing loss, both intrinsic and extrinsic to the VIIIth nerve and brainstem. Tables 10.3 and 10.4 (11) summarize the causes of retrocochlear hearing loss presenting at birth and in adult life respectively.

Auditory neuropathy plus peripheral neuropathy

Demyelinated axons have an impaired capacity to transmit trains of impulses explaining the absence of stapedius reflexes and loss of contralateral suppression of OAEs in patients with AN/AD. Demyelinated axons may also demonstrate 'cross-talk' (ephaptic transmission) between fibres, with one active fibre initiating

Table 10.3 Genetic and congenital causes of retrocochlear hearing loss

Genetic	Non-syndromal	Non-syndromal recessive auditory neuropathy due to mutations in the Otoferlin gene	
		Delayed maturation of auditory pathways	
	Syndromal	Degenerative conditions: with peripheral neuropathy	Hereditary sensory-motor neuropathy (HSMN), i.e. Charcot–Marie–Tooth
			Friedreich's ataxia
			Mutation on chromosome 8q24 in Roma (gypsy) families
			Neurofibromatosis type 2
			Refsum's disease
		without peripheral neuropathy	Arnold–Chiari
			Usher's syndrome
			Mitochondrial myopathies: • MELAS • Chronic progressive external ophthalmoplegia • Mohr–Tranebjaerg syndrome 'Deafness/dystonia peptide'
			Skeletal syndromes: • Branchio-otorenal • Wildervanck's
			Bone dysplasias: • Osteopetroses • Hyperostosis cranialis • Cammurati–Engelmann's disease
			Gaucher disease
Congenital	Toxic/metabolic		Perinatal risk factors: • Asphyxia • Respiratory distress syndrome • Low birth weight • Cerebral palsy • Hyperbilirubinaemia
			Thalidomide

From Davies (11).

Table 10.4 Acquired cause of retrocochlear hearing loss

Infection	Viral	Herpes zoster/herpes simplex Ramsay Hunt syndrome Bell's palsy Cytomegalovirus HIV/AIDS
	Bacterial	Basal meningitis • Pneumococcal • Meningococcal • Haemophilus • Tuberculosis
	Fungal	• Cryptococcosis • Coccidio-mycosis
	Spirochaetal	• Syphilis • Borrelia
Immune-mediated	Post-infective	Guillain–Barré syndrome
	Granulomatous/ vasculitic	Neuro-sarcoid, Behcet's disease
Demyelination		Multiple sclerosis affecting: • VIIIth nerve • Brainstem
Neoplasia/neoplasia related		Vestibular schwannoma Meningioma Other cerebellopontine angle lesions Carcinomatosis Radiotherapy induced
Metabolic/toxic		Uraemia Paget's disease Organic mercury Cisplatin Haemosiderosis
Vascular		Anterior inferior cerebellar artery (AICA) infarction involving the internal auditory artery Macrovascular: • Posterior fossa aneurysms • AV malformations • Vascular loop compressing VIIIth nerve

From Davies (11).

impulses in an adjacent fibre, possibly accounting in the auditory system for distortion in the coding complex of speech. However, in an axonal neuropathy, the reduced size of the nerve action potential due to the reduced number of functioning axons is likely to affect the low frequencies on the audiogram as the longest cochlear fibres extend to the apex of the cochlea.

In a recent series of 70 cases of auditory neuropathy (12), no aetiology was identifiable in 40% of affected individuals. Hereditary sensorimotor neuropathy (HSMN) was found in nine out of 70 patients, with three families providing all nine of these cases. The auditory neuropathy was typically bilateral and affected men and women equally. In general, auditory neuropathies have been considered to be an infrequent associate of peripheral neuropathies, and are less common than other cranial neuropathies, i.e. optic, trigeminal, and facial neuropathies. However, a peripheral neuropathy was identified in 26% of the

cases cited following clinical assessment of deep tendon reflexes at the ankle, vibration sense at 128 Hz in the foot and investigations with nerve conduction studies plus sural/peroneal nerve biopsy.

Several different genetic disorders may present with HSMN, and one Roma family from Slovenia (13) was shown to have a mutation on chromosome 8q24. In these patients, the peripheral neuropathy occurred first, and sural nerve biopsy demonstrated a mixed axonal and degenerative neuropathy, with hearing loss only developing later. These cases also had bilateral vestibular failure, presumably on the basis of VIIIth nerve involvement, and demonstrated a recessive mode of inheritance.

The neuropathy associated with Charcot–Marie–Tooth (CMT) type I is characteristically demyelinating, and that of CMT type II is axonal. The axonal neuropathy theoretically should not affect neural synchrony in the VIIIth nerve. However, as the axon and its

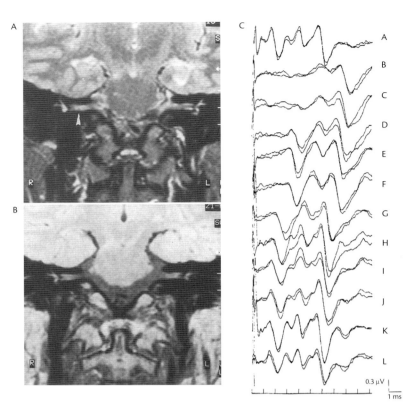

Fig. 10.8 (A) Coronal T$_2$ weighted MRI: mild enlargement of the right VIIIth nerve inside the internal auditory canal, and punctate area of hyperintense signal (arrow). (B) Coronal T2-weighted MRI: no lesion seen along the right VIIIth cranial nerve. (C) ABR recordings (rarefaction clicks, 65 dB SL (sensation level) intensity, 22.1 Hz frequency, C$_2$–A$_2$ electrodes) before (A), and after (B–L), right sudden hearing loss.

myelin sheath are so closely related, one cannot exist without the other, and an axonal neuropathy is often accompanied by signs of secondary demyelination, which would then be expected to impact on neural synchrony, as above.

Multiple sclerosis

The clinical diagnosis of multiple sclerosis (MS) rests upon the demonstration of two or more areas of demyelination in the central nervous system. Acoustic brainstem evoked response (ABR) audiometry has been used in patients presenting with a single lesion suggestive of MS, to detect other sites of demyelination. Wave V on the ABR trace is the most consistently abnormal wave in patients with MS and in approximately half of MS patients there is an ABR abnormality without clinical signs of brainstem MS. The presentation of multiple sclerosis with acute hearing loss is rare, and reported in only 1–3.5% of patients. Demyelinating lesions have been identified in the VIIIth nerve (Figure 10.8) (14), in the nerve root entry zone/cochlear nucleus, and in the pons.

Extrinsic and intrinsic tumours of the cerebellopontine angle

There are a number of tumours of the cerebellopontine angle (CPA) which can present with retrocochlear hearing loss and can be associated with vestibular dysfunction as a result of VIIIth nerve involvement: vestibular schwannoma (Figure 10.9) cerebellar medulloblastoma, neuroma, meningioma, cholesteatoma, ependymoma, jugular glomus tumour, and metastasis. In general, imaging will identify these tumours, and in the case of metastases, cerebrospinal fluid (CSF) lumbar puncture for cytological examination, or serological search for antineuronal antibodies (anti-ro,

anti-la, anti-RNP, anti-Jo-1, anti-SCL-70) will lead to the diagnosis. Cerebellar medulloblastomas are particularly common in childhood (25% of all intracranial neoplasia) where they tend to be midline, but in adulthood they tend to be located laterally and can present as CPA lesions.

Auditory processing disorders

Central auditory processing disorders (CAPDs) are neurological and thus beyond the remit of this chapter on otology, but suffice it to say that they are an important part of the differential diagnosis of hearing impairment. They may manifest in both children and adults with difficulties with recognition of words, environmental sounds or music, and with uncertainty about what the individual hears, despite the presence of normal hearing thresholds. Patients may experience difficulties listening in a background of noise or people conversing, difficulties in understanding degraded or rapid speech, following oral instructions, localizing sounds, or with the perception of music. They may also suffer from language and other disorders, professional and academic difficulties and behavioural, emotional, social, and other difficulties. The differential diagnosis is aided by a now well-recognized battery of specialist central auditory tests which allow further site of lesion identification in these disorders.

Conclusion

A detailed otological history, clinical assessment, and audiological test battery are the armamentarium of the neurologist faced with a patient with neuro-otological symptomatology. This chapter provides a framework for that otological assessment. An

Neurological ABR 2ch R-L

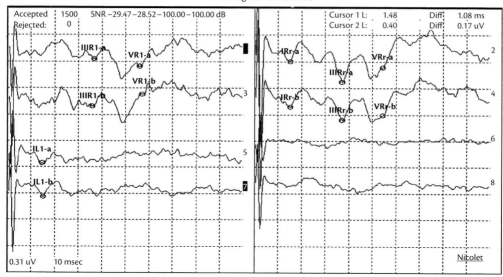

Fig. 10.9 Abnormal ABR found in a patient with a left vestibular schwannoma: the right ipsi- and contralaterally recorded ABRs demonstrate normal wave morphology with normal wave V latencies and wave I-V interwave intervals. On the left the waveforms beyond wave I on ipsilaterally recorded traces are absent, and no reproducible waveforms are seen on the contralaterally recorded traces.

anatomically-based classification can be used as an aide-memoire since the clinical presentation, the pattern of abnormalities on the auditory test battery, and likely aetiology, all vary according to the anatomical site of lesion. For detailed assessment and for the more complex patient, assistance can be sought from an audiovestibular physician, otorhinolaryngologist, or other clinician with a specialist interest in and access to audiovestibular testing.

References

1. British Society of Audiology (1981). Recommended procedures for pure tone audiometry using a manually operated instrument. *Br J Audiol*, 15, 213–16.

2. Davies RA (2003). Clinical assessment of hearing. In Luxon L (Ed) *Textbook of Audiological Medicine*, pp. 349–72. London: Martin Dunitz.

3. Kemp DT (1978). Stimulated acoustic emissions from within the human auditory system. *J Acoust Soc Am*, 64(5), 1386–91.

4. Van Camp G, Smith R (2011). Hereditary Hearing Loss Homepage. [Online] Available at http://hereditaryhearingloss.org.

5. Revised AAO-HNS guidelines (1995). Committee on Hearing and Equilibrium guidelines for the diagnosis and evaluation of therapy in Meniere's disease. *Otolaryngology Head and Neck Surgery*, 113, 181–5.

6. Andrews JC, Honrubia V (1996). Meniere's disease. In Baloh RW (Ed) *Disorders of the Vestibular System*, pp. 300–17. New York: Oxford University Press.

7. Overell J, Lindhall AA (2004). Neuro-otological syndromes for the neurologist. *J Neurol Neurosurg Psychiatry*, 75(suppl IV), 53–9.

8. Mccabe BF (1979). Auto-immune sensorineural hearing-loss. *Ann Otol Rhinol Laryngol*, 88(5), 585–9.

9. Schreiber BE, Agrup C, Haskard DO, Luxon LM (2010). Sudden sensorineural hearing loss. *Lancet*, 375(9721), 1203–11.

10. Hilger P, Paparella M, and Anderson RG (1984). Conductive hearing loss. In Meyerhoff WL (Ed) *Diagnosis and Management of Hearing Loss*, pp. 1–19. Philadelphia, PA: WB Saunders.

11. Davies RA (2004). Retrocochlear hearing disorders. In Gleeson M (Ed) *Scott Brown's Otolaryngology* (7th ed). London: Hodder.

12. Starr A, Sininger Y (2001). Preface. In Sininger Y, Starr A (Eds) *Auditory Neuropathy: A New Perspective on Hearing Disorders*, pp. ix–x. San Diego, CA: Singular.

13. Butinar D, Zidar J, Leonardis L, Popovic M, Kalaydjieva L, Angelicheva D, et al. Hereditary auditory, vestibular, motor and sensory neuropathy in a Slovenian Roma (Gypsy) kindred. *Ann Neurol*, 46, 36–44.

14. Bergamaschi R, Romani R, Zapoli, F, Versino M, Cosi C (1997). MRI and brainstem auditory evoked potential evidence of eighth cranial nerve involvement in multiple sclerosis. *Neurology*, 48, 270–2.

15. Ludman H (1998). Basic acoustics and hearing tests. In Ludman H, Wright T (Eds) *Diseases of the Ear* (6th ed), pp. 58–86. London: Arnold.

CHAPTER 11

Symptoms and Syndromes in the Patient with Dizziness or Unsteadiness

Adolfo M. Bronstein and Thomas Lempert

Symptoms in patients with balance disorders (see summary in Table 11.1)

Taking a good clinical history taking is the single most important component in the diagnosis of the dizzy and unsteady patient. Conditions such as benign paroxysmal positional vertigo (BPPV), vestibular neuritis, migrainous vertigo, Ménière's disease, vertebro-basilar transient ischaemic attacks (TIAs) and syncopal episodes are essentially diagnosed by the clinical history. The clinical and laboratory examinations will often confirm the diagnosis. In contrast, objective findings with no agreeing clinical history do not necessarily make a diagnosis of a disease. Neurological disorders of gait, which may present as unsteadiness or dizziness, such as cerebellar and Parkinsonian syndromes, can also be guessed from the history. Details of the symptoms of these disorders can be found in the specific sections of this book (see Chapter 9). Here we will present a description of the components that are common to several of these labyrinthine and neurological disorders and some practical help to differentiate them. In the second half of this chapter we will present a summary of the more frequent vestibular syndromes, namely the patient with a single acute vertigo attack, the patient with episodic dizziness or vertigo (including positional vertigo), and, finally, the patient with chronic symptoms of dizziness or unsteadiness.

Vertigo and dizziness

Vertigo is an illusion of movement. Rotational or 'true' vertigo, indicates disease of the semicircular canals or their central nervous system (CNS) connections. Patients with vertigo say that they themselves, or the room, spins around. When patients actually see the world spin around, it is very likely that they have nystagmus during the vertigo. Although some clinicians give less value to patients' reports of 'something spinning inside the head', patients with well-recognized vestibular disease such as BPPV can describe their vertigo in such way. Patients with 'true' vertigo usually have accompanying symptoms such as imbalance, unsteadiness, or veering of gait, nausea, and vomiting.

Dizziness and giddiness, are more difficult to define precisely both for patients and doctors alike. Other descriptions provided by patients are lightheadedness, feeling off balance, rocking sensations, 'walking on cotton wool'. They can indicate disease of the vestibular system, particularly in non-acute stages, but general medical (e.g. anaemia, hypoglycaemia, cardiac) or psychogenic disorders are also likely. It is useful to ask the patient to try to compare the symptom to anything that they may have experienced in everyday life. In doing so, patients often describe 'true' vertigo or vestibular mediated sensations, such as 'it's like the feeling one gets when lying down whilst drunk', or 'as coming off a merry-go-round', or 'on a boat on rough seas', or 'car sick'. Often, vague dizziness is a transitional state, between an acute vestibular episode and full recovery.

The diagnosis is often made not so much on the type or quality of the symptom, e.g. true vertigo as opposed to dizziness, but on its duration, presentation pattern, triggers, and accompanying symptoms as we will now see.

Duration: Vertigo duration is typically seconds in BPPV, hours in Ménière's disease (and some migraine patients), and days in vestibular neuritis. It is important to specify the duration of the actual rotational sensation or 'spinning' since patients tend to include the aftermath (malaise, nausea) in the total duration. This explains why so many patients with typical BPPV are adamant that their attacks last up to half an hour.

Presentation pattern: As soon as one sees a patient with dizziness it is critical to establish if the problem is: 1) a single, acute episode of vertigo, 2) recurrent or episodic vertigo, or 3) chronic sensations of unsteadiness or dizziness. The most frequent cause of single vertigo attack is vestibular neuritis; others are traumatic, infectious, ototoxic or vascular (peripheral or central) lesions. The one that needs to be ruled out is posterior fossa stroke (1). The most frequent causes of recurrent vertigo are BPPV and migrainous vertigo; others are Ménière's disease, vestibular paroxysms, vertebro-basilar TIAs, and episodic ataxias. Chronic dizziness can develop in any patient with difficulty in recovering fully from a single vertigo attack or from recurrent vertigo; other causes are general medical disorders, neurological gait disorders, or psychogenic dizziness.

Triggers: Of all possible triggers, head positioning is the most useful for diagnosis, but certain head positions are much more revealing than others. Given that the only way to achieve a new position of the head is by moving it and that the vestibular apparatus is the system specialized to detect head movements, it is hardly surprising that *any* change in position of the head will make *any* vestibular disorder worse. From this we can conclude that dizziness worsening on head movements is likely to be of vestibular origin. Therefore positional vertigo is not just getting dizzy on any head movement.

The specific situations that are useful for the diagnosis of positional vertigo, particularly BPPV, involve reorientation of the head with respect to the *gravity vector*. There are many instances involving such reorientation, for instance, looking up–down or standing up from the lying down position. However, the trigger situations most useful for diagnosing BPPV are lying down or turning over in bed. Patients with orthostatic blood pressure drops or neurological gait disorders report dizziness on standing up, but not on lying or turning over in bed. On the contrary, they feel better when getting in bed. A patient reporting dizziness on standing up from the sitting down position is more likely to have orthostatic hypotension than positional vertigo, since the head is not reoriented with respect to gravity from sitting to standing (Figure 11.1).

A common, related, misconception is that patients who report dizziness on moving the head suffer from poorly defined disorders such as 'vertebro-basilar insufficiency' or 'cervical vertigo'. Given that head movements are accomplished by neck movements, for the reasons outlined two paragraphs above, *most* vestibular disorders will become more symptomatic on neck movements. As a matter of fact, most patients referred to specialist dizzy clinics with provisional diagnoses of 'vertebro-basilar insufficiency' or 'cervical

vertigo' suffer from vestibular disorders. However, a few but well documented case reports of ischaemic induced vertigo brought about by vertebral artery occlusion during neck turning are available (3, 4). Usually a congenital hypoplasia of the other vertebral artery is present. 'Red flags' would be the fact that episodes tend to happen with head rotation whilst upright (unlike BPPV) and the presence of any associated aural or brainstem symptom. Detailed magnetic resonance angiography and/or angiography during neck movements are required. It has been estimated that, in highly specialized units, 15 such patients may be found in over 2000 cases of BPPV which points at the rarity of this condition (4).

There are other triggers which are very specific but rare, because the diseases they originate from are infrequent. Loud sounds and Valsalva manoeuvres can trigger vestibular symptoms (the Tullio phenomenon; see review (5)), including lateropulsion and oscillopsia, in the superior canal dehiscence syndrome. A labyrinthine fistula, with acute vertigo and unilateral deafness can be secondary to head trauma or strong Valsalva effort (e.g. heavy object lifting or cough attack). Alcohol or exercise can trigger vertigo in patients with episodic or paroxysmal ataxias.

Other triggers are encountered frequently but are not disease specific. In patients with chronic dizziness (secondary to previous or recurrent vestibular disorders), environments with repetitive visual patterns or visual motion can aggravate or trigger dizziness, sometimes called 'visual vertigo' (6) or visually-induced dizziness (7). In patients with psychogenic conditions, certain social situations or specific triggers (lifts, small rooms, airplanes) can trigger panic symptoms including dizziness.

Last but not least, one should enquire about common migraine triggers such as specific foods, e.g. association with chocolate or red wine ingestion, sleep deprivation, and the menstrual phase.

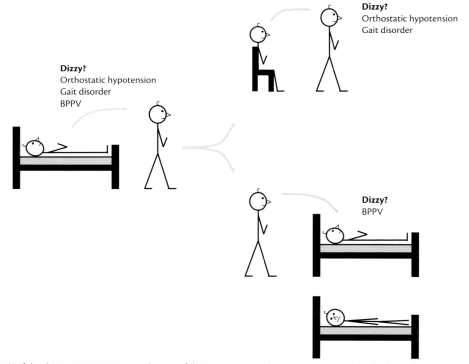

Fig 11.1 Differential diagnosis of the three more common syndromes of dizziness or unsteadiness on getting up from bed: gait disorders, orthostatic hypotension and BPPV. Adapted from Bronstein and Lempert (2).

Unsteadiness

During episodes of rotational vertigo patients are very unsteady. In acute and intense episodes, there is an irresistible tendency to fall in one direction, e.g. a BPPV episode whilst standing up ('hanging up clothes on the washing line'), the first day in vestibular neuritis, Ménière's attack, lateral medullary (Wallenberg) syndrome. Usually, this body lateropulsion is towards the hypoactive vestibular apparatus or nucleus but remember that BPPV and the initial phase of a Ménière's attack represent vestibular hyperactivity not hypoactivity. Extreme degrees of unsteadiness, where patients are physically unable to get out of bed to go to the toilet, are more suggestive of acute posterior circulation strokes.

A sense of lingering unsteadiness may persist in the chronic phase in most peripheral unilateral vestibular disorders. On specific questioning, however, most patients will acknowledge that this is only a subjective sensation and that friends, relatives, or colleagues have never noticed anything wrong.

Patients with bilateral vestibular disorders, when total or subtotal (see Chapter 26) report gait unsteadiness particularly when walking on irregular ground or in the dark. Note that bilateral vestibular failure can be insidious and idiopathic, so in a patient with unexplained gait unsteadiness always enquire about balance in the dark and about oscillopsia on walking (see later in chapter, and Chapters 13 and 26).

Patients with a variety of non-vestibular neurological disorders will report unsteadiness, sometimes leading to falls after trivial tripping over. The neurologist, but not necessarily ENT specialists will be familiar with these disorders. Except in cerebellar disease, where disordered cerebellar–vestibular interaction might provoke dizziness, most patients will acknowledge that there is no dizziness 'in the head' and that the trouble is 'in the legs'. So, specifically ask if the legs feel weak, heavy, clumsy, numb or with 'pins and needles' (see Chapter 9). Additional symptoms of sphincter dysfunction, memory loss, repetitive falls, vascular risk factors, or a family history of neurological disease can orient the diagnosis in the neurological direction.

Aural symptoms

It must be borne in mind that many common causes of vertigo do not produce hearing symptoms (e.g. BPPV, vestibular neuritis, migraine). Auditory symptoms helpful for diagnosis are not actually frequent in the clinic, except for Ménière's disease. Due to referral patterns, they are more conspicuous in ear, nose, and throat clinics than in neurology clinics.

In the emergency or acute admission wards, acute unilateral deafness in a patient with a first episode of vertigo should be taken very seriously. Severe cases of the peripheral condition called idiopathic sudden deafness can have vertigo; many specialists advocate acute steroid treatment so early diagnosis is important (8). The same applies for viral labyrinthitis, of known (e.g. mumps) or unknown aetiology. If the audio-vestibular symptoms develop after physical effort a labyrinthine fistula is almost certain and rest, observation and a possible middle ear exploration are indicated. These conditions are emergencies with respect to the outcome of the hearing loss. In contrast, a posterior circulation vascular episode giving rise to acute unilateral deafness (9), typically the anterior inferior cerebellar artery ('AICA') syndrome, has all the

potential life-threatening implications of any stroke. These vascular episodes usually add pathognomonic brainstem symptoms (diplopia, ataxia, numbness) but these should be actively elicited as patients can be overwhelmed by the vertigo and ignore the deafness or facial tingling.

Fluctuating aural pressure, tinnitus and hearing loss is reported in patients with Ménière's disease. However, it must be stressed that in an unselected clinical environment Ménière's disease is rare (10). In the context of repetitive vertebrobasilar TIA episodes patients may have tinnitus or hearing loss together with other brainstem symptoms. The presence of phono- (and photo-) phobia is useful for the diagnosis of migraine related vertigo. Although acoustic neuromas and other tumours usually do not cause vertigo or major unsteadiness, the presence of unilateral progressive tinnitus and deafness should raise a red flag.

Trivial and age-related aural symptoms are very common in the general population. When patients report that 'My wife/husband says that I put the TV too loud'; 'Yes, when I am quietly in bed I can hear a hissing sound in my ears' audiological investigations are usually unrevealing (but reassuring nevertheless). The label of Ménière's disease is so often stuck to the patient with vertigo and unrelated hearing symptoms such as presbycusis that one should refrain from suggesting this diagnosis to the patient until specialist investigations are completed.

Less frequent symptoms: disequilibrium, oscillopsia, brainstem symptoms, and loss of consciousness

Disequilibrium

Patients with balance disorders can be unsteady objectively ('they look unsteady') and subjectively ('they feel unsteady'). Patients with residual vestibular symptoms or patients with psychogenic dizziness can feel subjectively unsteady with no evidence from doctors, relatives, or colleagues that they are. Some patients with objective balance problems due to CNS disease may superficially describe the sensation that their balance is not right as dizziness. More commonly, however, patients who are objectively unsteady deny 'head' sensations such as dizziness, vertigo, or 'about to faint' feelings. This is called disequilibrium. When presented with the question 'Is the problem in the head or the legs?' patients with disequilibrium tend to acknowledge the latter. These patients may have a neurological disorder of gait including weakness, spasticity, numbness, slowness, shakiness, or incoordination of the legs due to lesions almost anywhere in the peripheral or central nervous system; some examples are polyneuropathy, spinal cord, brainstem, cerebellar, or hemispheric lesion, hydrocephalus, small-vessel white matter disease, parkinsonian or other movement disorders. Patients may have falls, indeed these are more common in patients with disequilibrium than in vestibular patients. The neurological and neuro-otological examination (in particular, abnormal eye movements and gait), will usually identify the non-peripheral vestibular origin of the problem (see Chapter 12). In essence, if a patient has normal gait (including gait with eyes open, closed, and tandem heel-to-toe) and normal eye movements it is unlikely that his/her unsteadiness is due to a neurological problem. Some of the neurological disorders causing disequilibrium and falls are reviewed in Chapter 9.

Visual symptoms

The main visual symptoms that can be associated with disorders of balance are diplopia, oscillopsia as well as photophobia and other migrainous phenomena. In addition some patients with vestibular disorders describe worsening or triggering of their dizziness in disorienting visual surroundings, a phenomenon called visual vertigo or visually-induced dizziness (see Chapter 13).

The presence of double vision in a patient with vertigo is worrying, particularly if the vertigo is acute, as these two symptoms combined are strongly suggestive of brainstem disease. Patients should be scanned by magnetic resonance imaging (MRI). Possible diagnoses, from the most acute to the slowly progressive conditions, are: posterior fossa stroke, inflammatory disease (demyelinating, vasculitis, viral encephalitis), extra axial (large acoustic neuroma), and intrinsic brainstem tumours. Occasionally, a patient with a large and acute peripheral unilateral vestibular lesion may report diplopia due to a degree of skew eye deviation (11) but this diagnosis must be reached after excluding brainstem lesions.

Oscillopsia is the illusion that the visual world is moving or oscillating. It must be mentioned that the specific illusion that the visual environment is rotating is usually called vertigo (or 'objective vertigo', as opposed to the illusion of self rotation or 'subjective' vertigo) but in German speaking countries it may be called oscillopsia. In Chapter 13 an approach to the differential diagnosis of oscillopsia is presented. Essentially, oscillopsia brought about by head movements indicates problems with the vestibulo-ocular reflex (VOR) whereas oscillopsia at rest is due to different forms of nystagmus. Hence, always ask your patient *when* the oscillopsia occurs.

Photophobia and migrainous symptoms

Patients with migraine report being bothered by loud sounds, strong smells, self- and visual movement, and, particularly, bright lights. This photophobia is what often takes patients to their bedrooms where they draw the curtains and lie down quietly in the dark. These 'phobias' are thought to represent cortical hyperexcitability to sensory stimuli which to a lesser extent is also present outside the migraine attack (12). The latter could also account for the increased motion sickness sensitivity observed in patients with migraine.

Visual auras are the more commonly observed just before a migrainous headache. Zig-zag lines, shimmering phosphenes, and scintillating scotomas, lasting 5–60 minutes, are well-recognized features even by the general public.

The presence of visual auras, photo-, and other sensory phobias should be actively enquired by the doctor in all patients with recurrent vertigo or dizziness. This is an important marker pointing at migraine as the most likely aetiology of such recurrent vestibular syndromes, indistinctly called migrainous vertigo or vestibular migraine. However, it must be borne in mind that vertigo can also trigger migraine in susceptible patients and it is not uncommon to see patients develop migrainous headaches and photophobia *after* a vertigo attack due to structural vestibular disease. Thus it is important to establish the chronology of headache, photophobia and dizziness as this may hold the key as to whether the vertigo is caused by migraine or vertigo has caused migraine (13). Finally, patients with the condition called basilar artery migraine have a more florid brainstem–occipital syndrome which may include vertigo, diplopia, facial paraesthesia, bilateral visual loss, and somnolence.

Brainstem symptoms

The presence of brainstem and cerebellar symptoms is the rule in patients with vertigo or imbalance due to vertebrobasilar strokes, TIAs, multiple sclerosis, or tumours. They include double vision, speech, limb or gait ataxia, swallowing difficulty, and facial numbness or weakness. The time course and presentation is directly related to the underlying disease, brief episodic in TIAs, relapsing–remitting in multiple sclerosis, progressive in tumours, and acute in strokes. Although the additional symptoms and signs in these conditions makes confusion with a vestibular disorder unlikely, acute small lesions in the intra-axial portion of the VIII nerve, vestibular nuclei or cerebellum can mimic the picture of a vestibular neuritis (14, 15). In vestibular neuritis, nystagmus and lateropulsion are expected. If in addition the eye movement examination is not quite normal, or if in doubt for any other reason, neuroimaging is warranted.

Loss of consciousness and fainting feelings

Loss of consciousness is rare amongst dizzy patients, except when the cause is haemodynamic. Thus, patients with syncope due to cardiac arrhythmia, vaso-vagal reactions, or autonomic nervous system disorders with orthostatic hypotension (pure autonomic failure, multiple system atrophy, polyneuropathy) often report dizziness or vertigo before they pass out. It is therefore important to enquire about previous heart history, palpitations, and tightness in the chest which would point to a heart disorder. Carotid sinus hypersensitivity can cause fainting during neck turns or compression. Needless to say that in the presence of these symptoms priority should be given to cardiological rather than neuro-otological investigations. However, always bear in mind that heart and vestibular disorders are very common and patients can have both.

Sweating, hot or cold bodily sensations, clammy hands, bilateral tinnitus, and 'greying out' of vision are reported by patients with hypotensive episodes as in vaso-vagal syncope and orthostatic hypotension. Witness can report that patients look pale, or the opposite, red and blushed, during the faints. Typically, patients regain consciousness within seconds of falling or lying down as brain irrigation is restored. With repeated episodes many patients learn to recognize the trigger situations and prevent the episodes by lying down or sitting with their heads lowered between their legs. Such situations can include hot and stuffy rooms, cognitive triggers (e.g. sight of blood), trivial pain, standing upright quickly or for long periods of time. Many patients only report dizziness and the accompanying symptoms described here, but do not faint. These presyncopal syndromes are difficult to diagnose, even with formal autonomic function tests. The clinician should therefore enquire actively about trigger situations, previous history of fainting episodes, and whether lying down has any beneficial effect.

Patients with hypoglycaemia, due to medication in diabetic patients or, more rarely, insulin-secreting tumours, can be dizzy and pass out. Most diabetic patients recognize this and can prevent the loss of consciousness with appropriate foods. Most patients with actual loss of consciousness would have been taken to a hospital emergency service and blood glucose measured but, if in doubt, measure it again.

Vestibular epilepsy is a not-well-defined entity. Since the work of Penfield, working with direct electrical stimulation of the cortex in awake patients, we know that rotational vertigo can be elicited by activation of the temporal lobe. We also know that isolated cases

Table 11.1 Symptoms in the dizzy patient

Symptom	Interpretation
Rotational vertigo	Semicircular canals or their central connections
Dizziness–giddiness	Vestibular, cardiovascular, metabolic, or psychological disorder
Duration	Seconds: BPPV, cardiac arrhythmia,
	Minutes: TIA, panic attacks
	Hours: migraine, Ménière's disease
	Days: vestibular neuritis
Dizziness presentation: (see Tables 11.2–11.5)	Single episode
	Recurrent vertigo and dizziness
	Chronic dizziness
Dizziness triggers	Standing up: orthostatic hypotension
	Lying down and turning in bed: BPPV
	Sleep deprivation: migrainous vertigo
	Situational triggers (supermarkets, crowds): visual vertigo, panic attacks
Other and associated symptoms	Fluctuating aural pressure and tinnitus: Ménière's disease
	Hearing loss: pan labyrinthitis, AICA infarct (with ataxia), Ménière's disease
	Migraine features: migrainous vertigo, basilar migraine
	V, VI, VII, long tracts: brainstem disorder, e.g. TIA, demyelination
	Leg weakness/incoordination: neurological gait disorders (e.g. cerebellar)
	Oscillopsia (see Chapter 13):
	Movement related: bilateral vestibular disorder
	Spontaneous: central nystagmus (e.g. downbeat nystagmus)
	Loss of consciousness: cardiac arrhythmia, vaso-vagal syncope

All tables modified from Bronstein and Lempert (2).

of acute vascular lesions of the temporal cortex producing vertigo have been reported and that patients with epilepsy can include brief vertigo in their aura. However, recurrent vertigo, without other epileptic phenomena, is not likely to be due to epilepsy. The term vestibular paroxysm or paroxysmia (Chapter 19) implies brief episodes of vertigo and/or oscillopsia due to irritation of the vestibular nerve or nuclei in the brainstem, and these patients do not lose consciousness.

Finally, some patients occasionally report that, during the intense vertigo in the acute phase of a vestibular neuritis or Ménière's disease, they 'think' they passed out. It is very difficult to know exactly what happens in these circumstances but one suspects that the combination of a new terrifying symptom, perhaps aggravated by panic or dehydration if vomiting has occurred, or syncope in the patient with a propensity, may be at play. When witnesses are available, they usually describe that communication with the patient was precarious but possible, indicating that no complete loss of consciousness was present.

Overview and summary of vestibular syndromes
See Tables 11.1 to 11.6.

Common dizziness and vertigo syndromes

In the following, we will delineate vertigo and dizziness syndromes according to their clinical presentation. This approach corresponds to clinical reasoning because the recognition of a characteristic presentation narrows the differential diagnosis down to a handful of common conditions. Identification of anatomical syndromes (e.g. unilateral loss of vestibular function or cerebellar syndrome) represents a step further ahead on the diagnostic path and will be discussed in the respective chapters of this volume.

Acute prolonged vertigo
This clinical pattern is usually encountered in the emergency room. Most patients present with a first episode of vertigo which persists at the time of examination. Decision-making is both difficult and critical in this situation, because there is no previous history to rely on and benign conditions, such as vestibular neuritis and vestibular migraine, have to be separated from serious disorders, such as brainstem or cerebellar stroke. Meticulous examination, particularly clinical VOR testing and the search for gaze-evoked nystagmus and skew deviation, will help to identify the latter (1; see Chapter 23). The most common causes of acute prolonged vertigo are listed in Table 11.2.

Other causes: perilymph fistula, labyrinthine infarction, bacterial labyrinthitis, drug/alcohol toxicity.

Recurrent vertigo and dizziness
Patients with recurrent vertigo and dizziness usually present in the symptom-free interval. Therefore, both clinical examination and vestibular testing is often negative. Diagnosis depends critically on accurate history taking, including attack duration and frequency, provoking factors and accompanying symptoms. Recurrent vertigo and dizziness are discussed separately, as they can be usually distinguished on the basis of the patient's account and reflect different pathophysiological mechanisms. The international classification of vestibular symptoms defines vertigo as the sensation of self-motion when no self motion is occurring or the false sensation that the visual surround is spinning or flowing. In contrast, dizziness is defined as the sensation of disturbed or impaired spatial orientation without a false or distorted sense of motion (7, see Chapter 16). As mentioned earlier, usually vertigo reflects a vestibular disturbance and dizziness a non-vestibular disorder. However, there

Table 11.2 Acute prolonged vertigo

Disorder	Key features
Vestibular neuritis	Acute onset of vertigo, nausea and imbalance. Spontaneous nystagmus towards healthy ear, unilateral VOR failure on head impulse testing, falls toward affected side. Improvement over days to weeks
Acute brainstem or cerebellar lesion (e.g. stroke, demyelination)	Vertigo with brainstem or cerebellar signs, particularly ocular motor abnormalities. Variable time course. MRI usually shows lesion affecting central vestibular pathways
First attack of vestibular migraine	Acute vertigo may last for days. Mostly central types of vestibular nystagmus and ataxia. History of migraine and often migrainous features during attack
First attack of Ménière's disease	Vertigo lasting hours may be isolated symptom in early Ménière's disease. Otherwise associated hearing loss, tinnitus and aural fullness

Table 11.3 Differential diagnosis of recurrent vertigo

Disorder	Key features
Vestibular migraine	Attacks of spontaneous or positional vertigo lasting minutes to days, history of migraine, migrainous symptoms during vertigo, migraine-specific precipitants provoking vertigo
Ménière's disease	Vertigo attacks lasting 20 min to several hours with concurrent hearing loss, tinnitus, and aural fullness. Progressive hearing loss over years
Vertebrobasilar TIA	Attacks of vertigo lasting minutes, often accompanied by ataxia, dysarthria, diplopia, or visual field defects, elderly patients with vascular risk factors
Vestibular paroxysmia (Vascular compression of the VIIIth nerve?)	Brief attacks (seconds) of vertigo several times per day with or without cochlear symptoms, response to carbamazepine
Perilymph fistula	Vertigo after head trauma, barotrauma, stapedectomy or provoked by coughing, sneezing, straining or loud sounds. Symptom duration variable

Table 11.4 Differential diagnosis of recurrent dizziness

Disorder	Key features
Orthostatic hypotension	Brief episodes of dizziness lasting seconds (to minutes) after standing up. Relieved by sitting/ lying down. Drop of systolic blood pressure of ≥20 mm after standing up
Cardiac arrhythmia	Dizziness lasting seconds. May be accompanied by palpitations. Can be caused by bradycardia <40/s or tachycardia >170/s
Psychogenic dizziness	Variable duration from minutes to permanent. Usually related to anxiety or depression. Often provoked by specific situations such as leaving the house, riding on buses or driving, height, crowds, lifts. Accompanied by choking, palpitations, tremor, heat, anxiety
Drug induced dizziness	Variable clinical presentation according to pharmacologic mechanism: sedation, vestibular suppression, ototoxicity, cerebellar toxicity, orthostatic hypotension, hypoglycaemia

are many exceptions to this rule, e.g. mild vestibular disturbance causing a giddy rather than spinning sensation. The differential diagnosis of the common causes of recurrent vertigo and recurrent dizziness is outlined in Tables 11.3 and 11.4.

Other causes of recurrent vertigo: autoimmune inner ear disease, syphilis of the inner ear, schwannoma of the 8th nerve, vestibular epilepsy, insufficient compensation of unilateral vestibular loss, otosclerosis, Paget's disease, episodic ataxia type 2.

Other causes of recurrent dizziness: sleep drunkenness, hypertension, metabolic disorders, height vertigo.

Positional vertigo

Identification of positional vertigo is straightforward from the history when the patient reports typical provoking situations such as lying down, turning over in bed, getting up from lying down, or reaching for a high shelf (see Chapter 20). However, positional vertigo can be overlooked when an elderly patient gives an imprecise account of his or her symptoms. Also, positional vertigo can be just one of several types of vertigo, e.g. in patients with vestibular migraine or when vestibular neuritis is complicated by subsequent BPPV. Table 11.5 lists common disorders causing positional vertigo.

Other causes: positional alcohol vertigo and nystagmus, perilymphatic fistula, macroglobulinaemia, amiodarone toxicity.

Chronic dizziness

Few disorders cause true chronic dizziness as most vestibular disorders manifest with attacks and because even permanent damage to the labyrinth is compensated by brain mechanisms. Neurological disorders that affect balance will cause symptoms when patients are standing or walking, but not when they are sitting or lying. Whenever a patient comes in and starts with 'Doctor, I am always dizzy' a clarification is necessary. Chronic unsteadiness affects mostly elderly patients and can be diagnosed by a standard neurological examination (Chapter 9) plus VOR clinical testing for detection of bilateral vestibulopathy. Computed tomography or MRI scans may be required for confirmation of normal pressure hydrocephalus, cerebral small-vessel disease,

Table 11.5 Disorders causing positional vertigo

Disorder	Key features
Posterior canal benign paroxysmal positional vertigo (PC-BPPV) (>70% of all positional vertigo)	Brief attacks (<30 s), provoked by turning in bed, lying down, sitting up from lying, head extension or bending over. Symptomatic episodes for weeks to months, remissions for years. Mainly torsional nystagmus toward the ground in lateral head-hanging position
Horizontal canal benign paroxysmal positional vertigo (20% of all positional vertigo)	Attacks mainly provoked by turning in bed. Usually alternates with episodes of PC-BPPV. Transient horizontal nystagmus toward the ground in either head lateral position (rare variants may show nystagmus away from the ground)
Migrainous vertigo	May present with predominant positional vertigo. History of migraine. Migrainous features during vertigo. Symptomatic episodes from minutes to days. Almost any type of nystagmus possible
Central positional vertigo	Duration of single attacks, provoking positions and nystagmus variable. Additional brainstem or cerebellar signs possible. May mimic single features of BPPV but not the whole syndrome
Disabling positional vertigo: vascular compression of the VIIIth nerve?	Brief attacks (seconds to minutes) of positional/spontaneous vertigo many times per day. Relief with carbamazepine

Table 11.6 Causes of chronic dizziness and unsteadiness

Disorder	Key features
Psychiatric dizziness syndromes	Constant dull or floating sensation. Occurs mostly with depressive syndromes, generalized anxiety disorders, or hypochondria. May superimpose organic vestibular disorder. Elderly fallers may develop gait disorder from fear of falling
Chronic vestibular migraine	Permanently enhanced sensitivity to head motion or visual motion in addition to attacks of spontaneous and positional vertigo. Psychiatric comorbidity common
Drug-induced dizziness	Permanent, fluctuating or episodic dizziness caused by various mechanisms: sedation, vestibular suppression, ototoxicity, cerebellar toxicity, orthostatic hypotension, hypoglycaemia
Effects of physiological aging	Chronic dizziness and imbalance due to age-related decline of vestibular, somatosensory, visual and motor function
Neurological disease	May cause dizziness and imbalance when sensory and motor systems are affected, e.g. by polyneuropathy, myelopathy, Parkinson's disease, cerebellar disease, cerebral small-vessel disease, normal pressure hydrocephalus
Bilateral vestibulopathy	Oscillopsia during head movements, imbalance in darkness. Bilateral VOR deficit on head impulse testing
Orthopaedic disorders	Hip, knee, and foot problems before and after surgery

or cervical spondylogenic myelopathy (see Chapter 24). Causes of chronic dizziness and unsteadiness are listed in Table 11.6.

References

1. Kattah JC, Talkad AV, Wang DZ, et al. (2009). HINTS to diagnose stroke in acute vestibular syndrome: three-step bedside oculomotor examination more sensitive than early MRI diffusion-weighted imaging. *Stroke*, 40, 3504–10.

2. Bronstein AM, Lempert T (2007). *Dizziness: A Practical Approach to Diagnosis and Management* (Cambridge Clinical Guides). Cambridge: Cambridge University Press.

3. Brandt T, Baloh RW (2005). Rotational vertebral artery occlusion: a clinical entity or various syndromes? *Neurology*, 65(8), 1156–7.

4. Noh Y, Kwon OK, Kim HJ, Kim JS (2011). Rotational vertebral artery syndrome due to compression of nondominant vertebral artery terminating in posterior inferior cerebellar artery. *J Neurol*, 258(10), 1775–80.

5. Kaski D, Davies R, Luxon L, Bronstein AM, Rudge P (2012). The Tullio phenomenon: a neurologically neglected presentation. *J Neurol*, 259, 4–21.

6. Bronstein AM (1995). Visual vertigo syndrome: clinical and posturography findings. *J Neurol Neurosurg Psychiatry*, 59(5), 472–6.

7. Bisdorff A, Von Brevern M, Lempert T, Newman-Toker DE (2009). Classification of vestibular symptoms: towards an international classification of vestibular disorders. *J Vestib Res*, 19(1–2), 1–13.

8. Labus J, Breil J, Stützer H, Michel O (2012). Meta-analysis for the effect of medical therapy vs. placebo on recovery of idiopathic sudden hearing loss. *Laryngoscope*, 120(9), 1863–71.

9. Mort DJ, Bronstein AM (2006). Sudden deafness. *Curr Opin Neurol*, 19(1), 1–3.

10. Alexander TH, Harris JP (2012). Current epidemiology of Meniere's syndrome. *Otolaryngol Clin North Am*, 43(5), 965–70.

11. Bronstein AM (2002). Under-rated neuro-otological symptoms: Hoffman and Brookler 1978 revisited. *Br Med Bull*, 63, 213–21.

12. van der Kamp W, Maassen VanDenBrink A, Ferrari MD, van Dijk JG (1996). Interictal cortical hyperexcitability in migraine patients demonstrated with transcranial magnetic stimulation. *J Neurol Sci*, 139, 106–10.

13. Murdin L, Davies RA, Bronstein AM (2009). Vertigo as a migraine trigger. *Neurology*, 73(8), 638–42.

14. Francis DA, Bronstein AM, Rudge P, du Boulay EP (1992). The site of brainstem lesions causing semicircular canal paresis: an MRI study. *J Neurol Neurosurg Psychiatry*, 55(6), 446–9.

15. Kim HA, Lee H (2012). Isolated vestibular nucleus infarction mimicking acute peripheral vestibulopathy. *Stroke*, 41(7), 1558–60.

CHAPTER 12

Clinical Bedside Examination

Amir Kheradmand, Adolfo Bronstein, and David S. Zee

The evaluation of patients with dizziness and imbalance is always challenging and often frustrating for patient and physician, but recent advances in both bedside and laboratory examinations have made outcomes more successful and gratifying. In this chapter we emphasize how to apply the latest physiological advances into practical bedside examination techniques that allow us to probe the function of individual components within the labyrinth. When coupled with laboratory testing of saccule function with cervical vestibular-evoked myogenic potentials (cVEMPs), utricular function with ocular vestibular-evoked myogenic potentials (oVEMPs), and lateral canal function with caloric irrigations, one can now test each of the vestibular end organs in isolation.

Taking the history from the dizzy patient is described in detail in Chapter 11. Here we address a few cardinal points and remind the reader that, like the bedside examination, the history probes the symptoms of the dizzy or imbalanced patient in the context of the functional requirements of the vestibular reflexes that help to maintain clear vision and stable posture.

Dizziness is a loosely used term and means different things to different people. It may describe sensations from a vestibular system gone awry, in which case there is often a component of movement. But it is also used to describe feeling faint, confused, unsteady, disconnected, anxious, or other discomforting sensations which can arise from nonvestibular causes such as cardiac, metabolic, and psychiatric disturbances. Likewise, alteration in visual and proprioceptive inputs as well as poor central integration of sensory signals can lead to symptoms described as dizziness. Recent research has emphasized that what patients mean by dizziness is often less reliable for diagnosis than what triggers or exacerbates their abnormal sensations and how long they last (1). A focused history and physical examination in a dizzy patient should address the following questions:

- Does the dizziness reflect an abnormality within the vestibular system including the more central areas of the brain that receive and process information from the labyrinth, or a more general medical cause such as: 1) hypoperfusion due to postural hypotension or cardiac arrhythmias, 2) metabolic causes such as hypoglycaemia, hypoxia, or hypercarbia, 3) side effects of medications, or 4) psychogenic factors, either primary, such as somatoform or panic disorders or secondary, such as phobias, anxiety, or depression due to longstanding vestibular dysfunction?

- If the symptoms suggest a vestibular aetiology, is it due to a peripheral problem in the labyrinth or VIIIth nerve, or to a central problem in the vestibular nuclei, vestibulocerebellum, or other parts of the brain that process vestibular information?

- If the symptoms are peripheral in aetiology, do they reflect an abnormality in processing of information from semicircular canals (SCCs) which can produce a sense of rotation of either the self or of the environment, or from the otolith organs which can produce a sense of tilt, translation, or vertical diplopia?

Physical examination

A careful 'bedside' clinical examination is vital for localizing and diagnosing the underlying cause of dizziness or imbalance, and becomes especially important when symptoms are vague or do not fall into easily recognized diagnostic categories. A comprehensive examination includes assessment of visual, vestibular, and ocular motor function as well as coordination, gait, and balance.

In this chapter, the ocular motor and vestibular examination at the bedside will be presented in the order in which they can be performed efficiently (Table 12.1). Although not reviewed here, a general physical and neurological examination including particular attention to all the cranial nerves is a must when evaluating a patient with dizziness or imbalance. It is also essential to measure the blood pressure both lying and standing in every patient as dizziness is a common complaint associated with orthostatic hypotension.

Physiological principles underlying the bedside examination

First we review important physiological properties that will guide the examination:

- Two fundamental reflexes assure clear vision during head motion. The rotational vestibulo-ocular reflex (VOR) produces an eye movement (the slow phase) that compensates for head rotation. The VOR stabilizes gaze when the head is rotated around the horizontal (yaw), torsional (roll), or vertical (pitch) axes. The translational vestibulo-ocular reflex (tVOR) produces a slow phase that compensates for head translation. The tVOR stabilizes gaze when the head is translated along the side-to-side (interaural), fore and aft (anterior–posterior), or up and down (vertical) axes. Both the VOR and the tVOR are

Table 12.1 Suggested order of ocular examination

Vision
Visual acuity with correction (monocular and binocular)
Dynamic visual acuity with head shaking
Pupil size and light reflex
Confrontational visual fields
Colour vision especially if an optic neuropathy is suspected
Binocular vision (stereopsis) especially if there is diplopia or ocular misalignment
Subjective visual vertical (bucket method)

Ophthalmoscopy
Nystagmus (occlusive ophthalmoscopy)
Ocular torsion
VOR

Ocular alignment
Range of motion (duction, version)
Symmetry of corneal reflex (Hirschberg test)
Cover testing
Red glass or Maddox rod

Gaze holding
Straight ahead fixation
Eye closure
Eccentric fixation (horizontal and vertical)

Eye movements
Convergence
Saccades (horizontal, vertical, diagonal)
Pursuit and VOR cancellation (horizontal, vertical)
OKN (horizontal, vertical)
Rotational VOR with slow passive head rotation (horizontal, vertical)
Rotational VOR with head impulse: horizontal and vertical (RALP, LARP)
Translational VOR or head heave

Provocative manoeuvres (Frenzel goggles)
Tragal compression
Valsalva (closed glottis, pinched nostrils)
Head shaking
Vibration (mastoid tips, vertex)
Hyperventilation (30–60 s)
Positional testing

LARP, left anterior, right posterior canals; RALP, right anterior, left posterior canals.

evaluated at the bedside by the amplitude and direction of eye motion relative to the motion of the head. Both the amplitude and direction are judged by the presence and direction of corrective saccades made during or after motion of the head to restore fixation on a stationary target.

- When the head of a healthy individual is still, the left and right vestibular nerves and the neurons to which they project to in the vestibular nuclei have equal resting discharge rates (vestibular tone). Movement of the head toward one side excites that labyrinth and inhibits the other. If the tone becomes relatively less on one side, for example, from a naturally occurring lesion or a simulated lesion as with a cold water caloric irrigation, a spontaneous nystagmus develops with slow phases directed toward, and quick phases directed away from the 'lesioned' side.

- The intensity of nystagmus usually depends on the position of the eye in the orbit. Nystagmus arising from a peripheral vestibular lesion is more intense (slow-phase velocity higher, usually with more frequent quick phases) or may only be evident when gaze is pointed in the direction of the quick phase (Alexander's law). With central lesions, for example, in the cerebellum or brainstem, the opposite may occur.

- The vestibular response to static tilts of the head is rudimentary in intact humans, largely because we are foveate and frontal-eyed which is optimal for high central acuity and stereopsis. The orientation of the fovea, for example, is little affected by static lateral head tilt (ear to shoulder), and in the case of static pitch forward (nose down) or backward (nose up) saccades can reorient the line of sight. Nevertheless, with disturbances in the otolith pathways, e.g. in Wallenberg syndrome or internuclear ophthalmoplegia (INO), a phylogenetically-old pattern of eye deviation to lateral tilt may emerge. Recall that in intact lateral-eyed animals the response to a lateral tilt of the body is a 'righting reflex' comprised of a compensatory tilt of the head toward the opposite (higher) ear and a readjustment of the vertical alignment of the eyes (physiological skew deviation), in which case the eye in the relatively lower orbit (lower ear) elevates and the eye in the higher orbit (upper ear) depresses. In pathological circumstances with an otolith imbalance in humans the ocular tilt reaction (OTR) emerges as if there is a compensatory response to a lateral head tilt. The OTR is analogous to the slow-phase response when there is an imbalance between the semicircular canals of the two labyrinths. The OTR consists of a lateral head tilt, vertical misalignment of the eyes (skew deviation with the eye being higher in the higher orbit), and ocular counter-roll (torsion of both eyes with the top poles rotating toward the side of lower eye) with a consequent tilt of the visual world.

- Disease can also lead to a dynamic imbalance during head rotation or translation producing a directional asymmetry during head movements that is superimposed on any imbalance in vestibular tone (Table 12.2). An example is Ewald's second law: excitatory stimuli produce a relatively greater vestibular response than inhibitory stimuli. This is best appreciated with high-acceleration, high-velocity, and high-frequency stimuli. Thus, in the case of a unilateral loss of labyrinthine function a greater response is elicited with rotation toward the intact side than toward the lesioned side. This can be detected at the bedside by performing brief, high-acceleration head rotations called head impulses. Similarly, a dynamic otolith imbalance can be elicited by brief, high-acceleration head translations called head heaves (both discussed later in this chapter).

- An important property of the vestibular nuclei is to improve the ability of the brain to faithfully sense low-frequency head motion, for example, when the rotation is prolonged and at a relatively unchanging speed. In other words, the vestibular nuclei improve upon the inherently unreliable low-frequency VOR response that is dictated by the physical properties of the cupula and endolymph. This central phenomenon, called 'velocity storage', extends the range of patterns of head motion that are accurately sensed by the brain. Velocity storage is important for understanding the significance and mechanism of post head-shaking nystagmus which will be discussed later in this chapter.

Table 12.2 Vestibular abnormalities

Static vestibular imbalance	
Canal-ocular	Spontaneous nystagmus
Otolith-ocular	Skew deviation
Dynamic vestibular imbalance	
Canal-ocular (rotational) or otolith-ocular(translational) VOR	Abnormal amplitude or direction

General features

The general appearance of the patient may yield diagnostic information. Usually, the acutely vertiginous patient will lie on one side with the affected ear uppermost. This position increases an inhibitory otolith influence upon the lowermost intact ear and will reduce any spontaneous horizontal nystagmus caused by the tone imbalance between the lateral semicircular canals in each labyrinth (2, 3). An abnormal tilt of the head when sitting suggests an OTR which reflects an imbalance in the otolith pathway. The head tilt can be toward or away from the side of the lesion depending upon the location of the lesion. Peripheral vestibular damage or lesions within the medulla or caudal pons (typically within the vestibular nuclei) cause a head tilt toward the affected side, and lesions within the rostral pons and midbrain (commonly in the medial longitudinal fasciculus (MLF)) usually cause a head tilt away from the affected side (4). Patients with a trochlear nerve palsy also commonly tilt their head, usually away from the side of the paretic eye. Other general findings may include lid nystagmus (e.g. with lesions in the medulla), lid-opening apraxia (e.g. in progressive supranuclear palsy), and facial synkineses due to aberrant regeneration following a lesion involving the facial nerve. Ptosis and a small pupil are signs of sympathetic defects (as in Wallenberg syndrome when the anisocoria is greater in dim illumination) or parasympathetic defects (as in an oculomotor palsy when the anisocoria is greater in bright illumination).

Vision

The vestibular and visual systems work together to keep objects in focus and stable on the retina (Chapter 13). Changes in different aspects of visual function including visual acuity, visual field, colour vision, and stereopsis can provide helpful clues to the primary source of symptoms in patients with dizziness. The best corrected visual acuity at distance (using corrective lenses or a pinhole) is measured using an acuity chart with each eye viewing alone. Testing of the visual fields by confrontation is a rapid screening though insensitive method for visual field defects. Binocular vision can be evaluated using stereoscopic acuity with the Titmus optical sterero-fly or Randot strereo tests especially when ocular misalignment is though to have its onset early in life. Colour vision can be assessed with Hardy–Rand–Rittler plates to screen for optic neuropathy (e.g. in patients with INO or monocular or asymmetrical pendular nystagmus).

Measures of visual acuity with the head moving (dynamic visual acuity (DVA)) are essential in patients with dizziness. Indeed the raison d'etre of the VOR is to see clearly when moving. Patients may complain of oscillopsia, an illusion of visual motion often described as blurred, jumping, or 'wobbly' vision. The vestibular system is usually involved when oscillopsia is brought on or exacerbated by motion of the head. DVA is measured by asking the patient to read the optotypes of a visual acuity chart with the head moving. The examiner first measures acuity with the head still (usually with both eyes viewing the target unless there is ocular misalignment when one eye should be covered) and then oscillates the head horizontally, vertically, and in the roll plane from ear to shoulder at a relatively high frequency of about two cycles per second. At this frequency visual tracking systems are too sluggish to contribute to gaze stability, and therefore the function of the VOR can be assessed acting alone. While oscillating the head, the patient should not be allowed to stop or slow down too much at the turnaround points to 'sneak' a look at the acuity chart. Normal individuals may lose one line of acuity with head rotation, whereas patients with vestibular abnormalities often lose more than two lines. Roll movements of the head (ear to shoulder) do not displace the fovea far from the visual target, and so cause smaller decreases in visual acuity even when vestibular function is completely lost. This dissociation can help detect malingering. DVA is more degraded by head motion at near than far viewing and diminishes with age especially in the vertical plane (5–7).

A tilt of the subjective visual vertical (SVV) is a sensitive sign of a disturbance in the otolith–ocular pathway (8). The otoliths act as gravito-inertial force sensors and contribute to the perception of the sense of verticality and uprightness. The SVV is a psychophysical measure of the angle between the perceptual and true (gravitational) vertical. In the upright position, normal individuals can position a visual linear marker in an otherwise completely dark room within 2° of true vertical. The values in patients with acute peripheral or central vestibular lesions, however, may deviate by several degrees from the true vertical. Most patients with acute vestibular neuritis show an ipsilateral deviation of the SVV (9, 10). As a topographic rule, lesions in the caudal pons and rostral medullary tegmentum of the brainstem cause ipsilateral tilts and lesions in the rostral pons and caudal mesencephalic tegmentum cause contralateral SVV tilts (11). Unilateral lesions of the thalamus or the vestibular cortex can cause either an ipsiversive or contraversive deviations of the SVV (12, 13).

The SVV can be measured reliably and quickly at the bedside using the bucket method (14) (Figure 12.1). In this test the subject estimates verticality by attempting to align a dark straight line visible on the bottom of a bucket that is randomly rotated to the right or left by the examiner. The field of vision of the subject should be covered completely by the rim of the bucket. On the outside, there is a plumb line on the bottom of the bucket that originates from the centre of a semicircle divided into degrees with the zero line adjusted to the dark line inside. With each adjustment by the subject the deviation from true vertical is recorded by the examiner. Ten adjustments are averaged to obtain the final SVV value. The bucket method can also be used to evaluate torsion in patients with vertical diplopia due to skew deviations or to ocular motor palsies. Patients with peripheral ocular motor lesions such as a trochlear nerve palsy may have a monocular tilt of the SVV (usually when viewing with the paretic eye) but a normal SVV with both eyes viewing (15).

Ophthalmoscopy

Ophthalmoscopy can detect subtle forms of nystagmus and other ocular oscillations. For example, the small-amplitude saccadic oscillations of microflutter are best detected during ophthalmoscopy (16, 17).

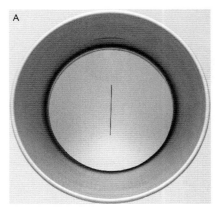 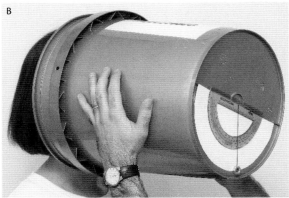

Fig. 12.1 The bucket method for bedside evaluation of subjective visual vertical (SVV). The subject estimates verticality in upright position by attempting to align a dark straight line visible on the inside bottom of a bucket (A) that is randomly rotated to the right or left by the examiner (B). On the outside bottom, there is a plumb line and a protractor adjusted to the dark line inside at zero. With each adjustment by the subject, the deviation from true vertical is recorded as the angle between the plumb line and the zero line on the protractor. Ten adjustments are averaged to obtain the final SVV value (14).

It is important to remove fixation (e.g. by alternately covering and uncovering the other eye) to see if any drift of the disc (or retina) is brought out or exacerbated by the removal of fixation. When viewing the fundus during ophthalmoscopy, the direction of any horizontal or vertical eye rotation will be opposite the direction of movement of the optic disc because the disc is behind the axis around which the globe is rotating. For torsion, however, the axis of rotation is around the line of sight, so the apparent direction of movement will change when looking at different parts of the retina. For example with a torsional nystagmus, there will be a vertical movement that will change sense when one compares the motion of a right versus a left part of the fundus. There will be a horizontal movement that will change sense when one compares the motion of a top versus a bottom part of the fundus. Abnormal ocular torsion, if large enough, can be also appreciated during ophthalmoscopy by the tilt of the imaginary line that connects the macula and the optic disc.

The VOR can be evaluated during ophthalmoscopy by observing the motion of the optic disc relative to the head, while the patient fixes on a distant target and oscillates the head horizontally or vertically at a frequency of about two cycles per second or above. At this frequency the pursuit system alone is unable to hold images stable on the retina so that gaze stability will depend mostly on the VOR. Alternatively, the fixating eye can be covered during the head shake to prevent pursuit. The patients must be instructed to imagine they are still looking at the target in front of them. If the VOR is intact, the optic disc does not move since the position of the eye with respect to the observer does not change as movement of the eye in the orbit is equal and opposite to the movement of the head on the body. If the disc appears to move in the opposite direction to the head, the reflex is hypoactive, and if it moves in the same direction, the reflex is hyperactive. If the disc drifts in one direction regardless of the direction of movement of the head, there is a directional preponderance caused by a vestibular imbalance. Note that if an individual habitually wears a far-sighted or near-sighted spectacle correction (but not contact lenses since they move with the eye), the amplitude of the VOR will increase or decrease in order to adapt to the new requirements for stable vision imposed by the magnification factor of the spectacles (18, 19). If this is the case, one can infer that the adaptive capability of the VOR is at least partially intact.

Ocular alignment

Careful examination of the alignment of the eyes is often neglected in dizzy patients, but it can provide important information about involvement of otolith–ocular pathways or the cerebellum. The examiner first establishes the range of motion with both eyes viewing (versions) and if there is any suspicion of misalignment, the range of motion of each eye viewing alone (ductions). One simple way of screening for ocular misalignment is looking at the symmetry of the corneal light reflex in both eyes (Hirschberg test). Further evaluation is performed subjectively with a red glass or Maddox rod, or objectively with cover testing. With the red glass method, the patient focuses on a pen light at different gaze positions with a red lens before one eye (by convention the right eye). With vertical misalignment, for example, a red and white light are seen one above the other. The higher image belongs to the lower eye and vice versa.

A Maddox rod is similar to the red glass except that it converts a point source of light into a thin bar making it easier for a patient to report the relative locations of the horizontal and vertical components of two separate images. A Maddox rod consists of small glass rods with a red filter such that if the small rods are oriented vertically before the right eye, the point of light becomes a horizontal red line. The vertical misalignment is then characterized by comparing the positions of the white light and the horizontal red line (Figure 12.2). Rotating the Maddox rod 90° makes the red line vertical so the method can be used to record horizontal deviations. A double Maddox rod, one red and one white, can be used to report differences in torsion between the two eyes (Figure 12.3C, D).

The cover tests demand less cooperation from patients as they only have to look at the light; however, it may be less reliable when fixation is interrupted by nystagmus or saccadic intrusions. With the cover tests ocular misalignment is detected by looking for a corrective movement when the occluder is immediately switched from one eye to the other (alternative cover test), or used to cover and uncover the same eye (cover uncover test). A misalignment with one eye viewing is a phoria and is detected with the cover test. Each eye takes up fixation when the cover is switched to the other eye. Phorias in the horizontal plane, exophoria (outward deviation), or esophoria (inward deviation), are often normal but phorias in the

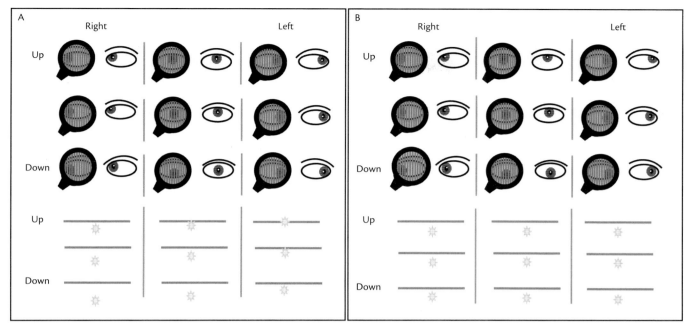

Fig. 12.2 (Also see Colour plate 9.) Evaluation of vertical ocular deviation with Maddox rod. A left hypertropia is shown. The Maddox rod is held vertically before the right eye and the positions of the white light (left eye) and the horizontal red line (right eye) are compared to evaluate vertical misalignment. In hypertropia due to a superior oblique palsy, the vertical misalignment is non-comitant and more marked on looking down and away from the affected eye (A). In hypertropia due to a comitant skew deviation, the vertical misalignment does not change in different gaze directions (B).

vertical plane, with one eye higher than the other (hyperphoria), are usually pathological. A misalignment with both eyes viewing is a tropia and is detected with the cover uncover test. The presence of a corrective movement of one eye that occurs when the cover is placed in front of the other eye tells the examiner that the eye was not fixing upon the target and hence there is a tropia. For example, using the alternative cover test with a left hyperphoria, when the occluder is switched to the right eye and the left eye is uncovered it moves down, and when the occluder is moved back to the left eye and the right eye is uncovered it moves up. When there is a left hypertropia with, for example, preferential fixation, with the left eye, the cover uncover test shows the following: when the left eye is covered the right eye moves up to take up fixation and when the left eye is uncovered the left eye moves down to take up fixation once again. When the right eye is covered and then uncovered again, there is no movement of the eyes because the left eye is always used for fixation. Therefore one must always perform the cover uncover test on both eyes to detect a tropia.

When there is a vertical misalignment the usual differential diagnosis is between a superior oblique palsy and a skew deviation. Skew deviation is a vertical misalignment of the eyes due to imbalance in tone in otolith–ocular pathways. The cause of the vertical misalignment can be differentiated further using the three steps of the Bielschowsky head tilt test. The first step determines which eye is higher, the second step determines whether the vertical separation is greater in right or left gaze, and the third step determines whether the separation increases in right head tilt or left head tilt. The hallmark of a superior oblique palsy is a vertical misalignment that is non-comitant, i.e. the degree of misalignment changes with direction of gaze. The affected eye is higher and the vertical misalignment is greatest with the affected eye adducted and depressed. The deviation is also greater when the head is tilted toward the side of

the higher eye (toward the side of the lesion). In contrast to superior oblique palsies, a skew deviation is usually relatively concomitant in which case the degree of misalignment changes little with different directions of gaze and is unaffected by head tilt (Figure 12.2). If the vertical deviation of a skew deviation is non-comitant (e.g. due to asymmetric involvement of vestibular pathways), and especially if the pattern of misalignment resembles that of an individual muscle palsy, it may be difficult to differentiate from a vertical extraocular muscle palsy (20, 21). In these cases, the relative direction of the torsion in the elevated eye (intorsion with skew and extorsion with a superior oblique palsy) is helpful in diagnosis (Figure 12.3A, B). The direction of torsion can be determined by examining the fundus with the ophthalmoscope, by the bucket test for SVV in each eye, or using visual field perimetry to detect the location of the blind spot relative to the fovea (14, 22). One can also check for torsion in both supine and upright positions as a skew deviation may decrease in the supine position while a superior oblique palsy should not (23). The vertical misalignment in skew deviation may also alternate its sense with horizontal eye position (e.g. right hypertropia on right gaze and left hypertropia on left gaze), a pattern that is common in cerebellar disease (24, 25).

Examination of eye movements

Gaze holding

The stability of gaze is evaluated by asking the patient to keep the head still and fix on a stationary target directly in front (commonly the nose of the examiner or a pencil point) and then about 30° eccentric in each direction. In straight ahead gaze, the examiner should look for abnormal movements such as pathological nystagmus and saccadic intrusions. The difference between nystagmus

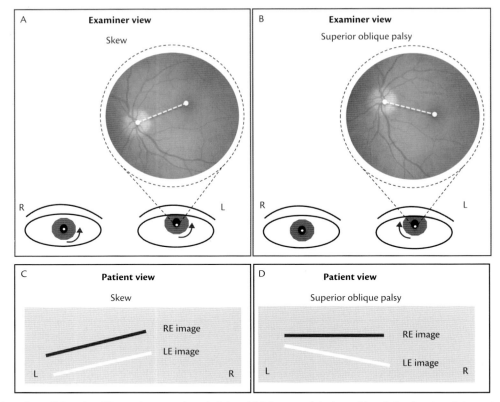

Fig. 12.3 (Also see Colour plate 10.) Superior oblique palsy versus skew deviation. A left hypertropia is shown. The relative direction of the torsion in the elevated eye (dashed white line between the macula and optic disc) from the examiner's view: intorsion with skew deviation (A) and extorsion with superior oblique palsy (B). Relative position of images from each eye as reported by the patient (with double Maddox rod): In skew deviation, there is no or little torsional diplopia (C). In superior oblique palsy, there is torsional diplopia with images pointing to side of the paretic eye (D). LE, left eye; RE, right eye.

and saccadic intrusions is in the initial eye movement that takes the line of sight away from the target. For nystagmus, the initial movement is a slow drift or 'slow phase' away from fixation and if there is a quick phase, it is corrective and brings the eye back to straight ahead fixation. This is known as a jerk nystagmus (Table 12.3). If the initial movement is an unwanted saccade taking the eye to an eccentric position, it is known as a saccadic intrusion.

Spontaneous jerk nystagmus is the hallmark of a tonic imbalance between the inputs from the semicircular canals of the two labyrinths. The slow phase is directed toward and the quick phase away from the weaker side. When nystagmus is peripheral in origin it is characteristically increased or only becomes apparent when fixation is eliminated. This may be detected with gentle eyelid closure, by observing movement of the corneal bulge, or by palpating the globes. Saccadic oscillations such as opsoclonus may also

Table 12.3 Evaluation of spontaneous nystagmus

Waveform of nystagmus (e.g. jerk or pendular)

Direction of nystagmus (horizontal, vertical, torsional, mixed, periodic alternating, elliptical)

Pattern of movement in each eye (dissociation of the nystagmus between two eyes)

Effect of removing fixation (occlusive ophthalmoscopy, Frenzel goggles)

Effect of convergence

Effect of eye in orbit and head position

Effect of provocative tests (Valsalva, tragal compression, head shaking, vibration, hyperventilation, and positional manoeuvres)

be brought out or exacerbated by eye closure. One can also determine the position of the eyes under closed lids by noting corrective movements when the patients open their eyes. In Wallenberg syndrome, for example, the eyes are often deviated toward the side of the lesion under closed lids so that when the eyes open there is a corrective saccade back to straight ahead fixation.

Because lid closure itself may affect nystagmus it is better to examine the effect of removing fixation using Frenzel goggles, or during occlusive ophthalmoscopy when one eye is covered and the fundus of the other eye observed for the appearance of drift or an increase in the amplitude of nystagmus. Frenzel goggles are fitted with magnifying glasses (+20 dioptres) and an internal lighting system. When used in an otherwise dark room, besides the well-illuminated and magnified view of the eyes, the goggles help to remove visual fixation as the patient cannot focus on any fixation target (see later 'Provocative tests' section, Figure 12.6A). One can also use a small +20 corrective lens alone placed in front of one eye and cover the other eye to eliminate fixation and still observe the eye but this method is less satisfactory than using the Frenzel goggles. Note that human beings have a relatively poor torsional fixation mechanism, so that the torsional component of a spontaneous nystagmus will be less suppressed by fixation than the horizontal or vertical components. Thus the true vector of a vestibular nystagmus can only be determined in the absence of fixation.

Using the anatomical arrangement of the semicircular canals within the labyrinth one can localize and interpret certain patterns of nystagmus more easily (Figure 12.4). Stimulation of a single

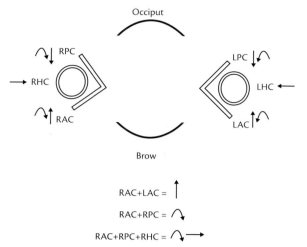

RAC+LAC = ↑

RAC+RPC = ⌒

RAC+RPC+RHC = ⌒→

Fig. 12.4 Slow-phase direction of nystagmus associated with stimulation of individual SCC (above) and combination of canals (shown for the right labyrinth, below). A pure vertical nystagmus can only arise from symmetrical involvement of two anterior or two posterior SCC and a pure torsional can only arise from symmetrical involvement of both the anterior and posterior SCC in one labyrinth. Involvement of all three canals in one labyrinth gives a mixed horizontal-torsional slow phase. AC, anterior canal; HC, horizontal canal; left; PC, posterior canal; R, right; L. Modified from Leigh and Zee (56).

semicircular canal leads to slow-phase eye movements that rotate the globe in a plane parallel to that of the stimulated canal. For the lateral SCC, this is predominantly horizontal motion and for the vertical SCC, a mixed vertical-torsional motion. A mixed horizontal-torsional nystagmus usually indicates a peripheral lesion. On the other hand, pure vertical nystagmus almost always has a central origin because it is rare that both anterior or both posterior SCC are involved alone, which is necessary if a peripheral lesion were to cause a pure spontaneous vertical nystagmus. Similarly, pure torsional nystagmus usually has a central origin because it is rare for the anterior and posterior SCC in one labyrinth alone, without the lateral canal, to be involved (Table 12.4). Note that the anterior SCC, lateral SCC, and utricle are innervated by the superior division of the vestibular nerve and the posterior SCC and saccule by the inferior division of the vestibular nerve.

Nystagmus on far eccentric gaze is a common finding and is not always abnormal. A gaze-evoked 'physiological' nystagmus in normal individuals is unaccompanied by other ocular motor or neurological abnormalities. It is usually short-lived and also disappears when the eyes are moved slightly toward the centre where they both

can see the target (the bridge of the nose is no longer in the way). In some normal individuals gaze-evoked nystagmus may have a slight torsional component. Horizontal nystagmus on eccentric gaze is more likely to be pathological when it is of high intensity, sustained, and persists even when the eyes are moved slightly toward the centre (Table 12.5). When a horizontal nystagmus only appears in one direction of eccentric gaze, the cause may be a unilateral peripheral vestibular lesion (see Alexander's law, discussed earlier). A strong downbeating component on lateral gaze implies central vestibular or cerebellar dysfunction (26), though occasionally normal subjects will have a slight downbeating component on far eccentric horizontal and downward gaze. Normal subjects may also show a small amount of nystagmus on far up gaze. Recall a common side effect of many sedatives, tranquilizers, and anticonvulsants is a gaze-evoked nystagmus.

After prolonged eccentric gaze, when the eyes return to the straight ahead position there may be a transient rebound nystagmus with slow phases directed toward the previously held eccentric position. This is commonly a sign of abnormal function of the cerebellar flocculus or paraflocculus (tonsil) (27, 28). If there is a spontaneous nystagmus in straight ahead gaze one should always look for a spontaneous change in its direction. Periodic alternating nystagmus changes its direction every few minutes and is a sign of abnormal function of the cerebellar nodulus (29, 30). The gaze-holding mechanism depends, in part, upon the vestibular nuclei and the vestibulocerebellum, so pathological gaze-evoked

Table 12.4 Features of peripheral vestibular and central nystagmus

Peripheral vestibular
Mixed horizontal-torsional
Quick phase away from the lesion
Slow phase with constant-velocity
Increased by removing fixation
Increased with gaze in the direction of the quick phase (Alexander's law)
May have characteristic pattern with changing head position (e.g. posterior canal BPPV)

Central vestibular
Horizontal, pure torsional or pure vertical (downbeat, upbeat)
Direction changing (gaze-evoked, periodic alternating nystagmus, rebound or centripetal beating nystagmus)
Poorly suppressed by fixation
Slow phase with constant, increasing or decreasing velocity
May increase with gaze away from quick phase
May change direction with convergence
May be dissociated between two eyes (e.g. with INO)
May change direction or intensity with change in eye or head position

INO, internuclear ophthalmoplegia.

Table 12.5 Features of physiological and pathological gaze-evoked nystagmus

	Physiological end-point nystagmus	**Pathological gaze-evoked nystagmus**
Amplitude	Low	High
Frequency	Low	High
Duration	Unsustained	Sustained
Direction	Horizontal on far lateral gaze upbeat on far upgaze	Vertical on lateral gaze
Rebound nystagmus	Absent	Present
Ocular motor examination	Normal	May be impaired

nystagmus due to brainstem or cerebellar lesions can also be accompanied by signs of vestibular imbalance. The combination may manifest as low-frequency, large-amplitude nystagmus on looking toward the lesion (due to defective gaze holding) and a high-frequency, small-amplitude nystagmus on looking away from the lesion (due to vestibular imbalance). This is called Bruns nystagmus and is typically seen with relatively large cerebellopontine angle tumours (31) (32).

Movements of the eyes can be divided into different functional subclasses and each needs to be examined separately (Table 12.1). These include vergence, saccades, pursuit, optokinetic nystagmus and vestibular eye movements. Convergence may expose, intensify, or alter the direction of some central forms of vestibular nystagmus. With convergence, congenital nystagmus is often diminished, acquired downbeat nystagmus is often accentuated, and upbeat nystagmus may change to downbeat nystagmus (33, 34).

Saccades

Saccades are the fastest eye movements with peak velocities as high as 600°/s for larger movements. Quick phases of nystagmus, although involuntary, are generated by the same premotor machinery in the brainstem. Saccades are best examined by instructing the patient to change fixation on command between two targets such as the tip of a pen held eccentrically and the examiner's nose. Both vertical and horizontal saccades should be examined and the time to initiate the movement, velocity, accuracy, and the conjugacy of the two eyes should be noted. Slow saccades with a full range of motion usually indicate brainstem disturbances. Selective slowing of horizontal saccades indicates pontine disease (pontine paramedian reticular formation), whereas selective slowing of vertical saccades suggests upper midbrain dysfunction (rostral interstitial nucleus of the MLF (riMLF)). Slowing of only one eye (e.g. the adducting eye) is seen with INO. If slowing of saccades occurs only in one plane of movement (horizontal or vertical), it can be easily appreciated when the patient attempts to make saccades between diagonally placed targets. This will cause saccades to be curved and sometimes appear L-shaped as the motion of the eyes in one plane finishes ahead of the movement of the eyes in the other plane.

Saccadic dysmetria can be inferred by the direction and size of corrective saccades needed to finally reach the target. Normal individuals may undershoot the target by a few degrees with large amplitude movements and saccadic overshoot may occur normally with centripetal, and especially, downward saccades. This 'normal' dysmetria often disappears with repetitive fixations between the same targets. Patients with cerebellar lesions may show various patterns of dysmetria, undershooting, overshooting, or inappropriately directed saccades, depending upon which parts of the cerebellum are affected (35). Undershooting occurs with lesions of the dorsal vermis and overshooting with bilateral lesions of the posterior fastigial nucleus. Delays in the initiation of saccades usually result from 'higher-level' cerebral cortical disorders producing so-called apraxia of eye movements in which more reflexive types of saccades such as quick phases are usually preserved (36–38). One can examine the ability of the patient to make reflexive saccades by eliciting quick phases of optokinetic nystagmus (OKN) with a striped pattern (see also 'Optokinetic nystagmus' section). OKN is a convenient way to elicit a number of saccades in succession making it easier, for example, to detect subtle degrees of disconjugacy

in INO when slowing of adducting saccades without limitation of range is an early sign.

Pursuit

Smooth pursuit eye movements allow clear vision of an object moving within the visual field. Patients are asked to track a slowly moving small target (at about 10°/s), such as a pencil tip, held a half metre or so in front of the eyes. Pursuit is perfect when the velocity of the eye matches the moving object. If smooth pursuit is slower than the target velocity, the patient will need corrective 'catch-up' saccades and if faster, corrective 'back-up' saccades (e.g. due to superimposed slow phases of vestibular nystagmus). A pursuit abnormality indicates central dysfunction but with the caveats that pursuit performance requires attention, declines with age, and is particularly susceptible to the influence of medications. Like saccades, pursuit abnormalities can be plane specific (horizontal or vertical) or in one direction (right or left). For example, cerebellar lesions involving one side of the dorsal vermis primarily impair ipsilateral pursuit (39).

During combined eye-head tracking of moving targets the VOR must be negated to allow smooth tracking of the target. This is accomplished by VOR cancellation which shares mechanisms with smooth pursuit made with the head stationary. To examine VOR cancellation, patients are asked to track a head-fixed, slowly moving target (e.g. a target attached to the end of a tongue depressor held between patient's teeth or a long pointer held on the patient's head), or instructed to hold up and follow their thumb as they are rotated en bloc (arm, head, and body). With these manoeuvres the eyes should remain motionless and fixed on the target. If VOR cancellation seems intact but smooth pursuit with the head still is inadequate one should suspect hypofunction of the VOR.

Optokinetic reflex

OKN represents the combined response of the smooth pursuit and optokinetic system. Optokinetic eye movements can be elicited at the bedside by asking the patients to follow moving stripes on a hand-held optokinetic drum or banded cloth. Even one's fingers can be used as an optokinetic stimulus. The patients are asked to look at each target as it moves in front of them. This will normally create a nystagmus with a slow phase in the direction of the moving stripes. Optokinetic responses can be used to detect asymmetries of pursuit (slow phase of OKN) or saccades (fast phase of OKN). Unilateral peripheral vestibular lesions, particularly during the acute phase, may also cause a directional preponderance of OKN (and pursuit), with a better response when the stimulus is moved toward the side of the lesion. OKN can also be used to detect aberrant regeneration with oculomotor palsies. For example, with horizontally moving stripes the normal eye will correctly make a horizontal nystagmus but the affected eye will make an inappropriately directed vertical nystagmus.

VOR examination

A perfect compensatory VOR produces a rotation of the eyes in the orbit of equal amplitude and exactly opposite to that of the head. The VOR should first be tested with relatively low-frequency (0.5 cycle per second) head rotations through the ocular motor range in the horizontal (yaw) and vertical (pitch) planes while the patient fixates on a target such as the examiner's nose. Corrective saccades

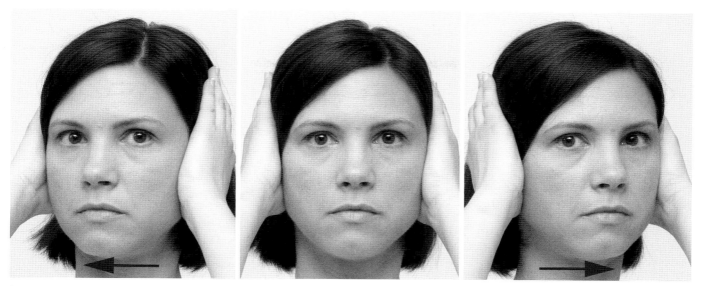

Fig. 12.5 Horizontal head impulse test for evaluation of the lateral SCC. The subject is instructed to fix on a target, usually the examiner's nose. The hands of the examiner are applied over the side of the head with the force being largely transmitted through the bottom of the palms over the temples. The amplitude of rotation in each direction should not be large but it must be abrupt and of high acceleration. In normal subjects the slow phase of the VOR compensates for the head rotation so the eyes remain on target. In patients with an underactive VOR there will be a corrective catch-up saccade opposite to the direction of head rotation.

opposite to the rotation of the head are a sign of a hypoactive VOR. As is the case for dynamic visual acuity, smooth pursuit can make up for a defective VOR when the head rotation is relatively low frequency, but when the loss of vestibular function is profound some catch-up saccades will be seen even during low-frequency oscillations in the light. An abnormally high amplitude of the VOR (e.g. from a cerebellar lesion) may result in slow phases that are too fast, requiring corrective backup saccades in the direction of head rotation (40). A superimposed gaze-evoked nystagmus may make assessment of the VOR difficult when the eyes are at the extremes of gaze. For rotation of the head around the anterior posterior axis (ear to shoulder), one can evaluate the torsional VOR by noting the torsional quick phases which are best seen by watching the movement of a blood vessel in the conjunctiva near the limbus. With a unilateral midbrain lesion that involves the riMLF quick phases of torsional nystagmus are absent when the head is tilted toward the side of the lesion (41).

A brief, high-acceleration head 'impulse' is the simplest bedside manoeuvre for detecting loss of labyrinthine function (42). The patient is instructed to fix on a target, usually the nose of the examiner, while the head is quickly turned from one position to another, horizontally or vertically. A comfortable range of head rotation should be established first with a slow rotation and one must be cautious in any patient with cervical disease and especially the elderly. The rotation need not be large (<15°), but should be abrupt and of high acceleration. The hands of the examiner are applied on the side of patient's head with the force being largely transmitted through the bottom of the palms over the patient's temples (Figure 12.5). Head-impulse testing is based upon Ewald's second law which states that a better response is elicited with excitatory than inhibitory stimulation. For the lateral semicircular canals the head impulse is applied horizontally, and for the vertical semicircular canals applied by turning the head about 30° to the right or left and then rotating to stimulate coplanar canals: right anterior, left posterior (RALP), or left anterior, right posterior (LARP)

(Videos 12.1–12.3). A corrective catch-up saccade (horizontally for the lateral canals and vertically for the vertical canals) is a sign of an underactive VOR response.

Occasionally with central, usually cerebellar lesions, the VOR will be hyperactive and the corrective saccade will be directed oppositely to the slow phase that is too fast. In some patients the VOR response may be inappropriately directed; for example, an upward slow-phase component followed by a downward corrective saccade with horizontal impulse testing. This sign is common with cerebellar lesions and reflects so-called 'cross-coupling' of the VOR (43). In patients with acute vestibular symptoms and a spontaneous nystagmus, a normal head impulse test suggests a central aetiology whereas an abnormal head impulse occurs with both peripheral and central lesions (44).

The head impulse test is most consistently positive when there is a complete loss of labyrinthine function involving the lateral canal. The

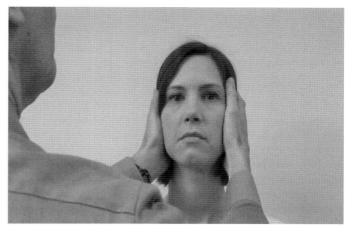

Video 12.1 Horizontal head impulse test. For the lateral SCC, the head impulse is applied horizontally starting from both central and eccentric gaze positions while the subject is instructed to look at the nose of the examiner.

132 OXFORD TEXTBOOK OF VERTIGO AND IMBALANCE

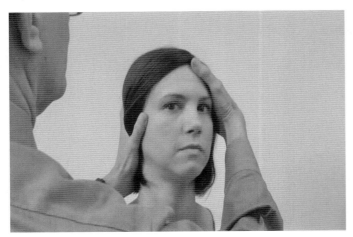

Video 12.2 Vertical head impulse test (RALP). For the right anterior and left posterior SCC, the head impulse is applied by turning the head about 30° to the right and then rotating in their corresponding plane while the subject is instructed to look at the nose of the examiner.

test, however, can be positive with a partial loss of function. Some normal subjects require a downward catch-up saccade in response to upward head impulses as downward slow phases may be slightly hypoactive. Similarly, many otherwise normal elderly individuals often show a small degree of VOR hypometria, particularly with high-acceleration head impulses, and they may make a catch-up saccade in both horizontal directions. Patients with chronic complete bilateral loss of labyrinthine function and occasionally patients with a long-standing unilateral loss may appear to have an intact impulse response because they have learned to trigger preprogrammed compensatory saccades, presumably by using information from neck proprioceptors. In well-adapted patients these corrective, 'covert' saccades are generated so early that they become embedded in the response during the head rotation and are complete by the time the head stops moving, making them hard to discern (45). The corrective saccades may be seen more easily and so become 'overt' by making the head impulse unpredictable in timing and amplitude. Again, note that with high accelerations the excursion of the head necessary to elicit the catch-up saccades need not be and should not be large.

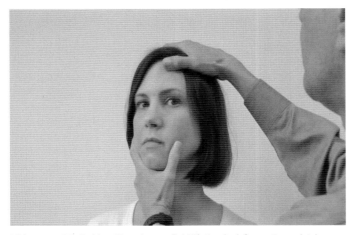

Video 12.3 Vertical head impulse test (LARP). For the left anterior and right posterior SCC, the head impulse is applied by turning the head about 30° to the left and then rotating in their corresponding plane while the subject is instructed to look at the nose of the examiner.

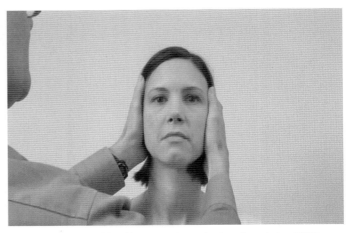

Video 12.4 Horizontal head heave test. For evaluation of translational VOR, an abrupt, high-acceleration lateral movement of the head is imposed while the subject is instructed to look at the nose of the examiner.

The head heave test, analogous to the head impulse test, is used to evaluate the translational VOR and in turn the function of utricle. In this test an abrupt, high-acceleration lateral movement of the head is imposed while the subject is instructed to look at the nose of the examiner (Video 12.4). A corrective catch-up saccade indicates the tVOR is hypoactive. Because normal individuals usually show a hypoactive tVOR in both directions of head motion and may require a corrective saccade, the finding of an asymmetric response to horizontal translation is more useful for identifying an abnormality. Unlike the head impulse sign, which is permanent if there is a complete loss of labyrinthine function, the head heave asymmetry is usually rapidly compensated and so only apparent in the first days after unilateral loss of function. A positive head heave sign, however, predicts a delayed or less complete recovery (46).

Provocative tests

A series of examinations can be performed at the bedside to elicit or modify nystagmus. This is best performed with the patient wearing Frenzel goggles to eliminate the effect of fixation on nystagmus (Figure 12.6A). In this way a peripheral vestibular nystagmus that is normally suppressed by fixation can become evident.

The Valsalva manoeuvre can induce nystagmus either by increasing intracranial pressure (straining against closed glottis as with lifting weights) or by increasing pressure in the middle ear (attempting to blow out against pinched nostrils) (Figure 12.6B). The nystagmus may be induced in patients with Ménière's disease, craniocervical junction anomalies such as Arnold–Chiari malformation, ossicular chain abnormalities, perilymph fistula, or superior canal dehiscence. In some patients jugular vein compression can induce nystagmus by increasing intracranial pressure. Tragal compression can also provoke nystagmus by changing the middle-ear pressure (Hennebert's sign). Increasing the pressure in the middle ear, however, is best done with a pneumatic otoscope.

Head-shaking induced nystagmus (HSN) is a useful sign of imbalance of dynamic vestibular function (47). To perform the head-shaking manoeuvre, after establishing a comfortable range of motion of the head and while wearing Frenzel goggles, the head of the patient is shaken at a frequency of about thee cycles per second for about 10 seconds from side to side (Video 12.5). Immediately afterwards

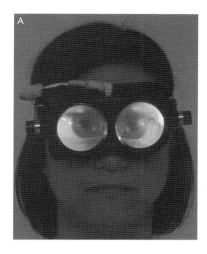
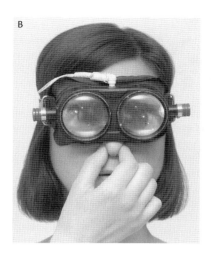
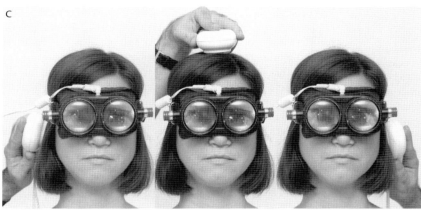

Fig. 12.6 Evaluation of nystagmus is best performed in a dark room with the subject wearing Frenzel goggles to eliminate the effect of fixation (A). Valsalva manoeuvre with blowing out against pinched nostrils (B). Vibration applied over the mastoid tips and the vertex to look for induced nystagmus (C).

an induced nystagmus is sought by the examiner. Normal individuals may have a beat or two of nystagmus. With a unilateral loss of vestibular function, a vigorous nystagmus with slow phases directed initially toward the affected side will usually appear followed by a reversal phase with slow phases directed toward the intact side. In patients with vestibular imbalance, there is an asymmetry of peripheral inputs during high-velocity head rotations (Ewald's second law), which leads to an unequal accumulation of activity in the central

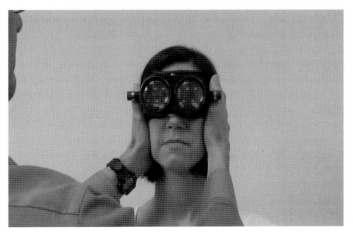

Video 12.5 Head-shaking manoeuvres: horizontal, vertical, and circular.

velocity-storage mechanism within the vestibular nuclei (48, 49). Immediately after head shaking, the initial phase of HSN appears as a result of a decay of activity within the velocity-storage mechanism. If one waits long enough, a reversal phase appears with slow phases directed toward the intact ear. This is accounted for by a short-term adaptation mechanism that balances out the initial nystagmus. HSN can be also induced in the vertical and roll planes (Video 12.5). With unilateral peripheral lesions, vertical head shaking may cause a small-amplitude horizontal nystagmus with slow phases directed toward the intact ear (away for the affected side). This oppositely-directed response likely reflects an asymmetry in the normal contribution of excitation of the posterior SCC to the horizontal VOR during vertical head shaking (49).

With circular head shaking (tracing out a circular path with the chin) normal individuals show a torsional nystagmus which is probably similar to a post-rotatory nystagmus when a subject is rotated in the roll plane (around the naso-occipital axis). Circular head shaking is a convenient way to confirm a suspicion of a profound loss of labyrinthine function. Patients with bilateral vestibular loss have a reduced or absent response (50). In the acute phases of a unilateral loss of labyrinthine function there may be no horizontal HSN. This is accounted for by a temporary disengagement of the velocity storage mechanism in the face of an acute vestibular imbalance. This phenomenon is similar to the loss of caloric sensitivity on the intact side in the first few days after a unilateral loss of labyrinthine function (see 'Bedside caloric testing' section).

Some patients with peripheral lesions may show horizontal HSN with slow phases directed away from the affected side. The mechanism may be related to 'recovery' nystagmus which refers to the appearance of a nystagmus with slow phases emanating from the lesioned ear. When there has been a prior adaptive rebalancing of vestibular tone after a unilateral lesion, and the tone from the paretic side is suddenly restored as peripheral function recovers, the new level of spontaneous activity on the paretic side becomes excessive relative to the central state of compensation. This leads to a new imbalance causing a spontaneous nystagmus with slow phases directed toward the intact year. The brain, however, catches up soon and rebalances vestibular tone to eliminate the 'recovery' nystagmus. The direction of HSN can be particularly confusing in Ménière's syndrome as it may be related to the excitatory phase, paretic phase, or the recovery phase. Finally, HSN may appear with central lesions, usually in the medulla and cerebellum (51). A cross-coupled HSN such as a vertical nystagmus following horizontal head shaking is almost always a sign of a central disturbance (52).

Vibration applied to the mastoid tip may bring out nystagmus in patients with unilateral loss of vestibular function and occasionally in other conditions such as superior canal dehiscence (53–55). In the case of a unilateral loss of function, vibration on either mastoid or over the vertex can elicit a nystagmus with a slow phase toward the paretic ear (Figure 12.6C). This direction of nystagmus usually is independent of the site of stimulation as the vibration impulses are transmitted through the skull nearly equally to both labyrinths. Because of this symmetry, normal individuals show little or no vibration-induced nystagmus. In patients with a unilateral loss of labyrinthine function, stimulating with a vibrator is comparable to a hot water caloric irrigation to the intact ear. When vibration elicits a vertical nystagmus a central lesion should be suspected.

Hyperventilation may induce a variety of symptoms is patients with anxiety and phobic disorders but usually does not produce nystagmus. Patients with demyelinating lesions of the vestibular nerve due to compression by a tumour (e.g. acoustic neuroma) or small blood vessels (microvascular compression) or with demyelination in central pathways (e.g. in multiple sclerosis) may develop nystagmus with hyperventilation (56–58). The alkalosis and change in ionized calcium caused by 30–60 seconds of hyperventilation can improve conduction on demyelinated axons leading to a recovery nystagmus (slow phases directed toward the intact ear). Hyperventilation may induce nystagmus in patients with history of a labyrinthitis (with the slow phase usually directed toward the paretic ear) which may reflect a decompensation of prior adaptive rebalancing of vestibular tone (59). Hyperventilation can also enhance spontaneous downbeat nystagmus in cerebellar patients which is likely mediated through metabolic effects on calcium channels of Purkinje cells (60). Moreover, hyperventilation may induce nystagmus by changing intracranial pressure in patients with craniocervical junction anomalies or with abnormal connections between the subarachnoid space and the inner ear as occurs with a perilymph fistula (56).

Positional testing

Positional testing is the essential part of the vestibular examination in all patients who complain of dizziness. Examination techniques are reviewed in detail by Nuti and Zee in Chapter 20. Here we briefly review the order in which the manoeuvres can be performed. The patient is first moved from the sitting position to the Hallpike position (the head is turned 45° to the left and then the patient is moved backward) to stimulate the left posterior SCC and look for a posterior canal positional nystagmus. The patient is then brought back again to the sitting position. This manoeuvre is then repeated with the right ear down to stimulate the right posterior SCC. Finally, the head is placed in the straight back hanging position to look for a vertical nystagmus and then the patient is turned 90° to the left ear down and then 180° to the right ear down positions to stimulate the lateral canals.

Bedside caloric testing

Bedside caloric testing often helps to determine the side of a peripheral vestibular lesion. To perform the test, after verifying that the tympanic membrane is intact, a small amount of ice water (about 0.3 ml) is used to assess the function of lateral SCC in each ear (61). The patient's head should be elevated 30° relative to earth-horizontal, to place the lateral SCC in a vertical position. Frenzel goggles or ophthalmoscopy with occlusion of the opposite eye should be used to eliminate fixation. If no response is elicited with the initial stimulus, a larger volume of ice water (up to about 10 ml) can be used. In a patient with an acute loss of vestibular function, the caloric response may be reduced temporarily on the intact side as well as lost on the lesioned side. This is due to adaptive mechanisms that rebalance the vestibular nuclei by suppressing activity in the vestibular nuclei on the intact side as well as restoring activity in the vestibular nuclei on the deafferented side. Caloric testing, as a low-frequency stimulus, can sometime detect vestibular impairment that may not be apparent during the high-frequency head impulse test.

Hearing

Hearing should be assessed in all dizzy patients. Simple methods such as thumb-finger rubbing or whispering numbers to each ear can be used to screen for asymmetric hearing loss at the bedside (62, 63). One can repeat these tests at different distances from the patient's ears to compare hearing thresholds on each side. If a hearing loss is detected it can be characterized further using 256- or 512-Hz tuning forks. Normally air conduction is greater than bone conduction. This is the basis for the Rinne test in which the vibrating tuning fork is first placed on the mastoid bone and then held next to the external auditory meatus. Patients with conductive hearing loss report louder bone conduction and the opposite is found in patients with sensorineural hearing loss. In the Weber test the vibrating tuning fork is placed on the middle of the forehead, chin, or on the vertex equidistant from the ears. Patients with unilateral conductive hearing loss hear the tuning fork louder in the affected ear and patients with unilateral sensorineural loss hear the tuning fork louder in the unaffected ear. In superior canal dehiscence, patients may report hearing the tuning fork when it is placed over the ankle (malleolus sign) (64). Note that bedside hearing examinations are relatively insensitive screening tests and an audiogram should be obtained in every patient who has any hearing symptoms and in all undiagnosed dizzy patients even without auditory complaints (see Chapter 10).

Sensorineural hearing loss can accompany vestibular dysfunction in Ménière's disease, inflammatory, ischaemic, and compressive lesions involving the VIIIth nerve. The hearing loss in association with ischemic and inflammatory processes is usually high frequency while with Ménière's disease and some inflammatory conditions, such as Susac's syndrome and Cogan's syndrome, the hearing loss is commonly low frequency. Conductive hearing loss can be associated with dizziness in otosclerosis or in destructive middle ear disease (cholesteatoma).

Posture, gait, and vestibulospinal reflexes

Unsteadiness and imbalance can be seen with a wide range of vestibular disorders. In patients with the complaint of dizziness, this part of the examination can be tailored to evaluate for underlying static or dynamic imbalance in vestibulospinal reflexes. A static imbalance mediated by the lateral SCC is best examined by having the patient perform tandem walking with both eyes open and closed, or with the Unterberger–Fukuda stepping test in which the patient closes their eyes and marches in place for 20–30 seconds. The imbalance is reflected in excessive turning to one direction. A static imbalance in vertical canal reflexes can be evaluated with various permutations of the Romberg test. A positive Romberg means that the patient shows a tendency to actually fall. The Romberg test is positives in the acute phase of a peripheral vestibular disorder, usually with a tendency to fall toward the same side of the lesion. The Romberg test is also positive in patients with dorsal column or severe peripheral polyneuropathy. With regard to unilateral vestibular hypofunction, the test is more sensitive when the patient stands in the tandem (heel-to-toe) position. The fundamental question is whether excessive anterior or posterior (pitch or sagittal component) or lateral (roll or coronal component) sway occurs when the patient stands in tandem with eyes closed (to remove visual cues) or when the somatosensory cues are minimized in the upright position (e.g. standing on a piece of foam rubber). Patients with significant hypofunction tend to lean ipsilesionally. Lateropulsion (i.e. falling to one side) is also seen in lateralized brainstem-cerebellar lesions whereas midline cerebellar-brainstem lesions can show retropulsion (i.e. falling backward). Of practical note, anyone who can stand on either foot unaided, with eyes closed, is unlikely to have any objective postural balance problem.

Static imbalance in otolith-spinal reflexes also leads to excessive postural sway (e.g. lateral head and body tilt with utriculospinal imbalance) and a sideways deviation on the stepping test. Past-pointing of the arms (or feet) to previously seen targets with eyes closed may also be a sign of acute vestibulospinal imbalance. For the arms, past-pointing is best elicited by having the patient repetitively raise both arms over the head with the index fingers extended and then bringing them down, with eyes closed, toward the examiner's index fingers held at waist level (without actually touching them).

Dynamic vestibulospinal function can be assessed by observing postural instability during rapid turns or in response to external perturbations imposed by the examiner (e.g. a gentle push forward, backward, or to the side). This can be done standing behind the patient to prevent anticipation of the precise timing and direction of the push to the shoulders. It is useful to see patients walk, first with eyes open and then with eyes closed. A number of peripheral and central neurological disorders can be detected during gait with open eyes, but most patients with vestibular disorders are normal unless in an acute vertiginous stage. Some patients with balance complaints exhibit a cautious or rather overcautious gait. The arms

of patients with a cautious gait reach out as if expecting to fall and step with apparently unnecessary care, giving the appearance of 'walking on ice'. Although a cautious gait can be part of a psychogenic gait disorder it can also be triggered by a vestibular episode. Sometimes this is the only finding in elderly patients. Walking with eyes closed in a straight line can reveal a previously unsuspected degree of unsteadiness or a cautious gait in patients with bilateral loss of vestibular function. In somatosensory ataxia, as in tabes dorsalis or severe polyneuropathies, this task is often impossible. In unilateral vestibular lesions, particularly in the acute stage, patients veer toward the side of the lesion. Just as for the VOR, tragal compression or the Valsalva manoeuvre can be used to elicit an increase in the postural sway in labyrinthine fistula syndromes.

A complete neurological examination is, of course, essential in the evaluation of any patient with oscillopsia and vertigo, dizziness, or imbalance. In addition to the cranial nerves, the examination should include motor strength, coordination, deep tendon reflexes, and sensory evaluation. Weakness of the legs can be documented by asking the patient to stand (or walk) on tiptoes and heels, or to crouch and rise. Identification of weakness of the ankle extensors is paramount as these muscles are responsible for toe clearance during the swing phase of the gait cycle. The tendon reflexes are exaggerated in pyramidal tract disease but depressed or absent in weakness due to root or peripheral nerve disease. Somatosensory function can be assessed with pin-prick stimuli, tuning fork, and joint position sense in the lower extremities.

References

1. Newman-Toker DE, Cannon LM, Stofferahn ME, Rothman RE, Hsieh YH, Zee DS (2007). Imprecision in patient reports of dizziness symptom quality: a cross-sectional study conducted in an acute care setting. *Mayo Clin Proc*, 82(11), 1329–40.
2. Fluur E, Mellstrom A (1970). Utricular stimulation and oculomotor reactions. *Laryngoscope*, 80(11), 1701–12.
3. Fluur E, Mellstrom A (1970). Saccular stimulation and oculomotor reactions. *Laryngoscope*, 80(11), 1713–21.
4. Brandt T, Dieterich M (1993). Skew deviation with ocular torsion: a vestibular brainstem sign of topographic diagnostic value. *Ann Neurol*, 33(5), 528–34.
5. Peters BT, Bloomberg JJ (2005). Dynamic visual acuity using 'far' and 'near' targets. *Acta Otolaryngol*, 125(4), 353–7.
6. Schubert MC, Herdman SJ, Tusa RJ (2002). Vertical dynamic visual acuity in normal subjects and patients with vestibular hypofunction. *Otolo Neurotol*, 23(3), 372–7.
7. Long GM, Crambert RF (1990). The nature and basis of age-related changes in dynamic visual acuity. *Psychol Aging*, 5(1), 138–43.
8. Dieterich M, Brandt T (1993). Ocular torsion and tilt of subjective visual vertical are sensitive brainstem signs. *Ann Neurol*, 33(3), 292–9.
9. Friedmann G (1970). The judgment of the visual vertical and horizontal with peripheral and central vestibular lesions. *Brain*, 93(2), 313–28.
10. Bohmer A, Rickenmann J (1995). The subjective visual vertical as a clinical parameter of vestibular function in peripheral vestibular disease. *J Vestib Res*, 5(1), 35–45.
11. Brandt T, Dieterich M (1994). Vestibular syndromes in the roll plane: topographic diagnosis from brainstem to cortex. *Ann Neurol*, 36(3), 337–47.
12. Dieterich M, Brandt T (1993). Thalamic infarctions: Differential effects on vestibular function in the roll plane (35 patients). *Neurology*, 43(9), 1732–43.
13. Brandt T, Dieterich M, Danek A (1994). Vestibular cortex lesions affect the perception of verticality. *Ann Neurol*, 35(4), 403–12.

14. Zwergal A, Rettinger N, Frenzel C, Dieterich M, Brandt T, Strupp M (2009). A bucket of static vestibular function. *Neurology*, 72(19), 1689–92.

15. Dieterich M, Brandt T (1993). Ocular torsion and perceived vertical in oculomotor, trochlear and abducens nerve palsies. *Brain*, 116(5), 1095–104.

16. Ashe J, Hain T, Zee D, Schatz N (1991). Microsaccadic flutter. *Brain*, 114(1), 461–72.

17. Shaikh AG, Miura K, Optican LM, Ramat S, Leigh RJ, Zee DS (2007). A new familial disease of saccadic oscillations and limb tremor provides clues to mechanisms of common tremor disorders. *Brain*, 130(11), 3020–31.

18. Cannon SC, Leigh RJ, Zee DS, Abel LA (1985). The effect of the rotational magnification of corrective spectacles on the quantitative evaluation of the VOR. *Acta Otolaryngol*, 100(1–2), 81–8.

19. Demer JL, Porter FI, Goldberg J, Jenkins HA, Schmidt K (1989). Adaptation to telescopic spectacles: vestibulo-ocular reflex plasticity. *Invest Ophthalmol Vis Sci*, 30(1), 159–70.

20. Donahue SP, Lavin PJ, Hamed LM (1999). Tonic ocular tilt reaction simulating a superior oblique palsy: diagnostic confusion with the 3–step test. *Arch Ophthalmol*, 117(3), 347–52.

21. Donahue SP, Lavin PJ, Mohney B, Hamed L (2001). Skew deviation and inferior oblique palsy. *Am J Ophthalmol*, 132(5), 751–6.

22. Versino M, Newman-Toker DE (2010). Blind spot heterotopia by automated static perimetry to assess static ocular torsion: centro-cecal axis rotation in normals. *J Neurol*, 257(2), 291–3.

23. Wong AMF (2010). Understanding skew deviation and a new clinical test to differentiate it from trochlear nerve palsy. *J AAPOS*, 14(1), 61–7.

24. Zee D (1996). Considerations on the mechanisms of alternating skew deviation in patients with cerebellar lesions. *J Vestib Res*, 6(6), 395–401.

25. Brodsky MC, Donahue SP, Vaphiades M, Brandt T (2006). Skew deviation revisited. *Surv Ophthalmol*, 51(2), 105–28.

26. Wagner JN, Glaser M, Brandt T, Strupp M (2008). Downbeat nystagmus: aetiology and comorbidity in 117 patients. *J Neurol Neurosurg Psychiatry*, 79(6), 672–7.

27. Bondar RL, Sharpe JA, Lewis AJ (1984). Rebound nystagmus in olivocerebellar atrophy: a clinicopathological correlation. *Ann Neurol*, 15(5), 474–7.

28. Lin CY, Young YH (1999). Clinical significance of rebound nystagmus. *Laryngoscope*, 109(11), 1803–5.

29. Kennard C, Barger G, Hoyt W (1981). The association of periodic alternating nystagmus with periodic alternating gaze: a case report. *J Clin Neuroophthalmol*, 1(3), 191–3.

30. Waespe W, Cohen B, Raphan T (1985). Dynamic modification of the vestibulo-ocular reflex by the nodulus and uvula. *Science*, 228(4696), 199–202.

31. Lloyd SK, Baguley DM, Butler K, Donnelly N, Moffat DA (2009). Bruns' Nystagmus in patients with vestibular schwannoma. *Otolo Neurotol*, 30(5), 625–8.

32. Croxson G, Moffat D, Baguley D (1988). Bruns bidirectional nystagmus in cerebellopontine angle tumors. *Clin Otolaryngol Allied Sci*, 13(2), 153–7.

33. Cox TA, Corbett JJ, Thompson HS, Lennarson L (1981). Upbeat nystagmus changing to downbeat nystagmus with convergence. *Neurology*, 31(7), 891–2.

34. Dickinson CM (1986). The elucidation and use of the effect of near fixation in congenital nystagmus. *Ophthalmic Physiol Opt*, 6(3), 303–11.

35. Versino M, Hurko O, Zee DS (1996). Disorders of binocular control of eye movements in patients with cerebellar dysfunction. *Brain*, 119(6), 1933–50.

36. Dehaene I, Lammens M (1991). Acquired ocular motor apraxia: A clinico-pathological study. *Neuro-Ophthalmology*, 11(2), 117.

37. Yee RD, Purvin VA (2007). Acquired ocular motor apraxia after aortic surgery. *Trans Am Ophthalmol Soc*, 105, 152–8.

38. Sharpe JA, Johnston JL (1989). Ocular motor paresis versus apraxia. *Ann Neurol*, 25(2), 209–10.

39. Ohtsuka K, Enoki T (1998). Transcranial magnetic stimulation over the posterior cerebellum during smooth pursuit eye movements in man. *Brain*, 121(3), 429–35.

40. Thurston SE, Leigh RJ, Abel LA, Dell'Osso LF (1987). Hyperactive vestibulo-ocular reflex in cerebellar degeneration. *Neurology*, 37(1), 53–7.

41. Helmchen C, Glasauer S, Bartl K, Buttner U (1996). Contralesionally beating torsional nystagmus in a unilateral rostral midbrain lesion. *Neurology*, 47(2), 482–6.

42. Halmagyi G, Curthoys I (1988). A clinical sign of canal paresis. *Arch Neurol*, 45(7), 737–9.

43. Walker MF, Zee DS (2005). Cerebellar disease alters the axis of the high-acceleration vestibuloocular reflex. *J Neurophysiol*, 94(5), 3417–29.

44. Newman-Toker DE, Kattah JC, Alvernia JE, Wang DZ (2008). Normal head impulse test differentiates acute cerebellar strokes from vestibular neuritis. *Neurology*, 70(24), 2378–85.

45. Weber K, Aw S, Todd M, McGarvie L, Curthoys I, Halmagyi G (2008). Head impulse test in unilateral vestibular loss. *Neurology*, 70(6), 454–63.

46. Mandalà M, Nuti D, Broman AT, Zee DS (2008). Effectiveness of careful bedside examination in assessment, diagnosis, and prognosis of vestibular neuritis. *Arch Otolaryngol Head Neck Surg*, 134(2), 164–9.

47. Hain TC, Spindler J (1993). Head-shaking nystagmus. In Sharpe JA, Barber HO (Eds) *The Vestibulo-Ocular Reflex and Vertigo*, pp. 217–28. New York: Raven Press.

48. Katsarkas A, Smith H, Galiana H (2000). Head-shaking nystagmus (HSN): the theoretical explanation and the experimental proof. *Acta Otolaryngol*, 120(2), 177–81.

49. Hain T, Fetter M, Zee D (1987). Head-shaking nystagmus in patients with unilateral peripheral vestibular lesions. *Am J Otolaryngol*, 8(1), 36–47.

50. Haslwanter T, Minor L (1999). Nystagmus induced by circular head shaking in normal human subjects. *Exp Brain Res*, 124(1), 25–32.

51. Choi KD, Oh SY, Park SH, Kim JH, Koo JW, Kim J (2007). Head-shaking nystagmus in lateral medullary infarction. *Neurology*, 68(17), 1337–44.

52. Minagar A, Sheremata WA, Tusa RJ (2001). Perverted head-shaking nystagmus: a possible mechanism. *Neurology*, 57(5), 887–9.

53. Hamann KF, Schuster EM (2000). Vibration-induced nystagmus-a sign of unilateral vestibular deficit. *ORL J Otorhinolaryngol Relat Spec*, 61(2), 74–9.

54. White JA, Hughes GB, Ruggieri PN (2007). Vibration-induced nystagmus as an office procedure for the diagnosis of superior semicircular canal dehiscence. *Otolo Neurotol*, 28(7), 911–16.

55. Perez N (2003). Vibration induced nystagmus in normal subjects and in patients with dizziness. A videonystagmography study. *Rev Laryngol Otol Rhinol*, 124(2), 85–90.

56. Leigh RJ, Zee DS (2006). *The neurology of eye movements* (4th ed). New York: Oxford University Press.

57. Minor LB, Haslwanter T, Straumann D, Zee DS (1999). Hyperventilation-induced nystagmus in patients with vestibular schwannoma. *Neurology*, 53(9), 2158–68.

58. Choi K, Kim J, Kim HJ, *et al.* (2007). Hyperventilation-induced nystagmus in peripheral vestibulopathy and cerebellopontine angle tumor. *Neurology*, 69(10), 1050–9.

59. Park HJ, Shin J, Lee Y, Park M, Kim J, Na B (2010). Hyperventilation-induced nystagmus in patients with vestibular neuritis in the acute and follow-up stages. *Audiol Neurotol*, 16(4), 248–53.

60. Walker MF, Zee DS (1999). The effect of hyperventilation on downbeat nystagmus in cerebellar disorders. *Neurology*, 53(7), 1576–9.

61. Nelson JR (1969). The minimal ice water caloric test. *Neurology*, 19(6), 577–85.

62. Torres-Russotto D, Landau W, Harding G, Bohne B, Sun K, Sinatra P (2009). Calibrated finger rub auditory screening test (CALFRAST). *Neurology*, 72(18), 1595–600.

63. Pirozzo S, Papinczak T, Glasziou P (2003). Whispered voice test for screening for hearing impairment in adults and children: systematic review. *BMJ*, 327(7421), 967–71.

64. Halmagyi GM, Aw ST, McGarvie LA, *et al.* (2003). Superior semicircular canal dehiscence simulating otosclerosis. *J Laryngol Otol*, 117(7), 553–7.

CHAPTER 13

Oscillopsia and Visuo-Vestibular Symptoms[1]

Adolfo M. Bronstein

In order to achieve clear vision, objects projecting onto the retina have to be stationary, otherwise vision is blurred. The vestibular and visual systems complement each other in eliciting slow-phase eye movements in order to stabilize moving visual images on the retina. Pursuit–optokinetic eye movements are elicited by visual motion whereas vestibular eye movements (vestibulo-ocular reflex,

VOR) are elicited by head motion. These two systems work synergistically when a person rotates with eyes open while gazing at the surrounding environment, for instance, a passenger looking out of a bus which is turning (Figure 13.1, top). However, they are said to be in conflict ('visuo-vestibular conflict') when a person looks at a visual object that rotates with him/her, e.g. a passenger reading

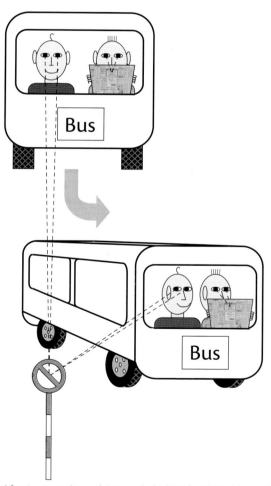

Fig. 13.1 In the passenger looking out of the bus and fixating upon the road sign, vestibular (VOR) and visual (pursuit) mechanisms cooperate to stabilize the eyes on the road sign as the bus turns round. In the passenger reading the newspaper, the VOR takes the eyes off the visual target (the newspaper) but pursuit eye movements are used to suppress the VOR. In the latter situation visual and vestibular inputs are said to be in conflict. From Bronstein and Lempert (67), with permission.

[1] This chapter is based on a previous publication (Bronstein AM (21)), appropriately updated.

a book on a bus (Figure 13.1, bottom). In this case, instead of collaborating with the VOR, the visual input actually suppresses the VOR (VOR suppression).

The vestibular and visual inputs also interact in pathological situations, e.g. in the presence of vestibular lesions. Figure 13.2, illustrates the fact that the first line of defence against a pathological nystagmus due to a labyrinthine lesion is to resort to VOR suppression mechanisms so that visual stability can be partly restored (Figure 13.2). Similarly, absent (1) or altered visual input as in congenital nystagmus (2) or external ophthalmoplegia (3) modifies vestibular function and perception. It is thus not surprising that vestibular lesions can cause visual symptoms and that visual input influences vestibular symptoms. The purpose of this chapter is to review some clinically relevant syndromes in which visuo-vestibular interaction is prominent. These are: 1) the presence of diplopia in vestibular lesions, 2) symptoms of oscillopsia, or illusory motion of the visual scene, and 3) the syndrome of 'visual vertigo' in which patients with vestibular disorders report worsening of their symptoms during visual motion stimuli (visually-induced dizziness) (4). Finally a brief comment on auditory-induced visuo-vestibular symptoms will be included.

Double vision in vestibular disorders

Diplopia arises when the image of an object falls on non-corresponding points in the two retinas. It is prudent to assume that, in principle, a lesion causing double vision has affected the nuclei or nerves of the IIIrd, IVth, or VIth cranial nerves or the neuromuscular apparatus (i.e. nuclear or infranuclear lesions). However, sometimes vertical and oblique ('skew') diplopia can be due to a skew ocular deviation which is a pre- or supranuclear eye movement disorder (5–8).

The vestibular system is a supranuclear mechanism controlling eye movements. Tilt of the head to an ear-down (i.e. coronal plane) side elicits the torsional VOR. In afoveated animals with laterally-placed eyes, like the rabbit, the torsional VOR

response includes a strong component of vertical ocular deviation, that is, the eye on the ear-down side moves up and the eye on the ear-up side moves down (9). This reflex eye movement is partly mediated by otolith (gravitational) and anterior and posterior semicircular canal input and supposedly contributes to preserving visual alignment with respect to earth horizontal (Figure 13.3). Unilateral vestibular lesions can cause severe imbalance in this mechanism, in turn leading to large vertical ocular misalignment in these animals (10). It has been postulated that the vertical misalignment observed in primates after unilateral vestibular nuclei lesions arises from imbalance in a similar 'vestigial' mechanism. Such vestigial mechanisms do exist in man since stimulation of the vertical (i.e. anterior and posterior) semicircular canals by rotation induces a physiological skew deviation of the eyes (11–13). Despite the fact that the otolith (gravitational) component of this normal skew deviation in man is smaller than the semicircular canal one (12), the pathways mediating this response are sometimes loosely labelled as 'graviceptive'.

In theory, any lesion involving the torsional VOR system in man could produce a skew eye deviation. Clinically, however, large skew deviations are due to lesions involving the brainstem vestibular pathways. Lesions in the region of the medullary vestibular nuclei are on the side of the lower (hypodeviated) eye whereas lesions in the midbrain, involving the interstitial nucleus of Cajal, tend to be on the side of the higher (hyperdeviated) eye (6, 14). This suggests that pathways subserving torsional and skew mechanisms cross the midline in the mid-upper pons. Cerebellar lesions can also induce skew deviations, probably by interfering with cerebellar control of vestibular nuclei activity (15, 16).

Peripheral lesions of the vestibular apparatus or nerve can sometimes induce diplopia and skew eye deviation, including after transtympanic gentamicin injections for Ménière's disease (8). Although exceptionally the ocular deviation is large and easily visible (5), patients with peripheral vestibular disorders typically show small skew deviations. It is not clear why some patients with identical

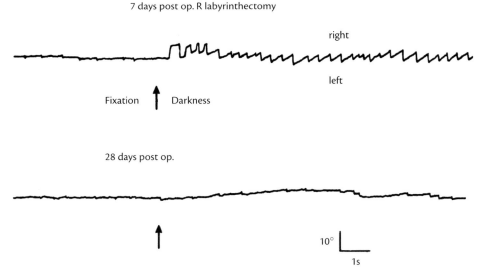

7 days post op. R labyrinthectomy

right

left

Fixation ↑ Darkness

28 days post op.

↑

10°

1s

Fig. 13.2 Horizontal eye movement recordings (electro-oculography technique) in a patient 7 days (top) and 1 month after a labyrinthectomy (bottom). Note that the nystagmus in the acute phase is almost exclusively seen in the dark—such suppression of the nystagmus by visual fixation is thought to be akin to normal VOR suppression.

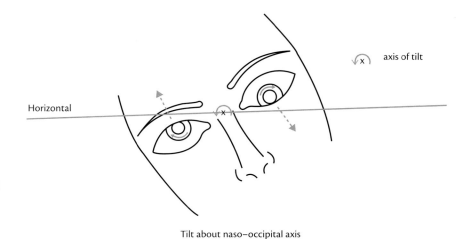

axis of tilt

Horizontal

Tilt about naso–occipital axis

Fig. 13.3 Diagram to illustrate the possible physiological mechanism underlying skew deviations in man. During right-ear-down tilt the eyes counter-rotate torsionally and diverge vertically so that they would tend to remain aligned with earth horizontal. Such eye movements exist in man but are stronger in response to vertical semicircular canal stimulation than to otolith-mediated static tilt (12). From Lopez et al. (18), with permission.

vestibular lesions (e.g. vestibular neurectomy) develop diplopia and skew deviation and some do not. It has been suggested that preoperative subclinical squints or extraocular muscle imbalances may predispose some subjects to develop a skew but this could not be confirmed in a controlled study pre- and post vestibular neurectomy (17). Instead, the appearance of a postoperative skew was related to the degree of ocular torsion induced, in turn related to the magnitude of the vestibular imbalance created, e.g. more likely to occur in patients with preoperatively preserved caloric function (17). In any case, the diplopia only lasted for a few days and was only present in about a third of the patients.

Other features are frequently associated with the skew deviation. These include a change in torsional eye position (eyes tilted or cycloverted in the direction of the lower eye) and, as a consequence, a tilt of subjective visual vertical in the same direction as the eye tilt (14). A torsional nystagmus beating opposite to the side of the lower eye is also common (18). In addition, patients often experience body lateropulsion, with a tendency to fall, and sometimes a head tilt towards the lower eye side. Conceptually, eyes and body are tilted in the same direction by a pathologically biased torsional vestibulo-ocular and -spinal systems.

Details of the clinical examination of these ocular features are covered in Chapter 12; however, the value of the alternate eye cover test in order to detect a small vertical skew deviation should be remembered. The most frequent differential diagnosis of an acquired skew deviation is a nuclear/infranuclear IIIrd, or more commonly, IVth nerve palsy (6). In principle, because they ultimately are a sign of a vestibular disorder, skew deviations occur in patients with severe postural imbalance and vertigo. Also, one expects a skew to be comitant (i.e. fairly constant with changes in gaze position) and a IVth nerve palsy to be incomitant (maximal with gaze deviation in the plane of the weakened muscle; e.g. for a left IVth palsy, maximal vertical ocular separation on right downward gaze deviation). Unfortunately, this is not a strict rule as some skews are partly incomitant and some trochlear palsies develop secondary comitancy. It should also be remembered that central lesions capable of producing these disorders (stroke, demyelination, brainstem gliomas, head injury) can involve nuclear, infranuclear, and prenuclear components simultaneously. Evidence of binocular ocular torsion, as measured from fundus photographs or separate eye subjective visual vertical settings, is strong indication that the disorder is prenuclear, i.e. a true skew (Chapter

12). In congenital strabismus, myasthenia gravis, chronic progressive extraocular ophthalmoplegia and orbital disorders, which can also induce a vertical ocular disconjugacy, there is a dearth of vestibular and brainstem symptoms. Details of how to differentiate these disorders from skew deviations should be sought elsewhere (see Chapter 12; 6, 19).

The treatment of a skew eye deviation is the treatment of the underlying condition and of the double vision. In peripheral vestibular disorders the diplopia is usually transient and requires no treatment. In brainstem lesions the disparity is usually large and, to a variable degree, permanent. In these cases, particularly when there is a high degree of comitancy, vertical prisms can help considerably but initially an eye patch may be required so that patients can progress in their general neurological rehabilitation. In the long term, squint surgery can be considered for individual patients.

Oscillopsia

The illusion that the visual surroundings are moving or oscillating is called oscillopsia. Patients with oscillopsia describe their problem in many different ways, so doctors should scrutinize patients' symptoms such as ' blurred vision', 'difficulty in focusing', 'shimmering vision' and ask directly if their vision is moving, oscillating, jumping, or 'wobbly' (20).

In order to diagnose the cause of the oscillopsia, it is practical to classify the various syndromes causing oscillopsia on the basis of specific questions to the patient. In particular one should ask *when* the oscillopsia occurs. Is the oscillopsia present *during* movements of the head? Is it *triggered* by certain movements of the head? Does it occur *at rest*? (See Table 13.1; slightly modified from (21).)

Oscillopsia during head movement

Typically, patients with absent vestibular function describe that while walking, running, or riding in a car, they are unable to recognize objects such as road signs or neighbours' faces. Often, they report that the blurring is actually bouncing up and down of the images. If they stop then they are able to see clearly and the oscillopsia disappears. This type of history should immediately prompt a diagnosis of bilateral severe vestibular failure. Oscillopsia induced by head (or whole-body) movements strongly suggests that the VOR is absent.

Table 13.1 Oscillopsia diagnostic algorithm. **When** does the oscillopsia occur?

1. **During** movements of the head:
   →Absent VOR: bilateral loss of vestibular function:
   - Postmeningitic
   - Ototoxicity
   - Idiopathic
   - Miscellaneous

2. **Triggered** by movements of the head:
   →Positional nystagmus: brainstem-cerebellar disease

3. **At rest** (not significantly associated to movement):
   Paroxysmal:
   - Sound-induced: Tullio phenomenon (superior canal dehiscence)
   - Vestibular paroxysms:
     - VIIIth nerve: vestibular paroxysmia
     - Vestibular nuclear lesions
   - Ocular flutter
   - Microflutter
   - Voluntary nystagmus
   - Monocular: superior oblique myokymia
   Continuous:
   - Nystagmus (brainstem-cerebellar lesion):
     - Pendular
     - Down/Up beat
     - Torsional
     - Others
   - Pseudonystagmus (head tremor + absent VOR)

There are several ways of identifying bilateral vestibular loss in the clinic (reviewed in Chapter 12). The general principle is that, in the absence of the VOR, the slow-phase compensatory eye movements generated during head movements will be absent or insufficient. The catch-up saccades generated to maintain fixation on a visual target, whilst the patient's head is moved by the doctor, can be seen during ophthalmoscopy (23) or by direct careful observation of the eyes during an imposed fast head movement (head thrust or head impulse test) (24, 25). Dynamic visual acuity is a clinical technique which does not rely so much on eye movement expertise; the principle is to compare a patient's visual acuity with and without imposed head oscillation (26) (Chapter 14). However, patients suspected of having bilateral vestibular loss should undergo objective rotational or caloric testing.

The more common causes of bilateral vestibular loss are meningitis, ototoxicity (mainly gentamicin), idiopathic bilateral vestibular loss, and miscellaneous causes (cranial neuropathies, degenerative conditions, severe head trauma) (27, 28). I would particularly like to draw attention to the high incidence of idiopathic cases of bilateral vestibular loss (up to 50% in some series). This condition is largely overlooked by clinical neurologists because the patient's unsteadiness is rarely pronounced and there is neither hearing loss nor major abnormalities on neurological examination. The only findings would be gait unsteadiness, particularly with eyes closed or during heel-to-toe walking, a bilaterally positive head thrust test (or broken up eye movements during doll's head movements), and loss of dynamic visual acuity (see preceding paragraph). Think of this condition in any patient with unexplained unsteadiness, particularly in the dark, or unexplained visual symptoms during movement. If in doubt, request formal vestibular tests. This syndrome is reviewed in Chapter 26.

Oscillopsia triggered by head position/positioning

These patients describe that in certain head positions the world seems to jump or flick, 'as if the vertical hold on the TV set has gone'. Patients may note that when they lie down in bed electrical appliances on the ceiling appear to move or 'flick'. A patient may be able to read his newspaper seated but not lying down, or more rarely, vice versa. Patients with this type of clinical history often have positional nystagmus, typically of central origin, since peripheral positional nystagmus (benign paroxysmal positional vertigo, BPPV) produces vertigo rather than oscillopsia. In all these cases, one should investigate patients with positional manoeuvres, such as the Hallpike manoeuvre. However, if a specific head position is the trigger for a particular patient this should be reproduced in the clinic under careful observation of the eyes (e.g. some patients have stronger nystagmus with the face prone) (29).

The most common central positional nystagmus is positional downbeat nystagmus. The associated positional oscillopsia is troublesome only in a small proportion of patients. The oscillopsia is often transient because the nystagmus usually lasts a few seconds—technically 'positioning' rather than positional nystagmus. In 50 patients with positional downbeat nystagmus, cerebellar degenerative disorders, including multiple system atrophy, were the most common cause (30). This was followed by vascular, demyelinating, and other miscellaneous disorders. Interestingly, although the Arnold–Chiari malformation is one of the frequent diagnoses for conventional downbeat nystagmus (i.e. present with the head upright) (31, 32), we did not encounter any Arnold–Chiari malformation in our 50 patients with only positional downbeat nystagmus.

Oscillopsia at rest

When patients report that the oscillopsia is largely unrelated to movement or position, the next important question is whether the oscillopsia is paroxysmal or continuous (see Table 13.1).

Paroxysmal oscillopsia

Paroxysmal oscillopsia usually reflects a transient paroxysmal nystagmus or ocular oscillation. Patients often report just a few seconds of shaking of visual images, but episodes may be very frequent. Extra-axial lesions impinging upon the vestibular nerve can cause paroxysmal oscillopsia with or without vertigo. This syndrome of 'vestibular paroxysmia' (33) is not uncommon but in many patients one cannot find a cause. Carbamazepine is a useful treatment and if the history sounds compatible a treatment trial is warranted.

If paroxysmal oscillopsia and unsteadiness are induced by loud sounds, either external or the patient's own voice, the patient has the Tullio phenomenon. This is vestibular activation by sound (or pressure) and is usually (but not always (34)) due to an internal fistula of the superior semicircular canal—the superior canal dehiscence syndrome which can be visualized on high-resolution bone computed tomography imaging (35).

A number of intra-brainstem irritative lesions such as arteriovenous malformations, tumours, and sequelae from vascular or inflammatory lesions can produce paroxysmal nystagmus and oscillopsia (36–38). Ocular flutter is a saccadic oscillatory disorder that can be observed in cerebellar or brainstem disease (reviewed in (38)); it is a disorder related to opsoclonus. In flutter there are back-to-back saccades selectively in the horizontal plane, often in paroxysms, whereas in opsoclonus the back-to-back saccades occur in all three planes in a fairly continuous fashion. Microflutter or microsaccadic oscillations can cause paroxysmal oscillopsia and be seen on ophthalmoscopy or high-resolution oculography; they often are not related to neurological disease (39).

Perhaps the most common cause of paroxysmal oscillopsia is 'voluntary nystagmus' or 'VN' (40). It consists of a horizontal fast saccadic oscillation (10–20Hz), sometimes associated with other ocular psychogenic conditions such as convergence spasm. Many normal subjects can generate VN (up to 8% according to (41), often via a conscious convergence effort. VN per se can be difficult to distinguish from ocular flutter and one has to resort to the general neurological and psychological context to reach a diagnosis.

Finally, if paroxysmal oscillopsia is monocular the diagnosis is almost certainly superior oblique myokymia. Vascular loops impinging on the IVth cranial nerve have been invoked as a cause but aetiology in an individual patient is often elusive (42, 43).

Continuous oscillopsia

When a patient experiences oscillopsia continuously, one must assume that the patient has spontaneous nystagmus in primary gaze, including downbeat nystagmus (31), upbeat nystagmus (29), pendular nystagmus (44), and torsional nystagmus (18). The majority of the diseases causing these various types of nystagmus have additional oculomotor and neurological signs and are usually diagnosed by magnetic resonance imaging; namely cerebellar atrophy, Arnold–Chiari malformation, intrinsic brainstem, or cerebellar lesions—chiefly multiple sclerosis, strokes, inflammation, and tumours. The most visually disabling nystagmus is pendular nystagmus with patients unable to read or watch TV.

Sometimes the nystagmus is of very low amplitude (<0.5°) and only visible with the ophthalmoscope. It must be kept in mind, however, that almost a quarter of normal subjects have a micro upbeat nystagmus (45) and that it can just be seen on fundoscopy (NB remember that directions of eye movements are inverted during fundoscopy because you are looking at the back of the eye).

A condition, not very common but capable of creating significant clinical confusion, is 'pendular pseudonystagmus' (46, 47). In this syndrome, patients report fairly continuous oscillopsia, sometimes aggravated by stress and relieved by resting or lying down. The origin of this syndrome is the chance combination in an individual of bilateral vestibular failure and head tremor. In the absence of VOR, the head tremor induces retinal image slippage and hence high-frequency oscillation (4–6Hz) of the visual world. Neurological examination shows mild to moderate postural unsteadiness (due to the bilateral vestibular failure) and head tremor which can be almost imperceptible. Ocular examination reveals 'pendular nystagmus' (but only during ophthalmoscopy) and a bilaterally positive head thrust test. If the head is rigidly immobilized, e.g. by an observer or by lying down with a firm head rest, the fundus oscillation and oscillopsia disappear.

Treatment of oscillopsia

Patients with bilateral absence of vestibular function can improve with vestibular rehabilitation and head–eye coordination exercises (47, 48). If an additional head tremor is aggravating the problem (pendular pseudonystagmus syndrome), propranolol or other treatments for tremor (including botulinum toxin) may help (46, 47).

A general review on the treatment of nystagmus and oscillopsia has been published but all evidence was classified as type 'C', since no double-blind trials are available (49). In patients with paroxysmal oscillopsia due to vestibular nerve or nuclei irritative lesions one should try carbamazepine in the first instance. Sometimes small amounts of the drug such as 100mg three times a day can produce good results. For more continuous cases of oscillopsia, as in pendular nystagmus, gabapentin, clonazepam, valproate, anti-parkinsonian anticholinergic drugs (e.g. biperiden, orphenadrine) and memantine can be tried. Different patients respond to different drugs so one should be used at a time but, eventually, a combination of drugs could be tried. Results are never spectacular. Downbeat nystagmus can respond to 3,4 diaminopiridine (3,4DAP) and to 4 aminopiridine (4AP) (50), in the author's opinion in approximately one-third of patients. 4AP is more effective probably due to its pharmacokinetic properties which provide a longer lasting effect (50).

Visual vertigo

The syndrome of visually-induced dizziness, as now defined by the International Committee on the Classification of Vestibular Disorders of the Barany Society, refers to the worsening or triggering of vestibular symptoms in certain visual environments (44). These patients dislike moving visual surroundings, as encountered in traffic, crowds, disco lights, and car-chase scenes in films. Typically, such symptoms develop when walking in busy visual surroundings such as supermarket aisles. The development of these symptoms in some patients with vestibular disorders has long been recognized (51, 52); (see (53) for review) and given various names such as visuo-vestibular mismatch (54), space and motion discomfort (55), or visual vertigo (56, 57). This syndrome should not be confused with oscillopsia. In oscillopsia there is oscillation of the visual world—the symptom is visual. In visual vertigo, the trigger is visual but the symptom is of a vestibular kind such as dizziness, vertigo, disorientation, and unsteadiness.

The symptoms of visual vertigo develop after a vestibular insult. A typical patient is a previously asymptomatic person who suffers an acute peripheral disorder (e.g. vestibular neuritis) and that after an initial period of recovery of a few weeks, he/she discovers that the dizzy symptoms do not fully disappear. Furthermore, symptoms are aggravated by looking at moving or repetitive images, as described earlier. Patients may also develop anxiety or frustration because symptoms do not go away or because medical practitioners tend to disregard this syndrome.

The origin and significance of the symptoms of visual vertigo in vestibular patients has been the subject of research. We know that tilted or moving visual surroundings have a pronounced influence on these patients' perception of verticality and balance, over and above what can be expected from an underlying vestibular deficit (56, 57). This increased responsiveness to visual stimuli is called 'visual dependency'. Patients with central vestibular disorders and patients combining vestibular disorders and congenital squints or squint surgery can also report visual vertigo and show enhanced visuo-postural reactivity (56).

Overall, these findings suggest that the combination of a vestibular disorder and visual dependence in a given patient is what leads to the visual vertigo syndrome. Ultimately, what makes some patients with vestibular disorders develop such visual dependence is not known. The role of the associated anxiety-depression, often observed in these patients, and whether this is a primary or secondary phenomenon is not known (see Chapter 30). The limited evidence so far does not indicate that anxiety or depression levels are higher in visual vertigo patients than in other patients seen in dizzy clinics (57, 58).

The more important differential diagnosis in these patients is, however, one of a purely psychological disorder or panic attacks (59). An accepted set of criteria to distinguish between psychological and vestibular symptoms is, however, not complete at this stage (28, 59, 60; see Chapter 30). However, a patient who has never had a clear history of vestibular disease, with no findings on vestibular examination and with visual triggers restricted to a single particular environment (e.g. only supermarkets) would be more likely to have a primary psychological disorder. Reciprocally, a patient with no premorbid psychological dysfunction who after a vestibular insult develops car tilting illusions when driving (61) or dizziness when looking at moving visual scenes (traffic, crowds, movies) is more likely to have the visual vertigo syndrome. A syndrome including migraine, dizziness, anxiety, and visual dependence, including interesting potential anatomical substrates, has been discussed by Furman et al. (62).

Treatment of visual vertigo

There are three aspects in the treatment of patients with the visual vertigo syndrome. The first is specific measures for the underlying vestibular disorder, e.g. Ménière's disease, BPPV, migraine and these will be found elsewhere in this book. However, a specific aetiological diagnosis cannot be confirmed in many patients with chronic dizziness.

Second, patients benefit from general vestibular rehabilitation with a suitably trained audiologist or physiotherapist. These exercise-based programmes can be either generic, like the original Cawthorne–Cooksey approach (63) or, preferably, customized to

the patient's needs. All regimes involve progressive eye, head, and whole-body movements (bending, turning) as well as walking exercises (64–66).

Finally, specific measures should be introduced in the rehabilitation programme in order to reduce their hyper-reactivity to visual motion. The aim is to promote desensitization and increase tolerance to visual stimuli and to visuo-vestibular conflict. Patients are therefore exposed, under the instruction of the vestibular physiotherapist, to optokinetic stimuli which can be delivered via projection screens, head-mounted virtual reality systems, video monitors, ballroom planetariums, or optokinetic rotating systems (67). Initially patients watch these stimuli whilst seated, then standing, walking, initially without and then with head movements, in a progressive fashion (Figure 13.4). Recent research has shown that these patients benefit from repeated and gradual exposure to such visual motion training programmes; both the dizziness and associated psychological symptoms improve over and above conventional vestibular rehabilitation (69).

Unusual audio-visuo-vestibular symptoms

Occasionally, some patients report that they can hear their own eye movements (70). There are two syndromes in which this unusual symptom is observed. The first one, gaze-evoked tinnitus, develops postoperatively in patients with cerebello-pontine angle surgery (71). Patients can describe a tonal tinnitus when looking towards the operated side. A patient 'could play a tune' with her eyes at different eccentricities (70). Gaze-evoked tinnitus was initially thought to be rare, but subsequently reported to be surprisingly common if actively enquired (prevalence 19–36% in one study of patients post vestibular schwannoma resection (72)). It has also been described in patients with cerebello-pontine angle meningioma, meningeal metastases of malignant melanoma, and sudden sensorineural hearing loss (72). It may develop months postoperatively, and is usually heard in, and caused by moving the eyes towards, the diseased ear. The exact mechanism is not known, but it has been postulated that neural plasticity mechanisms activated

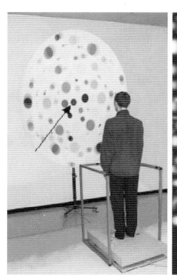 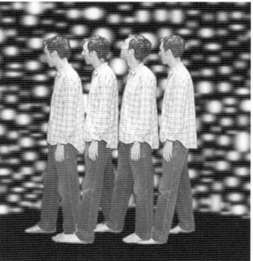 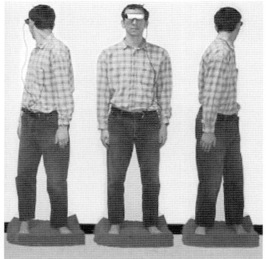

Fig. 13.4 Visual motion desensitization treatment for patients with vestibular disorders reporting visual vertigo symptoms. Left: roll (coronal) plane rotating optokinetic disk. Middle: planetarium-generated moving dots whilst the subject walks. Right: 'Eye-Trek' or head-mounted TV systems projecting visual motion stimuli. In this case, in advanced stages of the therapy, the patient moves the head and trunk whilst standing on rubber foam. Modified from Pavlou et al. (68) with permission.

by unilateral deafferentation result in cross-talk between neural elements controlling eye movements and the central auditory system. Functional imaging studies have shown anomalous activation of the auditory lateral pons and auditory cortex (73).

When, in addition to hearing their own eyes move, patients report being able to hear their own heart beats, bone taps, and footsteps the underlying condition is likely to be superior canal dehiscence. These patients also show the Tullio phenomenon, vestibular activation by loud sounds (74; 34, for review). Supranormal bone conduction thresholds, or so-called 'conductive hyperacusis', has been reported in this condition. The dehiscence may act as an alternative lower impedance pathway for sound energy (35), enabling these patients to hear the movements of their eyeballs within the bony sockets.

References

1. Seemungal BM, Glasauer S, Gresty MA, Bronstein AM. (2007). Vestibular perception and navigation in the congenitally blind. *J Neurophysiol*, 97(6), 4341–56.
2. Okada T, Grunfeld E, Shallo-Hoffmann J, Bronstein AM. (1999). Vestibular perception of angular velocity in normal subjects and in patients with congenital nystagmus. *Brain*, 122, 1293–303.
3. Grunfeld EA, Shallo-Hoffmann JA, Cassidy L, et al. (2003). Vestibular perception in patients with acquired ophthalmoplegia. *Neurology*, 60, 1993–5.
4. Bisdorff A, Von Brevern M, Lempert T, Newman-Toker DE (2009). Classification of vestibular symptoms: towards an international classification of vestibular disorders. *J Vestib Res*, 19, 1–13.
5. Halmagyi GM, Gresty MA, Gibson WP. (1979). Ocular tilt reaction with peripheral vestibular lesion. *Ann Neurol*, 6(1), 80–3.
6. Brodsky MC, Donahue SP, Vaphiades M, Brandt T. (2006). Skew deviation revisited. *Surv Ophthalmol*, 51(2), 105–28.
7. Vibert D, Hausler R, Safran AB, Koerner F. (1996). Diplopia from skew deviation in unilateral peripheral vestibular lesions. *Acta Otolaryngol*, 116(2), 170–6.
8. Ng D, Fouladvand M, Lalwani AK (2011). Skew deviation after intratympanic gentamicin therapy. *Laryngoscope*, 121, 492–4.
9. Barmack NH. (1981). A comparison of the horizontal and vertical vestibulo-ocular reflexes of the rabbit. *J Physiol*, 314, 547–64.
10. Magnus R (1924). *Korperstellung*. Berlin: Verlag-Springer.
11. Jauregui-Renaud K, Faldon M, Clarke A, Bronstein AM, Gresty MA (1996). Skew deviation of the eyes in normal human subjects induced by semicircular canal stimulation. *Neurosci Lett*, 23, 205(2), 135–7.
12. Jauregui-Renaud K, Faldon M, Clarke AH, Bronstein AM, Gresty MA. (1998). Otolith and semicircular canal contributions to the human binocular response to roll oscillation. *Acta Otolaryngol*, 118(2), 170–6.
13. Jauregui-Renaud K, Faldon ME, Gresty MA, Bronstein AM. (2001). Horizontal ocular vergence and the three-dimensional response to whole-body roll motion. *Exp Brain Res*, 136(1), 79–92.
14. Brandt T, Dieterich M. (1994). Vestibular syndromes in the roll plane: topographic diagnosis from brainstem to cortex. *Ann Neurol*, 36(3), 337–47.
15. Wong AM, Sharpe JA. (2005) Cerebellar skew deviation and the torsional vestibuloocular reflex. *Neurology*, 65, 412–19.
16. Mossman S, Halmagyi GM. (1997). Partial ocular tilt reaction due to unilateral cerebellar lesion. *Neurology*, 49(2), 491–3.
17. Riordan-Eva P, Harcourt JP, Faldon M, Brookes GB, Gresty MA. (1997). Skew deviation following vestibular nerve surgery. *Ann Neurol*, 41(1), 94–9.
18. Lopez L, Bronstein AM, Gresty MA, Rudge P, du Boulay EP (1992). Torsional nystagmus. A neuro-otological and MRI study of thirty-five cases. *Brain*, 115, 1107–24.
19. Leigh RJ, Zee D (1999). *The neurology of eye movements* (3rd ed). New York: Oxford University Press.
20. Bender MB (1965). Oscillopsia. *Arch Neurol*, 13, 204–13.
21. Bronstein AM (2004). Vision and vertigo. Some visual aspects of vestibular disorders. *J Neurol*, 251, 381–87.
22. Bronstein AM (2003). Vestibular reflexes and positional manoeuvres. *J Neurol Neurosurg Psychiatry*, 74, 289–93.
23. Zee DS (1978) Ophthalmoscopy in examination of patients with vestibular disorders. *Ann Neurol*, 3, 373–4.
24. Halmagyi GM, Curthoys IS (1988). A clinical sign of canal paresis. *Arch Neurol*, 45, 737–9.
25. Cremer PD, Halmagyi GM, Aw ST, et al. (1998). Semicircular canal plane head impulses detect absent function of individual semicircular canals. *Brain*, 121, 699–716.
26. Longridge NS, Mallinson AI (1987). The dynamic illegible E-test. A technique for assessing the vestibule-ocular reflex. *Acta Otolaryngol*, 103, 273–9.
27. Rinne T, Bronstein AM, Rudge P, Gresty MA, Luxon LM (1995) Bilateral loss of vestibular function. *Acta Otolaryngol Suppl*, 520, 247–50.
28. Brandt T (1996). Phobic postural vertigo. *Neurology*, 46, 1515–9.
29. Fisher A, Gresty MA, Chambers B, Rudge P (1983). Primary position upbeating nystagmus. A variety of central positional nystagmus. *Brain*, 106, 949–64.
30. Bertholon P, Bronstein AM, Davies RA, Rudge P, Thilo KV (2002). Positional down beating nystagmus in 50 patients: cerebellar disorders and possible anterior semicircular canalithiasis. *J Neurol Neurosurg Psychiatry*, 72, 366–72.
31. Bronstein AM, Miller DH, Rudge P, Kendall BE (1987). Downbeating nystagmus: magnetic resonances imaging and neuro-otological findings. *J Neurol Sci*, 81, 173–84.
32. Halmagyi GM, Rudge P, Gresty MA, Sanders MD (1983). Downbeating nystagmus. A review of 62 cases. *Arch Neurol*, 40, 777–84.
33. Brandt T, Dieterich M (1994). Vestibular paroxysmia: vascular compression of the eighth nerve? *Lancet*, 343, 798–9.
34. Kaski D, Davies R, Luxon L, Bronstein AM, Rudge P. (2012). The Tullio phenomenon: a neurologically neglected presentation. *J Neurol*, 259(1), 4–21.
35. Minor LB, Cremer PD, Carey JP, Della Santina CC, Streubel SO, Weg N (2001) Symptoms and signs in superior canal dehiscence syndrome. *Ann N Y Acad Sci*, 942, 259–73.
36. Bronstein AM, Pérennou DA, Guerraz M, Playford D, Rudge P (2003). Dissociation of visual and haptic vertical in two patients with vestibular nuclear lesions. *Neurology*, 61, 1260–2.
37. Lawden MC, Bronstein AM, Kennard C (1995). Repetitive paroxysmal nystagmus and vertigo. *Neurology*, 45, 276–80.
38. Radtke A, Bronstein AM, Gresty MA, et al. (2001) Paroxysmal alternating skew deviation and nystagmus after partial destruction of the uvula. *J Neurol Neurosurg Psychiatry*, 70, 790–3.
39. Ashe J, Hain TC, Zee DS, Schatz NJ (1991). Microsaccadic flutter. *Brain*, 114, 461–72.
40. Hotson JR (1984). Clinical detection of acute vestibulocerebellar disorder. *West J Med*, 140, 910–3.
41. Zahn JR (1978). Incidence and characteristics of voluntary nystagmus. *J Neurol Neurosurg Psychiatry*, 41, 617–23.
42. Yousry I, Dieterich M, Naidich TP, Schmid UD, Yousry TA (2002) Superior oblique myokymia: magnetic resonance imaging support for the neurovascular compression hypothesis. *Ann Neurol*, 51, 361–8.
43. Hashimoto M, Ohtsuka K, Hoyt WF (2001). Vascular compression as a cause of superior oblique myokymia disclosed by thin-slice magnetic resonance imaging. *Am J Ophthalmol*, 131, 676–7.
44. Lopez LI, Bronstein AM, Gresty MA, du Boulay EP, Rudge P (1996). Clinical and MRI correlates in 27 patients with acquired pendular nystagmus. *Brain*, 119, 465–72.

45. Bisdorff AR, Sancovic S, Debatisse D, Bentley C, Gresty MA, Bronstein AM (2000). Positional nystagmus in the dark in normal subjects. *Neuro-ophthalmology*, 24, 283–90.

46. Bronstein AM, Gresty MA, Mossman SS (1992). Pendular pseudonystagmus arising as a combination of head tremor and vestibular failure. *Neurology*, 42, 1527–31.

47. Yen MT, Herdman SJ, Tusa RJ (1999) Oscillopsia and pseudonystagmus in kidney transplant patients. *Am J Ophthalmol*, 128, 768–70.

48. Telian SA, Shepard NT, Smith-Wheelock M, Hoberg M (1991) Bilateral vestibular paresis: diagnosis and treatment. *Otolaryngol Head Neck Surg*, 104, 67–71.

49. Straube A, Leigh RJ, Bronstein A, *et al.* (2004) EFNS task force—therapy of nystagmus and oscillopsia. *Eur J Neurol*, 11, 1–7.

50. Strupp M, Schuler O, Krafczyk S, *et al.* (2003) Treatment of downbeat nystagmus with 3, 4-diaminopyridine: A placebo-controlled study. *Neurology*, 61, 165–70.

51. Hoffman RA, Brookler KH (1978). Underrated neurotologic symptoms. *Laryngoscope*, 88, 1127–38.

52. Hood JD (1980). Unsteadiness of cerebellar origin: an investigation into its cause. *J Laryngol Otol*, 94, 865–76.

53. Bronstein AM (2002). Under-rated neuro-otological symptoms: Hoffman and Brookler 1978 revisited. *Brit Med Bull*, 63, 213–21.

54. Longridge NS, Mallinson AI, Denton A (2002). Visual vestibular mismatch in patients treated with intratympanic gentamicin for Meniere's disease. *J Otolaryngol*, 31, 5–8.

55. Jacob RG (1988). Panic disorder and the vestibular system. *Psychiatr Clin North Am*, 11, 361–74.

56. Bronstein AM (1995). Visual vertigo syndrome: clinical and posturography findings. *J Neurol Neurosurgery Psychiatry*, 59, 472–76.

57. Guerraz M, Yardley L, Bertholon P, *et al.* (2001). Visual vertigo: symptom assessment, spatial orientation and postural control. *Brain*, 124, 1646–56.

58. Pavlou M, Davies RA, Bronstein AM. (2006). The assessment of increased sensitivity to visual stimuli in patients with chronic dizziness. *J Vestibular Res*, 16, 223–31.

59. Furman JM, Jacob RG (1997). Psychiatric dizziness. *Neurology*, 48, 1161–6.

60. Bronstein AM, Gresty MA, Luxon LM, Ron MA, Rudge P, Yardley L (1996). Phobic postural vertigo. *Neurology*, 46, 1515–9.

61. Page NG, Gresty MA. (1985). Motorist's vestibular disorientation syndrome. *J Neurol Neurosurg Psychiatry*, 48, 729–35

62. Furman JM, Balaban CD, Jacob RG, Marcus DA (2005). Migraine-anxiety related dizziness (MARD): a new disorder? *J Neurol Neurosurg Psychiatry*, 76, 1–8.

63. Cawthorne T (1952). The rationale of physiotherapy in vertigo and facial palsy. *Physiotherapy*, 38, 237–41.

64. Black FO, Pesznecker SC (2003). Vestibular adaptation and rehabilitation. *Curr Opin Otolaryngol Head Neck Surg*, 11, 355–60.

65. Pavlou M, Shummway-Cook A, Horak F, Yardley L, Bronstein AM (2004). Rehabilitation of balance disorders in the patient with vestibular pathology. In Bronstein AM, Brandt T, Woollacott M, Nutt J (Eds) *Clinical disorders of balance, posture and gait*, pp. 317–43. London: Edward Arnold Publishers.

66. Bronstein AM, Lempert T (2007). *Dizziness: a practical approach to diagnosis and management. Cambridge Clinical Guides.* Cambridge: Cambridge University Press, Cambridge.

67. Vitte E, Semont A, Berthoz A (1994). Repeated optokinetic stimulation in conditions of active standing facilitates recovery from vestibular deficits. *Exp Brain Res*, 102, 141–8.

68. Pavlou M, Lingeswaran A, Davies RA, Gresty MA, Bronstein AM. (2004). Simulator based rehabilitation in refractory dizziness. *J Neurol*, 251, 983–95.

69. Pavlou M, Bronstein AM, Davies RA (2012). Randomized Trial of Supervised Versus Unsupervised Optokinetic Exercise in Persons With Peripheral Vestibular Disorders. *Neurorehabil Neural Repair*, Oct 16, 2012.

70. Albuquerque W, Bronstein AM (2004). 'Doctor, I can hear my eyes': report of two cases with different mechanisms. *J Neurol Neurosurg Psychiatry*, 75, 1363–4.

71. Whittaker CK. (1982). Letter to the editor. *Am J Otol*, 4, 188.

72. Biggs NDW, Ramsden RT. (2002). Gaze-evoked tinnitus following acoustic neuroma resection: a de-afferentation plasticity phenomenon? *Clin Otolaryngol*, 27, 338–43.

73. Lockwood AH, Wack MA, Burkard RF, *et al.* (2001). The functional anatomy of gaze-evoked tinnitus and sustained lateral gaze. *Neurology*, 56, 472–80

74. Colebatch JG, Day DL, Bronstein AM, *et al.* (1998). Vestibular hypersensitivity to clicks is characteristic of Tullio phenomenon. *J Neurol Neurosurg Psychiatry*, 65, 670–8

CHAPTER 14

The Role of Vestibular Laboratory Testing

Neil Shepard, Kristen Janky, and Scott Eggers

Introduction

For consistency, the nomenclature used in this chapter will follow that suggested for the International Classification of Vestibular Disorders for the definitions of vertigo, dizziness, and unsteadiness, collectively referred to as vestibular symptoms (see Chapter 16 for details) (1).

Evaluation of the dizzy patient should be guided by the information required to make initial and subsequent management decisions. The goal of the evaluation is markedly different for the acutely vertiginous patient and the patient with longstanding symptoms. In the acute patient, the primary aim is to rule out significant cardio-vascular and neurological disorders, quiet symptoms, and determine a working diagnosis. Extensive laboratory testing is generally unnecessary in the acute patient since the presenting symptoms and office examination will primarily guide initial management decisions. In the chronic patient (defined as having symptoms that are intermittent or persistent for greater than 2 months) addressing the question of why natural central compensation has not taken place in a significant manner to reduce symptoms and establish a refined diagnosis and treatment programme would be the goals. While videonystagmography (VNG), especially caloric testing, can be of use in the acute patient, it is the exception that this would be used acutely. Therefore, for the purposes of this chapter, discussion will be limited to the evaluation of the chronic patient.

For the chronic patient a detailed neuro-otological history together with a comprehensive direct vestibular office examination are equally as important as in the acute patient. The reader is referred to Chapters 11 and 12 for discussions regarding the history and presenting symptoms along with the office examination, and to Chapter 10 for sociological aspects. In the chronic patient, a detailed pre-evaluation patient questionnaire combined with a focused history obtained at the start of laboratory testing can facilitate selection of appropriate laboratory tests and guide the examiner regarding what tests beyond a basic core series of tests are needed for any given patient. This use of a staged testing protocol effectively allows laboratory information to be collected prior to the clinician's direct office interview and examination so that all of the information can then be collectively analysed in the context of the history and presenting symptoms (2).

What are the roles of vestibular laboratory studies?

1. Determination of extent and site of lesion within the peripheral and central vestibular system.

2. Determination of the functional limitations in static and dynamic postural control (this may be related directly to gait abnormalities) and function performance of the vestibulo-ocular reflex (VOR).

3. Assessment of the status of the compensation process.

4. Along with symptom presentation, to aid prognosis and design of vestibular and balance rehabilitation.

The collective use of the information is most often in the confirmation of the suspected site of lesion and diagnosis, both derived from the patient's history and direct office vestibular evaluation with audiometric evaluation. This does not imply a prioritized order to the testing versus the office visit, as with chronic dizzy patients it can be very useful to triage them to laboratory evaluations prior to the office visit.

Practitioners' expectations from laboratory tests are often unrealistic. A common misconception is that the studies will render a specific diagnosis or at a minimum drive the remainder of the investigation and help determine levels of disability. However, when the various tests listed here are reviewed and correlated with high-level activities of daily living, virtually no significant relationships exist for the chronic dizzy patient (3, 4). Tests considered extent and site of lesion studies, such as electronystagmography (ENG) or VNG (5), rotational chair (6), and specific protocols in postural control assessment, (7), give results that cannot be used to predict symptom type, magnitude, or the level of disability of an individual patient. Conversely, patient complaints cannot be used to predict the outcomes of these tests. In a limited manner more functionally oriented evaluation tools such as computerized dynamic posturography (CDP) (8) and dynamic visual acuity (DVA) testing (9)

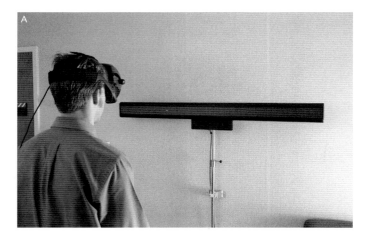

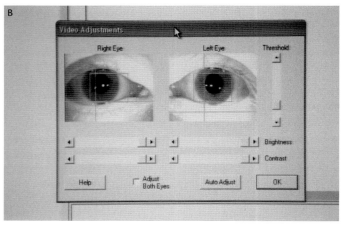

Fig. 14.1 The technique is shown for video recording of the eye movements used with pursuit, saccade, and graze stabilization testing. (A) shows the subject with binocular goggle system in place watching a moving target on the wall mounted light bar under computer control. (B) shows the video image of the subject's eyes as they are monitored and quantified by the computer system in the horizontal and vertical planes of motion. The system monitors directly the position of the eye in the orbit over time.

provide for correlation between test results, patient symptoms and functional limitations (10, 11). By adding to the testing specific or general health inventories such as the Dizziness Handicap Inventory, (12) predictive assessment of disability is improved but remains significantly limited (4). It is hypothesized that the reason for this dichotomy in test results versus functional disability and symptom complaints is the inability of the tests to adequately characterize the status of the central vestibular compensation process (10, 13, 14). In a number of cases the laboratory studies are confirmatory to the impressions of the detailed history and direct examination results. Also, it is rare that the laboratory studies return a specific aetiological diagnosis. Thus, vestibular laboratory testing is never a replacement for a detailed neuro-otological history and physical examination, but to be used in conjunction with the history and physical examination.

To summarize, the following are required elements to develop management decisions for the chronic dizzy patient: detailed neuro-otological history, office vestibular and physical examination, and formal audiometric testing given the inescapable anatomical relationship between the peripheral auditory and

vestibular systems. Laboratory vestibular and balance-function studies, neuroradiological evaluations, and serological tests all have important roles that are guided by the clinical context. It is important to realize that there will be patients for whom unexpected findings on any one of these latter studies will either completely alter management or add dimensions to the management not originally considered.

To establish how vestibular and balance studies may be utilized in a collective manner to assist in diagnosis and management and aid selection of the most useful tests for a given patient, a review of the specific rationale for each of the tests along with their performance at accomplishing that purpose is presented in the following section. These are abbreviated descriptions of the various tests. The reader seeking detailed descriptions of testing methodology and interpretations is referred to Jacobson and Shepard (15).

Routine tests of peripheral and central vestibular system function—ENG/VNG

Ocular motor testing

Ocular motor testing includes the grouping of pursuit, saccade, optokinetic, and gaze testing. Overall, these subtests provide an evaluation of central vestibulo-ocular and central ocular motor control function. The tests are performed using a computer-driven light bar or LCD projector for the visual stimulus with video or electrode recordings of the eye position in the orbit over time (Figure 14.1). For a more detailed description related to interpretations of this test grouping, the reader is referred to Leigh and Zee (16).

Pursuit tracking

The purpose of the pursuit tracking test is to assess the vestibulocerebellum and more generally, a variety of central ocular motor control pathways extending to regions above the cerebellum. Pursuit tracking is traditionally completed by asking the patient to track a moving target as it oscillates back and forth at variable frequencies, ranging from 0.2–0.7 Hz. The target is typically generated via a computerized system. The main outcome parameter is gain, which is calculated by dividing eye velocity by target velocity. Of all the ocular motor subtests, pursuit tracking has been demonstrated to be the most sensitive to central vestibular system abnormalities; however, does not provide the same site of lesion localization as the remaining ocular motor subtests (17).

Saccade testing

There are a variety of paradigms to assess saccade performance; however, the most widely used is the random saccade test. With the random saccade test the main outcome parameters are latency to onset of eye movement after the target movement, velocity of the eye movement, and accuracy in going to the target. In general, saccade accuracy is dictated by the cerebellar dorsal vermis and fastigial nucleus, with velocity influenced by the premotor burst neurons in the paramedian pontine reticular formation (horizontal saccades) and rostral interstitial nucleus of the medial longitudinal fasciculus (for vertical saccades) and latency determined by the frontal and parietal eye fields. Because these outcome parameters are engendered by different substrates, abnormalities of saccade latency, velocity, and accuracy can help to further determine site of lesion.

Gaze stability testing

The purpose of gaze testing is to assess for the presence of nystagmus during eccentric gaze. Gaze testing is completed by having patients direct their gaze in the centre position and then 20–30° to the right, left, up, and down and then in these same eye positions with visual fixation removed. Gaze-evoked nystagmus can originate from either the peripheral or the central vestibular system with differences in clinical presentation between the two. Nystagmus that is peripheral in origin will generally be direction-fixed and enhance with fixation removed and with gaze in the direction of the quick phases. Nystagmus is considered to be of central origin if it changes direction with change in gaze direction, if it is associated with rebound nystagmus (where the fast component of the nystagmus changes with the direction of the last eye movement), or if it enhances or does not change in intensity with fixation. In rare instances, eye movements can be consistent with both peripheral and central origin, such as Bruns' nystagmus from a combined unilateral peripheral vestibular and cerebellar lesion. A variety of other abnormalities may be evidenced during gaze testing such as congenital nystagmus and a variety of saccadic intrusions (special grouping of involuntary saccadic eye movements when visual fixation target is present), suggesting central vestibular system involvement.

Hyperventilation testing

The purpose of the hyperventilation test is to help diagnose, or unmask, disorders of the peripheral vestibular system and/or VIIIth cranial nerve (16, 18–21). Secondly, the test can suggest possible anxiety disorder via premature symptoms without nystagmus (22). The hyperventilation test is completed by first removing fixation, either by Frenzel lenses or infrared goggles, and then having the patient take one breath per second for 30 to 90 s. Nystagmus induced by hyperventilation is considered significant if it persists greater than 5 s and if the peak slow phase velocity is greater than 3–4°/s, subtracting out any pre-existing spontaneous nystagmus (16, 18). If no nystagmus is provoked but the patient becomes symptomatic within the first 20–30 s then anxiety issues are suspected (22).

Hyperventilation induced nystagmus can beat ipsilesionally (with the fast phase beating toward the side involved) or contralesionally (with the fast phase beating away from the side involved). As a general rule of thumb, hyperventilation induced nystagmus more often beats contralesionally in peripheral vestibular system lesions and ipsilesionally in VIII nerve or retrocochlear lesions; however this relationship is not mutually exclusive (23–25).

Headshake

The head shake test also helps uncover asymmetries in peripheral and central vestibular system function and serves as an indication of dynamic central compensation. The head shake test is completed by removing fixation. The patient's head is pitched downward 20–30° into the plane of the horizontal canal and shaken back and forth vigorously at approximately 2–4 Hz for 10–15 s. Post head-shake nystagmus is considered clinically significant if at least 3–5 consecutive beats of nystagmus are present directly following the head shake and if the nystagmus peak slow phase velocity is greater than 3–4°/s after subtracting out any pre-existing spontaneous nystagmus (21, 25, 26). Both vertical and horizontal head shaking can also be completed.

The head shake test has relatively low sensitivity (30–35%) but high specificity (90–95%) in peripheral vestibular disorders (21, 25,

27), with the incidence of post head-shake nystagmus increasing as the severity of caloric paresis increases (25, 28–30). Post head-shake nystagmus has also been documented in as many as 50% of normal controls (28) and in horizontal canal benign paroxysmal positional vertigo (BPPV) (31).

Vertical nystagmus in response to either a horizontal or vertical head shake is termed 'cross coupled nystagmus' and is frequently seen in central vestibulo-ocular disorders (21, 32, 33).

Testing for benign paroxysmal positional vertigo

The Dix–Hallpike and roll tests are a common part of the VNG; however the most common form of BPPV, posterior canal, cannot be recognized with the printouts of a typical two-dimensional recording system since the principal movement is torsional. Therefore, in reality these tests are clinical office tests where the examiner must watch and report the eye movements with typical recordings unnecessary. Video recording can be useful for reviewing eye movements during the Dix–Hallpike or roll tests.

Static positional testing

The purpose of static positional testing is to examine the effect of gravity on positional changes of the head–otolithic influence. Static positional testing is generally completed in the sitting, supine, body right, body left, and pre-caloric positions and additionally with the head turned right and left in the sitting, supine, and head hanging positions to examine the influence of the cervical region on symptoms and eye movements. Positional nystagmus is classified as either direction fixed (e.g. right beating in all positions) or direction changing (e.g. right beating in some positions and left beating in others). Direction changing nystagmus may be further categorized as geotropic (nystagmus beating towards the earth) or apogeotropic (nystagmus beating away from the earth). Positional nystagmus is the most common of the abnormalities on a VNG/ENG and is generally non-localizing, needing interpretation in the context of the ocular motor findings. Pure vertical nystagmus and nystagmus that changes direction in a fixed head position are of central origin and are the exceptions to the non-localizing aspect.

Caloric irrigation testing

The caloric test is an assessment of the horizontal semicircular canal and subsequently the superior branch of the VIIIth cranial nerve. One benefit of caloric testing is that it yields ear-specific information on the individual responsiveness of the horizontal canal to exogenous stimuli. Caloric testing can be completed with either air or water stimuli (Figure 14.2). With either method a cool (inhibiting) and warm (excitatory) stimulus is delivered to each ear (34–36). Sensitivity and specificity of the caloric test in response to air has been reported as 82% and 82% respectively and in response to water as 84% and 84% respectively (34). There are no other objective tests considered as sensitive as the caloric irrigation test in the frequency range it assesses (see later discussion on the head impulse test) to determine horizontal canal involvement so the use of presenting symptoms becomes the comparator of choice for these studies.

Vestibular-evoked myogenic potential

The purpose of the vestibular-evoked myogenic potential (VEMP) is to provide information regarding VIIIth nerve and otolith organ

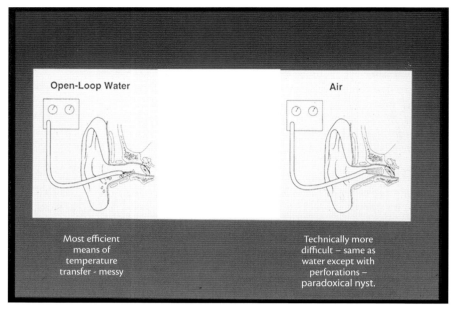

Fig. 14.2 Shown schematically are the two primary techniques for caloric irrigation testing, open-loop water (on the left) and air (on the right). As noted on the figure, while requiring a means for collecting the circulating water, the use of a liquid is the most efficient method of transferring temperature and less technically demanding compared to air. Also as noted, the situation in which air can produce a confusing result is when a tympanic membrane perforation of greater than 20% of the drum surface exists. In that case paradoxical nystagmus can be seen. This is where even though warm air is being used the nystagmus direction initially is what would be consistent with the cool air irrigation. This results from air blowing across the moist medial wall of the middle ear creating a cooling effect even though the air is warm. Once the evaporation occurs then the warm air heats the horizontal canal and the nystagmus direction reverses to that expected for the warm air irrigation.

function and to potentially separate superior from inferior vestibular nerve and likewise utricular from saccular involvement (37, 38). Like the caloric test, one benefit of the VEMP is that it provides ear specific information. There are two types of VEMP responses: the cervical VEMP (cVEMP) and the ocular VEMP (oVEMP). The cVEMP is measured at the sternocleidomastoid muscle and is a reflection of the ipsilateral vestibulo-collic reflex mediated by the ipsilateral saccule (39) (Figure 14.3). The oVEMP, on the other hand, is measured at the contralateral inferior oblique muscle (directly under the eye) and is a reflection of the VOR suggested to be mediated by the utricle (37, 38). VEMPs have demonstrated their effectiveness for aiding diagnosis in a variety of conditions. Most notably, VEMPs are part of a standard battery when diagnosing superior canal dehiscence syndrome and other third-window disorders (40, 41).

Non-routine test of peripheral and central vestibular system function

The following studies are most often found in highly subspecialized tertiary facilities dealing with widely diverse populations of patients with dizziness and balance disorder complaints.

On-axis total body rotation—rotational chair

The purpose of the test is to expand the investigation of the peripheral vestibular system by applying natural head movements and using three outcome parameters to characterize the peripheral vestibular system together with its central projections as to: 1) the timing relationship between eye movement and steady state (sinusoidal protocol) or transient (a step test) head movement; 2) the overall responsiveness of the system to the stimulus; and, 3) the

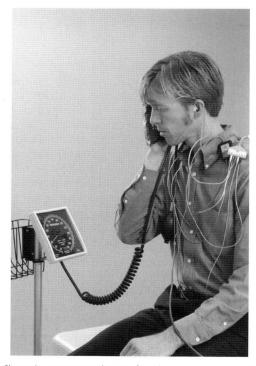

Fig. 14.3 Shown is one set up and means for achieving contraction of the sternocleidomastoid muscle (SCM) on the left in the recording of the cervical VEMP. The contraction strength is monitored via raw EMG activity along with the use of a blood pressure cuff with feedback to the patient to maintain the contraction at a constant and achieve the same level of contraction from right to left. Surface skin electrodes are attached over the left and right SCM (not visualized well in this photograph). This is the technique used in the development of the data for the VEMP threshold response curves noted in Figure 14.6 (49).

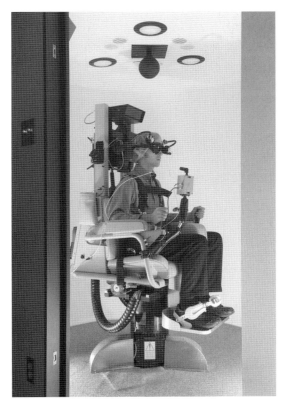

Fig. 14.4 The photograph shows a rotational chair system with video goggles for the recording of eye movements. The chair is within a light-tight enclosure (photograph taken through the open door). This particular system is able to shift the chair on the driving motor to change the alignment of the axis of rotation as is schematized in Figure 14.5.

responsiveness when rotating to the right versus the left. In this manner the test expands across frequency (beyond that of stimulation by caloric irrigations) the investigation of the function of the peripheral vestibular systems. This is the only test to investigate the extent of and verification of those with bilateral peripheral system hypofunction (42, 43). The test is administered by having the patient seated in a chair that is driving in a sinusoidal or fixed velocity trajectory by a motor affixed to the chair. The axis of rotation is vertical and passes through the centre of the patient's head (Figure 14.4).

Off-axis total body rotation—unilateral centrifugation

The class of off-axis rotational tests has been developed for assessing the otolith organs (43). Unilateral centrifugation is one protocol of the off-axis total body rotation test performed with rotary chair equipment. With unilateral centrifugation, the chair is translated laterally, which projects the vertical axis of rotation through the peripheral vestibular organ on the right or the left (Figure 14.5). The purpose of the test is to allow for evaluation of each utricular organ individually. Investigations to date show reliable detection of those with surgically confirmed utricular lesions. The interested reader is referred to a recent study that provides a review of work to date contained in the introduction (43, 44).

Head impulse test

Starting as the head thrust test for use in bedside evaluations (see Chapter 12) this test has expanded to be used with equipment and is referred to as the HIT (45). The test provides for a means of individually assessing the function of the VOR for the horizontal canals on the right and the left. It also provides for the assessment of the anterior and posterior canals individually. The assessment is in a different frequency range than that of the caloric test but there is a

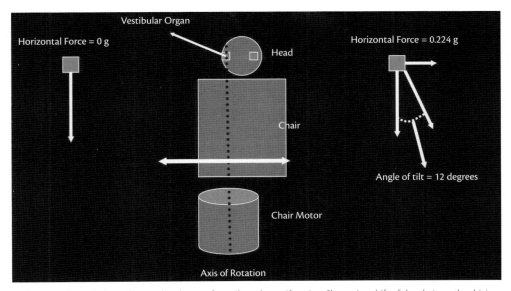

Fig. 14.5 The line drawing illustrates the technique discussed in the text for unilateral centrifugation. Shown is a shift of the chair on the driving motor to the left aligning the vertical axis of rotation through the right vestibular end organ. In this example the forces on the right utricle during rotation will only be that of the vertical pull of gravity as illustrated. The forces on the left utricle will be a combination of the pull of gravity and the horizontal force related to an approximate 8-cm radius from the axis of rotation and the speed of 300°/s angular rotation. These two forces give a resultant force at an angle to the left and the subject would have a sensation of tilting to the left at that equivalent angle causing an ocular counter roll of the eyes that can be measured with the video goggle system and via a change in the subject's perception of vertical. The change in perception is measured via a test call subjective visual vertical—simply the setting of a projected laser line to the subject's perceived sensation of vertical.

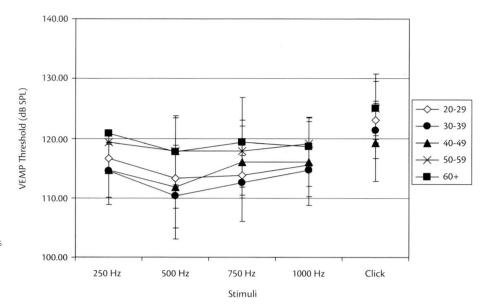

Fig. 14.6 The graph shows the threshold of the VEMP response in dB SPL peak as a function of the frequency of the toneburst stimuli over various age ranges. The graphic shows the tuning characteristics discussed in the text with most sensitive frequency at 500 Hz. Also illustrated is the reduction in those tuning properties as the subject population ages (49).

reasonable correlation between the caloric results and those of the clinical version (head thrust test) (46, 47). Recently after the addition of high-speed video recording devices and computer analysis the sensitivity of the test for identification and monitoring of the function of the six individual canals has been improved (45). This improvement comes from being able to calculate the actual gain of the eye movement for a specific head movement. This technique avoids problems with central nervous compensatory activity that cause difficulty in the simple identification of a corrective saccade when the eye is taken off the target with a head movement secondary to a deficient VOR (48).

VEMP threshold response curves

The cVEMP as previously discussed provides for an assessment of the status of the saccule. The function of the saccule varies over frequency. When plotting VEMP threshold across frequency, the saccule demonstrates specific tuning characteristic with the most sensitive frequency at 500 Hz (49) (Figure 14.6). It has been suggested (45, 50) that in an endolymphatic condition like that of Ménière's syndrome the most sensitive frequency shifts upward. Therefore, the use of the threshold response curve is being proposed as an independent study that may be able to assist in the diagnosis of Ménière's, or the more general condition of endolymphatic hydrops. A pilot study using this method showed sensitivity and specificity for identification of Ménière's to be 48–50% and 79–88% respectively, suggesting that while a negative test is not useful, a test showing the upward shift may add to the argument of the disorder being present (51).

Dynamic visual acuity and gaze stabilization test

All of the investigative tools discussed to this point would be classified as extent and site-of-lesion studies. Dynamic visual acuity (DVA) and gaze stabilization test (GST) however, are considered studies that provide information about the functional use of the VOR. These tests could be normal even in the presence of VOR abnormalities (i.e. caloric hypofunction) indicating the lack of functional impact of the physiological abnormality. Both studies assess

clarity of vision during head motion. For DVA, the head speed is fixed and the size of the target to be recognized is systematically changed, whereas with the GST, the target size is fixed and head speed is varied. These studies are primarily used within treatment programmes of vestibular and balance rehabilitation to help monitor progress and determine deficits on which to focus. However, in symptomatic individuals these studies have been shown to have sensitivity (64–71%) and specificity (88–93%) performance in identifying the involved peripheral system (52). The other purpose of these studies is to provide an objective quantification of a patient's complaint of oscillopsia.

Postural control assessment

For a given piece of laboratory equipment the purpose of the study will vary from strictly functional-based to strictly site of lesion-based contingent on the protocol used and the versatility of the equipment (53). Across most commercially available equipment a similar protocol is used for functional evaluation of maintaining of upright stance under changing sensory input conditions—Sensory Organization Test (SOT) (Figure 14.7). The outcome measure (independent of the details of the individual manufactures analysis) is body sway in two-dimensional space. The purpose of the SOT is to determine the individual's ability to utilize visual, proprioceptive/somatosensory, and vestibular cues for maintaining quiet stance. The test is performed by manipulating the visual and foot support surface cues in a systematic manner to reduce, or for vision eliminate, the cue forcing reliance on other than the normal combination. The outcome of the test is related to the patient's functional ability to maintain stance as the sensory input cues are varied. This information can be used for development and monitoring of treatment programmes. The information is descriptive not diagnostic, therefore the SOT is not a site-of-lesion test (54).

Four other principal protocols are used in postural control assessment, all of which fall into the category of extent and site-of-lesion studies with the exception of number 2: 1) reaction to

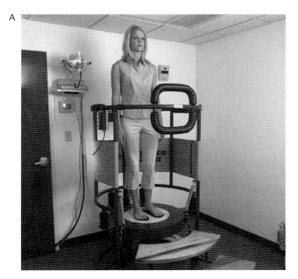

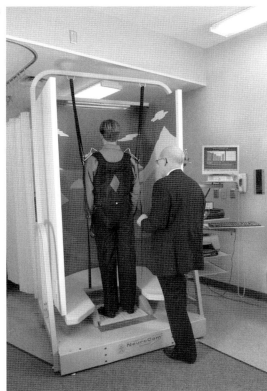

Fig. 14.7 The photographs show two commercial systems with different techniques for providing means for disrupting foot support surface cues and visual information. Both use a force plate system with the measured parameter floor reaction force. In (A) the force plate is suspended by springs while in (B) the force plate moved in the anterior/posterior plane via electric motors. While the analysis of the recorded information is analysed differently, both systems provide the means for performing the sensory organization protocol.

unexpected perturbation of the body's centre of mass through tilt or linear translations; 2) protocol to determine an individual's ability to adapt to changes in surface orientation; 3) recording of distal lower limb muscles in response to sudden toes up or down rotations around the ankle axis; and 4) quantifying an individual's sway response to changes in external auditory canal air pressure—focus

on investigation of perilymphatic fistulas including canal dehiscences. Details of these tests are beyond the scope of this chapter and the reader is referred to discussion by Shepard and Janky (55, 56) for descriptions and list of references.

Case examples

The previous sections give the reader a quick overview for the breadth of the laboratory testing that can be performed on the dizzy patient. The introduction set the stage as to some of the issues of the priority of the laboratory testing. Clearly not all of the studies are needed on all patients, and an organized approach as to a core set of studies with guidelines as to when further investigation is needed can be developed. A full discussion of the development of a staged protocol is beyond the scope of this chapter and can be found in the literature (2). The cases to follow provide examples of how the laboratory testing provides guidance with patient diagnosis and the confirmatory nature of the studies in the context of the history and physical.

Case 1

History

A 68-year-old woman presented for evaluation of 1year of episodic lightheadedness. Past history was notable for a lifelong history of episodic migraine headaches without aura (with associated nausea, vomiting, photophobia, phonophobia, osmophobia) that had largely resolved with menopause at age 53. She had no seizure risk factors, cardiovascular disease, or history of syncope.

Eight months ago she noticed reduced hearing in her left ear, and subsequent audiograms revealed stable moderate low-frequency up sloping to mild high-frequency sensorineural hearing loss on the left. Five months ago she had an intense episode of lightheadedness described as 'my whole head not working' that began abruptly and was accompanied by nausea and vomiting. Symptoms resolved after 3 hours. There was no accompanying vertigo, imbalance, headache, or other neurological or otological symptoms such as fluctuating aural fullness or tinnitus. She subsequently began having many episodes each week where she would feel 'lightheaded' for 3–4 h during which she was particularly nauseated by head motion such as turning, loading laundry, or looking for products on store shelves. Otherwise, symptoms were not positional or relieved by lying down. Despite repeated questioning, she never endorsed any illusion of self- or environmental motion (no vertigo) or unsteadiness during the episodes. Prior to referral, magnetic resonance imaging (MRI) of the brain with high-resolution internal auditory canal views, magnetic resonance angiography of the neck, computed tomography (CT) angiography of the head, electrocardiogram, transthoracic echocardiogram with bubble study, and extensive blood work had been unremarkable.

Physical examination

Pulse was 67 and regular, and blood pressure was normal, with no orthostatic hypotension. Neurological examination including tandem gait and tandem Romberg testing was normal. Otoscopic and general ENT exam were normal. Detailed ocular motor and vestibular examination including head impulse testing were also normal. Frenzel examination revealed mild right-beating nystagmus with left mastoid vibration. Hyperventilation for 30 s produced slow left-beating nystagmus that persisted for 1 min. There was no headshaking-induced or Valsalva-induced nystagmus.

Laboratory testing

VNG 1 week after office examination revealed mild spontaneous right-beating nystagmus that had not been apparent with occlusive ophthalmoscopy or Frenzel lenses. Bithermal caloric testing showed a 51% left-sided weakness and 43% right-beating directional preponderance. Sinusoidal rotary chair testing revealed an abnormal phase lead between 0.01–0.16 Hz, with left greater than right slow component velocity asymmetry, consistent with the caloric finding. Computerized platform posturography showed a vestibular pattern, with abnormalities on conditions 5 and 6 of the SOT. VEMP threshold response curves showed an upward shift in the most sensitive frequency for the left ear.

Discussion

Diagnosis: based heavily on the vestibular testing and audiogram, this patient was given a diagnosis of Ménière's disease.

Although a detailed history and careful physical examination are generally the most important factors to guide neuro-otological diagnosis, this case illustrates the utility of vestibular laboratory testing when the history is ambiguous and the examination is inconclusive. Though episodic 'lightheadedness' does not generally suggest a vestibular disorder, this patient's coexisting nausea, motion intolerance, and associated low-frequency hearing loss raised suspicion of one. A lifelong migraine history might also cause vestibular migraine to be considered, though this would not be expected to cause hearing loss or significant vestibular hypofunction. Mastoid vibration-induced and hyperventilation-induced nystagmus with Frenzel lenses suggested a possible left vestibular lesion.

Ocular motor testing (electro-or video-oculography): in this case the presence of spontaneous right beating nystagmus in several gaze and head positions suggested an uncompensated asymmetry within the vestibular system (left hypofunction or right irritability). Normal saccades, smooth pursuit, antisaccades, and VOR suppression argue against a central nervous system (CNS) lesion.

Caloric testing: demonstrating a significant unilateral caloric weakness was helpful in several ways. It provided evidence of peripheral vestibular dysfunction even when bedside head impulse testing did not. This occasional disparity between caloric testing and head impulse testing likely reflects the different frequency ranges over which each test evaluates (low frequency for caloric testing, high frequency for head impulse testing). In this case, the left caloric weakness is consistent with the right-beating spontaneous and vibration-induced nystagmus as an uncompensated vestibular weakness.

Rotary chair testing: the phase lead lends additional support to the presence of peripheral dysfunction. The severity of the phase lead, as well as the degree of asymmetry, can help differentiate unilateral from bilateral vestibular hypofunction, especially when the absolute caloric responses are borderline low.

Computerized posturography: though not capable of precisely localizing lesions, computerized posturography was useful here to demonstrate a specific vestibular pattern of imbalance. Though she performed normally on conditions 1 through 4 of the SOT, she performed abnormally and had fall reactions on conditions 5 and 6, which disrupt both proprioceptive and visual cues in order to test the ability to use vestibular input to maintain balance.

VEMPs: cervical VEMPs are a measure of saccular function. In this setting, VEMP threshold response curves were determined in order to measure the most sensitive frequency during stimulation to each ear. The shift up in most sensitive frequency has been associated as discussed earlier with conditions of endolymphatic hydrops and Ménière's.

Summary

Although completely normal vestibular function testing should not prohibit a diagnosis of Ménière's disease in the proper clinical setting, this case illustrates how several components of laboratory testing can reveal characteristic abnormalities to support a Ménière's diagnosis when the history and physical examination are unclear.

Case 2

History

A 16-year-old girl developed nearly daily occipital headaches at age 10 and underwent a reportedly normal head CT. These headaches improved with puberty at age 13 but would still sometimes awaken her. She reports minor problems with balance and coordination in the past year but continues to play on the tennis team. When she tosses the tennis ball and tips her head back to serve, she develops a sudden feeling that her body is swaying, making her feel unsteady. She may then have up to a minute where she has difficulty focusing her vision. She also experiences occasional oscillopsia when looking far laterally to either side. She denies any tinnitus or other otological or neurological symptoms.

Physical examination and laboratory testing

Both careful office examination and video-oculography revealed moderate gaze-evoked nystagmus in lateral (left and right beating with a dominant down beat) and downward gaze, with associated rebound nystagmus upon return to primary gaze. Pursuit eye movements were moderately impaired in all directions, and attempted VOR cancellation was similarly choppy. Optokinetic nystagmus was poorly formed. Primary gaze fixation, saccadic eye movements, caloric testing, positioning, and other provocative manoeuvres were all normal. Head impulse testing was normal. Ocular alignment was normal except for a small oesophoria at distance. The rest of the neurological examination was notable only for mild difficulty with tandem gait and tandem Romberg testing. Clinical test of sensory integration on balance (CTSIB) was normal. Rotary chair testing showed an increased phase lead across all frequencies—a finding associated with central vestibular system involvement or bilateral peripheral involvement.

Discussion

Diagnosis: based on her symptoms and laboratory examination findings, a brain MRI was obtained that demonstrated a 3-cm Chiari malformation with basilar invagination producing compression of the cerebellar tonsils and kinking at the cervical medullary junction.

Ocular motor testing: beyond a careful office examination, vestibular laboratory testing may be useful to identify signs of CNS dysfunction. Ocular motor abnormalities in this case that point toward CNS, most typically cerebellar, dysfunction include gaze-evoked and rebound nystagmus, impaired smooth pursuit, impaired VOR cancellation, and poor optokinetic nystagmus.

Many additional CNS signs can be detected with oculography. Abnormal saccadic intrusions such as macrosquare-wave jerks, ocular flutter, and opsoclonus can be recognized. Nystagmus types pointing to a CNS cause include primary position pure vertical or torsional nystagmus, pendular nystagmus, periodic alternating nystagmus, see-saw nystagmus, perverted nystagmus (e.g. downbeat nystagmus following horizontal headshaking), congenital nystagmus waveforms, or pure vertical nystagmus with positional testing.

Most vestibular laboratories analyse binocular saccadic eye movements during a horizontal random saccade paradigm, measuring latency, velocity, and accuracy. Thus, central disorders of saccadic accuracy (hypometria, hypermetria, or lateropulsion), velocity (conjugate slowing, adduction slowing of internuclear ophthalmoplegia), or prolonged latency can be identified.

Case 3

History

A 57-year-old man with chronic noise exposure began to develop slowly progressive hearing loss in his 30s. At age 37 he sustained a prolonged loss of consciousness in a motor vehicle accident but made a complete recovery. In the past 5 years he has now developed slowly progressive imbalance, particularly in the dark or on uneven surfaces but does not require gait aids. He also reports that his visual acuity declines and the world seems to bounce while he is walking or riding in the car, so that he may have to stop moving in order to restore normal vision. His hearing loss has worsened considerably in the past 5 years, requiring amplification. His sense of smell is also reduced.

Physical examination

Gait was brisk and narrow-based but mildly ataxic with occasional stumbling, and tandem gait was quite impaired. Romberg test produced only mild swaying. Visual acuity was 20/20 but fell to 20/200 during passive vertical or horizontal 2-Hz head rotation. Ocular motor examination was normal, including alignment, fixation, gaze-holding, saccades, pursuit, convergence, optokinetic responses, VOR cancellation, and slow oculocephalic testing. Head impulse testing produced moderately sized catch-up saccades in all six semicircular canal planes as well as with lateral head translations (head heaves). The rest of the examination was normal.

Laboratory testing

Video-oculography revealed normal fixation, gaze holding, saccades, pursuit, and positional testing. Bithermal caloric testing with warm and ice water irrigations demonstrated bilateral vestibular hypofunction, generating no more than 2°/s of nystagmus with either stimulus. Rotary chair testing revealed abnormally increased phase lead and reduced gain across all sinusoidal frequencies as well as shortened time constants with step testing at 60°/s. Computerized posturography was abnormal, with an SOT composite score of 40 (normal >70) and abnormalities on conditions 3 through 6 and consistent fall reactions on conditions 5 and 6. Cervical VEMPs were normal.

Discussion

Diagnosis: based on the progressive ataxia, hearing loss, and anosmia in the setting of prior trauma, a brain MRI was obtained that demonstrated a rim of haemosiderin deposition on the surface of the brainstem, cerebellar folia, and Sylvian fissures consistent with superficial siderosis. Spinal fluid examination confirmed xanthochromia. Further evaluation revealed a post-traumatic cervical spine meningocoele at an area of old fracture dislocation, which was surgically repaired.

Patients with progressive gait ataxia in the absence of vertigo are often referred to neurologists for evaluation. This patient had been thought to have a progressive cerebellar ataxia. However, his head motion-induced oscillopsia, head impulse sign, and ocular motor evaluation supported a vestibular instead of cerebellar cause. Romberg test was insensitive at detecting sensory ataxia. Vestibular testing confirmed severe bilateral vestibular hypofunction but did not show any ocular motor signs of cerebellar or other CNS dysfunction despite siderosis on the cerebellum.

Ocular motor testing: if this patient had significant cerebellar dysfunction, ocular motor evaluation would be expected to show one or more of the following: square wave jerks, downbeat nystagmus, gaze evoked nystagmus, impaired pursuit, saccadic dysmetria, impaired VOR cancellation, or impaired optokinetic nystagmus.

Consistent with bilateral peripheral hypofunction, DVA testing showed inability to stabilize a visual target with the head in motion, yet visual stabilization was normal with the head held stationary.

Caloric testing: warm and cool irrigations produced virtually no measurable response, indicating several bilateral vestibular hypofunction. When this is the case, ice water caloric can also be used as a stronger stimulus in attempt to elicit any response.

Rotary chair testing: as a physiological bilateral stimulus, rotary chair testing is particularly useful for evaluating suspected bilateral vestibular dysfunction since the range of absolute caloric responses is wide among individuals and can provide misleading results in bilateral cases regarding the extent of the lesion.

VEMPs: normal VEMPs in this case suggest an intact pathway from the saccule to inferior vestibular nerve to brainstem despite the fact that head impulse and laboratory testing show severe impairment of all semicircular canal function.

The SOT test was abnormal in more conditions than expected for a bilateral hypofunction case where the two conditions (5 and 6) that force reliance on the vestibular system cues would be deficient. However, we find that bilateral hypofunction patients will routinely have more diffuse difficulty until they have started vestibular and balance rehabilitation therapy with specific work on balance and gait.

Closing opinions

Collectively, the authors believe, especially for the patient with chronic dizziness and balance complaints, that vestibular laboratory studies are useful in helping determine the diagnosis and treatment path, even if the outcome is simply confirmatory. There are examples, in addition to the cases discussed, where routine laboratory studies are essential. First, in the determination of whether a canal dehiscence identified on high-resolution CT is actively an open fistula possibly responsible for the patient's symptoms. In this situation, aside from a possible low-frequency air-bone gap on an audiogram in the presence of a normally functioning middle ear, the use of either ocular or cervical VEMPs are of significant importance in providing objective indicators of the status of openness of a known dehiscence. Secondly, patients suspected of having chronic subjective dizziness syndrome, visual vertigo, or postural phobic vertigo (57) (Chapters 13 and 30) require full use of the studies noted earlier, including assessment for otolith function in order to rule out a neurotologic basis that is active and a reasonable cause for the ongoing symptoms.

The key in the use of the various laboratory studies at one's disposal is the realistic expectation of what the studies can provide and the critical understanding that the findings of the laboratory studies need to be used in concert with each other, not in isolation, and in the context of a well developed and detailed presenting history.

References

1. Bisdorff A, Von Brevern M, Lempert T, Newman-Toker DE (2009). Classification of vestibular symptoms: Towards an international classification of vestibular disorders. *J Vestib Res*, 19(1–2), 1–13.

2. Ruckenstein MJ, Shepard NT (2000). Balance function testing – a rational approach. *Oto-Laryngol Clin North Am*, 33, 507–18.

3. Stephens SD, Hogan S, Meredith R (1991). The dis-synchrony between complaints and signs of vestibular disorders. *Acta Oto-Laryngol*, 111, 188–92.

4. Shepard NT, Gavies S, Goldenrod N, et al. (1997). Assessment of activities of daily living in balance disorder patients—comparison to routine balance function studies and patient perceptions. Abstract midwinter ARO meeting, St Petersburg Beach, FL.

5. Handelsman JA, Shepard NT (2008). Electronystagmography and videonystagmography, In Goebel J (Ed) *Practical management of the dizzy patient* (2nd ed), pp. 137–52. Philadelphia, PA: Lippincott Williams & Wilkins.

6. Handelsman JA, Shepard NT (2008). Rotational chair testing. In Goebel J (Ed) *Practical management of the dizzy patient* (2nd ed), pp. 137–52. Philadelphia, PA: Lippincott Williams & Wilkins.

7. Shepard NT (2000). Clinical utility of the motor control test (MCT) and postural evoked responses (PER). *A NeuroCom® Publication Rev*, 8, 3–19.

8. Monsell EM, Furman JM, Herdman SJ, et al. (1997). Technology assessment: Computerized dynamic platform posturography, *Otolaryngol Head Neck Surg*, 117, 394–8.

9. Herdman SJ, Tusa RJ, Blatt P, et al. (1998). Computerized dynamic visual acuity test in the assessment of vestibular deficits, *Am J Otol*, 19, 790.

10. Jacobson GP, Newman CW, Hunter L, Balzer G (1991). Balance function test correlates of the dizziness handicap inventory, *J Am Acad Audiol*, 2, 253–60.

11. Robertson DD, Ireland DJ (1995). Dizziness handicap inventory correlates of computerized dynamic Posturography, *Otolaryngol Head Neck Surg*, 24, 118–24.

12. Jacobson GP, Newman CW (1990). The development of the dizziness handicap inventory, *Arch Otolaryngol Head Neck Surg*, 116, 424–7.

13. Shepard NT, Telian SA (1996). *Practical management of the balance disorder patient*. San Diego, CA: Singular Publishing Group, Inc.

14. Zee DS (2000). Vestibular Adaptation. In Herdman SJ (Ed) *Vestibular rehabilitation*, pp. 77–90. Philadelphia, PA: FA Davis Co.

15. Jacobson GP, Shepard NT (2008). *Balance function assessment and management*. San Diego, CA: Plural.

16. Leigh R, Zee D (2006). *The Neurology of Eye Movements*. New York: Oxford University Press.

17. Shepard NT, Schubert M (2008). Interpretation and usefulness of ocular motility testing. In Jacobson GP, Shepard NT (Eds) *Balance function assessment and management*, pp. 147–70. San Diego, CA: Plural.

18. Robichaud J, DesRoches H, Bance M (2002). Is hyperventilation-induced nystagmus more common in retrocochlear vestibular disease than in end-organ vestibular disease? *J Otolaryngol*, 31, 140–3.

19. Park HJ, Shin JE, Lee YJ, et al. (2010). Hyperventilation-induced nystagmus in patients with vestibular neuritis in the acute and follow-up stages. *Audiol Neurootol*, 16, 248–53.

20. Choi KD, Kim JS, Kim HJ, et al. (2007). Hyperventilation-induced nystagmus in peripheral vestibulopathy and cerebellopontine angle tumor. *Neurology*, 69, 1050–9.

21. Cherchi M, Hain TC (2010). Provocative maneuvers for vestibular disorders. In Eggers DZ, Zee DS (Eds) *Vertigo and imbalance: Clinical neurophysiology of the vestibular system*, pp. 111–34. New York: Elsevier.

22. Papp LA, Klein DF, Gorman JM (1993). Carbon dioxide hypersensitivity, hyperventilation, and panic disorder. *Am J Psychiatry*, 150(8), 1149–57.

23. Minor LB, Haslwanter T, Straumann D, et al. (1999). Hyperventilation-induced nystagmus in patients with vestibular schwannoma. *Neurology*, 53, 2158–68.

24. Bance ML, O'Driscoll M, Patel N, et al. (1998). Vestibular disease unmasked by hyperventilation. *Laryngoscope*, 108, 610–14.

25. Harvey SA, Wood DJ, Feroah TR (1997). Relationship of the head impulse test and head-shake nystagmus in reference to caloric testing. *Am J Otol*, 18, 207–13.

26. Perez P, Llorente JL, Gomez JR, et al. (2004). Functional significance of peripheral head-shaking nystagmus. *Laryngoscope*, 114, 1078–84.

27. Angeli SI, Velandia S, Snapp H (2011). Head-shaking nystagmus predicts greater disability in unilateral peripheral vestibulopathy. *Am J Otolaryngol*, 32, 522–7.

28. Hall SF, Laird ME (1992). Is head-shaking nystagmus a sign of vestibular dysfunction? *J Otolaryngol*, 21, 209–12.

29. Mandala M, Nuti D, Broman AT (2008). Effectiveness of careful bedside examination in assessment, diagnosis, and prognosis of vestibular neuritis. *Arch Otolaryngol Head Neck Surg*, 134, 164–9.

30. Iwasaki S, Ito K, Abbey K (2004). Prediction of canal paresis using head-shaking nystagmus test. *Acta Otolaryngol*, 124, 803–6.

31. Gananca FF, Gananca CF, Caovilla HH (2009). Active head rotation in benign positional paroxysmal vertigo. *Braz J Otorhinolaryngol*, 75, 586–92.

32. Lee JY, Lee WW, Kim JS (2009). Perverted head-shaking and positional downbeat nystagmus in patients with multiple system atrophy. *Mov Disord*, 24, 1290–5.

33. Walker MF, Zee DS (1999). Directional abnormalities of vestibular and optokinetic responses in cerebellar disease. *Ann N Y Acad Sci*, 871, 205–20.

34. Zapala DA, Olsholt KF, Lundy LB (2008). A comparison of water and air caloric responses and their ability to distinguish between patients with normal and impaired ears. *Ear Hear*, 29, 585–600.

35. Maes L, Dhooge I, De VE (2007). Water irrigation versus air insufflation: a comparison of two caloric test protocols. *Int J Audiol*, 46, 263–9.

36. Zangemeister WH, Bock O (1980). Air versus water caloric test. *Clin Otolaryngol Allied Sci*, 5, 379–87.

37. Manzari L, Tedesco A, Burgess AM (2010). Ocular vestibular-evoked myogenic potentials to bone-conducted vibration in superior vestibular neuritis show utricular function. *Otolaryngol Head Neck Surg*, 143, 274–80.

38. Curthoys IS, Iwasaki S, Chihara Y, et al. (2011). The ocular vestibular-evoked myogenic potential to air-conducted sound; probable superior vestibular nerve origin. *Clin Neurophysiol*, 122, 611–16.

39. Colebatch JG, Halmagyi GM (1992). Vestibular evoked potentials in human neck muscles before and after unilateral vestibular deafferentation. *Neurology*, 42, 1635–6.

40. Welgampola MS, Myrie OA, Minor LB, et al. (2008). Vestibular-evoked myogenic potential thresholds normalize on plugging superior canal dehiscence. *Neurology*, 70, 464–72.

41. Brantberg K, Bergenius J, Tribukait A (1999). Vestibular-evoked myogenic potentials in patients with dehiscence of the superior semicircular canal. *Acta Otolaryngol*, 119, 633–40.

42. Brey RH, McPherson JL (2008). Technique, interpretation and usefulness of whole body rotational testing. In Jacobson GP, Shepard NT (Eds) *Balance function assessment and management*, pp. 281–317. San Diego, CA: Plural.

43. Furman JM (2010). Rotational testing: background, technique and interpretation. In Eggers DZ, Zee DS (Eds) *Vertigo and imbalance: Clinical neurophysiology of the vestibular system*, pp. 141–9. Elsevier, New York.

44. Janky K, Shepard NT (2011). Unilateral centrifugation: Protocol comparison. *Otol Neurotol*, 32(1), 116–21.

45. Aw ST, Todd MJ, Halmagyi MG (2010). Head impulse testing: angular vestibulo-ocular reflex (VOR). In Eggers DZ, Zee DS (Eds) *Vertigo and imbalance: Clinical neurophysiology of the vestibular system*, pp. 150–64. Elsevier, New York.

46. Shepard NT (1998). Caloric weakness needed to achieve a positive head thrust test. XX Barany Society Meeting, Wurzburg, Germany.

47. Perez N, Rama-Lopez J (2003). Head-impulse and caloric tests in patients with dizziness. *Otol Neurotol*, 24, 913–17.

48. Schubert MC, Migliaccio AA, Della Santina CC (2006). Modification of compensatory saccades after aVOR gain recovery. *J Vestib Res*, 16, 285–91.

49. Janky KL, Shepard NT (2010). Vestibular evoked myogenic potential (VEMP) testing: Normative threshold response curves and effects of age. *J Am Acad Audiol*, 20, 514–22.

50. Rauch SD, Zhou G, Kujawa SG, Guinan JJ, Herrmann BS (2004). Vestibular evoked myogenic potentials show altered tuning in patients with Meniere's disease. *Otol Neurol*, 25, 333–8.

51. Shepard NT, McPherson JP (2011). Sensitivity/specificity performance of VEMP threshold response curves in identification of Ménière's syndrome. Oral presentation, American Balance Society Annual Meeting, March, Scottsdale, AZ.

52. Goebel JA, Tungsiripat N, Sinks B, Carmody J (2006). Gaze stabilization test: A new clinical test of unilateral vestibular dysfunction. *Otol Neurol*, 28, 68–73.

53. Allum JHJ, Shepard NT (1999). An overview of the clinical use of dynamic posturography in the differential diagnosis of balance disorders. *J Vestib Res*, 9, 223–52.

54. Shepard NT (2008). Interpretation and usefulness of computerized dynamic posturography. In Jacobson GP, Shepard NT (Eds) *Balance function assessment and management*, pp. 359–78. San Diego, CA: Plural.

55. Shepard NT, Janky K (2008). Background and technique of computerized dynamic posturography. In Jacobson GP, Shepard NT (Eds) *Balance function assessment and management*, pp. 339–57. San Diego, CA: Plural.

56. Shepard NT, Telian SA, Niparko JK, Kemink JL, Fujita S (1992). Platform pressure test in identification of perilymphatic fistula. *Am J Otol*, 13(1), 49–54.

57. Staab JP, Ruckenstein MJ (2007). Expanding the differential diagnosis of chronic dizziness. *Arch Otolaryngol Head Neck Surg*, 133, 170–6.

CHAPTER 15

Imaging of Vertigo and Labyrinthine Disorders

M. Radon and T. A. Yousry

Introduction

Vertigo is a common complaint with a lifetime prevalence of approximately 7% (1) with acute vertigo, prompting urgent care, having been estimated at approximately 3.5% (2). The relatively high incidence of misdiagnosis (3) and the risk of a potentially serious underlying disorder (such as stroke) require careful assessment, both clinically and radiologically.

Imaging techniques

The techniques available for imaging of the labyrinthine structures are mainly computed tomography (CT) and magnetic resonance imaging (MRI). In essence, these two modalities are complementary, rather than alternatives. The strength of CT resides in the assessment of the bony labyrinth at increasingly higher resolution. Modern multislice CT scanners now routinely offer submillimetre isotropic imaging which is ideally suited for multiplanar reconstruction. The excellent bone detail revealed by CT also makes it the test of choice for assessment of middle ear pathology. However, what CT offers in terms of bony detail resolution, it loses in terms of soft-tissue contrast. In particular, for lesions of the facial and vestibulocochlear nerves, CT has only a limited role; these structures cannot be visualized directly. Nevertheless, indirect assessment is possible by being attentive to changes in the calibre of the internal auditory meatus or canal, such as widening by the presence of slow-growing tumours (4) or narrowing in the case of nerve hypoplasia.

The strength of MRI resides in the assessment of the soft tissue, especially the vestibulocochlear nerves and the brainstem. The favoured sequences for imaging the brainstem are high-resolution T2 fast spin-echo or T2*-weighted sequences. For imaging the vestibulocochlear nerves and the labyrinthine structures three-dimensional (3D) sequences with very high cisternographic contrast are used. Historically, the use of 3D constructive interference in the steady state (CISS) was pioneered by Casselman et al. (5), and offered a dramatic improvement of the visualization of the vestibulocochlear nerve. Since then, a number of sequences with imaging characteristics similar to CISS have been developed;

including driven equilibrium (DRIVE) and fast imaging employing steady state acquisition (FIESTA). These sequences provide excellent contrast and spatial resolution (as low as 0.5 mm on 3 Tesla scanners), enabling optimal visualization of the cisternal segment of the facial and vestibulocochlear nerves as well as the labyrinth, and has led to them becoming the current standard for examination of the cranial nerves III–XII (6). Nevertheless, the demanding nature of imaging the small labyrinthine structures requires optimized equipment. In comparison to 1.5 T MR scanners, 3 T scanners provide a greater signal-to-noise ratio resulting in significantly improved image quality with high spatial resolutions, giving reliable demonstration of semicircular canals, cochlear modiolus, and nerves VII/VIII (7). The small size of the membranous labyrinth has largely precluded direct imaging of its internal structure, with most imaging limited to demonstration of the endolymphatic fluid signal. However, at 3 T, it has proven possible to demonstrate the utricular macula, with optimized sequences (8).

Additional sequences, such as 3D fluid attenuated inversion recovery (3D-FLAIR) sequences have also been reported as having fewer artefacts and better sensitivity for impairment of the blood–labyrinthine barrier (9).

While the high-resolution techniques described are suitable for assessment of peripheral causes of vertigo, consideration should also be given to the need to assess the brain parenchyma for evidence of central causes. Vertebrobasilar stroke is an important differential diagnosis in acute vertigo and clinical suspicion of a central cause should prompt dedicated brain imaging with CT and/or MRI. In the case of suspected infarction, the high sensitivity of diffusion-weighted imaging (DWI) makes MRI the examination of choice.

While neuroimaging enables a variety of diagnoses to be made in the context of vertigo, as with investigation in general, the yield and clinical benefit of imaging depends upon the selection of patients and the suspected clinical diagnosis. Where this has been examined, the conclusion has been that imaging is not routinely warranted for most cases of 'dizziness'. The major exceptions are acute vertigo in patients with increased vascular risk; patients with associated hearing loss or other clinical suspicion of CNS or invasive disease, for example, cranial nerve deficits (10). However, even where imaging referrals are screened with referral guidelines, imaging yields may still be low (approximately 2% with contemporary criteria) (11). Given the progressively improving access to high-quality imaging techniques, particularly MRI which does not impose an ionizing radiation burden, and lack of other similarly accurate diagnostic tests, this diagnostic yield may be acceptable.

Imaging anatomy of the vestibular system

Overview

The vestibular system begins peripherally with the labyrinth, which contains the primary sensory epithelium and its sensory hair cells. From these arise the vestibular nerve which enters the brainstem, and terminates at the vestibular nuclei. The vestibular nuclei show complex interconnection with the cerebellum and other brainstem nuclei. However, they also have ascending efferent projections to the ventral posterior nucleus complex of the thalamus, and from there to the parieto-insular cortex. For optimal examination of each component of the pathway, a dedicated technique is required.

The labyrinth

The labyrinth can be divided into the membranous and bony components. The membranous labyrinth is the endolymphatic-fluid filled structure comprising several interconnected chambers which contains the sensory epithelium. The membranous labyrinth is, itself, surrounded by perilymphatic fluid, which lies within a matching set of cavities in the temporal bone, known as the bony labyrinth.

The labyrinth comprises three main regions: the vestibule, semicircular canals, and cochlea. The vestibule is the central component and lies medial to the middle ear cleft. The three semicircular canals, the lateral, posterior, and superior semicircular canals are arranged orthogonally to each other, and lie superiorly and lateral to the vestibule. They communicate with the vestibule at each end.

High-resolution multidetector CT can clearly delineate the major components (Figure 15.1).

At present, clinical imaging techniques for directly imaging the distribution of endolymph and perilymph are unsatisfactory. Enhancement of the perilymph can be obtained by the use of a triple-dose of gadolinium-containing contrast media (12), and endolymph distribution can be imaged by direct intratympanic injection of contrast media (13). However, the increasing recognition of adverse effects of high-dose gadolinium-containing agents (14), and the invasiveness of intratympanic administration mean that these techniques are not in routine clinical use.

The vestibular nerves

The primary vestibular neurons are of the bipolar type, with cell bodies located in Scarpa's ganglion which lies within the internal auditory canal. Scarpa's ganglion contains two masses, separated by a narrow isthmus, and these give rise to the superior and inferior divisions of the vestibular nerve. The superior division of the vestibular nerve primarily receives input from the superior and lateral semicircular canals, whereas the inferior division receives input from the posterior semicircular canal. Both divisions lie posteriorly within the internal auditory canal (IAC) before fusing with the cochlear nerve to form the vestibulocochlear nerve, which then enters the brainstem (15).

The nerves within the IAC are best imaged with a cisternographic MRI sequence, such as the CISS 3D technique (Figure 15.2). Imaging at 3 T is preferable to 1.5 T, as the higher spatial resolution is helpful in discriminating the individual nerve branches (Figure 15.3) (16).

Brainstem nuclei and tracts

Nuclei

The axons of the vestibular nerves terminate primarily in the medial, inferior, and superior vestibular nuclei within the brainstem. The lateral vestibular nucleus receives only a minority of primary afferent fibres; as a result, it has previously been described as being, functionally, a cerebellar nucleus. A minority of fibres project, via

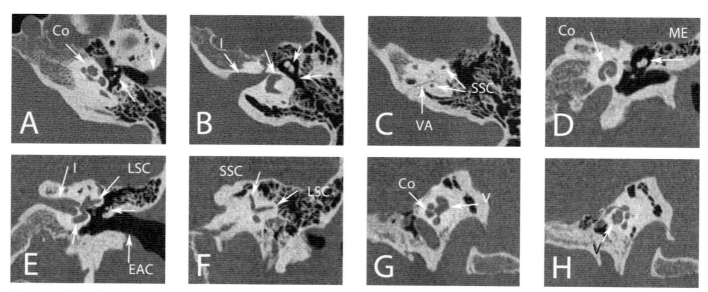

Fig. 15.1 Axial (A–C), coronal (D–F), and sagittal CT (G, H) sections through the left petrous bone. Co, cochlea; EAC, external auditory canal; I, internal auditory canal; LSC, lateral semicircular canal; ME, middle ear cleft; SSC, superior semicircular canal; V, vestibule; VA, vestibular aqueduct.

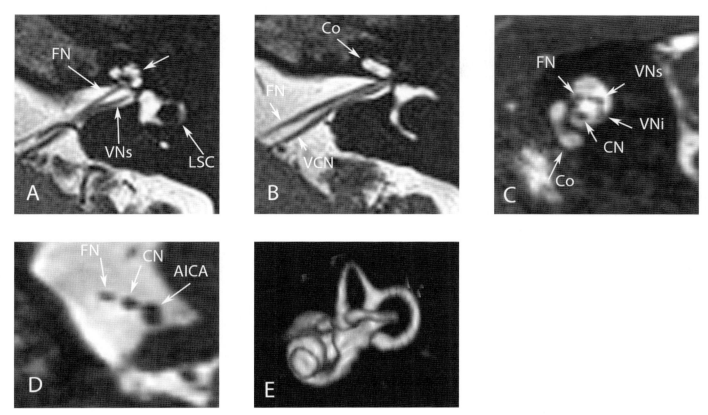

Fig. 15.2 Axial (A, B) and sagittal (C, D) 3D CISS MRI at 3 T of the left internal auditory canal. AICA, anterior inferior cerebellar artery; Co, cochlea; CN, cochlear nerve; FN, facial nerve (VII); LSC, lateral semicircular canal; VCN, vestibulocochlear nerve (VIII); VNi, inferior division of vestibular nerve; VNs, superior division of vestibular nerve. 3D volume rendered image of the membranous labyrinth from the same source data (E).

the vestibulocerebellar tract, directly to the flocculonodular lobe (FNL) of the cerebellum. The vestibular nuclei also receive a variety of inputs from the cerebellum (primarily the FNL and fastigial nucleus) and from multiple other brainstem nuclei, spinal cord, and midbrain nuclei.

The vestibular nuclei lie at the ponto-medullary junction, in the floor of the fourth ventricle, with the larger lateral vestibular nucleus extending superiorly into the pons. The vestibular nuclei cannot be visualized directly at 1.5 T and at 3 T. However, their approximate locations can be determined on clinical imaging. The location of the vestibular region can be inferred as a bulge projecting into the fourth ventricle from the medulla at the level of the inferior olivary nuclei. Nevertheless, high-field MRI microscopy of cadaveric specimens has been able to demonstrate the individual vestibular nuclei (Figure 15.4).

In the clinical context, however, the brainstem can be adequately imaged with a T2-weighted fast spin-echo sequence. It should be noted that cisternographic sequences, such as CISS 3D, lack the parenchymal contrast needed.

Tracts

The brainstem contains a number of white matter tracts which interconnect between the various brainstem nuclei, cerebellum, midbrain, and spinal cord. A number of these are relevant to the vestibular system. The medial longitudinal fasciculus (MLF) is a pair of white matter tracts, located centrally within the brainstem, containing multiple individual pathways linking the oculomotor nuclei (cranial nerves III, IV, and VI) with multiple other

brainstem, spinal and cerebellar nuclei. In particular, the MLF contains the vestibulo-oculomotor fibre bundles which provide afferents to the oculomotor nuclei from the vestibular nuclei, and which are responsible for the vestibulo-ocular reflex, with additional fibre bundles from the FNL of the cerebellum, and head and neck proprioceptors, inputs which are integrated to assist with gaze. The classic manifestation of MLF injury is internuclear opthalmoplegia (INO), caused by interruption of the pathways linking the individual oculomotor nuclei; this disorder of conjugate gaze causing impaired adduction of the ipsilateral eye and contralateral dissociated nystagmus is quite characteristic. If present, therefore, it is a useful sign, as its presence implies a central lesion. The MLF's position in the brainstem is close to the midline in the dorsal pons, extending from the basis pontis to the tegmentum (Figure 15.4). Like the vestibular nuclei, it is not visible as an individual structure on conventional clinical imaging, and the location must be inferred from the gross anatomy.

Vestibulothalamic projections arise from the vestibular nuclei and project to the ventral posteromedial nucleus of the thalamus and the lateral geniculate nucleus (LGN). As the LGN is a major relay station within the visual pathway, this multimodality sensory integration, may explain some aspects of the conscious perception of vertigo (17).

Cerebellum

The FNL and the vermis (lingua and uvula) together form the vestibulocerebellum. Phylogenetically, this region of the cerebellum is

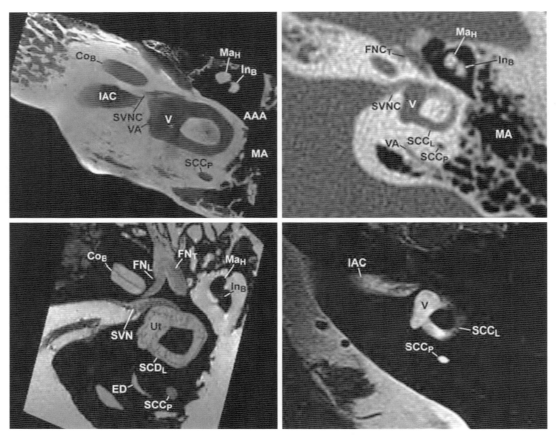

Fig. 15.3 The relations of the vestibule (V) and utricle (Ut) to the IAC and superior vestibular nerve (SVN)/superior vestibular nerve canal (SVNC) are clearly demonstrated on these multimodality series of axial images. Top left—*ex vivo* micro CT. Top right—*in vivo* MDCT. Bottom left—*ex vivo* 9.4 T Micro MR. Bottom right—*in vivo* 3 T MR. Image from Lane and Witte (59).

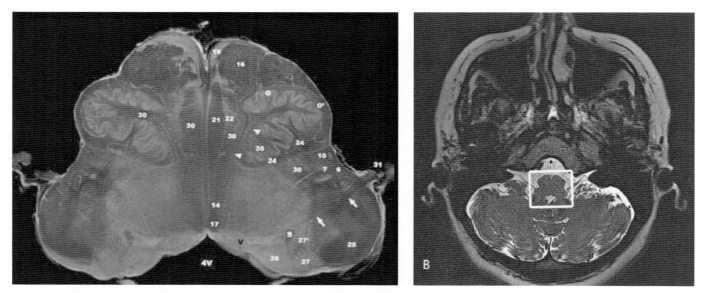

Fig. 15.4 Axial section through the mid-medulla at the level of the dorsal accessory olivary nucleus and the vestibular nuclei. (A) 9.4 T MRI of postmortem specimen (from Naidich et al. (60)); 26: Medial vestibular nucleus; 27: lateral vestibular nucleus; 4V: fourth ventricle; 17: medial longitudinal fasciculus. (B) Equivalent section using 3 T clinical imaging (3D CISS). The box illustrates the region imaged in (A). Detection of the vestibular nuclei is limited to the small bulges on the dorsal surface of the medulla.

the most ancient. By its control of proximal muscles and limb extensors, it provides maintenance of balance and postural equilibrium.

The FNL receives direct input from the vestibular labyrinth, with efferents returning to the vestibular nuclei. The FNL, particularly the lateral component, the flocculus, can be easily seen as small cerebellar protrusion into the cerebellopontine angle (CPA) (Figure 15.5).

The vermis receives proprioceptive input from the trunk and neck via the dorsal columns, visual inputs (via cortico-ponto-cerebellar pathways), extraocular muscle afferents from the oculomotor nuclei, and the vestibular nuclei. This integrative function of the vermis underlies smooth pursuit eye movements. The bulk of the vermian efferents are via the fastigial nucleus, and project to the vestibular nuclei (and thence to the vestibulospinal pathways), reticulospinal pathways, the colliculi, ventral posterior lateral, and ventral lateral nuclei of the thalamus. The vermis can be identified as a discrete component of the cerebellum at the midline (Figure 15.5).

Cortical regions

The primary vestibular cortex was first described in non-human primates. Clinical studies based on patients with acute lesions, giving vestibular syndromes have provided the initial evidence that there is an analogous region in humans. Initial functional imaging with isotope studies provided corroborative evidence (18). More recently, Eickhoff et al. performed a detailed functional MRI (fMRI) and cytoarchitechtonic analysis localizing the primary vestibular cortex to a region of the posterior parietal operculum (Figure 15.6) (19).

Imaging pathology

Choice of imaging technique

The choice of imaging technique depends on the clinical question and the expected site of pathology. In peripheral disorders imaging is concentrated on the labyrinth and the vestibular nerves. CT is the first choice if the lesion is likely to be related to bone, such as in known middle ear disease, e.g. infection or cholesteatoma, trauma, or a primary osseous disorder. However, in the unselected population with vertigo, these cases are in the minority. MRI with its high contrast for the nerves and membranous labyrinth, should therefore usually be the first choice. In 'central' vestibular disorders, the whole brain should be imaged, preferably with MRI.

Peripheral disorders

The labyrinth

Congenital malformations

Vertigo and sensorineural hearing loss (SNHL) are common presentations of congenital malformations of the labyrinth. These usually present during childhood, although milder forms may not become symptomatic until early adulthood.

Dilated vestibular aqueduct syndrome is the most common congenital malformation (20), and commonly presents with progressive SNHL with vestibular dysfunction a common associated feature (21). This is often found in conjunction with other labyrinthine malformations. However, it is easily recognized on imaging both with CT and MR (3D CISS or equivalent) (Figure 15.7). Based on population measurements using high-resolution CT, diameters greater than 1 mm at the midpoint of the aqueduct, or 2 mm at the operculum have been suggested as indicating dilatation (22). The posterior semicircular canal has a similar diameter, and can provide a convenient point of reference.

Endolymphatic hydrops

In endolymphatic hydrops failure of absorption of endolymphatic fluid in the endolymphatic sac leads to raised pressure within the endolymphatic system with subsequent dilatation of the endolymphatic spaces. There are congenital, acquired, and idiopathic forms (23). Congenital labyrinthine and cochlear malformations, as well as a number of acquired conditions, including trauma and infection

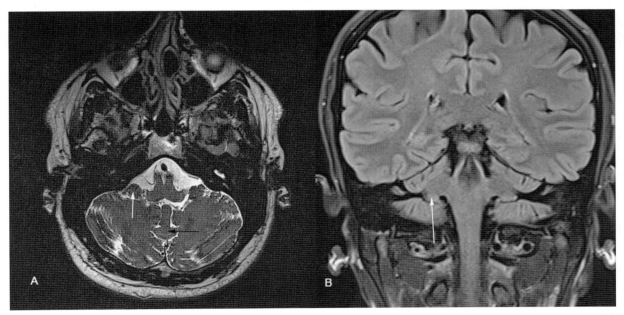

Fig. 15.5 (A) Axial CISS image through the medulla and cerebellum, showing the flocculus of the cerebellum (white arrow) and inferior vermis (black arrow). (B) Coronal FLAIR image showing the flocculus (arrow)

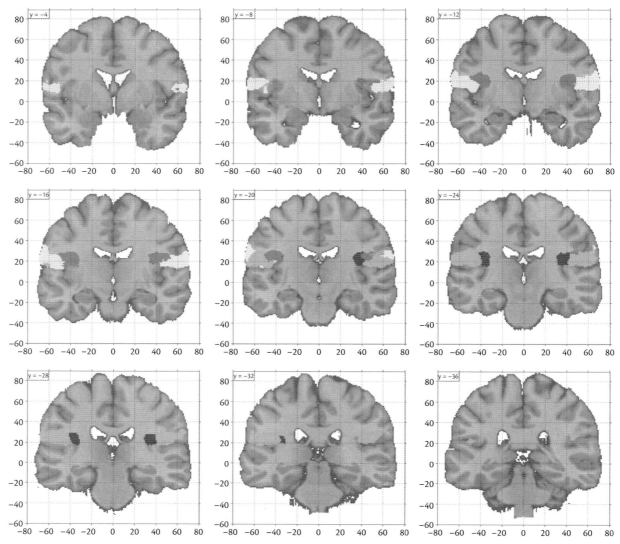

Fig. 15.6 (Also see Colour plate 11.) Cytoarchitectonic maximum probability maps showing the location of the four cytoarchitectonic divisions within the parietal operculum. Region OP2, the region that has been identified as localizing most closely with the primary vestibular cortex, is labelled in blue. Figure reproduced from Eickhoff et al. (61).

can be assessed by CT and MR (24). However, the most well known idiopathic form, *Ménière's disease*, has no specific imaging abnormalities. The role of imaging is therefore confined to excluding alternative diagnosis. Occasionally, enhancement of the endolymphatic sac can be observed, most probably reflecting an underlying inflammatory process, possibly a viral infection (25).

Canal dehiscence and perilymph fistula
Canal dehiscence is an abnormal connection between the vestibular system and surrounding structures, where there is a defect in the bone around one, usually the superior, of the semicircular canals (Figure 15.8). This abnormal communication disrupts the normal fluid dynamics of the inner ear, particularly with regard to abnormal pressure transmission, resulting in the typical clinical features of episodic vertigo and oscillopsia triggered by loud noise (Tullio's phenomenon), pressure changes in the ear canal, or Valsalva manoeuvres (26). Superior canal dehiscence is thought to be a developmental condition, even though it tends to present in adulthood, as the condition can remain asymptomatic until the

dura or remaining bone becomes sufficiently compliant to permit pressure transmission. Lateral canal dehiscence is less common, but has been attributed to chronic otitis media and cholesteatoma. Posterior canal dehiscence is rare, but has been seen in association with superior canal dehiscence. Perilymphatic fistulas are an abnormal communication between the perilymph space and the middle ear which can lead to symptoms similar to those of canal dehiscence. Causes include trauma, cholesteatoma, and previous middle-ear surgery, but also more subtle abnormalities such as abnormalities of the stapes footplate and air bubbles.

Labyrinthitis
Labyrinthitis refers to an inflammatory process involving the membranous labyrinth. Most frequently, this is a viral illness, but bacterial and autoimmune conditions are also recognized, as well as a post-traumatic complication. A perilymphatic fistula, as might occur in cholesteatoma, can also provide a route for subsequent spread of infection into the labyrinth. CT may therefore have a role if a complication of a middle ear disorder is possible.

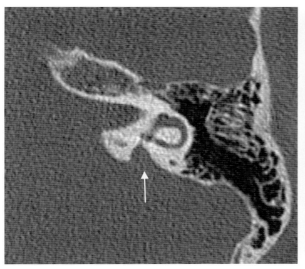 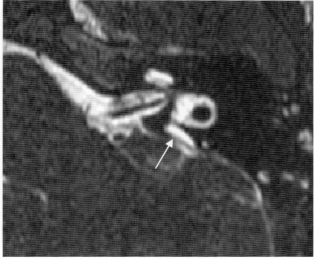

Fig. 15.7 Dilated vestibular aqueduct syndrome. (A) Axial CT through the left petrous bone showing the dilated vestibular aqueduct. (B) Axial CISS MRI of the left petrous bone in a different patient confirms the presence of fluid signal within the aqueduct (arrow). Both canal dehiscence and perilymphatic fistula can be diagnosed by CT (Figure 15.8) which can provide high-resolution images of the bone structure. The sensitivity and specificity are dependent on the performance of the CT equipment. Optimal diagnostic information is obtained at a slice thickness of 0.5 mm, whereas a slice thickness of 1 mm has demonstrably poorer positive predictive value (62).

On MRI, labyrinthitis can be associated with a signal that is mildly higher than CSF on T1-weighted (T1W) images, a lower signal than CSF on T2-weighted (T2W) images and a high signal on FLAIR images. Enhancement of the labyrinth following contrast injection can be seen during the acute phase. While these imaging features are frequently due to labyrinthitis, they are relatively non-specific (27). The sequelae of inflammatory disease are of fibrosis and calcification, termed labyrinthitis ossificans (Figure 15.9). Once present, the obliteration of the labyrinthine fluid and replacement by fibrous or calcified tissue enhancement can be no longer detected and the FLAIR signal normalizes. An MR imaging protocol for the diagnosis of labyrinthitis would include high resolution T1W (± contrast) and T2W sequences, FLAIR, and 3D CISS sequences centred on the IAC.

Labyrinthine tumours

Intralabyrinthine schwannomas are a benign neoplasm originating within the labyrinth (usually the cochlea) (Figure 15.10). These have been generally regarded as being extremely rare, but accurate incidence rates are not known. Nevertheless, they are increasingly identified on high resolution imaging, with prevalence rates of up

to 0.4% in MRI series (28). They are well demonstrated on MRI as filling-defects within the membranous labyrinth on T2W or CISS sequences. As do other schwannomas, they avidly enhance after contrast administration. An MR imaging protocol would include a 3D CISS sequence centred on the IAC, and a high-resolution T1W sequence (± contrast).

The cerebellopontine angle

A wide variety of lesions can affect the CPA. Neoplasia, granulomatous, and inflammatory lesions, haematomas, cholesterol granulomas, lymphoid, and vascular malformations are all frequently reported.

The overwhelming majority of CPA lesions are vestibular schwannomas, followed by meningiomas (6%) and epidermoids (5%) (29).

Vestibular schwannomas

Vestibular schwannomas are the most common tumour arising within the IAC. They are frequently called acoustic neuroma, although this is a misnomer, as the vast majority arise from the

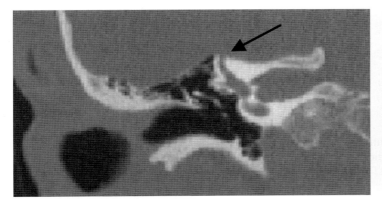 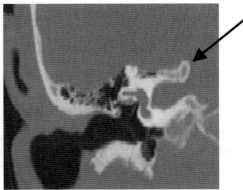

Fig. 15.8 Superior canal dehiscence—coronal CT sections through the right petrous bone. (A) The superior semicircular canal can be seen approaching the superior margin of the bone (arrow). (B) The superior semicircular canal is seen as a shallow indentation in the bone with no bony covering (arrow).

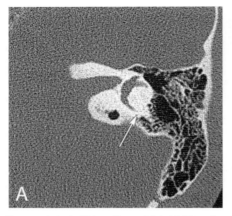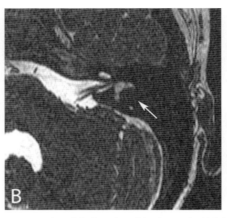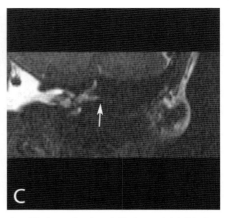

Fig. 15.9 Labyrinthitis ossificans. (A) Axial CT section shows attenuation of the lateral semicircular canal which is replaced by bone density calcified material. Axial 3D CISS (B) and coronal reformat (C) shows loss of the normal fluid signal of the lateral semicircular canal (arrows).

vestibular nerve. They tend to occur in people aged over 40 years and have an incidence of approximately 1/100,000 person-years (30).

MRI is exceptionally useful for the detection and follow-up of these lesions. High-resolution 3D CISS imaging is capable of detecting small, intracanalicular lesions and, for small tumours, distinguishing which nerve branch the tumour arises from. The gold standard imaging technique is post-contrast T1W imaging (31). This is particularly important for the follow-up of these lesions, as it permits clear delineation of the lesion's borders and an estimate of its dimensions.

Additionally, imaging is important for surgical planning; where the tumour is demonstrably separate from the cochlea, the surgeon can use a hearing preserving surgical approach, reserving the use of the translabyrinthine approach for those patients at higher risk of postoperative deafness (Figure 15.11).

In the context of screening for vestibular schwannoma in the patient with SNHL, and the low incidence in this population, the use of a CISS or equivalent sequence alone is less costly and likely to be as effective (32).

Meningiomas

Meningiomas are neoplastic lesions arising from the cap cells near arachnid villi. The overwhelming majority are benign (World Health Organization grade I), with approximately 5–7% benign atypical, and 1–3% overtly malignant (33). Approximately 2% of meningiomas involve the CPA.

Meningiomas are readily detected by both CISS and post-contrast T1 imaging, with the post-contrast images being more sensitive due to the usually avid contrast enhancement shown by meningiomas. Post-contrast T1 sequences are therefore ideal for follow-up, in much the same way as for schwannomas. Meningiomas do have several imaging features that may help with their identification: the dural attachment, resulting in the tumour forming obtuse angles to the surface of the petrous bone, an enhancing dural tail, calcification (seen on CT) and high vascularity evidenced as multiple flow-voids within the tumour.

Epidermoids

These are congenital lesions, arising from rests of ectodermal tissue containing stratified squamous epithelium. Despite their congenital nature, the peak age of presentation is 20–50 years.

MRI is highly accurate at the diagnosis of intracranial epidermoids. These lesions characteristically appear hypointensense on T1W images, isointense, or slightly hyperintense, to CSF on T2W sequences (34) and may contain some internal structure, visible as heterogeneity particularly on FLAIR sequences. These appearances are similar to those of arachnoid cysts. However, the hyperintensity on DWI reflecting restricted diffusion are markedly different, and

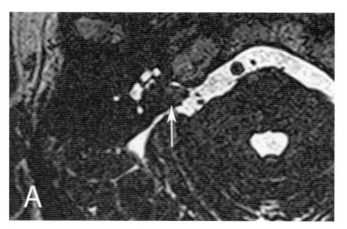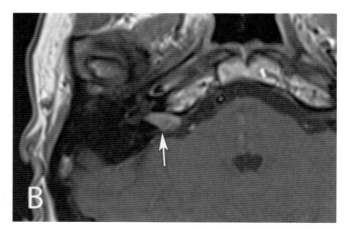

Fig. 15.10 Intracanalicular vestibular schwannoma. (A) Axial 3D CISS. There is loss of the normal CSF signal within the IAC (arrow), consistent with a mass lesion. (B) Post-gadolinium axial T1. There is enhancement of the soft-tissue within the IAC, permitting more accurate assessment of the lesion's size.

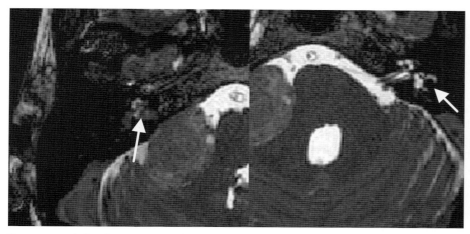
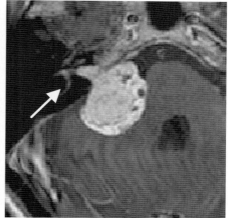

Fig. 15.11 Vestibular schwannoma with labyrinthine extension. (A) Axial CISS section through the right petrous bone. A large vestibular schwannoma is present within the CPA. However, there is loss of the normal fluid signal within the membranous labyrinth, including vestibule and basal turn of cochlea (arrow). (B) Axial CISS of the left petrous bone of the same patient for comparison. Normal fluid signal is visible within the membranous labyrinth. (C) Axial T1 post-gadolinium section shows enhancing soft tissue within the lateral semicircular canal, consistent with intralabyrinthine tumour.

in a significant proportion of cases, the only specific imaging finding (35). This property is also useful in the radiological follow-up.

A CPA tumour imaging protocol would include in addition to the normal brain protocol (T1W, T2W/FLAIR), high resolution T1W (± contrast), T2W and if the lesion is small 3D CISS sequences centred on the CPA. In case of suspected epidermoid, contrast is not needed and a DWI sequence should be added.

Superficial siderosis

This rare syndrome results from chronic iron deposition in superficial CNS parenchymal tissues. The most common reported cause is chronic subarachnoid haemorrhage, often from arteriovenous malformations, dural arteriovenous fistulae, or traumatic or iatrogenic injury to venous structures (36). The syndrome consists of several key symptoms with SNHL, ataxia, and pyramidal signs being among the most common.

MRI can detect the characteristic T2W-hypointense rim of haemosiderin on the surface of the neural parenchyma. However, greatly

increased sensitivity can be achieved with the addition of T2*-weighted imaging, or susceptibility weighted imaging (37) (Figure 15.12). MRI is the usual method of diagnosis, even when the CSF examination is normal. The imaging protocol would include T1W, T2W, and T2* or susceptibility weighted sequences of the brain.

Inflammatory and granulomatous conditions

There are a wide range of granulomatous conditions which may affect the CPA. Petrous apicitis (Gradenigo's syndrome) can cause localized meningeal inflammation, manifesting as meningeal thickening and enhancement on MRI. In the event that the IAC is involved, auditory or vestibular symptoms may result.

Direct involvement of the vestibulocochlear nerve can occur with certain organisms, notably herpes zoster (Ramsay–Hunt syndrome), syphilis, and Lyme disease. Localized enhancement of the meninges and/or the VII/VIII nerves (38) are the usual imaging findings, although labyrinthine enhancement has also been reported in the context of Ramsay–Hunt syndrome (10).

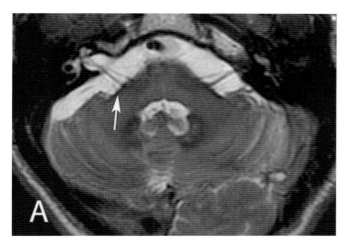
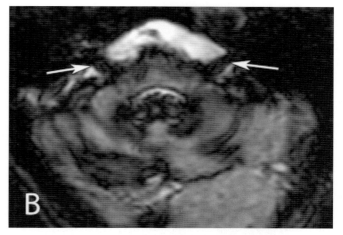

Fig. 15.12 Superficial siderosis in an 80-year-old man presenting with progressive unsteadiness, ataxia with disequilibrium, and bilateral sensorineural hearing loss. (A) Axial T2W MRI showing siderotic rim over the middle cerebellar peduncles (arrow). (B) Axial T2*W MRI revealing the greater sensitivity of T2*W sequences for haemosiderin. Hypointensity, indicative of siderosis is more conspicuous over the middle cerebellar peduncles and cerebellar folia. There is also direct evidence of involvement of the VII/VIII nerve complexes (arrows).

The imaging protocol would include T1W (± contrast), T2W/FLAIR sequences of the brain and the same sequences dedicated to the CPA.

Vascular compression

An increasingly recognized syndrome is that of vestibular paroxysmia. This manifests as episodic vertigo, motion intolerance and hearing loss, which often responds well to anticonvulsant treatment, and has been attributed to neurovascular compression (39), in the same way as the more established diagnosis of neurovascular compression in trigeminal and glossopharyngeal neuralgias and in hemifacial spasm. Occasionally, similar symptoms have been reported through compression of the nerve by other lesions, such as arachnoid cysts.

In recent studies (40, 41), positive findings on MRI have been described, notably the presence of a vascular loop within the IAC. However, it should be pointed out that these loops can be seen in up to 30% of healthy controls (42). They are best visualized using 3D CISS sequences.

Central disorders

Stroke

Vertigo is a common symptom of cerebellar stroke, with studies reporting vertigo as a presenting symptom in up to 87% of cerebellar hemispheric strokes (43).

Occlusion of major intracranial arteries or large branches tends to cause a series of well-defined syndromes. However, small, non-territorial cerebellar infarcts can also cause severe symptoms, which include vertigo, but which may not include the classically described constellation of symptoms.

Imaging of vertebrobasilar stroke

Where stroke is suspected, imaging should be performed as soon as possible. In most centres, due to its availability, the modality of choice is CT. While CT is satisfactory for the exclusion of acute intracranial haemorrhage, its sensitivity within the posterior fossa, particularly for small infarcts, is reduced. CT images are frequently degraded by artefacts attributable to the dense bone of the skull base.

The supplementation of unenhanced CT with CT angiography can visualize the extracranial arteries and major intracranial branch arteries, including the trunk of the posterior inferior cerebellar arteries (PICA), anterior inferior cerebellar arteries (AICA), and superior cerebellar arteries (SCA). Unfortunately, the branches of these smaller arteries are frequently too small to be adequately imaged.

MRI has an excellent sensitivity for detecting infarctions, particularly when DWI is performed. DWI is capable of detecting infarctions within 30 min of time of ictus, with close to 100% sensitivity. DWI can be performed very rapidly on modern equipment (<60 s), and therefore adds little to the cost and resource requirements for an MRI study. For vascular assessment, MR angiography (MRA) is an alternative to CTA. While the greater availability of CT means that it may frequently be obtained as the initial imaging modality, in CT negative cases where clinical suspicion of stroke remains, MRI is indicated as the next step.

Vertigo can be seen as a symptom in several classical posterior fossa vascular syndromes; notably the lateral medullary syndrome, due to PICA and AICA territory infarctions.

In the case of PICA territory infarction, the vertigo can be attributed to injury to the brainstem vestibular nuclei (Figure 15.13), and also to infarction of the FNL. In these contexts, the phenomenon of 'pseudo-acute peripheral vestibulopathy' can be recognized, due to damage to very early central vestibular pathways (44).

Haemorrhagic stroke

Posterior fossa haemorrhage, accounting for approximately 10% of intracranial haemorrhages, can often present with vertigo. CT is the technique of choice in this potentially life-threatening situation.

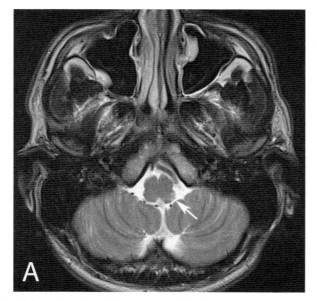 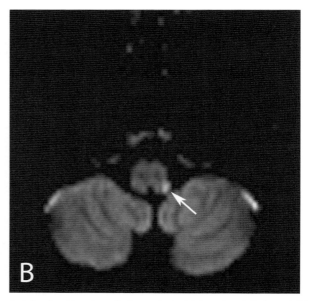

Fig. 15.13 (A) T2W MRI in a patient presenting with abrupt-onset vertigo suspected to be infarction. Hyperintensity is seen in the left lateral medulla (arrow). (B) DWI hyperintensity in the left lateral medulla (arrow), corresponding to the lesion seen in B, with restricted diffusion confirmed on ADC map (not shown).

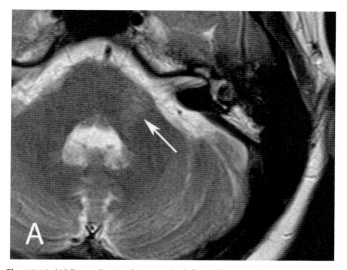
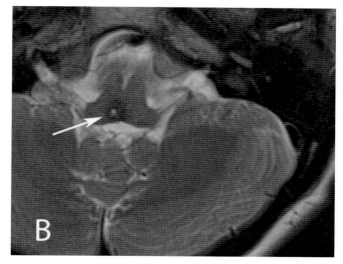

Fig. 15.14 (A) Demyelinating lesion in the left middle cerebellar peduncle (arrow) in a patient with multiple sclerosis. (B) Medullary cavernous angioma in a different patient. The hypointense haemosiderin rim and central hyperintensity is characteristic.

Vasculitic syndromes

Inflammatory syndromes which are typically associated with vestibular involvement include Cogan and Susac syndromes.

Cogan syndrome is characterized by ocular involvement with interstitial keratitis, and sometimes conjunctivitis, subconjunctival haemorrhage and iritis; and audiovestibular involvement causing progressive hearing loss of period of up to 6 months, with occasional systemic cardiovascular involvement. MRI findings of abnormal enhancement of the membranous labyrinth have been reported during the acute phase of the illness (45), with decreased or obliterated labyrinthine fluid in the chronic phase.

Susac syndrome (retinocochleocerebral vasculopathy) is a rare angiitis affecting the arterioles of the retina, cochlea, and brain. It follows a relapsing-remitting course causing variable symptoms including visual loss, hearing loss and encephalopathy. There is a characteristic MRI pattern of supratentorial white matter lesions, involving the corpus callosum, deep grey matter and posterior fossa. The appearances are similar to demyelination, except for the central involvement of the corpus callosum, rather than the callososeptal interface (46).

Additionally, a number of systemic inflammatory syndromes can be associated with audiovestibular syndromes, such as systemic lupus erythematosus (SLE), Behçet's disease, Churg–Strauss syndrome, Wegener's granulomatosis, and giant cell arteritis.

Migrainous vertigo

Vertigo is a common symptom in patients with migraine, reported by up to 77% of patients with migraine (47). However, the pathophysiological mechanism by which it occurs remains unknown. Diagnostic criteria for migrainous vertigo (48) include recurrent vestibular symptoms of moderate or severe intensity, a diagnosis of migraine, coincident migrainous and vertiginous symptoms, and lack of an alternate diagnosis.

The majority of patients with migraine have normal neuroimaging. An increased incidence of cerebral white matter hyperintense lesions at MRI has been reported (49), as has an increased incidence of cerebellar infarctions (50).

Other central disorders

In addition to the relatively specific syndromes already described, any CNS disease involving the vestibular pathways, cerebellum or insular cortex, can, by virtue of its location, result in vertiginous symptoms. More generalized inflammatory diseases, demyelination, neoplastic diseases (both primary and secondary), as well as a variety of miscellaneous conditions are all potential causes (Figure 15.14).

Specific clinical syndromes and their imaging protocols

Acute vertigo

Acute vertigo (especially when abrupt) can be caused by central ischaemia (51), and central defects should be examined for, even in the absence of clear additional signs of infarctions. Peripheral causes include labyrinthitis and vestibular neuronitis, but acute presentations are recognized from almost all causes, including CPA disorders.

In the context of isolated acute vertigo, the whole-brain (T2W, T1W, DWI) and the IAC and CPA (3D CISS or equivalent) should be imaged.

Central nystagmus

Downbeat nystagmus (DBN) is the most common primary gaze nystagmus, thought to be caused by damage to the FNL (52), as occurs in Chiari malformation, cerebellar degeneration and less commonly multiple sclerosis (53, 54). The imaging protocol should therefore include in addition to the usual brain protocol (T1W, T2W, FLAIR), sagittal and/or coronal sequences to assess the position and the volume of the cerebellum.

Positional nystagmus and vertigo

Benign paroxysmal positional vertigo (BPPV) is the most common positional vertigo syndrome. Imaging in BPPV is usually normal and therefore only performed to exclude other disorders.

In one series, however, semicircular canal abnormalities (stenoses and occlusions) have been demonstrated in a high proportion of patients with intractable BPPV (55).

Vestibular paroxysmia

Vestibular paroxysmia is a rare cause of positional vertigo. Neurovascular compression by a vascular loop can be demonstrated with 3D CISS or equivalent sequences (56).

Positional DBN is an occasional manifestation of DBN where nystagmus is not present in primary gaze. CNS lesions are frequent in this group, notably multisystem atrophy and cerebellar degeneration, but not the Chiari malformation. However, in one series, 25% of cases were idiopathic, although some had middle ear and labyrinthine abnormalities (57).

Bilateral vestibular failure

Bilateral vestibular failure (BVF) is a relatively uncommon cause of disequilibrium, unsteadiness, and oscillopsia. Reported causes include antibiotic toxicity, ontological neoplasianeoplastic disease (bilateral acoustic neuromas, skull base tumours, leptomeningeal metastases), cerebellar degeneration, cranial or peripheral neuropathies, and sequelae of meningitis (58). The imaging protocol should include the usual brain protocol (T1W, T2W, FLAIR) including a sagittal T1W sequence as well as the IAC/CPA protocol (3D CISS or equivalent).

Conclusion

The high resolution offered by modern CT and MRI has the ability to demonstrate both labyrinthine, CPA, and central anatomy in great detail, and identify a wide gamut of pathologies. Though the majority of patients presenting with vertigo have normal imaging, in a number of conditions, imaging does play an indispensable role in the diagnosis and follow-up of these diseases.

References

1. Neuhauser HK, von Brevern M, Radtke A, et al. (2005). Epidemiology of vestibular vertigo: A neurotologic survey of the general population. *Neurology*, 65(6), 898–904.
2. Crespi V (2004). Dizziness and vertigo: an epidemiological survey and patient management in the emergency room. *Neurol Sci*, 25(Suppl 1), S24–25.
3. Lawson J, Johnson I, Bamiou DE, Newton JL (2005). Benign paroxysmal positional vertigo: clinical characteristics of dizzy patients referred to a falls and syncope unit. *OJM*, 98, 357–64.
4. Salzman KL, Davidson HC, Harnsberger HR, et al. (2002). Dumbell schwannomas of the internal auditory canal. *AJNR Am J Neuroradiol*, 22, 1368–76.
5. Casselman JW, Kuweide R, Deimling M, et al. (1993). Constructive interference in steady state–3DFT MR imaging of the inner ear and cerebellopontine angle. *AJNR Am J Neuroradiol*, 14, 47–57.
6. Yousry I, Camelio S, Schmid UD, et al. (2000). Visualization of cranial nerves I–XII: value of 3D CISS and T2-weighted FSE sequences. *Eur Radiol*, 10(7), 1061–7.
7. Lane JI, Ward H, Witte RJ, et al. (2004). 3-T imaging of the cochlear nerve and labyrinth in cochlear-implant candidates: 3D fast recovery fast spin-echo versus 3-D constructive interference in the steady state techniques. *AJNR Am J Neuroradiol*, 25, 618–22.
8. Lane J, Witte RJ, Bolster B, et al. (2008). State of the art: 3T Imaging of the membranous labyrinth. *AJNR Am J Neuroradiol*, 29, 1436–40.
9. Naganawa S, Nakashima T (2009). Cutting edge of inner ear MRI. *Acta Oto-Laryngol*, 2009 129, 15–21.
10. Gizzi M, Riley E, Molinari S (1996). The diagnostic value of imaging the patient with dizziness. A Bayesian approach. *Arch Neurol*, 53(12), 1299–304.
11. Vandervelde C, Connor SEJ (2009). Diagnostic yield of MRI for audio-vestibular dysfunction using contemporary referral criteria: correlation with presenting symptoms and impact on clinical management. *Clin Radiol*, 64(2), 156–63.
12. Naganawa S, Koshikawa T, Nakamura T, Fukatsu H, Ishigaki T, Aoki I (2003). High-resolution T1-weighted 3D real IR imaging of the temporal bone using triple-dose contrast material. *Eur Radiol*, 13, 2650–8.
13. Fiorino F, Pizzini FB, Beltramello A, Barbieri F (2011). MRI performed after intratympanic gadolinium administration in patients with Meniere's disease: correlation with signs and symptoms. *Eur Arch Otorhinolaryngol*, 268(2), 181–7.
14. Thomsen H (2009). Nephrogenic systemic fibrosis: history and epidemiology. *Radiol Clin North Am*, 47(5), 827–31.
15. Nieuwenhuys R, Voogd J, van Huijzen C (2008). *The Human Central Nervous System*. New York: Springer.
16. Fisbach F, Müller M, Bruhn H (2009). High-resolution depiction of the cranial nerves in the posterior fossa (N III-N XII) with 2D fast spin echo and 3D gradient echo sequences at 3.0 T. *Clin Imaging*, 33(3), 169–74.
17. Lopez C, Blanke O (2011). The thalamocortical vestibular system in animals and humans, *Brain Research Reviews*, 67(1–2), 119–46.
18. Brandt T, Dietrich M. The vestibular cortex. Its locations, functions and disorders. *Ann NY Acad Sci* 1999. 871:297–312.
19. Eickhoff SB, Weiss PH, Amunts K, Fink GR, Zilles K (2006). Identifying human parieto-insular vestibular cortex using fMRI and cytoarchitechnoic mapping. *Hum Brain Mapp*, 27(7), 611–21.
20. Madden C, Halsted M, Benton C, et al. (2003). Enlarged vestibular aqueduct syndrome in the pediatric population. *Otol Neurotol*, 24, 625–32.
21. Berrettini S, Forli F, Bogazzi F, et al. (2005). Large vestibular aqueduct syndrome: audiological, radiological, clinical, and genetic features. *Am J Otoaryngol*, 26, 363–71.
22. Vijayasekaran S et al. (2007). When is the vestibular aqueduct enlarged? A statistical analysis of the normative distribution of vestibular aqueduct size. *AJNR*, 28: 1133–8.
23. Schuknecht HF, Gulya AJ (1983). Endolymphatic hydrops. An overview and classification. *Ann Otol Rhinol Laryngol Suppl*, 106, 1–20.
24. Hauser R, et al. (1996). Meniere's disease in children *Am J Otol*, 17, 724–9.
25. Fitzgerald DC, Mark AS (1996). Endolymphatic duct/sac enhancement on gadolinium magnetic resonance imaging of the inner ear: preliminary observations and case reports. *Am J Otol*, 17, 603–6.
26. Minor LB, Solomon D, Zinreich JS, Zee DS (1998). Sound- and/or pressure-induced vertigo due to bone dehiscence of the superior semicircular canal. *Arch Otolaryngol Head Neck Surg*, 124, 249–58.
27. Dubrulle F, Kohler R, Vincent C, Puech P, Ernst O (2010). Differential diagnosis and prognosis of T1-weighted post-gadolinium intralabyrinthine hyperintensities. *Eur Radiol*, 20(11), 2628–36.
28. Deux JF, Marsot-Dupuch K, Ouayoun M, et al. (1998). Slow-growing labyrinthine masses: contribution of MRI to diagnosis, follow-up and treatment. *Neuroradiology*, 40, 684–9.
29. Moffat DA, Ballagh RH (1995). Rare tumours of the cerebellopontine angle. *Clin Oncol*, 7, 28–41.
30. Gal T, Shinn J, Huang B (2010). Current epidemiology and management trends in acoustic neuroma. *Otolaryngol Head Neck Surg*, 142(5), 677–81.
31. Sidman JD, Carrasco VN, Whaley RA, Pillsbury HC 3rd (1989). Gadolinium. The new gold standard for diagnosing cerebellopontine angle tumors. *Arch Otolaryngol Head Neck Surg*, 115(10), 1244–7.
32. Fortnum H, O'Neill C, Taylor R, et al. (2009). The role of magnetic resonance imaging in the identification of suspected acoustic neuroma: a

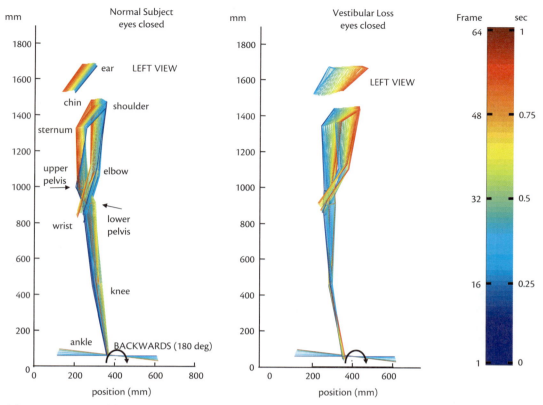

Colour plate 1 Stick figure representation of the movements of a normal and a bilateral vestibular loss (BVL) subject following a 7.5°, 60°/s backwards rotation of the support surface. Both subjects stood with eyes closed. Eighteen infrared Optotrak markers were placed on the body and 3 on the rotating support surface to track movements. The 64 time frames, recorded over 1 s, are indicated by the colour code. Blue frames mark the start of the recording, red the end. The platform rotation started at frame 6. To create the stick figure, marker movements in response to 8 identical stimuli were averaged, and then marker positions on a segment were joined. Note the backwards falling tendency in the vestibular loss subject and contrast this with the forward leaning of the normal subject. Data from Allum et al. (12).

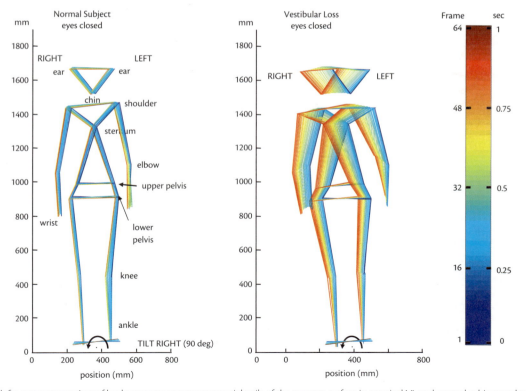

Colour plate 2 Stick figure representatives of body segment movements to right tilt of the support-surface in a typical VL and control subject under eyes closed conditions. For details of the figure refer to the legend of Figure 4.6. The views are from in front of the subjects. Note the similar arm and leg positions for the two subjects prior to tilt and tendency of the BVL subject to fall to the right. Data from Allum et al. (12).

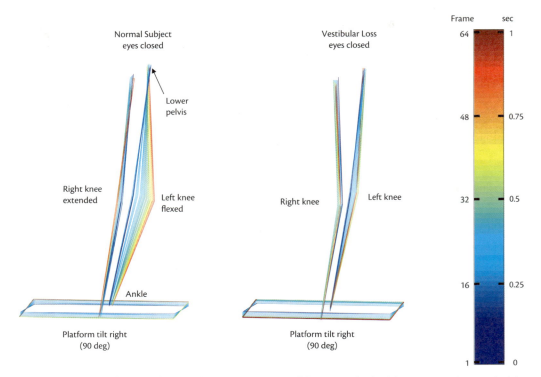

Colour plate 3 Stick figure representations of the knee flexion and extension movements following a right tilt of the support surface. On the left a normal subject and on the right a BVL subject, both standing with eyes closed. The views in the figures are from slightly in front (8°), slightly raised (4°) and from the right. Note the normal uphill knee flexion and downhill knee extension is reduced in the BVL subject. Same subjects as in Figure 4.9. For further details refer to the legend of Figure 4.6. Data from Allum et al. (12).

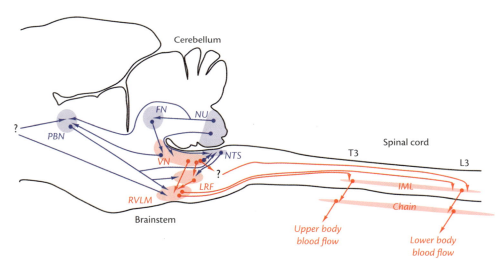

Colour plate 4 Schematic diagram of the circuitry producing vestibulosympathetic responses, transposed on a sagittal section of the cat brainstem and spinal cord. Areas and connections that play a primary role in generating these responses are indicated in red, and those that modulate the responses are indicated in blue. Vestibulosympathetic responses are mediated by the caudal regions of the medial and inferior vestibular nuclei (*VN*), which provide direct inputs to bulbospinal neurons in the rostral ventrolateral medulla (*RVLM*) as well as indirect inputs conveyed through the lateral portions of the caudal medullary reticular formation (*LRF*). The RVLM plays a critical role in relaying vestibular signals to sympathetic preganglionic neurons in the intermediolateral cell column (*IML*), which spans from the third thoracic (*T3*) to the third lumbar (*L3*) spinal cord segments. In turn, sympathetic preganglionic neurons provide inputs to sympathetic postganglionic cells positioned in the sympathetic chain (*chain*). Vestibulosympathetic responses are patterned, as indicated by the observation that vestibular stimulation produces opposite changes in forelimb and hindlimb blood flow. Since RVLM neurons respond similarly to vestibular stimulation despite their level of projection in the spinal cord, it is likely that additional areas of the brainstem that are presently unidentified also participate in relaying vestibular signals to sympathetic preganglionic neurons. The responses of RVLM neurons to vestibular stimulation are blunted in conscious animals, suggesting that the responses are modulated by higher brain regions that are currently unidentified. Descending influences of forebrain neurons on cardiovascular regulation may also be mediated through the parabrachial nucleus (*PBN*). Vestibulosympathetic responses are also altered by damage of the nodulus-uvula (*NU*) region of the caudal cerebellar vermis, which influences the activity of neurons in the caudal VN both directly and indirectly through connections in the cerebellar fastigial nucleus (*FN*). It has been proposed that NU indirectly influences the activity of neurons in nucleus tractus solitarius, presumably through relays in PBN or the caudal VN. These connections may participate in adjusting the gain of the baroreceptor reflex in accordance with body position in space or behavioural context.

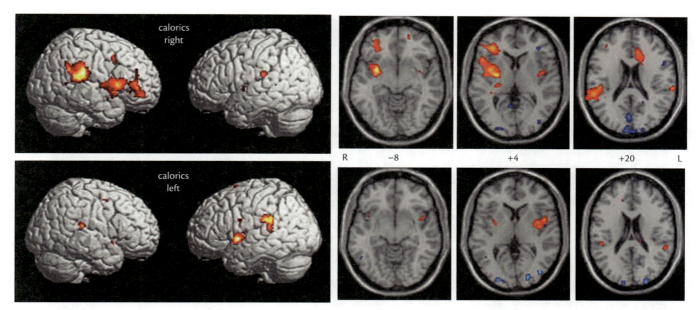

Colour plate 5 Illustration of the normal activation–deactivation pattern during unilateral vestibular stimulation in healthy volunteers (activations in yellow-red, deactivations in blue). For comparison, a schematic drawing is given of a monkey brain with the neurophysiologically determined multisensory vestibular areas 6, 3aV, 2v, 7a,b, PIVC and VTS (top left). Note that the locations of the activated areas during galvanic stimulation of the vestibular nerve in humans (fMRI; top right) are similar to those in monkey. During caloric irrigation of the right ear in healthy right-handers, activations ($H_2^{15}O$-PET) occur in the temporo-parieto-insular areas of both hemispheres, but there is a dominance of the non-dominant right hemisphere (middle: surface view of the right and left hemispheres; bottom: transverse sections Z = −10, +10, +20 mm). Deactivations are located in areas of the visual cortex bilaterally. Modified after (13).

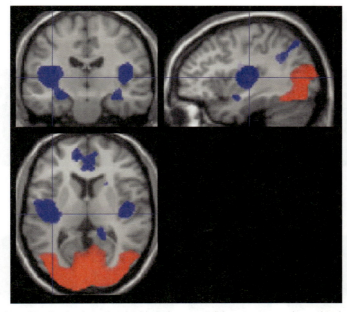

Colour plate 6 Activated areas during visual optokinetic stimulation in 7 healthy volunteers. While activations are located in the visual cortex bilaterally, areas with BOLD signal decreases are found in the temporal, insular and parietal cortex areas and the anterior cingulate cortex (p for activations: ≤0.001, p for deactivations: ≤0.0001).

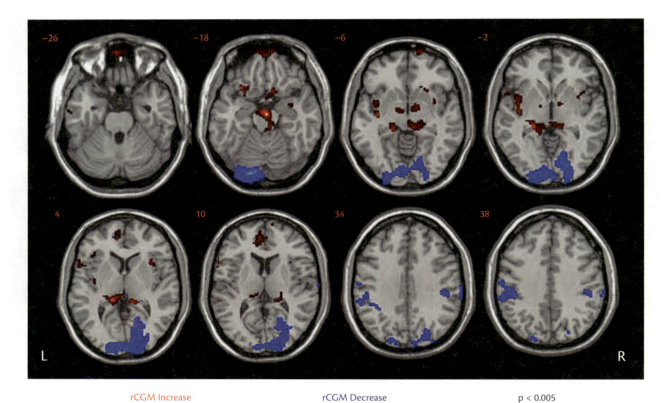

rCGM Increase   rCGM Decrease   p < 0.005

Colour plate 7 Statistical group analysis of five patients with vestibular neuritis of the right ear versus the control condition 3 months later (eyes closed, without stimulation). A significant increase (red) of regional cerebral glucose metabolism (rCGM) is seen in the contralateral left vestibular cortex, left superior temporal gyrus, hippocampus, thalamus bilaterally; it is also pronounced in the anterior cingulate gyrus. Simultaneously rCGM decreases (blue) are located in the visual and somatosensory cortex bilaterally. For illustrative purposes, voxels above a threshold of p ≤0.005, uncorrected, are shown.

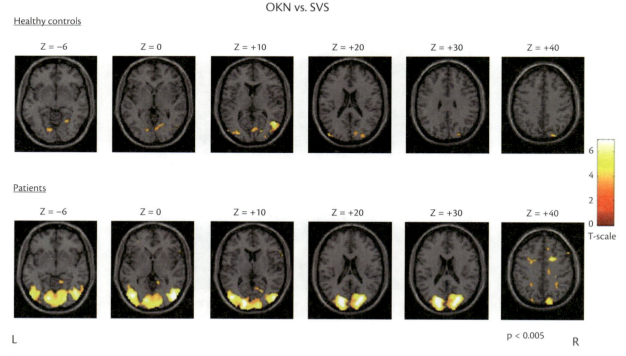

Colour plate 8 Head-to-head display of the activation in the t-contrast optokinetic nystagmus (OPK) vs. stationary visual stimulus (SVS) condition in fMRI for BVF patients (bottom) and the age-matched healthy control group (top). For illustrative purposes, voxels above a threshold of p < 0.005, uncorrected, are shown. Modified after Dieterich et al. (42).

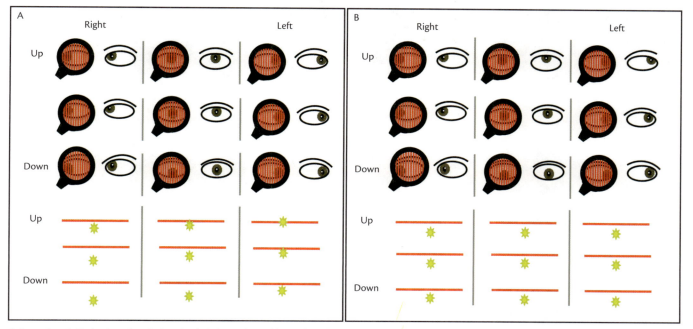

Colour plate 9 Evaluation of vertical ocular deviation with Maddox rod. A left hypertropia is shown. The Maddox rod is held vertically before the right eye and the positions of the white light (left eye) and the horizontal red line (right eye) are compared to evaluate vertical misalignment. In hypertropia due to a superior oblique palsy, the vertical misalignment is non-comitant and more marked on looking down and away from the affected eye (A). In hypertropia due to a comitant skew deviation, the vertical misalignment does not change in different gaze directions (B).

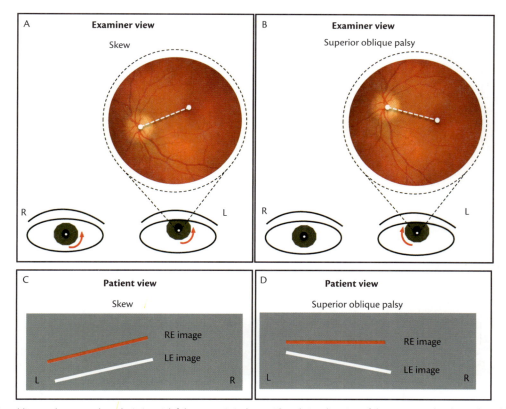

Colour plate 10 Superior oblique palsy versus skew deviation. A left hypertropia is shown. The relative direction of the torsion in the elevated eye (dashed white line between the macula and optic disc) from the examiner's view: intorsion with skew deviation (A) and extorsion with superior oblique palsy (B). Relative position of images from each eye as reported by the patient (with double Maddox rod): In skew deviation, there is no or little torsional diplopia (C). In superior oblique palsy, there is torsional diplopia with images pointing to side of the paretic eye (D). LE, left eye; RE, right eye.

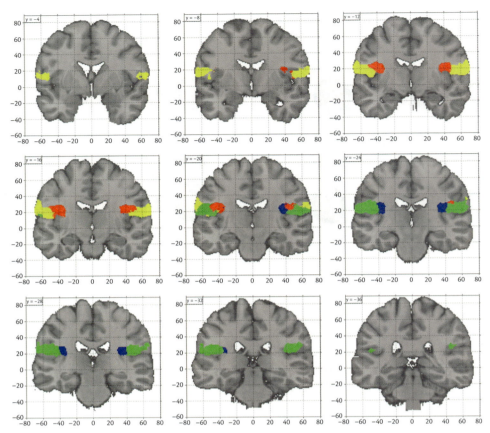

Colour plate 11 Cytoarchitectonic maximum probability maps showing the location of the four cytoarchitectonic divisions within the parietal operculum. Region OP2, the region that has been identified as localizing most closely with the primary vestibular cortex, is labelled in blue. Figure reproduced from Eickhoff et al. (61).

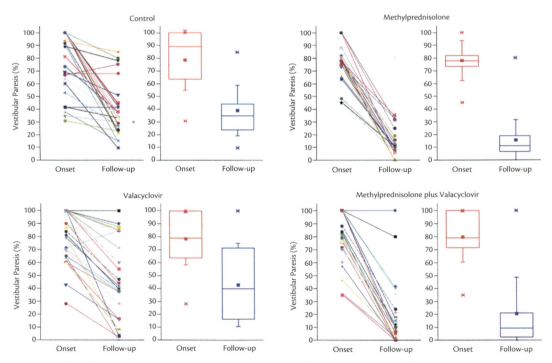

Colour plate 12 Unilateral vestibular failure within 3 days after symptom onset and after 12 months. Vestibular function was determined by caloric irrigation, using the 'vestibular paresis formula' (which allows a direct comparison of the function of both labyrinths) for each patient in the placebo (upper left), methylprednisolone (upper right), valacyclovir (lower right), and methylprednisolone plus valacyclovir (lower left) groups. Also shown are box plot charts for each group with the mean (■) ± standard deviation (SD), and 25% and 75% percentile (box plot) as well as the 1% and 99% range (x). A clinically relevant vestibular paresis was defined as greater than 25% asymmetry between the right-sided and the left-sided responses (28). Follow-up examination showed that vestibular function improved in all four groups: in the placebo group from 78.9 ± 24.0 (mean ± SD) to 39.0 ± 19.9, in the methylprednisolone group from 78.7 ± 15.8 to 15.4 ± 16.2, in the valacyclovir group from 78.4 ± 20.0 to 42.7 ± 32.3, and in the methylprednisolone plus valacyclovir group from 78.6 ± 21.1 to 20.4 ± 28.4. Analysis of variance revealed that methylprednisolone and methylprednisolone plus valacyclovir caused significantly more improvement than placebo or valacyclovir alone. The combination of both was not superior to steroid monotherapy. From (96).

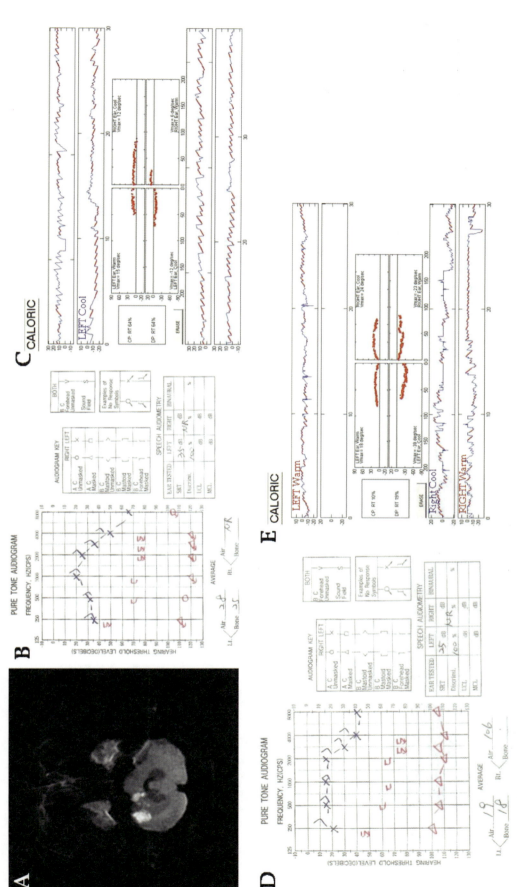

Colour plate 13 MRI and progress of audiovestibular dysfunction in a patient with AICA territory infarction who had profound hearing loss at initial and last follow-up. (A) Axial diffusion-weighted MRI demonstrates acute infarcts involving the right middle cerebellar peduncle and right anterior cerebellar hemisphere. (B) Initial pure tone audiogram reveals profound hearing loss on the right side. Hearing levels in decibels (dB) (American National Standards Institute, 1989) are plotted against stimulus frequency on a logarithmic scale. (C) Initial video-oculographic recordings of bithermal caloric tests showed a right CP (64%). (D) Follow-up testing performed 6 years after the onset of symptoms showed persistent hearing loss with no interval change. (E) Follow-up caloric test performed 6 years after the onset of symptoms showed normal caloric responses on the right side. AICA, anterior inferior cerebellar artery; CP, canal paresis; Vmax, maximal velocity of slow phase of nystagmus.

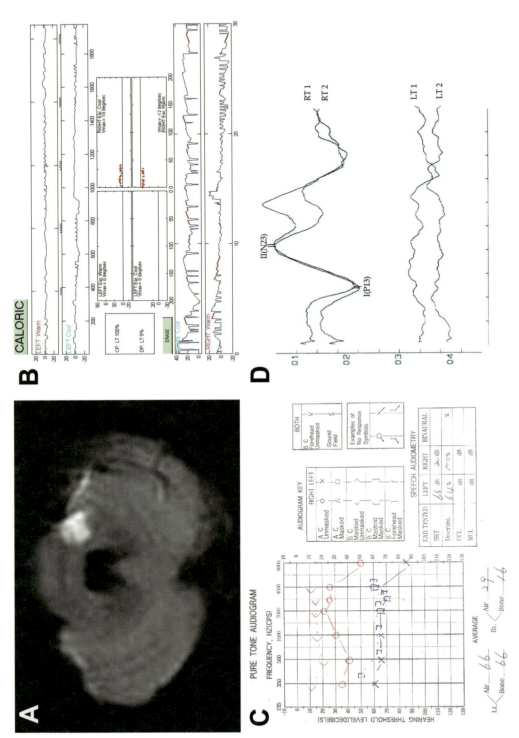

Colour plate 14 MRI, audiovestibular function tests, and cervical VEMP in a patient (patient 2) with AICA territory infarction. (A) Axial diffusion-weighted MRI demonstrates acute infarcts involving the left middle cerebellar peduncle. (B) Video-oculographic recordings of bithermal caloric tests disclose the left CP of 100%. (C) PTA reveals severe degree of hearing loss of 66 dB with 64% speech discrimination in the left ear. Hearing levels in decibels (dB) (American National Standards Institute, 1989) are plotted against stimulus frequency on a logarithmic scale. (D) Recording of cervical VEMP shows no wave formation in the ipsilesional side. AICA, anterior inferior cerebellar artery; CP, canal paresis; PTA, pure tone audiogram; VEMP, vestibular evoked myogenic potential; Vmax, maximal velocity of slow phase of nystagmus.

systematic review of clinical and cost effectiveness and natural history. *Health Technol Assess*, 13(18), 1–176.

33. Louis DN, Scheithauer BW, Budka H, *et al.* (2000). *World Health Organization Classification of Tumours. Pathology and Genetics of Tumours of the Nervous System.* Lyon: IARC Press.

34. Osborn A, Preece M (2006). Intracranial cysts: Radiologic-pathologic correlation and imaging approach. *Radiology*, 239, 650–64.

35. Hu XY, Hu CH, Fang XM, Cui L, Zhang QH (2008). Intraparenchymal epidermoid cysts in the brain: diagnostic value of MR diffusion-weighted imaging. *Clin Radiol*, 63(7), 813–18.

36. Fearnley JM, Stevens JM, Rudge P (1995). Superficial siderosis of the central nervous system. *Brain*, 118, 1051–66.

37. Wang J, Gong X (2011). Superficial siderosis of the central nervous system: MR findings with susceptibility-weighted imaging. *Clin Imaging*, 35(3), 217–21.

38. Martin-Duverneuil N, Sola-Martínez MT, Miaux Y, *et al.* (1997). Contrast enhancement of the facial nerve on MRI: normal or pathological? *Neuroradiology*, 39, 207–12.

39. Jannetta PJ (1975). Neurovascular cross-compression in patients with hyperactive dysfunction symptoms of the eighth cranial nerve. *Surg Forum*, 26, 467–9.

40. Hufner K, Barresi D, Glaser M, *et al.* (2008). Vestibular paroxysmia: Diagnostic features and medical treatments. *Neurology*, 71, 1006–14.

41. Brackmann DE, Kesser BW, Day JD (2001). Microvascular decompression of the vestibulocochlear nerve for disabling positional vertigo: the House ear clinic experience. *Otol Neurotol*, 22, 882–7.

42. De Carpentier J, Lynch N, Fisher A, Hughes D, Willatt D (1996). MR imaged neurovascular relationships at the cerebellopontine angle. *Clin Otolaryngol Allied Sci* 21(4), 312–16.

43. Ye BS, Kim YD, Nam HS, *et al.* (2010). Clinical manifestations of cerebellar infarction according to specific lobular involvement. *Cerebellum*, 9(4), 571–9.

44. Kim HA, Lee H (2010). Isolated vestibular nucleus infarction mimicking acute peripheral vestibulopathy. *Stroke*, 41(7), 1558–60.

45. Helmchen C, Jäger L, Büttner U, Reiser M, Brandt T (1998). Cogan's syndrome. High resolution MRI indicators of activity. *J Vestib Res*, 8, 155–67.

46. Susac JO, Murtagh FR, Egan RA, *et al.* (2003). MRI findings in Susac's syndrome. *Neurology*, 61(12), 1783–87.

47. Kayan A, Hood JD (1984). Neuro-otological manifestations of migraine. *Brain*, 107(4), 1123–42.

48. Furman JM, Marcus DA, Balaban CD (2003). Migrainous vertigo: development of a pathogenetic model and structured diagnostic interview. *Curr Opin Neurol*, 16, 5–13.

49. Swartz RH, Kern RZ (2004). Migraine is associated with magnetic resonance imaging white matter abnormalities: a meta-analysis. *Arch Neurol*, 61(9), 1366–8.

50. Kruit MC, van Buchem MA, Hofman PA, *et al.* (2004). Migraine as a risk factor for subclinical brain lesions. *JAMA*, 291(4), 427–34.

51. Zhang Y, Chen X, Wang X, *et al.* (2011). A clinical epidemiological study in 187 patients with vertigo. *Cell Biochem Biophys*, 59(2), 109–12.

52. Pierrot-Deseilligny C, Milea D (2005). Vertical nystagmus: clinical facts and hypotheses. *Brain*, 128(6), 1237–46.

53. Halmagyi G, Rudge P, Gresty MA, Sanders MD (1983). Downbeating nystagmus. A review of 62 cases. *Arch Neurol*, 40(13), 777–84.

54. Bronstein A, Miller DH, Rudge P, Kendall BE (1987). Down beating nystagmus: magnetic resonance imaging and neuro-otological findings. *J Neurol Sci*, 81(2–3), 173–84.

55. Horii A, Kitahara T, Osaki Y, *et al.* (2010). Intractable benign paroxysmal positioning vertigo: long-term follow-up and inner ear abnormality detected by three-dimensional magnetic resonance imaging. *Otol Neurotol*, 31(2), 250–5.

56. Naraghi R et al. (2007). Classification of neurovascular compression in typical hemifacial spasm: three-dimensional visualization of the facial and the vestibulocochlear nerves. *J Neurosurg*, 107(6), 1154–63.

57. Bertholon P, Bronstein AM, Davies RA, Rudge P, Thilo KV (2002). Positional down beating nystagmus in 50 patients: cerebellar disorders and possible anterior semicircular canalithiasis. *J Neurol Neurosurg Psychiatry*, 72, 366–72.

58. Rinne T, Bronstein AM, Rudge P, Gresty MA, Luxon LM (1998). Bilateral loss of vestibular function: clinical findings in 53 patients. *J Neurol*, 245, 314–21.

59. Lane J, Witte R (2010). *The Temporal Bone: An Imaging Atlas*. New York: Springer.

60. Naidich TP, Duvernoy HM, Delman BN, Sorensen AG, Kollias SS, Haacke EM (Eds) (2009). *Duvernoy's Atlas of the Human Brain Stem and Cerebellum*. Berlin: Springer.

61. Eickhoff SB, Amunts K, Mohlberg H, Zilles K (2006). The human parietal operculum. II. Stereotaxic maps and correlation with functional imaging results. *Cerebral Cortex*, 16, 268–79.

62. Belden CJ, Weg N, Minor LB, Zinreich SJ (2003). CT evaluation of bone dehiscence of the superior semicircular canal as a cause of sound- and/or pressure-induced vertigo. *Radiology*, 226, 337–43.

CHAPTER 16

Vestibular Symptoms, Balance, and Their Disorders: How Will We Classify Them?

Alexandre R. Bisdorff, Jeffrey P. Staab, and David E. Newman-Toker

Introduction

Early efforts to classify diseases go back to Paracelsus (born Theophrastus von Hohenheim, 1493–1541) and later to Swedish naturalist Carolus Linnaeus (1707–1778), best known for his botanical classifications, including his treatise *Genera morborum*. A contemporary of his, François Bossier de Lacroix (1706–1777), better known as Sauvages, published the first attempt to classify diseases systematically under the title *Nosologia methodica*. The later 19th century was a period of change in the statistical reporting of diseases. In 1900, the French government convened the first international conference to revise and promote the International Classification of Causes of Death (ICD) by Bertillon. Successive conferences continued standardization and development of a central family of classifications. In 1946, the International Health Conference entrusted the World Health Organization (WHO) with the responsibility for the sixth revision of the International Lists of Diseases and Causes of Death and expanded the classification to include non-fatal diseases (1).

Symptom and disease definitions are a fundamental prerequisite for professional communication in clinical, research, and public health settings. The WHO's International Classification of Diseases has influenced numerous healthcare-related political decisions. Some medical disciplines have developed their own, much more detailed ICD extensions such as the International Classification of Diseases for Oncology (ICD-O), International Classification of External Causes of Injuries (ICECI), International Classification of Primary Care (ICPC), and the ICD-10 Classification of Mental and Behavioural Disorders.

Efforts to build a formalized classification system, uniform definitions, or explicit diagnostic criteria vary somewhat by discipline. The need for structured criteria for epidemiological, diagnostic, and therapeutic research is more obvious for disciplines that rely heavily on symptom-driven syndromic diagnosis, such as psychiatry and headache, where there are currently no histopathological, radiographic, physiological, or other confirmatory diagnostic tests available. However, diagnostic standards and classifications are also crucial in areas of medicine such as epilepsy and rheumatology, where, although confirmatory tests do exist, there is substantial overlap in clinical features or biomarkers across syndromes. Interestingly, not only scientific and therapeutic progress but also public awareness of psychiatric and headache disorders has vastly increased after the introduction of the Diagnostic and Statistical Manual of Mental Disorders (DSM) by the American Academy of Psychiatry (2) and the International Classification of Headache Disorders (ICHD) by the International Headache Society (IHS) (3).

Although numerous advances in basic vestibular research have been made over the past several decades, there is mounting evidence that progress in the field may have been hampered by the lack of explicit and uniform criteria for the description of symptoms, syndromes, and clinical disorders. Vestibular nomenclature remains in its infancy. Other than the definition of Ménière's disease by the American Academy of Otolaryngology—Head and Neck Surgery (AAOHNS) (4) and the Classification of Peripheral Vestibular Disorders by the Spanish Society of Otorhinolaryngology (5), there appear to have been no systematic efforts to create widely accepted classification criteria prior to the current initiative by the Bárány Society. A 2005 expert summary from the National Institute for Deafness and Communication Disorders (NIDCD) at the National Institutes of Health (NIH) pointed to lack of consistency in terminology and classification as a major barrier to population-level epidemiological research related to vestibular disorders:

> The balance and vestibular field lags significantly behind other NIDCD components in epidemiological research. In order to move forward, epidemiologically significant common language to describe vestibular symptoms needs to be developed. In particular, the distinction between vertigo, disequilibrium, and presyncope is often lost in standard American Medical Association Current Procedural Terminology (CPT*) code based population epidemiology, yet it is critical for understanding symptoms as they may relate to organ systems and disease processes in the population setting. Therefore, standardized definitions are necessary to share and compare data between studies, and validation work needs to be completed with these definitions. (6)

Specific examples include the ongoing controversy surrounding the distinction between 'vestibular migraine' and 'vestibular Ménière disease' (7) or the varied use of the terms 'vestibular neuritis', 'cochleovestibular neuritis', 'labyrinthitis', 'cochleolabyrinthitis', and 'acute peripheral vestibulopathy' in the medical literature. There continue to be problems of terminology used for describing core vestibular symptoms such as dizziness and vertigo. Even when studied in a single, English-speaking country, the term 'vertigo' has been shown to have diverse meanings for patients (8), generalist physicians (9), and even otologists (10). We describe recent advances in developing a standardized terminology for vestibular and balance disorders as part the International Classification of Vestibular Disorders (ICVD) initiative.

Goals and scope for the ICVD Initiative

The goal of the ICVD initiative is to enhance research and improve the quality of clinical care for patients with vestibular and balance disorders by: 1) developing robust definitions for vestibular symptoms, signs, syndromes, and diseases, 2) establishing reporting standards for diagnostic certainty, causation, and functional outcomes of vestibular diseases, and 3) promoting terminological consistency internationally. An iterative, staged process has been proposed for developing the ICVD (Table 16.1). Achieving these aims will require the concerted efforts of dozens of content experts, frequent cross-disciplinary interactions (especially with groups developing related terminological standards), and, ultimately, strong political advocacy (e.g. to align clinical billing and coding procedures with new disease terminology). It is expected that the

Table 16.1 Planned stages for developing the ICVD-I

Stage	Name	Description
I	Classification	Create ICVD-I
IA	Symptoms	Develop definitions for vestibular symptoms
IB	Nosology	Establish rubric for classifying vestibular disorders
IC	Disorders	Define diagnostic criteria for vestibular diseases or syndromes
ID	Harmonization	Unify diagnostic criteria into cohesive compendium (ICVD-I)
II	Dissemination	Promulgate use of these criteria for research purposes (e.g. publication, endorsement of relevant professional societies)
III	Renewal	Establish a mechanism for knowledge maintenance and periodic updates to the criteria with evolving scientific knowledge.

first edition of the ICVD will be used predominantly to guide investigators conducting clinically-oriented vestibular research. The hope is that, over time, well-honed research criteria will gradually spread to use in the clinical domain, as has occurred in other areas such as headache disorders. The volume of work to be done is large, and it will take years to build the first complete draft of the ICVD. It is anticipated that component parts will be published as they are completed and vetted.

The term 'vestibular disorders' strictly refers to disturbances arising from the vestibular system, but the definition of the vestibular system itself can be understood broadly or narrowly. The vestibular system contributes to gait, stance, locomotion, balance, vision, spatial orientation, navigation, and spatial memory because of the widespread use of vestibular information in the brain. Furthermore, brain dysfunction of almost any cause, whether primary or secondary, may adversely affect balance. It is therefore necessary to limit the scope of problems classified within the ICVD as 'vestibular disorders', although some such decisions may ultimately seem arbitrary.

The ICVD will include diseases of the inner ear affecting the labyrinth, conditions arising from lesions of the connections of the labyrinth to the brain at the brainstem, cerebellum, subcortical structures, and the vestibular cortex. For these 'vestibular' conditions, it is expected that the ICVD will become the principal reference for standardized definitions of symptoms, signs, syndromes, diseases, and causes. The ICVD will also include illnesses that are primarily the province of other specialties, but produce symptoms that mimic vestibular disorders. The ICVD will focus on the vestibular presentations of these conditions, but will not seek to redefine or reclassify the primary non-vestibular disorder. Examples include syncope, seizures, stroke, headache disorders, cerebellar ataxia syndromes, extrapyramidal movement disorders, and behavioral disorders that are already defined by other groups. The classification will eventually include controversial and emerging entities such as cervical vertigo (11), in the hope that identifying limits of current scientific knowledge will prompt research to fill these gaps.

Genesis of the ICVD initiative and the critical role of the Bárány Society

The Bárány Society was founded in 1960 by Dr C. S. Hallpike and Professor C. O. Nylen, in order to honor the memory of Robert Bárány, who was professor of Otorhinolaryngology at the University of Uppsala, Sweden, from 1926–1936. Professor Bárány was awarded the Nobel Prize in Physiology or Medicine in 1915 for his fundamental work on the physiology and pathology of the vestibular apparatus. The Bárány Society is an international, interdisciplinary society bringing together clinicians and basic scientists with an interest in vestibular disorders (12).

The Committee for Classification of Vestibular Disorders of the Bárány Society was inaugurated at its 24th biannual meeting in Uppsala, Sweden, in 2006. Its charge is to promote the development of an implementable ICVD. Building the ICVD is currently the main activity of the Bárány Society between its biannual meetings. Dedicated sessions of the Classification Committee are planned for each Bárány Society meeting to update the membership on progress with the ICVD and discuss ongoing work. The first of these sessions was held at the XXVI Congress in Reykjavik in 2010.

In order to achieve the goal of building an ICVD that is widely accepted, the Bárány Society is actively seeking the input of members from other associations dealing with vestibular disorders, such as the Société Internationale d'Otoneurologie and the Comisión de Otoneurología de la Sociedad Española de Otorrinolaringología in Europe, and the American Academy of Otolaryngology—Head and Neck Surgery (AAO-HNS) in the United States, as well as from the international vestibular community at large. For this purpose the Bárány Society's website now offers an online discussion forum on specific topics related to classification.

Beyond cooperation with individuals and associations within the vestibular community, the Bárány Society is also seeking cooperation and consensus with scientific associations from related disciplines, if there are important aspects of diseases that touch more than one society. One example is vestibular migraine, which is considered to be an important entity in the vestibular community, but is not recognized in the current edition of the ICHD. The IHS is in the process of revising its second version of the ICHD and discussions are underway to find a mutually acceptable way to define the interface of migraine and episodic vestibular symptoms.

Methodology and process for developing the ICVD

In 2006 the Classification Committee convened its first meeting to begin structuring the approach to developing the ICVD. It was recognized early on that initial definitions would have to rely on consensus expert opinion, since 'gold standard' tests for most vestibular disorders are lacking. The group needed to develop a conceptual framework, a list of initial topics, and a process for consensus building. To permit terminological consistency in defining vestibular disorders as part of the ICVD, it was decided early on to first define key vestibular symptoms and build consensus around these formalized definitions; the product of this initial work has already been published (13). The conceptual framework and structure for the ICVD is described in the section that follows. Initial topics (e.g. Ménière's disease, vestibular migraine, benign paroxysmal positional vertigo) were chosen for their frequency and importance to the vestibular disorders community. Because of large numbers of tasks, their complexity, and the need for multiple perspectives, a working group structure was developed to manage the process.

In this process, difficult and controversial issues are delegated to working groups in charge of well-defined tasks with predetermined guidelines and time frames. The working groups report to the Classification Committee for comments and suggestions to ensure that all the parts of the classification are coherent with each other. Every working group needs the approval of the Classification Committee before its work is submitted for publication. Working groups have a coordinator designated by the Classification Committee. The coordinator is a member of the Bárány Society and selects the members of his/her own working group, although rules have been established to insure adequate international representation and diversity of perspectives. Each working group must include members from three continents. At least one clinician must have an otolaryngology training background and one a neurology background. Clinicians and scientists from other fields are included, based on the committees' needs for additional expertise. Each member of a working group is expected to contribute to the group's endeavors to the extent that he or she qualifies for

authorship of the group's products. The goal is to encourage small, efficient working groups.

Workflow is to progress in a series of steps. Each work group is tasked with reviewing relevant literature in its assigned area to become familiar with existing nomenclature worldwide. The groups then prepare written drafts of standardized definitions and diagnostic criteria, presenting them initially to the Classification Committee and Bárány Society membership. The groups revise drafts based on feedback from the Classification Committee and general membership and then solicit input from other professional societies and individual experts worldwide using an internet based discussion forum on the Bárány Society's website (12). This feedback is used to prepare a final revision of definitions and diagnostic criteria to be approved by the Classification Committee, before publication of the final product in an international journal.

The Classification Committee expects the ICVD to be compatible and coherent with established international diagnostic nomenclature and the latest versions of the ICD (14), ICHD (3), and DSM (2). The ICD, ICHD, and DSM are presently undergoing revisions, so affected subcommittees are expected to stay abreast of proposed changes and, if possible, exchange information with the respective working groups of the other societies as they write content for the ICVD.

ICVD structure

It was recognized that a conceptual framework was essential to developing a robust ICVD. The guiding principles in developing this framework were as follows: 1) the approach should be face valid, intuitive, and usable; 2) it should minimize the use of new terminology and deviations from current clinical or research practice; 3) it should be consistent or compatible with other classification systems (ICD, ICHD, DSM, etc.); 4) it must addresses the full spectrum of relevant clinical and research problems related to vestibular disorders, recognizing that the maturity of science varies from topic to topic; and 5) it should leave room for expansion, revision, and evolution with new science, allowing flexibility for rigorous scientific validation.

The proposed structure of the ICVD currently includes four layers: Layer I—symptoms and signs, Layer II—clinical syndromes, Layer III-A—diseases and disorders, and Layer III-B—pathophysiological mechanisms (Figure 16.1). Each layer contains elements (e.g. specific symptoms or diseases) that are important in their own right, but are also important in their links to other elements. This structure will allow the ICVD to depict conceptual connections between elements within layers (e.g. disease comorbidity in Layer III-A) and across layers (e.g. epidemiological relationship between disease in Layer III-B and clinical syndrome in Layer II). Since knowledge of these connections is incomplete, it is recognized that some links may also 'skip' layers.

A multilayer approach was considered essential to accommodate the breadth of clinical and research applications, now and in the future. Some clinicians and researchers must organize their approach beginning with signs and symptoms, whereas others must lead with a primary focus on specific diseases or pathophysiological mechanisms. While the focus varies depending on the clinical or research application (e.g. individual case formulation, developing a diagnostic care pathway, or researching a new mechanism-based therapy), the need is universal. For example, clinical definitions

ICVD Proposed Multi-Layer Classification Structure

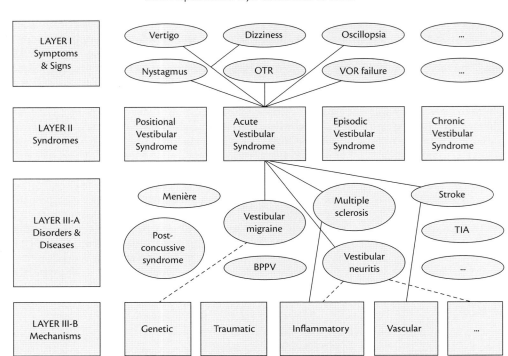

Fig. 16.1 This figure outlines the proposed four-layer architecture for the ICVD. Connections between diagrammed components depict a specific 'use case' of the ICVD for a single clinical syndrome (acute vestibular syndrome) that could be utilized for clinical care or diagnostic research. Solid lines represent well-established scientific relationships between conceptual components; dashed lines represent less certain links.

are crucial even for those whose scientific pursuits may, to casual inspection, seem entirely non-clinical (e.g. searching for genetic polymorphisms in patients with vestibular migraine, where the precise definition for vestibular migraine heavily determines the source population for 'cases' as opposed to 'controls', and, ultimately, the scientific result).

The structure is designed with the intent to be equally useful when approached from any starting point in the hierarchy. For example, a clinical epidemiologist studying associations of vestibular signs and symptoms in the general population might focus on vertigo and dizziness (Layer I) to determine a link to episodic versus chronic vestibular syndromes (Layer II). A clinical administrator seeking to improve the emergency care of vestibular patients might build a plan around a single syndrome such as the acute vestibular syndrome (Layer II) to ensure that clinicians assess relevant clusters of symptoms and signs (Layer I) in order to efficiently and effectively diagnose critical diseases and disorders in the emergency department (Layer III-A) (15). By contrast, a vestibular geneticist might focus on phenotypic variation (Layers I, II, III-A) associated with a single genotype (Layer III-B).

ICVD Layer I—symptoms and signs

Layer I of the ICVD, which includes definitions for specific vestibular symptoms, has been completed and published (13). This layer was addressed first because it was considered foundational to the development of all subsequent definitions, the vast majority of

which will be based on clinical phenomena. It was decided to limit the scope of this work to defining cardinal vestibular symptoms, representing the primary clinical symptoms typically resulting from vestibular disorders. Secondary symptoms such as nausea, fatigue, or anxiety, even if frequent accompaniments in patients with vestibular disturbances, were not included. Additional terms will likely be added as they arise in the construction of syndrome and disease definitions. A future working group will develop technical specifications for individual clinical signs.

The principles followed for developing symptom definitions were as follows:

- No 'vestibular' symptom has a totally specific meaning in terms of topology or nosology and its pathogenesis is likely to be incompletely understood.

- Symptom definitions should be as purely phenomenological as possible without reference to a theory on pathophysiology or a particular disease.

- Definitions for symptoms are clearest if they are non-overlapping and non-hierarchical but allow one or more symptoms to coexist in a particular patient.

- English will be the primary language of the ICVD, but consideration should be given in choice of terminology to ease of translation into languages beyond English, given current word usage patterns (13).

The ICVD describes four categories of cardinal vestibular symptoms: 1) vertigo, 2) dizziness, 3) vestibulo-visual symptoms, and

4) postural symptoms, including subtypes for each (Table 16.2) (13). The new nomenclature distinguishes *vertigo* (a false sense of motion) and *dizziness* (disturbed spatial orientation without a false sense of motion), which represents an important departure from typical US practice which considers vertigo a subtype of dizziness along with presyncope, unsteadiness, and other 'non-specific' sensations (9). It defines subtypes of vertigo as either 'spinning' or 'non-spinning' and clarifies the difference between an internal percept of motion (*internal vertigo*) and the external visual sense of directional world motion (*external vertigo*). By default, use of the term vertigo without specification is considered internal vertigo.

While vertigo and dizziness are distinguished from one another, neither is considered specific in its link to underlying vestibular pathology. Both symptoms are frequently encountered in patients with either vestibular or non-vestibular disorders, whether acute or chronic (8, 16). Vertigo and dizziness are each divided into two categories, spontaneous and triggered. The triggers listed for both symptoms are the same (Table 16.2). An important distinction is made between head motion vertigo/dizziness and positional vertigo/dizziness. Head motion vertigo/dizziness occurs during the head motion, whereas positional vertigo/dizziness is triggered by and occurring *after* a change of head position in space relative to gravity.

A separate category on vestibulo-visual symptoms was developed, since vestibular dysfunction can result in a range of visual disturbances. In part, grouping these symptoms together was an explicit attempt to promote awareness around this issue. Because 'internal' and 'external' vertigo are sometimes dissociated clinically (e.g. in a patient who sees the world spinning or rotating from jerk nystagmus but feels no spinning with eyes closed), the visual sense of motion could not simply be incorporated into the definition of vertigo, and the term 'external vertigo' was listed among the vestibulo-visual symptoms. Although some prior studies (17) have called this sense of visual flux 'oscillopsia', group consensus was that oscillopsia should be restricted to describing a bidirectional, oscillating visual motion that incorporates complaints such as 'jumping' or 'bouncing' vision. Other terms such as 'objective vertigo', 'visual vertigo', and 'vertigopsia' were proposed but rejected in favour of 'external vertigo' for various reasons (13).

The ICVD definitions for postural balance symptoms use *unsteadiness* as the preferred descriptive term for upright postural instability (when sitting, standing, or walking), rather than the more linguistically ambiguous terms 'disequilibrium' or 'imbalance'. If the unsteadiness has a particular directional bias, the term *directional pulsion* should be used and the direction specified (e.g. lateropulsion to the right).

These definitions require some clinical judgement to be applied correctly in their present form, especially in languages other than English. Once clinicians become comfortable with the new terminological distinctions, it is anticipated that they will classify patient symptoms accordingly, making necessary modifications to their medical history interviewing questions in their local language or dialect as appropriate. As has occurred with the DSM, the development of validated, structured interview instruments to identify specific symptoms or symptom clusters through direct patient interview is expected in the future.

ICVD Layer II—syndromes

Layer II, syndromes, offers an intermediate layer of syndromic classification that bridges between constellations of symptoms and signs (e.g. vertigo, nausea, vomiting, head motion intolerance, gait unsteadiness, and nystagmus in the 'acute vestibular syndrome') and underlying causes (e.g. vestibular neuritis or acute cerebellar infarction). Currently proposed are four specific syndromes comprising the bulk of all vestibular presentations: 1) positional vestibular syndrome (e.g. due to benign paroxysmal positional vertigo (BPPV), central positional syndromes); 2) acute vestibular syndrome (e.g. due to vestibular neuritis or acute stroke); 3) episodic vestibular syndrome (e.g. due to Ménière's disease, vestibular migraine, or transient ischemic attack); and 4) chronic vestibular syndrome (e.g. due to bilateral vestibular failure or cerebellar degeneration). Layer II will facilitate the development of clinical care pathways and standardized inclusion criteria for research studies focused on accurate diagnosis. A syndromic definitions working group has recently been formed to generate these definitions.

ICVD Layer III—disorders and diseases

Layer III-A contains the diseases and disorders and seeks to be relatively comprehensive. It is this layer where the need for coherence and compatibility with other classifications is most evident and requires the most coordination. The ICVD will use existing terms for vestibular disorders and diseases wherever possible and only introduce new terms for conditions not included in previous

Table 16.2 Synopsis of ICVD definitions of vestibular symptoms (14)

Symptom	Definition	Subtypes
Vertigo	Sensation of motion of self when no motion is present or altered sensation of motion when motion occurs. The motion sensation may be rotary, translational, or tilt. A similar sensation of motion of the environment is a vestibulo-visual symptom (external vertigo)	Spontaneous vertigo Triggered vertigo: • Positional vertigo • Head-motion vertigo • Visually-induced vertigo • Sound-induced vertigo • Valsalva-induced vertigo • Orthostatic vertigo • Other triggered vertigo
Dizziness	A disturbed or altered sensation of spatial orientation without false or altered movement	Spontaneous dizziness Triggered dizziness: • Positional dizziness • Head-motion dizziness • Visually-induced dizziness • Sound-induced dizziness • Valsalva-induced dizziness • Orthostatic dizziness • Other triggered dizziness
Vestibulo-visual symptoms	Visual symptoms that result from vestibular pathology or visual-vestibular interactions. Symptoms arising from ocular pathology are not included	External vertigo Oscillopsia Visual lag Visual tilt Movement-induced blur
Postural symptoms	Balance-related symptoms that occur while in an upright posture. For example, unsteadiness is a sensation of swaying or rocking when sitting, standing, or walking. Symptoms that occur only when changing positions (e.g. standing up from sitting) are classified as orthostatic, not postural	Unsteadiness Directional pulsion Balance-related near fall Balance-related fall

classifications. If several words are used to describe the same condition, the most suitable one will be included in the ICVD classification system. Other terms will be designated as 'terms not used in this nomenclature'.

For most diseases no pathognomonic or definitive, confirmatory tests are available. In such cases, the definitions will use operational criteria for symptom dimensions (e.g. type, timing, or triggers) or symptom clusters and ancillary test results, as appropriate. Both supporting and negating criteria will be considered. Criteria will generally be graded to define the certainty of a particular diagnosis from most specific to most sensitive as *definite*, *probable*, or *possible*. Denoting a degree of diagnostic certainty is important for both clinical care and research. For example, clinicians will likely apply a high-risk therapy (e.g. vestibular neurectomy) only to patients with 'definite' disease, while they may be willing to apply a low-risk therapy (e.g. dietary modification) even to a patient with only 'possible' disease. Likewise, the highest degree of diagnostic certainty (e.g. 'definite') may be necessary for exploratory, early-stage diagnostic or therapeutic research, whereas lesser degrees of certainty may be preferred (e.g. 'definite or probable') for later-stage investigations where generalizability to a broader population or large-scale dissemination is intended to maximize public health impact.

The Classification Committee established the first four disease-oriented working groups to address the definitions and diagnostic criteria for diseases where consensus is most urgently needed because of their epidemiological importance or ongoing controversy. These working groups are focused on Ménière's disease, BPPV, vestibular migraine, and behavioural neuro-otological conditions. The Ménière's working group seeks to build on the AAO-HNS definition of Ménière's disease, which has been used worldwide since its publication in 1995 (4). Greater precision will be needed in some aspects, particularly regarding diagnostic overlap with other conditions also presenting with episodic vestibular syndrome, mainly vestibular migraine. The BPPV working group has already presented detailed definitions of symptoms and signs for all variations of canalolithiasis and cupulolithiasis currently described in the medical literature. These definitions have reached the stage in which they are posted on the Bárány Society's website for online comments from members and non-members of the Bárány Society throughout the world. Once finalized, these criteria will be a ready reference for all forms of BPPV, including rare and emerging manifestations of that disorder. The vestibular migraine and behavioural disorders groups have more challenging tasks because they are charged with developing definitions of clinical entities for which there are no agreements about terminology, no pathognomonic signs or symptoms, and no laboratory or neuroimaging biomarkers. In addition, these disorders must resonate with extant classifications (ICHD and DSM).

The vestibular migraine working group began by choosing *vestibular migraine* as the preferred term over 'migrainous vertigo', 'migraine-related vertigo', 'migraine-related dizziness', and other similar terms. Vestibular migraine stresses that vestibular symptoms (whether vertigo, dizziness, or other vestibular complaint) may be the predominant manifestation of migraine and should be regarded as a special subcategory of migraine, similar to retinal migraine. Draft criteria were based on the definitions of definite and probable vestibular migraine first proposed by Neuhauser, et al. in 2001 (18) and later formalized by Furman, et al. (19). *Definite* vestibular migraine will now likely require five, rather than two, vestibular episodes accompanied by migraine headaches. Criteria for *probable* vestibular migraine (i.e. recurrent spells of vestibular symptoms with migrainous features, triggers, or treatment response) will likely change little. *Possible* vestibular migraine will likely be added to prior criteria. Additional details may be found in Chapter 21).

The behavioural subcommittee was the last of the current working groups to be formed and met for the first time in August 2010 in Reykjavik during the 26th Bárány Society meeting. That subcommittee is currently in the process of writing draft criteria for behavioural conditions that are commonly encountered in neuro-otology. The committee's goal is to identify a small number of the most important behavioural phenomena for otologists and neuro-otologists and prepare definitions that can easily be implemented by clinicians and researchers who have minimal training or experience in psychiatry. This task is complicated by the fact that the current psychiatric nomenclature, the DSM-IV-TR (2), is undergoing a major revision to DSM-5, scheduled for publication in 2013. One of the parts most applicable to otology and neuro-otology, the somatoform disorders section, is being completely restructured for the DSM-5 (20). Fortunately, these proposed changes appear to be aligned with current thinking for the ICVD, offering new and modified psychiatric diagnoses that are more compatible with behavioural neuro-otology than existing DSM-IV-TR disorders (15). Additional insights are offered in Chapter 30).

ICVD Layer III-B—mechanisms

Layer III-B contains the pathoanatomical, pathophysiological, and aetiological mechanisms underlying vestibular disorders. It is anticipated that this layer will be developed last and will be the most incomplete in the first iteration of the ICVD, but will expand and grow the most with future scientific discovery. This layer has been created with the knowledge that eventually, clinical phenomena (i.e. symptoms and signs) may be linked directly to mechanistic understanding (e.g. genetic mutation) for the purposes of diagnosis and treatment, skipping intermediate steps in the diagnostic process that are unavoidable at present (e.g. 'diagnosis' of Ménière's disease).

ICVD functional outcomes

Finally, it is recognized that the functional impact of vestibular and balance disorders is substantial and that a schema for standardized assessment of disability or handicap is needed. The 2005 NIDCD summary included the following statement, 'The field also needs to develop vestibular and balance related quality of life instruments that are sensitive to change in order to assess improvement, if any, after patients are treated for vestibular and balance disorders' (6). A diagnosis alone itself does not provide information about functional consequences for the affected individual. Coding of diagnostic entities linked to ICVD will need to be complemented by routine assessment of disability or handicap, as is prescribed by the DSM. WHO has created the International Classification of Functioning, Disability and Health (ICF), which describes the adverse effect of disease on daily activities and makes the various diseases comparable in this respect. Some groups have begun to address this topic (21). As the ICVD evolves, this aspect of classification is expected to develop in parallel.

Conclusions

An initiative under the aegis of the Committee for Classification of Vestibular Disorders of the Bárány Society is currently underway to develop a comprehensive classification structure and formal definitions for vestibular symptoms, syndromes, diseases, causes, and functional consequences. The success of the ICVD initiative will depend on its ability to improve communication among scientists, clinicians, patients, policy-makers, and the general public. It is envisioned that initial success of the ICVD will lead to an ongoing renewal and growth process in which identifiable gaps or inconsistencies in the ICVD structure, terminology, or definitions will spur related research, and that advances in research will, in turn, be reflected in reciprocal changes to ICVD.

References

1. History of ICD: http://www.who.int/classifications/icd (accessed 1 May, 2011).

2. American Psychiatric Association (2000). *Diagnostic and Statistical Manual of Mental Disorders, 4th ed, Text Revision*. Washington, DC: American Psychiatric Association.

3. Headache Classification Committee (2004). The International Classification of Headache Disorders. *Cephalagia*, 24(Suppl 1), 9–160.

4. Monsell EM, Balkany TA, Gates GA, Goldenberg RA, Meyerhoff W, House JW (1995). Committee on Hearing and Equilibrium guidelines for the diagnosis and evaluation of therapy in Meniere's disease. *Otolaryngol Head Neck Surg*, 113, 181–5.

5. Morera C, Pérez H, Pérez N, Soto A (2008). Peripheral Vertigo Classification. Consensus Document. Otoneurology Committee of the Spanish Otorhinolaryngology Society (2003–2006). *Acta Otorrinolaringol Esp*, 59(2), 76–9.

6. National Institute of Deafness and other Communication Disorders. NIDCD Workshop on Epidemiology of Communication Disorders. 25–30 March, 2005, Bethseda, MD. http://www.nidcd.nih.gov/funding/programs/ep/Pages/episummary.aspx

7. Boyev KP (2005). Meniere's disease or migraine? The clinical significance of fluctuating hearing loss with vertigo, *Arch Otolaryngol Head Neck Surg*, 131(5), 457–9.

8. Newman-Toker DE, Cannon LM, Stofferahn ME, Rothman RE, Hsieh YH, Zee DS (2007). Imprecision in patient reports of dizziness symptom quality: a cross-sectional study conducted in an acute-care setting, *Mayo Clin Proc*, 82(11), 1329–40.

9. Stanton VA, Hsieh YH, Camargo CA Jr, *et al.* (2007). Overreliance on symptom quality in diagnosing dizziness: results of a multicenter survey of emergency physicians. *Mayo Clin Proc*, 82(11), 1319–28.

10. Blakley BW, Goebel J (2001). The meaning of the word 'vertigo'. *Otolaryngol Head Neck Surg*, 125(3), 147–150.

11. Brandt T, Bronstein AM (2001). Nosological entities?: Cervical vertigo. *J Neurol Neurosurg Psychiatry*, 71, 8–12.

12. Bárány Society website: http://www.baranysociety.nl (accessed 1 May, 2011).

13. Bisdorff A, von Brevern M, Lempert T, Newman-Toker DE (2009). Classification of vestibular symptoms: towards an international classification of vestibular disorders. *J Vestib Res*, 19(1–2), 1–13.

14. World Health Organization. *International Statistical Classification of Diseases and Related Health Problems, 10th Revision, Version for 2007*. Available at: http://apps.who.int/classifications/apps/icd/icd10online/ (accessed 1 May, 2011).

15. Staab J, Newman Toker DE, Bisdorff A (in press). Progress in the development of an international classification of vestibular disorders. *Otol Neurotol*.

16. Newman-Toker DE, Dy FJ, Stanton VA, Zee DS, Calkins H, Robinson KA (2008). How often is dizziness from primary cardiovascular disease true vertigo? A systematic review. *J Gen Intern Med*, 23(12), 2087–94.

17. Neuhauser HK, von Brevern M, Radtke A, *et al.* (2005). Epidemiology of vestibular vertigo: a neurotologic survey of the general population. *Neurology* 65(6), 898–904. Erratum in: *Neurology*, 2006, 67(8), 1528.

18. Neuhauser H, Leopold M, von Brevern M, Arnold G, Lempert T (2001). The interrelations of migraine, vertigo, and migrainous vertigo. *Neurology*, 56, 436–41.

19. Furman J, Marcus DA, Balaban CD (2003). Migrainous vertigo: development of a pathogenetic model and structured diagnostic interview. *Curr Opin Neurol*, 16(1), 5–13.

20. American Psychiatric Association. *Proposed Draft Revisions to DSM Disorders and Criteria*. Available at: http://www.dsm5.org (accessed 6 March, 2011).

21. Grill E, Cieza A. *Functioning and quality of life in vertigo and balance disorders*. http://www.klinikum.uni-muenchen.de/IFB-Schwindel/en/Research_projects/Full_research_projects/index.html (accessed 1 May, 2011).

CHAPTER 17

The Principles of Balance Treatment and Rehabilitation

Marousa Pavlou and Di Newham

Introduction

This chapter intends to bridge the gap between clinical neurologists, ear, nose, and throat specialists and physiotherapists. It aims to provide: 1) an understanding of the balance components that should be assessed and potentially included within a balance rehabilitation programme; 2) an understanding of various types of exercises that can be practised according to individual impairments and symptoms; 3) a brief review of the evidence for balance rehabilitation for specific patient populations.

Principles of balance physiology

Key to balance assessment and rehabilitation is understanding that postural control and spatial orientation are interlinked and emerge from an interaction of many musculoskeletal and neural systems. These are organized in accordance with the stability requirements inherent in the task being performed, and constrained by the environment. The central processes mediating both spatial orientation and postural control are dependent on the same sources of peripheral sensory inputs, mostly arising from the visual, proprioceptive, and vestibular systems. The following is a very brief, grossly simplified overview of balance function. Please refer to Chapters 4 and 7 for in-depth reading.

The vestibular system detects angular (semicircular canals) and linear (otoliths: utricle and saccule) head movements. This input is centrally processed to control balance through: 1) low-level reflexes such as vestibulo-spinal or vestibulo-ocular (VOR) reflexes, 2) higher-order motor responses interacting with voluntary motor control (1), and 3) the generation of conscious awareness of head orientation and movement.

Somatosensory receptors, including muscle spindles, Golgi tendon organs, joint receptors, and cutaneous mechanoreceptors located throughout the body, provide information about the relative location of body segments to one another and the body's position and movement in relation to the support surface. Patients with somatosensory loss display greater and more permanent postural dysfunction and disability than patients with peripheral vestibular loss, even those with bilateral vestibular failure. However, many patients with somatosensory loss compensate through increased sensitivity to available sensory input and adaptive strategies such as stiffer body posture (2–5).

The visual system provides information about body movements and postural sway in relation to surrounding objects and influences postural alignment by providing a reference for verticality. It also has a unique property as a tele-receptor (distance) for anticipation, obstacle avoidance, and navigation, etc. Vision reduces postural sway because the optic flow generated by head sway generates fairly automatic, subconscious postural corrections, e.g. the motion of retinal visual images when a person sways to the left will trigger a posture correction to the right. However, cognitive processes play a significant role in modulating these primitive responses (6). Vestibular, proprioceptive, and visual inputs usually generate congruent postural reactions, such that if a person standing upright is pushed forwards, head acceleration (vestibularly-mediated), soleus stretch (proprioceptive) and visual inputs will indicate forwards body motion and thus generate an integrated corrective postural response in the opposite direction.

Musculoskeletal balance components include adequate strength, joint range of movement, and muscle tone. Muscle tone depends on both neural and non-neural components, including activation of the stretch reflex and a muscle's intrinsic stiffness (7). Muscle tone, referring to the tonic activity of antigravity muscles primarily in the limbs, trunk, and neck, depends on postural reflexes including the myotatic stretch loop, tonic labyrinthine, and tonic neck reflexes. Adequate strength and range of movement is required to generate sufficient muscular activity to counteract the force of gravity and prevent a fall when the base of support (BOS) exceeds stability limits (8).

Numerous additional properties, such as sensory reweighting, promote adaptability to changing environmental and task conditions and neural plasticity induced by peripheral or central lesions. Sensory reweighting occurs when other sensory inputs are centrally upregulated in response to a particular sensory input being reduced, absent, or unreliable. For instance, when standing on an uneven surface in darkness, the efficiency of vestibular responses increases, whereas unavailable or unreliable visuo-proprioceptive responses are downregulated. Patients with a vestibular disorder may develop increased perceptual and postural responses to visual motion stimuli (9). Physiological compensation and clinical recovery depend on the adaptive, plastic properties of the postural control system. However, the mechanisms mediating sensory reweighting in postural control remain poorly understood (10).

Additional higher-order balance mechanisms include anticipatory postural adjustments—motor phenomena primarily triggered to counteract the destabilizing consequences of a voluntary movement prior to its initiation. One example is step initiation which involves anticipatory postural adjustments that propel body mass forward and laterally before the first step. Finally, motor learning and adaptation are widespread in the motor system and many studies have documented this in the postural and locomotor systems (11–13).

Balance assessment

This section describes the rehabilitation assessment required for patients with balance disorders, which involves identifying: 1) functional limitations, 2) underlying impairments affecting balance control, and 3) symptoms.

Functional assessment

The functional assessment aims to determine a patient's objective and perceived ability to perform various tasks requiring balance. The objective component is partly incorporated into the clinical examination (e.g. Romberg test, gait assessment). However, it may be useful to observe the patient through sequential or dual-tasking actions (e.g. walking while carrying a cup of water) which can be rated or timed using objective assessment scales that simultaneously assess falls risk. This information will help establish functional ability and limitations, and provide a quantitative baseline measurement of performance.

The Berg balance scale (14), one of the most widely used scales, was originally designed to assess balance and falls risk in community-dwelling older adults. It has subsequently been validated in patients after stroke (15), with Parkinson's disease (PD; 16), and multiple sclerosis (MS; 17) and can differentiate fallers from non-fallers in patients with Huntington's Disease (18). The scale's validity in patients with peripheral vestibular disorders is questionable with studies showing normal scores (19, 20). Cohen and Kimball (19) recommend that when computerized dynamic posturography (see 'Sensory function assessment' section) is unavailable, combining the Berg with a commonly used gait test (i.e. Dynamic Gait Index) may increase sensitivity for detecting a vestibular impairment. This combination may be a useful initial screening tool outside of tertiary care settings where facilities may be limited and non-physician health professionals see patients (19).

Other commonly used tests include the 'Get Up and Go' with or without a timing component (21, 22), Tinetti Balance and Mobility Scale (23), Functional (24) or Multi-Directional Reach Tests (25). Tests such as the Dynamic Gait Index (26), 'Stops Walking When Talking Test' (27), and Functional Gait Assessment (28) assess higher-level gait control involving various levels of multitasking

(further discussion see 'Cognition' section), and the ability to modify and adapt gait according to environmental and task demands.

The Dynamic Gait Index and Functional Gait Assessment are both valid falls risk predictors in older adults and patients with vestibular dysfunction (28–30). The former has been validated in patients with MS (31), PD (32), and stroke (33). The Functional Gait Assessment, however, includes tasks patients with vestibular disorders find more challenging and has clear decision rules for scoring, avoiding the ceiling effect noted with the Dynamic Gait Index (28). Based on the authors' clinical experience it is the better gait assessment tool for vestibular patients. Further tests for assessing balance within specific patient groups are also constantly emerging such as the Postural Assessment Scale for Stroke Patients (34).

Self-report measures quantify a patient's perceptions regarding the impact of balance problems on daily activities. The most widely used test is the Activities of Balance Confidence scale which asks patients to rate their level of confidence in their ability to perform 16 activities of daily living (ADLs; e.g. indoor and outdoor walking activities, reaching-oriented activities) without falling (35, 36). It is validated in older community-dwelling adults and to a lesser extent for distinct patient groups including vestibular disorders (37), stroke (38, 39), MS (17), and PD (40). ADL scales for specific client groups have also been developed, i.e. The Vestibular Disorders ADL Scale (41). Table 17.1 lists commonly used objective and subjective tests.

Balance assessment scales should show good feasibility and provide meaningful information. Tests are chosen according to the patient's abilities and their sensitivity in detecting functional limitations within the test population to avoid a ceiling or floor effect (26). We believe they are useful for providing a baseline quantitative measure of performance, as stated earlier, and evaluating the need and effectiveness of interventions. However, they are unable to guide treatment as their primary aim is to screen for potential balance problems and predict falls risk, rather than identify underlying balance impairments. Additional tests, including a conventional neurological, vestibular, and/or musculoskeletal examination, provide insight into the underlying impairments limiting functional independence.

Impairment-based assessment

Motor function

This assessment includes observation of postural alignment and the ability to generate and coordinate the multijoint movements necessary for balance. Changes in verticality perception can lead to abnormal alignment of body segments with respect to each other and the BOS. Postural alignment with respect to vertical and adjacent body segments should be observed in sitting and standing. A plumb line and grid can be used to quantify alignment with photographs or video. Therapists can assess a patient's internal sense of vertical by passively moving them off vertical in stance or sitting and asking them to voluntarily realign to vertical. In standing, posturography or two weighing scales can be used to measure centre of pressure and assess for any discrepancy between the two sides (26, 42).

Controlling body position for balance and orientation requires motor coordination processes that organize muscles throughout the body into coordinated movement strategies. The main strategies used to recover balance in the anterior/posterior and lateral directions are the ankle, hip, and stepping strategies (43, 44;

Table 17.1 Commonly used objective and subjective tests for balance assessment

Type	Assessment Tool	Purpose
Self Perception Scales	Activities-Specific Balance Confidence Scale (Powell and Myers, 1995)	Quantifies a person's confidence in their balance during various tasks
	Falls Efficacy Scale (Tinetti et al., 1990)	Quantifies fear of falling
	Vestibular Activities of Daily Living Scale (Cohen and Kimball, 2000)	Quantifies perceived impairments in daily activities due to dizziness
	Dizziness Handicap Inventory (Jacobson, Newman, 1990)	Quantifies perceived handicap due to dizziness or postural instability
	Vertigo Symptom Scale (Yardley et al., 1992)	Quantifies frequency of vestibular and autonomic symptoms
	Situational Characteristics Questionnaire (Jacob et al., 1994; Guerraz et al., 2001)	Quantifies the severity of visual vertigo symptoms
Balance/Gait assessment	Timed "Up & Go" (Posdiadlo and Richardson, 1991)	Functional gait and falls risk assessment
	Performance-Oriented Mobility Assessment POMA) (Tinetti et al., 1986)	Function gait, balance, and falls risk assessment
	Dynamic Gait Index (Shumway-Cook et al.,1997)	Functional gait and falls risk assessment
	Functional Gait Assessment (Wrisley et al., 2004)	Functional gait and falls risk assessment
	Berg Balance Scale (Berg et al., 1995)	Multifactorial balance assessment
	Five times sit to stand (Csuka and McCarty, 1985)	Functional assessment of balance and strength
Use of sensory inputs	Sensory Organization Test of Computerized Dynamic Posturography (Nashner, 1982)	Assessment of the ability to use sensory information for standing balance
	Clinical Test of Sensory Interaction and Balance (Shumway-Cook and Horak, 1986)	Assessment of the ability to use sensory information for standing balance
Multi-impairment based tests	BESTest	Multiple balance subsystems assessment
	Short Form Physiological Profile Assessment	Quantifies falls risk by identifying impairments in key physiological measurements

Figure 17.1). Healthy adults respond to a small perturbation in the anterior/posterior direction by swaying predominantly about the ankles and laterally by using hip abduction/adduction. The ankle joints should carefully be observed for tibialis anterior activity in both legs in response to backward body sway; knee and hip motion should be minimal during compensatory ankle sway movements. Larger displacements to standing posture cause a greater hip and trunk response, i.e. a hip strategy, as the subject attempts to maintain the centre of mass (COM) within the BOS. Large or fast displacements may result in a stepping response (Figure 17.1).

Combinations of these strategies are used according to environmental and task demands as well as internal biomechanical and neural factors including joint range of movement, muscle strength, attention to task, and availability and accuracy of sensory input (2, 45). Various clinical protocols can assess movement strategies, including self- or externally-initiated postural sway, and anticipatory postural adjustments accompanying a potentially destabilizing limb movement, e.g. lifting a heavy object.

Many patients with central nervous system (CNS) deficits show improperly timed and uncoordinated movement strategies for postural control that cannot be classified as an ankle, hip,

or stepping strategies, e.g. excessive knee flexion, asymmetric leg movements, excessive trunk or arm movements. However, peripheral vestibular patients usually show normally coordinated lower limb and trunk muscle activation (46–49); but postural responses can be hypo- or hypermetric and cervical and trunk muscles often exhibit abnormal co-contraction that stiffens joints. Age-related changes have been observed for movement strategies; older adults tend to adopt the hip rather than ankle strategy even when the latter is appropriate (50, 51). A combination of reduced vestibular, somatosensory, and musculoskeletal function together with reduced central integrative and executive function has been suggested as a possible cause for the changes noted in older adults (51). Progressive deterioration with age in virtually all sensorimotor functions necessary for postural control and mobility is well documented and is a major falls risk factor (52, 53). Older adult literature focuses primarily on women (54, 55) but men also demonstrate reduced musculoskeletal function, balance, reaction times, and general mobility in their 60s (56) which is before attention is usually paid to ageing effects. Balance disorders can occur at any age; however, some are more prevalent in older adults (PD, stroke) or show increased prevalence with age, i.e. peripheral vestibular disorder

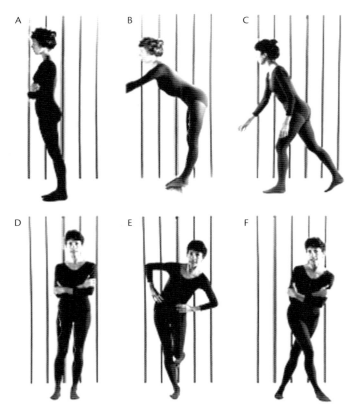

Fig. 17.1 Three movement strategies for recovery of balance; an ankle, hip, and stepping strategy for the anterior/posterior direction (top) and for the lateral direction (bottom) (113). Vertical orientation of the trunk is preserved in an ankle strategy but compromised in a hip strategy while the hips or lumbothoracic spine actively moves the centre of mass. In a stepping strategy, the base of support moves under the falling centre of body mass.

(57). Therefore, therapists must consider the normal effects of ageing during the assessment.

Sensory function assessment

Sensory function assessment begins by evaluating the individual senses important to postural control. Lower limb somatosensation is usually assessed by vibration and joint position sense tests. Vestibular function examination is briefly discussed in section 'Symptoms assessment'; please refer to Chapters 12, 14, and 15 for in-depth reading.

The type and degree of information used for postural control varies even between individuals with normal sensory function. A person may be over-reliant on a particular sense for balance and continue to rely on it even when it is unavailable or inaccurately reporting self-motion. Examples include an over-reliance on proprioceptive cues for orientation (surface dependence) causing difficulty when walking on uneven, soft surfaces or when changing between different floor surface types. Assessment involves asking patients to stand and walk on unstable or compliant surfaces (e.g. tilt board and foam cushions respectively).

Patients with chronic vestibular disorders, stroke, and older adult fallers (58–60) are visually dependent and may complain of discomfort, symptom exacerbation, and postural instability in challenging visual environments, i.e. supermarkets, busy roads. This phenomenon is referred to as visually-induced dizziness (61) and can be identified by asking specific questions about symptom triggers; the severity can

be subjectively quantified using a shortened version of the Situational Characteristics Questionnaire (9, 62; Table 17.2). However, an increased visual reliance may be beneficial and encouraged in patients with PD, i.e. visual cueing strategies (63, 64), proprioceptive deficit due to peripheral neuropathy (PN), or dorsal root or column disease.

The Sensory Organization Test of computerized dynamic posturography (65) and the modified Clinical Test of Sensory Interaction and Balance (42) were developed to quantify one's ability to use and reweigh sensory information for standing balance under altered surface and/or visual conditions. In patients with a peripheral vestibular disorder, studies comparing dynamic posturography scores and functional ability, measured objectively (gait velocity, tandem/single leg stance, etc.) or subjectively (questionnaires) show results varying from a positive to poor or no relationship (66–68). Many vestibular rehabilitation studies use the Sensory Organization Test as an outcome measure for functional performance (69–72). It can reliably assess pre–post treatment change in standing balance function, the minimal clinically significant difference is 10 points (73) and can distinguish malingerers (74, 75) and individuals with secondary gain, e.g. worker's compensation, pending lawsuits (76) from those with true disability. It also differentiates between type 2 diabetes mellitus patients with and without peripheral neuropathy with the former group showing poorer composite and individual condition scores for those assessing the somatosensory system (77). However, approximately 30% of patients with a peripheral vestibular disorder show normal scores (20, 72).

Perception of the gravitational vertical

Peripheral vestibular and somatosensory systems and/or CNS pathology can affect the ability to detect and process gravitational input resulting in asymmetric reflex mechanisms, e.g. VOR and vestibulo-spinal, or impaired verticality perception. The body's orientation relative to the gravito-inertial force has been named the *behavioural vertical* (78, 79), i.e. an implicit representation of verticality used to control balance, which in quiet stance usually corresponds to the direction of the longitudinal body axis. It can be clinically observed and measured by movement analysis systems (79). Additionally, several sensory channels convey relatively independent gravitational inputs that can be measured individually and provide additional useful information. These are the subjective *visual* (SVV), *haptic* (derived from the sense of touch), and *postural* (the position of the head or body with respect to true vertical) *vertical*.

Subjective vertical assessments are performed in darkness to eliminate the contribution of environmental visual vertical cues, e.g. buildings, walls, people standing. For the SVV, subjects visually adjust a luminous rod to the estimated vertical normally within 1° (80; Figure 17.2A); for the haptic vertical the bar is set using tactile sensation (81; Figure 17.2B); and for postural vertical the subject is seated on a tilted chair and must indicate at which point he/she perceives him/herself vertical (82, 83; Figure 17.2C). The SVV has been widely assessed in vestibular and stroke patients (84–87). In stroke patients, a strong correlation was found between longitudinal body axis and SVV tilt, suggesting that weight-bearing asymmetry following stroke results not only from motor weakness, somatosensory deficits, and muscle tone asymmetry but also spatial cognitive disorders (88). They suggest longitudinal body axis rehabilitation, which can be started in supine and should include appropriate sensory stimulations, i.e. vestibular, may be a useful component within weight-bearing asymmetry retraining (88).

Table 17.2 A copy of the Situational Characteristics Questionnaire which measures thefrequency of visually induced dizziness symptoms. It yields a normalized score between 0–4 bydividing the total sum by 19— 0.7/4 indicate abnormal scores.
Dizziness is the term used for symptoms which patients often describe as feelings of unusual disorientation, giddiness, lightheadedness or unsteadiness. Please ring a number to indicate the degree to which each of the situations listed below provokes feelings of dizziness, or makes your dizziness worse. If you have never been in one of the situations then for that item ring "N.T" for "Not Tried".
The categories are:

0	1	2	3	4		N.T.	
Not at all	**Very slightly**	**Somewhat**	**Quite a lot**	**Very much**		**Not tried**	
Riding as a passenger in a car on straight, flat roads				0	1	2	3	4	N.T.
Riding as a passenger in a car on winding or bumpy roads				0	1	2	3	4	N.T.
Walking down a supermarket aisle				0	1	2	3	4	N.T.
Standing in a lift while it stops				0	1	2	3	4	N.T.
Standing in a lift while it moves at a steady speed				0	1	2	3	4	N.T.
Riding in a car at a steady speed				0	1	2	3	4	N.T.
Starting or stopping in a car				0	1	2	3	4	N.T.
Standing in the middle of a wide open space (e.g. large field or square)				0	1	2	3	4	N.T.
Sitting on a bus				0	1	2	3	4	N.T.
Standing on a bus				0	1	2	3	4	N.T.
Heights				0	1	2	3	4	N.T.
Watching moving scenes on the T.V. or at the cinema				0	1	2	3	4	N.T.
Travelling on escalators				0	1	2	3	4	N.T.
Looking at striped or moving surfaces (e.g. curtains, Venetian blinds, flowing water)				0	1	2	3	4	N.T.
Looking at a scrolling computer screen or microfiche				0	1	2	3	4	N.T.
Going through a tunnel looking at the lights on the side				0	1	2	3	4	N.T.
Going through a tunnel looking at the light at the end				0	1	2	3	4	N.T.
Driving over the brow of a hill, around bends, or in wide open spaces				0	1	2	3	4	N.T.
Watching moving traffic or trains (e.g. trying to cross the street, or at the station)				0	1	2	3	4	N.T.

Cognition

Many daily activities involve maintaining balance while performing at least one other concurrent task, e.g. standing or walking and talking, whereby attentional resources must be appropriately divided between maintaining postural control and cognitive performance. Dual-tasking postural control is the norm rather than the exception in daily life. Studies consistently show that while younger adults are able to generally perform both tasks effectively, older people show decreased performance, presumably because of increased competition for central processing resources (89, 90). Cognitive deficits affecting memory, attention, and executive functions as a result of age, disease, or both can increase reaction times on a secondary task, decrease gait speed and step length during dual-tasking, and are associated with an increased falls risk (91–97). The most commonly used testing technique compares baseline performance on individual tasks to performance when two tasks are practised simultaneously. Secondary tasks can be motor (carrying an object), cognitive (answering questions such as in the 'Stops walking when talking test'; 27), or a combination. The effect may vary according to task type and difficulty; therefore a variety of dual-task situations should be assessed.

Clinical tools to measure impairments

As previously discussed, postural control involves many systems and subsystems. Recently, tools aiming to systematically assess multiple subsystems underlying balance deficits have been developed. The Balance Evaluation Test (BESTest) was devised to assess six balance domains including biomechanical constraints, stability limits/

verticality, anticipatory postural adjustments, postural responses, sensory orientation, and gait stability (98). A shorter version covering four of the six original domains was also developed (99). Both versions can discriminate fallers in people with PD (100).

The Short-Form Physiological Profile Assessment (101) aims to assess falls risk in older adults by identifying impairments in key physiological measurements (edge contrast sensitivity, hand reaction time, knee joint proprioception, maximal isometric quadriceps strength, and postural sway) which individually act as predictors for multiple falls (102, 103). However some individuals able to complete the postural sway test receive a higher falls risk score than those unable to complete it, questioning the test's clinical validity (104).

Symptoms assessment

A bedside vestibular function assessment includes examination of spontaneous, gaze-evoked, and positional nystagmus and head thrust tests (105, 106). The patient's history will provide information regarding symptom severity, frequency, duration, and triggers, and may provide insight into the possible cause of symptoms. Validated questionnaires can aid in quantifying this information (Table 17.1). Eye, head, and body movements or positions and challenging environments, e.g. visually rich or unstable surroundings, compliant floors, which provoke symptoms, must be identified to design an appropriate exercise programme.

Approximately 20–40% of patients with vertigo have benign paroxysmal positional vertigo (BPPV). Posterior semicircular canal

A
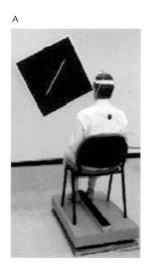

B
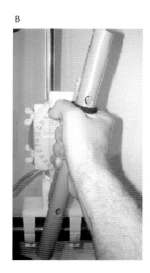

C
1
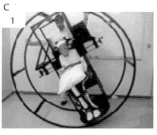

2
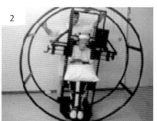

3
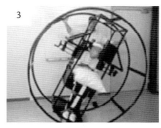

4
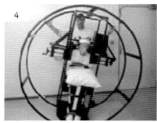

Fig. 17.2 The three modalities of verticality perception, subjective (A) (208), haptic (B) (209), and postural (C) (210). (C) shows the wheel paradigm for measuring the postural vertical whereby the subject is randomly tilted to either side of true vertical between 15° to 45°. The wheel is then rolled immediately in the opposite direction until the subject reports having reached an upright position. The figure shows a patient with a right hemisphere stroke (photo 1, 2) and left lateropulsion (photo 3, 4). (1) starting position on the right, the patient feels upright in (2), and (3) starting position on the left, the patient feels upright in (4) (210).

BPPV is the most common type accounting for 85–95% of patients (107). In-depth information regarding BPPV types, presentation, and treatment may be found in Chapter 20. Balance problems and dizzy symptoms often persist after BPPV resolution (108) and many patients may benefit from balance rehabilitation after repositioning treatments. Some patients with non-positional vertigo may have an underlying labyrinthine disorder and may require full vestibular and audiometric testing; rehabilitation can usually proceed in the meantime.

Additional factors that may affect outcome

Many patients with neurological deficits, peripheral vestibular disorders, and older adult fallers experience increased anxiety, depression, and fear of falling which may impact on the patient's willingness or ability to participate in rehabilitation, impede clinical recovery, and lead to decreased activity levels and changes in spatiotemporal gait parameters which further increase falls risk (109, 110). Every effort should be made to identify and act on these negative factors, referring the patient for counselling and/or adding psychopharmacological medication as appropriate.

Other factors, i.e. orthostatic hypotension, that may delay vestibular compensation and balance rehabilitation are shown in Table 17.3. However we would like to briefly mention the possible impact of visuo-motor symptoms on rehabilitation outcome. For patients with oscillopsia ('wobbly' vision) due to a unilateral or, more commonly, bilateral vestibular failure, treatment is based on eye–head exercises within a vestibular rehabilitation programme. When oscillopsia results from CNS disease, usually due to a nystagmus, drug treatment is required (111). Recently pilot data from the Departments of Ophthalmology and Neuro-Otology at the National Hospital for Neurology and Neurosurgery, London showed that patients with binocular vision abnormalities and a peripheral vestibular disorder experience worse baseline subjective symptoms (vestibular, visually induced dizziness, psychological state) and objective balance test

Table 17.3 Factors that may delay vestibular compensation

Fluctuating vestibular disorder (i.e. Meniere's disease)
Additional disorder:
CNS
Peripheral nerve
Cervical spine
Visual (reduced visual acuity, modified optics (e.g. cataract operation), strabismus, diplopia)
Age
Lack of mobility (orthopaedic problem, forced bedrest, psychological/fear
Medication (antivertiginous drugs)
Psychosocial
"Visual vertigo"

(posturography, functional gait assessment) scores and poorer outcomes after vestibular rehabilitation. Further work is needed to identify the relationship between ocular abnormalities and vestibular rehabilitation outcome.

Balance rehabilitation

Balance rehabilitation is impairment and symptom based. It aims to: 1) resolve, reduce, or prevent impairments, 2) develop effective strategies for recovery of functional skills despite potentially permanent impairments, 3) retrain functional tasks in a wide variety of environmental contexts, and 4) improve symptoms.

Retraining postural alignment and movement strategies

The goal when retraining alignment is to develop an initial position which maximizes stability, is appropriate for the specified task, and efficient with regards to muscle activity requirements. Verbal and manual cues, mirrors, and kinetic or force feedback devices have been used to retrain vertical posture. Patients learn to maintain an upright posture during progressively more difficult tasks including eyes closed and standing on compliant surfaces, e.g. foam, with progressively reduced feedback about position.

The goal when retraining movement strategies is to develop those successful in moving the COM relative to a stationary BOS (ankle or hip strategy) and changing the BOS relative to the COM (stepping strategy). Retraining a coordinated ankle or hip strategy involves practising voluntary anteroposterior and lateral sway, without taking a step. Facilitating a hip strategy involves faster and larger displacements than an ankle strategy and may include activities such as tandem or single-leg stance. Retraining externally-induced postural responses involves pushes or pulls of various amplitudes, speed, and direction applied at the hips or shoulders, or the use of moving surfaces.

Stepping can be practised by shifting the patient's weight to one side and then quickly bringing the COM back towards the unweighted leg, or in response to large anteroposterior or lateral perturbations. Multidirectional stepping, stepping over a visual target or obstacle can also be practised. In PD, practising multidirectional stepping with rhythmic auditory stimulation can improve functional gait and balance (112).

Activities requiring a subtle shift of the COM prior to the voluntary movement, i.e. reaching, lifting, and throwing, help patients develop strategies for anticipatory postural control. A hierarchy of tasks should be included as the level of required anticipatory postural activity is directly related to the speed, effort, degree of external support, and task complexity, e.g. lifting the foot onto a stool while touching a chair with one hand. External support should progressively decrease while movement speed and task complexity (i.e. patient simultaneously holds a cup of water; see section 'Retraining cognitive strategies') increase.

As musculoskeletal impairments can contribute to problems in postural alignment and effective use of movement strategies, they should be treated using appropriate progressive resistive strengthening exercises, stretching, and passive and active joint movements. Modalities such as heat, biofeedback, and ultrasound can also be used.

Retraining sensory strategies

Sensory strategy retraining aims to help patients learn to effectively select appropriate sensory information for balance in various environments. Treatment focuses on maintaining balance during progressively more difficult static and dynamic balance exercises while the availability and accuracy of sensory input is systematically varied.

Patients who over-rely on somatosensory cues for orientation, i.e. difficulty when walking on uneven surfaces, changing between different types of floor surface, practise tasks while sitting, standing, or walking on surfaces with disrupted somatosensory cues such as compliant foam, moving platforms or tilt boards. Visually-dependent patients should practise exercises where visual cues are absent (eyes closed), reduced (blinders) or inaccurate (glasses smeared with petroleum jelly) for orientation. Advanced techniques include exposure to optokinetic stimuli or moving rooms (20, 113). 'Busy' moving images (i.e. tunnel or boat scenes; Figure

A   HORIZONTAL BOAT SCENE

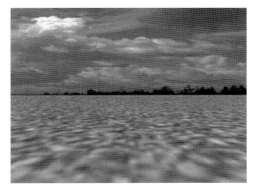

B   CLOCKWISE BOAT TILT SCENE

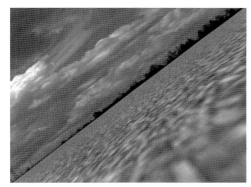

C   TUNNEL SCENE

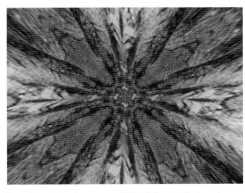

Fig. 17.3 Examples of 'busy' visual motion scenes (211). (A) and (B) show images from a moving boat scene either in a horizontal position or tilted clockwise. (C) shows images from a moving tunnel scene. The true visual motion stimuli are viewed in colour. Patients can be asked to focus on the centre of the moving scene while watching the stimuli with head stationary or while practising vertical or horizontal head movements in sitting, standing, or walking.

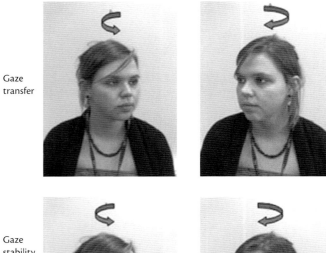

Gaze transfer

Gaze stability (VOR)

Fig. 17.4 Gaze transfer and adaptation exercises (212) included within a vestibular rehabilitation programme. During 'gaze transfer' (A), the normal head and eye movement required for transferring gaze from one object to another is practised. The exercise can initially be practised without head movements with objects placed approximately 40 cm apart at eye level. During adaptation exercises (B), the vestibulo-ocular reflex (VOR) is being stimulated which is responsible for maintaining a steady gaze on a fixated object with progressively faster head movements.

17.3A, B), some computer games, moving cardboard posters with vertical/horizontal lines, or a DVD including visual stimulation recorded from the clinical equipment, i.e. optokinetic test in neuro-otology departments (72, 114) can be used. Exposure should be gradual and progressive. We have noted that many patients with visual dependency focus on the ground while walking. If this occurs, a gait exercise instructing the patient to look out at the horizon rather than at the ground should be included within the initial exercise programme. To increase the use of vestibular cues for orientation, exercises with visual and proprioceptive cues absent and/or inaccurate are prescribed, e.g. standing on foam with eyes closed.

Learning to adapt strategies to changing contexts

Functional independence requires the ability to modify sensory and movement strategies according to environmental and task demands. As postural stability improves, exercises must progressively increase in complexity and difficulty and be practised under varied conditions so the patient may learn to maintain balance when faced with new or changing environments and tasks. A hierarchy of tasks with progressively greater postural demands are used to develop adaptive capacities including maintaining balance with a reduced BOS, while changing head and trunk orientation, and/or practising upper limb activities.

Retraining cognitive strategies

Dual-task training involves practising progressive balance exercises, e.g. tandem standing or walking with or without upper limb activities, while simultaneously performing a secondary task such as counting backwards by three, recounting daily activities (115). During training patients are asked to either constantly maintain attention on both tasks or focus attention on one of them.

Motor, sensory, and cognitive strategy retraining should occur in parallel rather than sequentially. Balance exercises must be practised safely, i.e. parallel bars, standing near a wall or corner, with a chair in front of patient—at least initially.

Vestibular exercises

Vestibular rehabilitation should be based on the eye (i.e. 'gaze transfer', Figure 17.4A), head, and postural exercises that provoke a patient's symptoms. Adaptation exercises (116; Figure 17.4B) incorporating gaze fixation and head movements and postural exercises are prescribed to promote recovery of VOR and vestibulo-spinal reflex function. Gaze fixation exercises are practised with varying target distances (i.e. 2 m, 1 m, 0.5 m) since VOR gain varies with target distance (closer targets require higher gains; 117). Fixation exercises are given to patients with oscillopsia and/or decreased VOR gain, most often seen in peripheral vestibular disorders. Table 17.4 includes examples of commonly prescribed exercises, which can be viewed on a DVD (106). A total of four or

Table 17.4 Examples of commonly prescribed exercises in vestibular rehabilitation

Head exercises
(performed with eyes open and eyes closed)
Bend head backwards and forwards
Turn head from side to side
Eye movement exercises
Head stationary follow movement of finger left and right/ up and down
Head stationary, look back and forth between two targets; repeat with head movements
Visual fixation exercises
Perform head exercises while fixating stationary target
Perform head exercises while fixating moving target
Positioning exercises
(performed with eyes open and closed)
While seated, bend down to touch the floor
While seated, turn to look over shoulder both to left and right
Bend down with head turned first to one side and then the other
Lying down, roll from one side to the other
Sit up from lying supine and on each side
Postural exercises
(performed eyes open; eyes closed under supervision)
Practice static stance with feet as n circles, pivot turns, up slopes, stairs, around obstacles
Stand and walk in environments with altered surface and/or visual conditions with and without head and fixation exerclose together as possible
Practice standing on one leg, and heel-to-toe
Repeat head and fixation exercises while standing and then walking
Practice walking icises

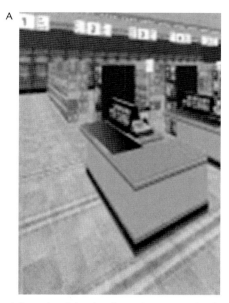 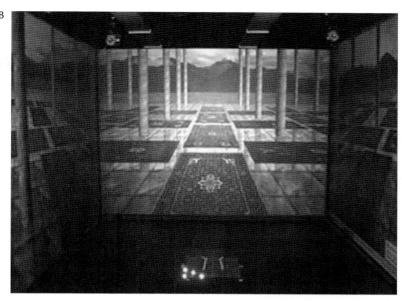

Fig. 17.5 Examples of virtual reality motion scenes whereby the experience is one of being immersed within a realistic environment with textural context and optic flow. The University of Pittsburgh Balance Nave Virtual Environment (A) (119) depicting a supermarket scene whereby patients can 'navigate' walking through aisles and searching for specific items on the shelves. (B) (120) is from the virtual reality environment at Temple University depicting columns which again can be navigated while simultaneously viewing complex floor patterns and a landscape in the distance. Patients can either stand stationary, walk on a treadmill, or real-time walk within a full-field virtual reality environment. Limited field-of-view virtual reality head mounted devices are also available.

five exercises are prescribed to be practised for approximately 1–2 minutes each, twice daily initially at a slow speed which gradually increases as symptoms improve.

In our experience of treating patients with migraine-associated dizziness, particularly prior to effective migraine management with prophylactic medication, an initial exercise programme including fewer exercises, i.e. three maximum, will be better tolerated and adhered to. These should be practised only once daily initially and gradually increased to twice daily. As symptoms and tolerance improve, the number and total duration of daily exercises progressively increases.

In patients with a peripheral vestibular disorder or migraine-associated dizziness (which combines both peripheral and central vestibular components; 118) who experience visual-induced dizziness, it is important for improvement to be noted with exercises such as those in Table 17.4 before progressing to the inclusion of optokinetic stimuli.

General characteristics of vestibular rehabilitation include specificity, repetition, progression, and patient education, e.g. initially symptoms may worsen, and improvement may be uneven. Patients should be aware that even after symptoms have largely resolved, a temporary reoccurrence may occur during periods of stress, fatigue, or illness. Patients should be advised to stop exercising and seek advice if they experience neck pain, loss of consciousness or vision, sensations of numbness, weakness or tingling in the face or limbs, or increased migraine frequency.

Novel and supplementary techniques

Various authors have discussed the potential benefit of virtual reality as a therapeutic tool to improve postural stability and symptoms in situations closely reflecting conditions found in everyday environments, e.g. supermarket aisles, crowded square (Figure 17.5A, B; 119, 120). Two studies using a limited field-of-view head-mounted device noted improvements in VOR gain and symptoms in patients

with a peripheral vestibular disorder (121, 122). In stroke, limited evidence exists showing virtual reality can improve balance and gait function (123, 124) while in patients with PD no significant differences were noted between virtual reality and conventional balance training (125). Virtual reality is a novel tool with a potentially promising future in balance rehabilitation but future work needs to demonstrate its clinical efficacy.

Whole-body vibration (WBV; Figure 17.6) is a relatively new technique, currently fashionable in commercial gyms. While a number of claims have been made about its ability to increase muscle strength and power, good evidence exists only for an effect on bone strength (reviewed in 126). There appears to be an age-related effect of WBV on balance with little or no improvements seen in healthy younger individuals although few studies have investigated this. In older people, unchallenged balance also appears little changed (127) but improvements have been reported during more challenging balance tasks and those involving a dynamic component (126, 128). Improvements of 5–35% have been reported in all studies utilizing appropriate control groups (129–134), but only during single-leg standing and dynamic balance tests. The large variability in improvement amount is probably explained by the very different vibration frequencies and amplitudes used and study durations. WBV may have a greater effect on those with poorer initial balance ability (134). Current evidence suggests it may be most beneficial for older and untrained individuals (128, 135). No studies to date have specifically involved subjects with vestibular disorders.

Improved balance may also be due to the learning effect required to maintain a stable position on the platform (134, 136) rather than a direct effect of vibration on the CNS. Effective dampening reduces the transmission of vibrations through the feet at each body segment and even at the highest frequencies there is little vibration above the knee, and virtually none at the head (137) although the visual disturbance is obvious.

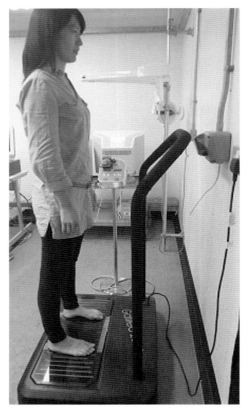

Fig. 17.6 Whole-body vibration equipment (Centre of Human and Aerospace Physiological Sciences, King's College London). The person stands on the platform, at varying vibration frequencies and amplitudes, stationary or while progressively performing various balance tasks and altering base of support.

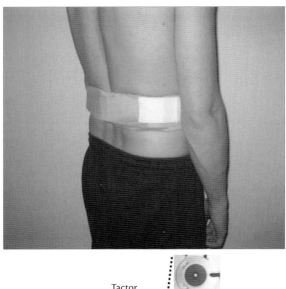

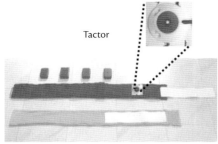

Tactor

Fig. 17.7 Example of a balance prostheses (Balance Belt; 138) which provides vibrotactile tilt feedback of a person's body motion in the anteroposterior and mediolateral directions.

Other exciting advances include the use of balance prostheses which provide information regarding head and/or body orientation through vibrotactile cues delivered to the trunk (138, 139; Figure 17.7) head (140), or tongue (141, 142). The prostheses work by translating information normally sensed by the vestibular system into a proprioceptive cue which is then integrated with remaining sensory information for postural control. Findings vary with some studies showing improvements in standing balance and gait, and reduced falls risk in individuals with vestibular disorders or post-stroke (138–142) while others show no effect (143). Most studies have brief training sessions, are uncontrolled and carryover of improvements to performance without the tactile device is not assessed. Currently, no randomized controlled trials have investigated the clinical usefulness of balance prostheses.

Falls prevention

Patients with neurological and/or vestibular disorders have an increased falls risk (29, 144, 145). Specific questions about frequency, circumstances, location, preceding symptoms, e.g. dizziness, injuries sustained, 'long lie', and ability to get up after a fall must be asked. Appropriate techniques for getting up after a fall should be taught and/or an alarm pendant to alert emergency services provided. Patients should be educated about common falls risks, e.g. loose rugs, wet leaves, and walking barefoot or in socks or poorly-fitting slippers at home (146). An environmental home hazards assessment and recommendations for appropriate

modifications, e.g. clearance of obstructive objects, grab rail installation by an occupational therapist, may be useful although patient compliance is about 50% (147).

Assistive devices, such as a stick or walking frame, are an option for people with a high falls risk. They should not be prescribed instead of exercise training but in addition to it. Benefits rely upon prescription of the most appropriate walking aid according to individual needs. Patients after stroke who do not load more than 40% of their body weight on the paretic lower limb may benefit from using a stick (148). A four-point stick increases stability of moderately severe hemiparetic patients during stance more than a single-point stick, and the shift of weight toward the walking aid does not adversely affect weight bearing on the paretic limb (149). The use of a walking frame is less common in stroke patients but in some PD patients, wheeled walking frames may be considered. Those without wheels are not recommended as their use requires sequential actions patients with PD find difficult (150). Likewise, walking sticks usually provide little help and can become a distracting source of dual-task interference.

Efficacy of balance rehabilitation in neurological disorders

This section summarizes the literature in the most common balance disorders although some can be overlooked; the most common cause of vertigo in MS is BPPV (151). Peripheral vestibular disorders are extremely common, particularly in older and less mobile populations, and the existing diagnosis may not explain all symptoms.

Peripheral and central vestibular disorders

Vestibular rehabilitation, in the form of appropriate movements and sensory exposure is currently the standard of care for patients with peripheral vestibular disorders (discussed in 'Balance rehabilitation' section). Customized programmes provide greater benefit than generic ones (Cawthorne–Cooksey) with significant improvements in subjective symptoms, dynamic visual acuity, gait, and postural stability regardless of age and symptom duration (71, 152–155).

Some studies report similar responses for patients with peripheral, central, and mixed pathology, but others claim poorer outcomes for the latter two groups. Differing results may be due to individual study variations regarding treatment duration (patients with central deficits are expected to require a longer duration for improvement), extent and location of central deficit, and any additional cognitive or neuromuscular deficits (156–158). Cerebellar and vascular disease, migraine, and traumatic brain injuries (including concussion) are examples of central vestibular disorders associated with dizziness. Vestibular rehabilitation may improve dizziness, gait, and postural stability after concussion (159). The involvement of cerebellar dysfunction appears to reduce the effect of rehabilitation (158). Patients with migraine associated dizziness, benefit significantly from a vestibular rehabilitation programme, particularly when on antimigraine medication (160). Patients with vestibular migraine or migraine history and a peripheral vestibular disorder can also tolerate and benefit from customized vestibular rehabilitation incorporating optokinetic exposure; surprisingly, migraineurs report significantly greater improvements for visually-induced dizziness compared to non-migraineurs (72). It has been suggested medication may help control visually-induced dizziness symptoms in migraineurs enabling them to better tolerate the exercises leading to greater improvement (160,161).

Stroke

Guidelines state that patients with significant balance impairments after stroke should be offered intensive, progressive balance rehabilitation (162) although many receive traditional therapy which is unlikely to develop the dynamic balance reactions needed for an active lifestyle. Stroke consequences are highly variable as different sized lesions can occur in any CNS area and the primary sensorimotor consequences result from the affected neurological function. Balance can be impaired if basic reflexes (e.g. vestibulo-spinal pathways in Wallenberg syndrome), cerebellar coordination, muscle power, extrapyramidal mechanisms, sensory and high-order perception (neglect, 'pusher') mechanisms have been involved. Balance can be further compromised by secondary developments, i.e. muscle spasticity or flaccidity.

In chronic stroke affecting a single cerebral hemisphere the main causes of balance problems are visual dependency and sensorimotor organization deficits (60, 87, 163). Balance rehabilitation should focus on movement strategy re-training, decreasing visual dependency, improving sensory integration, and include progressively more difficult functional and dual-task activities (see 'Balance rehabilitation' section). Recent studies show promising results (164–168). Little knowledge exists regarding optimal training type and dose (169) or long-term retention.

Polyneuropathies

Older adults with PN experience particular problems on uneven walking surfaces and in low-light conditions (170) and therefore need education about falls risk and strategies for use in challenging environments. Patients with PN often develop various adaptive balance control strategies (171) which require careful assessment as in peripheral vestibular disorders. Light touch, visual reliance training, assistive devices (169, 172, 173) and active orthoses may be helpful but further research is required for clear recommendations to be made about these (174) or other balance rehabilitation interventions.

Weight-bearing exercises appear to be safe for those with diabetes-related polyneuropathy (175). Leg-strengthening and/or functional balance exercises improve physical function (175, 176) and a pilot study found Tai Chi significantly improved plantar sensation and postural sway in older adults (177).

Parkinson's disease and other movement disorders

Balance and gait nearly always become impaired as PD progresses (178). Medication and exercise are frequently prescribed concurrently to improve mobility. Combination strategies incorporating strengthening, endurance, and balance exercises show greater improvements in walking speed, transfers, and balance in patients with mild to moderate PD (179,180).

Balance training focuses on optimizing movement and sensory strategies (see sections 'Retraining postural alignment and movement strategies' and 'Retraining sensory strategies') (181, 182). Exercises progressively challenging sensorimotor control of dynamic balance and gait may delay mobility disability (183). Progression involves changes in movement speed and amplitude, dual-tasking, and learning to adapt strategies to changing contexts, e.g. quick direction changes in tight spaces (see sections 'Learning to adapt strategies to changing contexts' and 'Retraining cognitive strategies'). Targeted activities, i.e. tango dancing and boxing, show improvements in balance, ADLs, and gait function (184, 185).

Patients with severe PD (186) or freezing of gait (187) show multiple lateral anticipatory postural adjustments in response to a backward translation resulting in slower step latencies, reduced step length, and an increased number of steps to recover balance, increasing falls risk (187). Compensatory stepping may improve with training; however traditional postural weight-shifting (see section 'Retraining postural alignment and movement strategies') may not be beneficial for this client group (187). Patients should learn to step quickly and take bigger steps in responses to postural perturbations, without initial weight-shifting which impairs stepping ability (187).

Long-term retention of gains, optimal dose and exercise components at different disease stages, and the role of exercise in other movement disorders remain unknown. Despite the lack of evidence, balance training has been recommended to improve falls risk in patients with Huntington's disease and progressive supranuclear palsy (188, 189).

The effects of deep-brain stimulation (DBS) on posture and gait are unclear. A recent meta-analysis showed that when on medication, DBS improves posture and gait to a greater extent compared to medication alone (190). However, subthalamic nucleus DBS provides worse long-term outcome compared to DBS in the globus pallidus interna (190).

Multiple sclerosis

In patients with relapsing-remitting or secondary progressive MS, studies incorporating progressive vestibular exercises, sensorImotor strategy retraining, and dual-tasking improve ability on functional balance tests (see 191–193; 'Balance rehabilitation' section). Recently customized vestibular rehabilitation was shown to improve fatigue, balance function, and perceived disability due to unsteadiness and/or dizziness compared to control groups receiving strength and endurance training or usual medical care (194). These results are not surprising as one study reported 86% of patients with MS tested had vestibular pathology of peripheral aetiology in all except one person (195).

Balance exercises are safe and improve ataxia caused by cerebellum lesions, by small amounts (191, 192, 196) but effects may be transient (197). Strengthening exercises alone are ineffective (198). A meta-analysis of studies using aerobic, strengthening and flexibility training showed a small improvement in walking ability (199). As always, individually tailored rehabilitation is advised. Further research is required (199, 200).

Cerebellar disorders

Motor learning is possible with cerebellar damage (201); therefore exercise aimed at promoting neural plasticity may be beneficial. Balance rehabilitation for ataxia and dizziness in cerebellar disease is discussed in sections 'Peripheral and central vestibular disorders' and 'Multiple sclerosis'. Exercises challenging static and dynamic balance, facilitating sensory integration and retraining motor strategies may improve gait velocity, postural sway, and activity limitations (see sections 'Re-training postural alignment and movement strategies' and 'Re-training sensory strategies'; 156, 158) although the evidence is modest and should be interpreted with caution (202).

Conclusion

Balance disorders are common in patients with peripheral or CNS deficits. Balance rehabilitation should be informed by assessment and individually designed as evidence showing improvements in postural stability, ADLs, and dizziness is constantly increasing. Further work is needed regarding neural plasticity and recovery after CNS lesions, optimum interventions and long-term efficacy, and the potential benefit of novel techniques, i.e. virtual reality.

References

1. Münchau A, Corna S, Gresty MA, et al. (2001). Abnormal interaction between vestibular and voluntary head control in patients with spasmodic torticollis. *Brain*, 24(Part 1), 47–59.
2. Horak FB, Nashner LM, Diener HC (1990). Postural strategies associated with somatosensory and vestibular loss. *Exp Brain Res*, 82(1), 167–77.
3. Bloem BR, Allum JH, Carpenter MG, Verschuuren JJ, Honegger F (2002). Triggering of balance corrections and compensatory strategies in a patient with total leg proprioceptive loss. *Exp Brain Res*, 142(1), 91–107.
4. Horak FB, Hlavacka F (2002). Vestibular stimulation affects medium latency postural muscle responses. *Exp Brain Res*, 144(1), 95–102.
5. Stål F, Fransson PA, Magnusson M, Karlberg M (2003). Effects of hypothermic anesthesia of the feet on vibration-induced body sway and adaptation. *J Vestib Res*, 13(1), 39–52.
6. Guerraz M, Gianna CC, Burchill PM, Gresty MA, Bronstein AM (2001). Effect of visual surrounding motion on body sway in a three-dimensional environment. *Percept Psychophys*, 63(1), 47–58.
7. Basmajian JV, De Luca CJ (1985). *Muscles alive: their function revealed by electromyography* (5th ed). Baltimore, MD: Williams and Wilkins.
8. Horak FB (1987). Clinical measurement of postural control in adults. *Phys Ther*, 67(12), 1881–5.
9. Guerraz M, Yardley L, Bertholon P, et al. (2001). Visual vertigo: symptom assessment, spatial orientation and postural control. *Brain*, 124(Pt. 8), 646–56.
10. Mahboobin A, Loughlin PJ, Redfern MS, Sparto PJ (2005). Sensory re-weighting in human postural control during moving-scene perturbations. *Exp Brain Res* 167(2), 260–7.
11. Horak FB, Diener HC (1994). Cerebellar control of postural scaling and central set in stance. *J Neurophysiol*, 72(2), 479–93.
12. Fransson P-A, Magnusson M, Johansson R (1998). Analysis of adaptation in anteroposterior dynamics of human postural control. *Gait Posture*, 7(1), 64–74.
13. Ivey FM, Hafer-Macko CE, Macko RF (2008). Task-oriented treadmill exercise training in chronic hemiparetic stroke. *J Rehabil Res Dev*, 45(2), 249–59.
14. Berg KO, Wood-Dauphinee SL, Williams JI, Maki B (1992). Measuring balance in the elderly: validation of an instrument. *Can J Public Health*, 83(Suppl 2), 7–11.
15. Blum L, Korner-Bitensky N (2008). Usefulness of the Berg Balance Scale in stroke rehabilitation: a systematic review. *Phys Ther*, 88(5), 559–66.
16. Landers MR, Backlund A, Davenport J, et al. (2008). Postural instability in idiopathic Parkinson's disease: discriminating fallers from non-fallers based on standardized clinical measures. *J Neurol Phys Ther*, 32, 56–61.
17. Cattaneo D, Jonsdottir J, Repetti S (2007). Reliability of four scales on balance disorders in persons with multiple sclerosis. *Disabil Rehabil*, 29(24), 1920–5.
18. Busse ME, Wiles CM, Rosser AE (2009). Mobility and falls in people with Huntington's disease. *J Neurol Neurosurg Psychiatry*, 80(1), 88–90.
19. Cohen HS, Kimball KT (2008). Usefulness of some current balance tests for identifying individuals with disequilibrium due to vestibular impairments. *J Vestib Res*, 18(5–6), 295–303.
20. Pavlou M, Lingeswaran A, Davies RA, Gresty MA, Bronstein AM (2004). Simulator based rehabilitation in refractory dizziness. *J Neurol*, 251(8), 983–95.
21. Mathias S, Nayak U, Issacs B (1986). Balance in elderly patients: the 'Get-up and Go' test. *Arch Phys Med Rehabil*, 67(6), 387–9.
22. Podsiadlo D, Richardson S (1991). The timed 'Up &Go': a test of basic functional mobility for frail elderly persons. *J Am Geriatr Soc*, 39(2), 142–8.
23. Tinetti ME (1986). Performance-oriented assessment of mobility problems in elderly patients. *J Am Geriatr Soc*, 34(2), 119–26.
24. Duncan PW, Weiner DK, Chandler J, Studenski S (1990). Functional reach: a new clinical measure of balance. *J Gerontol*, 45(6), 192–95.
25. Newton RA (2001). Validity of the multi-directional reach test: a practical measure for limits of stability in older adults. *J Gerontol A Biol Sci Med Sci*, 56(4), 248–52.
26. Shumway-Cook A, Woollacott MH (2007). *Motor control: Translating research into clinical practice* (3rd ed). Philadelphia, PA: Lippincott, Williams, and Wilkins.
27. Lundin-Olsson L, Nyberg L, Gustafson Y (1997). 'Stops walking when talking' as a predictor of falls in elderly people. *Lancet*, 349(9052), 617.
28. Wrisley DM, Marchetti GF, Kuharsky DK, Whitney SL (2004). Reliability, internal consistency, and validity of data obtained with the functional gait assessment. *Phys Ther*, 84(10), 906–18.
29. Whitney SL, Hudak MT, Marchetti GF (2000a). The dynamic gait index relates to self-reported fall history in individuals with vestibular dysfunction. *J Vestib Res*, 10(2), 99–105.
30. Wrisley DM, Kumar NA (2010). Functional gait assessment: concurrent, discriminative, and predictive validity in community-dwelling older adults. *Phys Ther*, 90(5), 761–73.

31. McConvey J, Bennett SE (2005). Reliability of the Dynamic Gait Index in individuals with multiple sclerosis. *Arch Phys Med Rehabil*, 86(1), 130–3.

32. Dibble LE, Lange M (2006). Predicting falls in individuals with Parkinson disease: a reconsideration of clinical balance measures. *J Neurol Phys Ther*, 30(2), 60–7.

33. Jonsdottir J, Cattaneo D (2007). Reliability and validity of the dynamic gait index in persons with chronic stroke. *Arch Phys Med Rehabil*, 88(11), 1410–5.

34. Benaim C, Pérennou DA, Villy J, Rousseaux M, Pelissier JY (1999). Validation of a standardized assessment of postural control in stroke patients: the Postural Assessment Scale for Stroke Patients (PASS). *Stroke*, 30(9), 1862–8.

35. Powell LE, Myers AM (1995). The activities-specific balance confidence (ABC) scale. *J Gerontol*, 50A(1), M28–M34.

36. Myers AM, Fletcher PC, Myers AH, Sherk W (1998). Discriminative and evaluative properties of the activities-specific balance confidence (ABC) scale. *J Gerontol*, 53(4), M287–94.

37. Whitney SL, Hudak MT, Marchetti GF (1999). The activities-specific balance confidence scale and the dizziness handicap inventory: a comparison. *J Vestib Res*, 9(4), 253–9.

38. Botner EM, Miller WC, Eng JJ (2005). Measurement properties of the Activities-specific Balance Confidence Scale among individuals with stroke. *Disabil Rehabil*, 27(4), 156–63.

39. Salbach NM, Mayo NE, Hanley JA, Richards CL, Wood-Dauphinee S (2006). Psychometric evaluation of the original and Canadian French version of the activities-specific balance confidence scale among people with stroke. *Arch Phys Med Rehabil*, 87(12), 1597–604.

40. Peretz C, Herman T, Hausdorff JM, Giladi N (2006). Assessing fear of falling: Can a short version of the Activities-specific Balance Confidence scale be useful? *Mov Disord*, 21(12), 2101–5.

41. Cohen HS, Kimball KT (2000). Development of the vestibular disorders activities of daily living scale. *Arch Otolaryngol Head Neck Surg*, 126(7), 881–7.

42. Shumway-Cook A, Horak F (1986). Assessing the influence of sensory interaction on balance. *Phys Ther*, 66(10), 1548–50.

43. Nashner LM (1976). Adapting reflexes controlling the human posture. *Exp Brain Res*, 26(1), 59–72.

44. Horak F, Nashner L (1986). Central programming of postural movements: Adaptation to altered support surface configurations. *J Neurophysiol*, 55(6), 1369–81.

45. Brown LA, Shumway-Cook A, Woollacott MH (1999). Attentional demands and postural recovery: the effects of aging. *J Gerontol A BiolSci Med Sci*, 54(4), M165–71.

46. Di Fabio RP, Badke MB, McEvoy A, Ogden E (1990). Kinematic properties of voluntary postural sway in patients with unilateral primary hemispheric lesions. *Brain Res*, 513(2), 248–54.

47. Horak FB, Shupert CL, Dietz V, Horstmann G (1994). Vestibular and somatosensory contributions to responses to head and body displacements in stance. *Exp Brain Res*, 100(1), 93–106.

48. Allum JH, Bloem BR, Carpenter MG, Honneger F (2001). Differential diagnosis of proprioceptive and vestibular deficits using dynamic support-surface posturography. *Gait Posture*, 14(3), 217–26.

49. Carpenter MG, Allum JH, Honegger F (2001). Vestibular influences on human postural control in combinations of pitch and roll planes reveal differences in spatiotemporal processing. *Exp Brain Res*, 140(1), 95–111.

50. Mackey DC, Robinovitch SN (2005). Postural steadiness during quiet stance does not associate with ability to recover balance in older women. *ClinBiomech*, 20(8), 776–83.

51. Okada S, HirakawaK, Takada Y, Kinoshita H (2001). Age-related differences in postural control in humans in response to a sudden deceleration generated by postural disturbance. *Eur J Appl Physiol*, 85(1–2), 10–8.

52. Lord SR, Lloyd D, Sek Keung LI (1996). Sensori-motor function, gait patterns and falls in community-dwelling women. *Age Ageing*, 25(4), 292–9.

53. Lord SR, Rogers MW, Howland A, Fitzpatrick R (1999). Lateral stability, sensorimotor function and falls in older people. *J Am Geriatr Soc*, 47(9), 1077–81.

54. Isles RC, Low Choy NL, Steer M, Nitz JC (2004). Normal values of balance tests in women aged 20–80. *J Am Geriatr Soc*, 52(8), 1367–72.

55. Low Choy NL, Brauer SG, Nitz JC (2007). Age-related changes in strength and somatosenstaion during midlife rationale for targeted preventive intervention programs. *Ann N Y Acad Sci*, 1114, 180–93.

56. Nolan M, Nitz J, Choy NL, Illing S (2010). Age-related changes in musculoskeletal function, balance and mobility measures in men aged 30–80 years. *Aging Male*, 13(3), 194–201.

57. Agrawal Y, Carey JP, Della Santina CC, Schubert MC, Minor LB (2009). Disorders of balance and vestibular function in US adults: data from the National Health and Nutrition Examination Survey, 2001–2004. *Arch Intern Med*, 169(10), 938–44.

58. Redfern MS, Furman JM (1994). Postural sway of patient with vestibular disorders during optic flow. *J Vestib Res*, 4(3), 221–30.

59. Sundermier L, Woollacott MH, Jensen JL, Moore S (1996). Postural sensitivity to visual flow in aging adults with and without balance problems. *J Gerontol*, 51(2), M45–52.

60. Bonan IV, Colle FM, Guichard JP, et al. (2004). Reliance on visual information after stroke. Part I: balance on dynamic posturography. *Arch Phys Med Rehabil*, 85(2), 268–73.

61. Bisdorff A, Von Brevern M, Lempert T, Newman-Toker DE (2009). Classification of vestibular symptoms: towards an international classification of vestibular disorders. *J Vestib Res*, 19(1–2), 1–13.

62. Pavlou M, Davies RA, Bronstein AM (2006). The assessment of increased sensitivity to visual stimuli in patients with chronic dizziness. *J Vestib Res*, 16(4–5), 223–31.

63. Lewis GN, Byblow WB, Walt SE (2000). Stride length regulation in Parkinson's disease: the use of extrinsic, visual cues. *Brain*, 123(Pt 10), 2077–90.

64. vanWegen E, Lim I, de Goede C, et al. (2006). The effects of visual rhythms and optic flow on stride patterns of patients with Parkinson's disease. *Parkinsonism Relat Disord*, 12(1), 21–7.

65. Nashner LM (1982). Adaptation of human movement to altered environments. *Trends Neurosci*, 5, 358–61.

66. El-Kashlan HK, Shepard NT, Asher AM, Smith-Wheelock M, Telian SA (1998). Evaluation of clinical measures of equilibrium. *Laryngoscope*, 108(3), 311–19.

67. O'Neill DE, Gill-Body KM, Krebs DE (1998). Posturography changes do not predict functional performance changes. *Am JOtol*, 19(6), 797–803.

68. Gill-Body KM, Beninato M, Krebs DE (2000) Relationships among balance impairments, functional performance, and disability in people with peripheral vestibular dysfunction. *Phys Ther*, 80(8), 748–58.

69. Horak F, Jones-Rycewicz C, Black FO, Shumway-Cook A (1992). Effects of vestibular rehabilitation on dizziness and imbalance. *Otolaryngol Head Neck Surg*, 106(2), 175–80.

70. Gillespie MB, Minor LB (1999). Prognosis in bilateral vestibular hypofunction. *Laryngoscope*, 109(1), 35–41.

71. Black FO, Angel CR, Peszecker SC, Gianna C (2000). Outcome analysis of individualized vestibular rehabilitation protocols. *Am J Otol*, 21(4), 543–51.

72. Pavlou M, Bronstein AM, Davies RA (2009). Advances in vestibular rehabilitation: high-tech vs. low-tech optokinetic stimulation and the role of supervision and migraine on outcome (abstract). In: *Program and Abstracts of the 19th conference of the international Society for Posture and Gait Research*; Bologna, Italy, p. 107.

73. Broglio SP, Ferrara MS, Sopiarz K, Kelly MS (2008). Reliable change of the sensory organization test. *Clin J Sport Med*, 18(2), 148–54.

74. Goebel, JA, Sataloff, RT, Hanson, JM. Nashner LM, Hirshout DS, Sokolow CC (1997). Posturographic evidence of nonorganic sway patterns in normal subjects, patients, and suspected malingerers. *Otolaryngol Head Neck Surg*, 117(4) 293–302.

75. Krempl GA, Dobie RA (1998). Evaluation of posturography in the detection of malingering subjects. *Am J Otol*, 19(5), 619–27.

76. Gianoli G, McWilliams S, Soileau J, Belafsky P (2000). Posturographic performance in patients with the potential for secondary gain. *Otolaryngol Head Neck Surg*, 122(1), 11–18.

77. Emam AA, Gad AM, Ahmed MM, Assal HS, Mousa SG (2009). Quantitative assessment of posture stability using computerised dynamic posturography in type 2 diabetic patients with neuropathy and its relation to glycaemic control. *Singapore Med J*, 50(6), 614–18.

78. Luyat M, Ohlmann T, Barraud PA (1997). Subjective vertical and postural activity. *Acta Psychol*, 95(2), 181–93.

79. Pérennou DA, Amblard B, Laassel el M, Benaim C, Hérisson C, Pélissier J (2002). Understanding the pusher behavior of some stroke patients with spatial deficits: a pilot study. *Arch Phys Med Rehabil*, 83(4), 570–5.

80. Mann C, Berthelot-Berry N, Dauterive H (1949). The perception of the vertical: I. Visual and non-labyrinthine cues. *J Exp Psychol*, 39(4), 538–47.

81. Bauermeister M, Werner H, Wapner S (1964). The effect of body tilt on tactual-kinesthetic perception of verticality. *Am J Psychol*, 77, 451–6.

82. Witkin HA, Asch SE (1948). Studies in space orientation. III. Perception of the upright in the absence of a visual field. *J Exp Psychol*, 38(5), 603–14.

83. Bisdorff AR, Wolsley CJ, Anastasopoulos D, Bronstein AM, Gresty MA (1996). The perception of body verticality (subjective postural vertical) in peripheral and central vestibular disorders. *Brain*, 119(Pt 5), 1523–34.

84. Brandt T, Dieterich M, Danek A (1994). Vestibular cortex lesions affect the perception of verticality. *Ann Neurol*, 35(4), 403–12.

85. Kerkhoff G, Zoelch C (1998). Disorders of visuospatial orientation in the frontal plane in patients with visual neglect following right or left parietal lesions. *Exp Brain Res*, 122(1), 108–20.

86. Anastasopoulos D, Bronstein AM (1999). A case of thalamic syndrome: somatosensory influences on visual orientation. *J Neurol Neurosurg Psychiatry*, 67(3), 390–4.

87. Yelnik AP, Kassouha A, Bonan IV, et al. (2006). Postural visual dependence after recent stroke: assessment by optokinetic stimulation. *Gait Posture*, 24(3), 262–9.

88. Barra J, Oujamaa L, Chauvineau V, Rougier P, Pérennou D (2009). Asymmetric standing posture after stroke is related to a biased egocentric coordinate system. *Neurology*, 72(18), 1582–7.

89. Maylor EA, Wing AM (1996). Age differences in postural stability are increased by additional cognitive demands. *J Gerontol B Psychol Sci Soc Sci*, 51(3), 143–54.

90. Li KZ, Krampe RTH, Bondar A (2005). An ecological approach to studying aging and dual-task performance. In Engle RW, Sedek G, von Hecker U, McIntosh DN (Eds) *Cognitive limitations in aging and psychopathology*, pp. 190–218. Cambridge: Cambridge University Press.

91. Yardley L, Papo D, Bronstein A, et al. (2002). Attentional demands of continuously monitoring orientation using vestibular information. *Neuropsychologia*, 40(4), 373–83.

92. Rochester L, Hetherington V, Jones D, et al. (2004). Attending to the task: interference effects of functional tasks on walking in Parkinson's disease and the roles of cognition, depression, fatigue, and balance. *Arch Phys Med Rehabil*, 85(10), 1578–85.

93. Parker TM, Osternig LR, Lee HJ, Donkelaar P, Chou LS (2005). The effect of divided attention on gait stability following concussion. *Clin Biomech*, 20(4), 389–95.

94. Plummer-D'Amato P, Altmann LJ, Saracino D, et al. (2008). Interactions between cognitive tasks and gait after stroke: a dual task study. *Gait Posture*, 27(4), 683–8.

95. Paul L, Ellis BM, Leese GP, McFadyen AK, McMurray B (2009). The effect of a cognitive or motor task on gait parameters of diabetic patients, with and without neuropathy. *Diabet Med*, 26(3), 234–9.

96. Kalron A, Dvir Z, Achiron A (2010). Walking while talking – difficulties incurred during the initial stages of multiple sclerosis disease process. *Gait Posture*, 32(3), 332–5.

97. Plummer-D'Amato P, Altmann LJ (2012). Relationships between motor function and gait-related dual-task interference after stroke: A pilot study. *Gait Posture*, 35(1), 170–2.

98. Horak FB, Wrisley DM, Frank J (2009). The Balance Evaluation Systems Test (BESTest) to differentiate balance deficits. *Phys Ther*, 89(5), 484–98.

99. Franchignoni F, Horak F, Godi M, Nardone A, Giordano A (2010). Using psychometric techniques to improve the Balance Evaluation Systems Test: the mini-BESTest. *J Rehabil Med*, 42(4), 323–31.

100. Leddy AL, Crowner BE, Earhart GM (2011). Utility of the Mini-BESTest, BESTest, and BESTest sections for balance assessments in individuals with Parkinson disease. *J Neurol Phys Ther*, 35, 90–7.

101. Lord SR, Menz HB, and Tiedemann A (2003). A physiological profile approach to falls risk assessment and prevention. *Phys Ther*, 83, 237–52.

102. Lord SR, Sambrook PN, Gilbert C, et al. (1994). Postural stability, falls and fractures in the elderly: results from the Dubbo Osteoporosis Epidemiology Study. *Med J Aust*, 160, 684–5, 688–91.

103. Lord, SR, Clark RD, Webster IW (1991) Physiological factors associated with falls in an elderly population. *J Am Geriatr Soc*, 39(12), 1194–200.

104. Liston, M, Pavlou, M, Martin FVM (2008). 'An exploratory investigation of the Physiological Profile Assessment data from the Southwark and Lambeth falls clinics.' Poster presentation at British Geriatric Society, 9th International Conference on Falls and Postural stability, York, UK.

105. Bronstein AM (2003). Vestibular reflexes and positional manoeuvres. *J Neurol Neurosurg Psychiatry*, 74(3), 289–93.

106. Bronstein AM, Lempert T (2007). *Dizziness: a practical approach to diagnosis and management*, Cambridge Clinical Guides. Cambridge: Cambridge University Press.

107. Parnes LS, Agrawal SK, Atlas J (2003). Diagnosis and management of benign paroxysmal positional vertigo (BPPV). *CMAJ*, 169(7), 681–93.

108. Blatt PJ, Georgakakis GA, Herdman SJ, Clendaniel RA, Tusa RJ (2000). The effect of the canalith repositioning maneuver on resolving postural instability in patients with benign paroxysmal positional vertigo. *Am J Otol*, 21(3), 356–63.

109. Gillen R, Tennen H, McKee TE, Gernert-Dott P, Affleck G (2001). Depressive symptoms and history of depression predict rehabilitation efficiency in stroke patients. *Arch Phys Med Rehabil*, 82(12), 1645–9.

110. Chamberlin ME, Fulwider BD, Sanders SL, Medeiros JM (2005). Does fear of falling influence spatial and temporal gait parameters in elderly persons beyond changes associated with normal aging? *J Gerontol A Biol Sci Med Sci*, 60(9), 1163–7.

111. Straube A, Leigh RJ, Bronstein A, et al. (2004). EFNS task force-therapy of nystagmus and oscillopsia. *Eur J Neurol*, 11(2), 83–9.

112. Kadivar Z, Corcos DM, Foto J, Hondzinski JM (2011). Effect of step training and rhythmic auditory stimulation on functional performance in Parkinson patients. *Neurorehabil Neural Repair*, 25(7), 626–35.

113. Shumway-Cook A, Horak F (1990). Rehabilitation strategies for patients with vestibular deficits. *Neurol Clin*, 8(2), 441–57.

114. Wrisley DM, Pavlou M (2005). Physical therapy for balance disorders. *Neurol Clin*, 23(3), 855–74, vii–viii.

115. Silsupadol P, Shumway-Cook A, Lugade V, et al. (2009). Effects of single-task versus dual-task training on balance performance in older adults: a double-blind, randomized controlled trial. *Arch Phys Med Rehabil*, 90(3), 381–7.

116. Tusa RJ, Herdman SJ (1983). Vertigo and disequilibrium. In Johnson R, Griffin J (Eds) *Current therapy in neurological disease* (4th ed), p. 12. St Louis, MO: Mosby Yearbook.

117. Crane BT, Demer JL (1998). Gaze stabilization during dynamic posturography in normal and vestibulopathic humans. *Exp Brain Res*, 122(2), 235–46.

118. von Brevern M, Zeise D, Neuhauser H, Clarke AH, Lempert T (2005). Acute migrainous vertigo: clinical and oculographic findings. *Brain*, 128(Pt 2), 365–74.

119. Whitney SL, Sparto PJ, Hodges LF, Babu SV, Furman JM, Redfern MS (2006). Responses to a virtual reality grocery store in persons with and without vestibular dysfunction. *Cyberpsychol Behav*, 9(2), 152–6.

120. Keshner EA, Kenyon RV (2009). Postural and spatial orientation driven by virtual reality. *Stud Health Technol Inform*, 145, 209–28.

121. Viirre E, Draper M, Gailey C, Miller D, Furness T (1998). Adaptation of the VOR in patients with low VOR gains. *J Vestib Res*, 8(4), 331–4.

122. Viirre E, Sitarz R (2002). Vestibular rehabilitation using visual displays: preliminary study. *Laryngoscope*, 112(3), 500–3.

123. Kim JH, Jang SH, Kim CS, Jung JH, You JH (2009). Use of virtual reality to enhance balance and ambulation in chronic stroke: a double-blind, randomized controlled study. *Am J Phys Med Rehabil*, 88(9), 693–701.

124. Walker ML, Ringleb SI, Maihafer GC, *et al.* (2010). Virtual reality-enhanced partial body weight-supported treadmill training poststroke: feasibility and effectiveness in 6 subjects. *Arch Phys Med Rehabil*, 91(1), 115–22.

125. Yen CY, Lin KH, Hu MH, Wu RM, Lu TW, Lin CH (2011). Effects of virtual reality-augmented balance training on sensory organization and attentional demand for postural control in people with Parkinson disease: a randomized controlled trial. *Phys Ther*, 91(6), 862–74.

126. Rittweger J (2010). Vibration as an exercise modality: how it may work, and what its potential might be. *Eur J Appl Physiol*, 108(5), 877–904.

127. Verschueren SMP, Roelants M, Delecluse C, Swinnen S, Vanderschueren D, Boonen S (2004). Effect of 6-month whole body vibration training on hip density, muscle strength, and postural control in postmenopausal women: A randomized controlled pilot study. *J Bone Miner Res*, 19(3), 352–9.

128. Torvinen S, Kannus P, Sievanen H, *et al.* (2003). Effect of 8-month vertical whole body vibration on bone, muscle performance, and body balance: A randomized controlled study. *J Bone Miner Res*, 18(5), 876–84.

129. Bautmans I, Van Hees E, Lemper J-C, Mets T (2005). The feasibility of whole body vibration in institutionalised elderly persons and its influence on muscle performance, balance and mobility: a randomised controlled trial [ISRCTN62535013]. *BMC Geriatr*, 5, 17.

130. Bruyere O, Wuidart MA, Di Palma E, *et al.* (2005). Controlled whole body vibration to decrease fall risk and improve health-related quality of life of nursing home residents. *Arch Phys Med Rehabil*, 86(2), 303–7.

131. Cheung WH, Mok HW, Qin L, Sze PC, Lee KM, Leung KS (2007). High-frequency whole-body vibration improves balancing ability in elderly women. *Arch Phys Med and Rehabil*, 88(7), 852–7.

132. Furness TP, Maschette WE (2009). Influence of whole body vibration platform frequency on neuromuscular performance of community-dwelling older adults. *J Strength Cond Res*, 23(5), 1508–13.

133. Kawanabe K, Kawashima A, Sashimoto I, Takeda T, Sato Y, Iwamoto J (2007). Effect of whole-body vibration exercise and muscle strengthening, balance, and walking exercises on walking ability in the elderly. *Keio J Med*, 56(1), 28–33.

134. Rees SS, Murphy AJ, Watsford ML (2009). Effects of whole body vibration on postural steadiness in an older population. *J Sci Med Sport*, 12(4), 440–4.

135. Rehn B, Lidstrom J, Skoglund J, Lindstrom B (2007). Effects on leg muscular performance from whole-body vibration exercise: a systematic review. *Scand J Med Sci Sports*, 17(1), 2–11.

136. Schuhfried O, Mittermaier C, Jovanovic T, Pieber K, Paternostro-Sluga T (2005). Effects of whole-body vibration in patients with multiple sclerosis: a pilot study. *Clin Rehabil*, 19(8), 834–42.

137. Pollock RD Woledge RC, Mills KR, Martin FC, Newham DJ (2010). Muscle activity and acceleration during whole body vibration: effect of frequency and amplitude. *Clin Biomech*, 25(8), 840–6.

138. Wall C III, Weinberg MS (2003). Balance prostheses for postural control. *IEEE Eng Med Biol Mag*, 22(5), 84–90.

139. Peterka RJ, Wall C III, Kentala E (2006). Determining the effectiveness of a vibrotactile balance prosthesis. *J Vestib Res*, 16(1–2), 45–56.

140. Goebel JA, Sinks BC, Parker BE Jr, Richardson NT, Olowin AB, Cholewiak RW (2009). Effectiveness of head-mounted vibrotactile stimulation in subjects with bilateral vestibular loss: a phase 1 clinical trial. *OtolNeurotol*, 30(2), 210–16.

141. Danilov YP, Tyler ME, Skinner KL, Hogle RA, Bach-y-Rita P (2007). Efficacy of electrotactile vestibular substitution in patients with peripheral and central vestibular loss. *J Vestib Res*, 17(2–3), 119–30.

142. Badke MB, Sherman J, Boyne P, Page S, Dunning K (2011). Tongue-based biofeedback for balance in stroke: results of an 8-week pilot study. *Arch Phys Med Rehabil*, 92(9), 1364–70.

143. Asseman F, Bronstein AM, Gresty MA (2007). Using vibrotactile feedback of instability to trigger a forward compensatory stepping response. *J Neurol*, 254(11), 1555–61.

144. Herdman SJ, Blatt P, Schubert MC, Tusa RJ (2000). Falls in patients with vestibular deficits. *Am J Otol*, 21(6), 847–51.

145. Thurman DJ, Stevens JA, Rao JK (2008). Practice parameter: Assessing patients in a neurology practice for risk of falls (an evidence-based review): report of the Quality Standards Subcommittee of the American Academy of Neurology. *Neurology*, 70(6), 473–9.

146. Menz HB, Morris ME, Lord SR (2006). Footwear characteristics and risk of indoor and outdoor falls in older people. *Gerontology*, 52(3), 174–80.

147. Cumming RG, Thomas M, SzonyiG, *et al.* (1999). Home visits by an occupational therapist for assessment and modification of environmental hazards: a randomized trial of falls prevention. *J Am Geriatr Soc*, 47(12), 1397–402.

148. Guillebastre B, Rougier PR, Sibille B, Chrispin A, Detante O, Pérennou DA (2012). When might a cane be necessary for walking following a stroke? *Neurorehabil Neural Repair*, 26(2), 173–7.

149. Laufer Y (2003). The effect of walking aids on balance and weight-bearing patterns of patients with hemiparesis in various stance positions. *Phys Ther*, 83(2), 112–22.

150. Morris ME (2006). Locomotor training in people with Parkinson disease. *Phys Ther*, 86(10), 1426–35.

151. Frohman EM, Zhang H, Dewey RB, Hawker KS, Racke MK, Frohman TC (2000). Vertigo in MS: utility of positional and particle repositioning maneuvers. *Neurology*, 55(10), 1566–9.

152. Brown KE, Whitney SL, Wrisley DM, Furman JM (2001). Physical therapy outcomes for persons with bilateral vestibular loss. *Laryngoscope*, 111(10), 1812–17.

153. Whitney SL, Wrisley DM, Marchetti GF, Furman JM (2002). The effect of age on vestibular rehabilitation outcomes. *Laryngoscope*, 112(10), 1785–90.

154. McGibbon CA, Krebs DE, Parker SW, Scarborough DM, Wayne PM, Wolf SL (2005). Tai Chi and vestibular rehabilitation improve vestibulopathic gait via different neuromuscular mechanisms: preliminary report. *BMC Neurol*, 5(1), 3.

155. Schubert MC, Migliaccio AA, Clendaniel RA, Allak A, Carey JP (2008). Mechanism of dynamic visual acuity recovery with vestibular rehabilitation. *Arch Phys Med Rehabil*, 89(3), 500–7.

156. Gill-Body KM, Popat RA, Parker SW, Krebs DE (1997). Rehabilitation of balance in two patients with cerebellar dysfunction. *Phys Ther*, 77(5), 534–52.

157. Gurr B, Moffat N (2001). Psychological consequences of vertigo and the effectiveness of vestibular rehabilitation for brain injury patients. *Brain Inj*, 15(5), 387–400.

158. Brown KE, Whitney SL, Marchetti GF, Wrisley DM, Furman JM (2006). Physical therapy for central vestibular dysfunction. *Arch Phys Med Rehabil*, 87(1)76–81.

159. Alsalaheen BA, Mucha A, Morris LO (2010). Vestibular rehabilitation for dizziness and balance disorders after concussion. *J Neurol Phys Ther*, 34(2), 87–93.

160. Whitney, SL, Wrisley, DM, Brown, KE, Furman JM (2000b). Physical therapy for migraine-related vestibulopathy and vestibular dysfunction with history of migraine. *Laryngoscope*, 110(9), 1528–34.

161. Johnson GD (1988). Medical management of migraine-related dizziness and vertigo. *Laryngoscope*, 108(1 Pt2), 1–28.

162. Royal College of Physicians (2008). *National Clinical Guidelines for Stroke* (3rd ed). London: RCP.

163. Smania N, Picelli A, Gandolfi M, Fiaschi A, Tinazzi M (2008). Rehabilitation of sensorimotor integration deficits in balance impairment of patients with stroke hemiparesis: a before/after pilot study. *Neurol Sci*, 29(5), 313–19.

164. Marigold DS, Eng JJ, Dawson AS, Inglis JT, Harris JE, Gylfadóttir S (2005). Exercise leads to faster postural reflexes, improved balance and mobility, and fewer falls in older persons with chronic stroke. *J Am Geriatr Soc*, 53(3), 416–23.

165. Salbach NM, Mayo NE, Robichaud-Ekstrand S, Hanley JA, Richards CL, Wood-Dauphinee S (2005). The effect of a task-oriented walking intervention on improving balance self-efficacy poststroke: a randomized, controlled trial. *J Am Geriatr Soc*, 53(4), 576–82.

166. Bayouk JF, Boucher JP, Leroux A (2006). Balance training following stroke: effects of task-oriented exercises with and without altered sensory input. *Int J Rehabil Res*, 29(1), 51–9.

167. Yelnik AP, Le Breton F, Colle FM, *et al.* (2008). Rehabilitation of balance after stroke with multisensorial training: a single-blind randomized controlled study. *Neurorehabil Neural Repair*, 22(5), 468–76.

168. Kang HK, Kim Y, Chung Y, Hwang S (2011). Effects of treadmill training with optic flow on balance and gait in individuals following stroke: randomized controlled trials. *Clin Rehabil*, 26(3), 246–55.

169. French B, Thomas LH, Leathley MJ, *et al.* (2009). Repetitive task training for improving functional ability after stroke. *Stroke* 40, e98–e99.

170. DeMott TK, Richardson JK, Thies SB, Ashton-Miller JA (2007). Falls and gait characteristics among older persons with peripheral neuropathy. *Am J Phys Med Rehabil*, 86(2), 125–32.

171. Bunday KL, Bronstein AM (2009). Locomotor adaptation and aftereffects in patients with reduced somatosensory input due to peripheral neuropathy. *J Neurophys*, 102(6), 3119–28.

172. Dickstein R, Shupert C, Horak F (2001). Fingertip touch improves postural stability in patients with peripheral neuropathy. *Gait Posture*, 14(3), 238–47.

173. Tusa RJ (2007). Non-vestibular dizziness and imbalance: From disuse disequilibrium to central degenerative disorders. In Herdman SJ (Ed) *Vestibular rehabilitation* (3rd ed), pp. 433–43. Philadelphia, PA: FA Davis.

174. Hijmans JM, Geertzen JH, Dijkstra PU, Postema K (2007). A systematic review of the effects of shoes and other ankle or foot appliances on balance in older people and people with peripheral nervous system disorders. *Gait Posture*, 25(2), 316–23.

175. Lemaster JW, Mueller MJ, Reiber GE, Mehr DR, Madsen RW, Conn VS (2008). Effect of weight-bearing activity on foot ulcer incidence in people with diabetic peripheral neuropathy: feet first randomized controlled trial. *Phys Ther*, 88(11), 1385–98.

176. Bulat T, Hart-Hughes S, Ahmed S (2007). Effect of a group-based exercise program on balance in elderly. *Clin Interv Aging*, 2(4), 655–60.

177. Richerson S, Rosendale K (2007). Does Tai Chi improve plantar sensory ability? A pilot study. *Diabetes Technol Ther*, 9(3), 276–86.

178. Bloem BR, Beckley DJ, van Dijk JG, Zwinderman AH, Remler MP, Roos RA (1996). Influence of dopaminergic medication on automatic postural responses and balance impairment in Parkinson's disease. *Mov Disord*, 11(5), 509–21.

179. Goodwin VA, Richards SH, Taylor RS, Taylor AH, Campbell JL (2008). The effectiveness of exercise interventions for people with Parkinson's disease: a systematic review and meta-analysis. *Mov Disord*, 23(5), 631–40.

180. Dibble LE, Addison O, Papa E (2009). The effects of exercise on balance in persons with Parkinson's disease: a systematic review across the disability spectrum. *J Neurol Phys Ther*, 33(1), 14–26.

181. Hirsch MA, Toole T, Maitland CG, Rider RA (2003). The effects of balance training and high-intensity resistance training on persons with idiopathic Parkinson's disease. *Arch Phys Med Rehabil*, 84(8), 1109–17.

182. Ashburn A, Fazakarley L, Ballinger C, Pickering R, McLellan LD, Fitton C (2007). A randomised controlled trial of a home based exercise programme to reduce the risk of falling among people with Parkinson's disease. *J Neurol Neurosurg Psychiatry*, 78(7), 678–84.

183. King LA, Horak FB (2009). Delaying mobility disability in people with Parkinson disease using a sensorimotor agility exercise program. *Phys Ther*, 89(4), 384–93.

184. Combs SA, Diehl MD, Staples WH (2011). Boxing training for patients with Parkinson disease: a case series. *Phys Ther*, 91(1), 132–42.

185. Duncan RP, Earhart GM (2012). Randomized controlled trial of community-based dancing to modify disease progression in Parkinson disease. *Neurorehabil Neural Repair*, 26(2), 132–43.

186. King LA, St George RJ, Carlson-Kuhta P, Nutt JG, Horak FB (2010). Preparation for compensatory forward stepping in Parkinson's disease. *Arch Phys Med Rehabil*, 91(9), 1332–8.

187. Jacobs JV, Nutt JG, Carlson-Kuhta P, Stephens M, Horak FB (2009). Knee trembling during freezing of gait represents multiple anticipatory postural adjustments. *Exp Neurol*, 215(2), 334–41.

188. Steffen TM, Boeve BF, Mollinger-Riemann LA, Petersen CM (2007). Long-term locomotor training for gait and balance in a patient with mixed progressive supranuclear palsy and corticobasal degeneration. *Phys Ther*, 87(8), 1078–87.

189. Zinzi P, Salmaso D, De Grandis R, *et al.* (2007). Effects of an intensive rehabilitation programme on patients with Huntington's disease: a pilot study. *Clin Rehabil*, 21(7), 603–13.

190. St George RJ, Nutt JG, Burchiel KJ, Horak FB (2010). A meta-regression of the long-term effects of deep brain stimulation on balance and gait in PD. *Neurology*, 75(14), 1292–9.

191. Lord SE, Wade DT, Halligan PW (1998). A comparison of two physiotherapy treatment approaches to improve walking in multiple sclerosis: a pilot randomized controlled study. *Clin Rehabil*, 12(6), 477–86.

192. Armutlu K, Karabudak R, Nurlu G (2001). Physiotherapy approaches in the treatment of ataxic multiple sclerosis: a pilot study. *Neurorehabil Neural Repair*, 15(3), 203–11.

193. Cattaneo D, Jonsdottir J, Zocchi M, Regola A (2007b). Effects of balance exercises on people with multiple sclerosis: a pilot study. *Clin Rehabil*, 21(9), 771–81.

194. Hebert JR, Corboy JR, Manago MM, Schenkman M (2011). Effects of vestibular rehabilitation on multiple sclerosis-related fatigue and upright postural control: a randomized controlled trial. *Phys Ther*, 91(8), 1166–83.

195. Zeigelboim BS, Arruda WO, Mangabeira-Albernaz PL, *et al.* (2008). Vestibular findings in relapsing, remitting multiple sclerosis: a study of thirty patients. *Int Tinnitus J*, 14(2), 139–45.

196. Mills RJ, Yap L, Young CA (2007). Treatment for ataxia in multiple sclerosis. *Cochrane Database Syst Rev* 1, CD005029.

197. Wiles CM, Newcombe RG, Fuller KJ, *et al.* (2001). Controlled randomised crossover trial of the effects of physiotherapy on mobility in chronic multiple sclerosis. *J Neurol Neurosurg Psychiatry*, 70(2), 174–9.

198. DeBolt LS, McCubbin JA (2004). The effects of home-based resistance exercise on balance, power, and mobility in adults with multiple sclerosis. *Arch Phys Med Rehabil*, 85(2), 290–7.

199. Snook EM, Motl RW (2009). Effect of exercise training on walking mobility in multiple sclerosis: a meta-analysis. *Neurorehabil Neural Repair*, 23(2)108–16.

200. Asano M, Dawes DJ, Arafah A, Moriello C, Mayo NE (2009). What does a structured review of the effectiveness of exercise interventions for persons with multiple sclerosis tell us about the challenges of designing trials? *Mult Scler*, 15(4), 412–21.

201. Matsumura M, Sadato N, Kochiyama T, *et al.* (2004). Role of the cerebellum in implicit motor skill learning: A pet study. *Brain Res Bull*, 63(6), 471–83.

202. Martin CL, Tan D, Bragge P, Bialocerkowski A (2009). Effectiveness of physiotherapy for adults with cerebellar dysfunction: a systematic review. *Clin Rehabil*, 23(1), 15–26.

203. Jacobson GP, Newman CW (1990). The development of the Dizziness Handicap Inventory. *Arch Otolaryngol Head Neck Surg*, 116(4), 424–7.

204. Yardley L, Masson E, Verschuur C, Haacke N, Luxon L (1992). Symptoms, anxiety and handicap in dizzy patients: development of the vertigo symptom scale. *J Psychosom Res*, 36(8), 731–41

205. Tinetti ME, Richman D, Powell L (1990). Falls efficacy as a measure of fear of falling. *J Gerontol*, 45(6), P239–43.

206. Tinetti ME (1986). Performance-oriented assessment of mobility problems in elderly patients. *J Am Geriatr Soc*, 34(2), 119–26.

207. Csuka M, McCarty DJ. Simple method for measurement of lower extremity muscle strength. *Am J Med*, 78(1), 77–81.

208. Bray A, Subanandan A, Isableu B, Ohlmann T, Golding JF, Gresty MA (2004). We are most aware of our place in the world when about to fall. *Curr Biol*, 14(15), R609–10.

209. Schuler JR, Bockisch CJ, Straumann D, Tarnutzer AA (2010). Precision and accuracy of the subjective haptic vertical in the roll plane. *BMC Neurosci*, 11, 83.

210. Pérennou DA, Mazibrada G, Chauvineau V, *et al.* (2008). Lateropulsion, pushing and verticality perception in hemisphere stroke: a causal relationship? *Brain*, 131(Pt 9), 2401–13.

211. Pavlou M, Quinn C, Murray K, Spyridakou C, Faldon M, Bronstein AM (2011). The effect of repeated visual motion stimuli on visual dependence and postural control in normal subjects. *Gait Posture*, 33(1), 113–18.

212. Bronstein AM, Lempert T, Seemungal BM (2010). Chronic dizziness: a practical approach. *Pract Neurol*, 10(3), 129–39.

CHAPTER 18

The Epidemiology of Vertigo and Imbalance

Hannelore K. Neuhauser

Introduction

Epidemiological findings on vertigo and imbalance are a valuable resource for evidence-based clinical decision-making and patient care. Epidemiological studies systematically analyse patterns of disease in defined populations and provide clinicians with probabilistic expectations on disease frequency (1), as well as on outcome and prognosis. Additionally, epidemiology can contribute to understanding the causes of disorders leading to vertigo and imbalance through observational studies on risk factors.

Compared to cardiovascular or cancer epidemiology, the epidemiology of vertigo and imbalance is still a small and emerging field. However, its potential impact on patient care is rather large. For example, the awareness of vestibular migraine (VM) as a vestibular syndrome causally linked to migraine was promoted by epidemiological observation indicating a more than chance association of migraine with vertigo and dizziness and not by pathophysiological hypotheses (2–5). Moreover, as robust data on the population-wide high prevalence of dizziness and vertigo and their specific underlying disorders accumulate, a need for improved recognition and therapy of these diseases beyond specialized dizziness clinics and neuro-otological training programmes becomes evident.

This book chapter will focus on the frequency and distribution of dizziness, vertigo, and imbalance and of selected vestibular disorders and will report recent findings on associated risk factors and personal and healthcare impact. A few definitions and comments on epidemiological concepts may facilitate the reading. It is essential to understand that the clinical value of most epidemiological findings reported here is not dictated by their statistical significance, i.e. by their precision, but by minimization of bias in the study design, i.e. minimization of systematic error that may affect the validity of the study (the ability to measure the truth), the reliability (the ability to reproduce the results) and the generalizability (does this study result apply to my patient?). Bias cannot be corrected for in the analysis, no matter how statistically sophisticated this is. There are two main types of biases, both of which are common in epidemiological studies on vertigo and imbalance. *Selection bias* occurs when study participants are systematically different from the group about which

the study wants to make an inference. Examples are prevalence estimates or prognostic studies from specialized dizziness clinics (which may not apply to more unselected patients). For example, the relative frequency of Ménière's disease (MD) of 5–11% in specialized care setting (4, 6, 7) is almost certainly due to selection bias and considerably overestimates the prevalence in the community. Sometimes however, these studies give the best (and only) information available at the time. *Information bias* due to misclassification of both symptoms and diagnoses is a particular concern for dizziness studies at two levels: misclassification by study participants who are given options of describing their subjective symptoms and have to choose among them, and misclassification by investigators who have to interpret standardized (or non-standardized) symptom descriptions and assign medical terms and diagnoses based on insufficiently operationalized diagnostic criteria or criteria which have been modified for study purposes without validation. Patient descriptions may be unclear, inconsistent, and unreliable (8), and there are language-specific linguistic issues. Moreover, patients are more likely to misclassify their symptoms when they are not offered enough options that cover the entire range of specific subcategories and appear to be equally valued by the investigators. On the other hand, even physicians do not agree on the meaning of the word 'vertigo' (9) and investigators tend to diagnose conditions that they know about or are interested in ignoring others (10, 11). Patients and many physicians tend to use the terms vertigo and dizziness interchangeably while dizziness experts use vertigo as a vestibular symptom, defined as a sensation of self-motion when no self-motion is occurring (12, 13). As a general rule, unless the term dizziness and vertigo and individual diagnoses have been explicitly defined and reported, they may be imprecise and not comparable between studies or even within studies (11). The recently published classification of vestibular symptoms by the Committee for the Classification of Vestibular Disorders of the Bárány Society (12), is a very valuable basis for future studies but has not been applied yet, so most of the findings reported in this chapter don't refer to the exact terms and definitions of this classification. In this chapter the term vertigo denotes a vestibular symptom but the exact definition varies among studies. Measures of disease frequency in the population are incidence (proportion of newly developed—incident—disease over a specific period of time) and prevalence (proportion of an existing disease, either at one point in time—point prevalence—or during a given period, i.e. period prevalence, e.g. 1-year prevalence). Lifetime prevalence denotes the cumulative lifetime frequency of a disease to the present time, i.e. the proportion of people who have had the event at any time in the past.

Symptom epidemiology: dizziness, vertigo, and imbalance

Prevalence, incidence, and demographic factors

Dizziness (used as an umbrella term that includes vertigo) ranks among the most common complaints in medicine, affecting 15% to 35% of the general population (14–19). A 12-month incidence of 3% has been reported among unselected adults (20). This high prevalence and incidence contrasts with low (or no) estimates of population prevalences (not frequencies in specialized settings) of underlying disorders, some of which are largely underdiagnosed such as benign paroxysmal positional vertigo (BPPV) and VM (21–24). Surprisingly, *rotatory* dizziness, which may be interpreted as vestibular vertigo, has also been reported in up to 20–30% of adults in population-based questionnaire studies (15–17, 25), but various methodological factors may lead to this high prevalence, foremost the suggestibility of a rotatory sensation when no or not enough alternative descriptions of symptoms are offered.

An estimate of the proportion of vestibular symptoms among dizziness complaints was achieved by means of a population survey with validated neuro-otological interviews carried out in Germany (26). This study combined a screening of a representative National Health Survey general population sample (n = 4869) for moderate or severe dizziness or vertigo with detailed validated neuro-otological interviews (n = 1003) which included an interactive part similar to a clinical situation and detailed standardised questions. Each participant was classified by at least two raters. Vestibular vertigo was defined as rotational vertigo (illusion of self-motion or object motion), positional vertigo (vertigo or dizziness precipitated by changes of head position, such as lying down or turning in bed), or recurrent dizziness with nausea and oscillopsia or imbalance. The lifetime prevalence of vertigo in adults aged 18–79 was 7.4%, the 1-year prevalence 4.9% and the 1-year incidence 1.4% (Table 18.1). VM accounted for almost a quarter (24%) of dizziness/vertigo cases

in the community. For the definition of vestibular vertigo the study emphasized specificity over sensitivity, therefore the prevalence and incidence of vestibular vertigo may actually be even higher in reality. The study confirmed previous findings of a marked female preponderance among individuals with vertigo (1-year prevalence ratio male to female 1:2.7) and showed that vertigo is almost three times more frequent in the elderly compared to young adults (Figure 18.1). By design of the study, non-vestibular dizziness was investigated only in participants without vestibular vertigo. More than half of participants with non-vestibular dizziness had orthostatic dizziness with reported provocation by postural changes on standing up from a supine or sitting position and a duration of seconds to 5 min. The 12-month population prevalence of orthostatic dizziness was 11% (women 13%, men 8%) (27).

Data on dizziness and vertigo in children is scarce and based on unvalidated questionnaires with limited power to exclude provoked physiological vertigo during playing and to understand and discriminate terms like 'rotational' or 'imbalance'. Three population-based studies with a number of methodological differences that hamper comparability report prevalences of 6% to 18% of dizziness (mostly 'rotatory') in children (28–30). A rough estimation of the frequency of dizziness in paediatric care is given by a report from a large database of paediatric encounters from the US where ICD-9 codes related to vestibular and balance disorders accounted for 0.45% of diagnoses (31). This is, as expected, considerably less than the 3.4% and 8.3% reported from adult and geriatric general practice databases (32, 33).

Imbalance and unsteadiness

Epidemiological data on unsteadiness and imbalance is scarce. In a population-based study from Sweden, the 1-year prevalence of self-reported unsteadiness without a sense of rotation among a sample of 2547 adults was 9.2% (17). As part of a larger population study, only six questions on dizziness/unsteadiness were included with no definition of unsteadiness given, leading to a potential overestimation of the prevalence of unsteadiness through misclassification of patients who actually suffered from dizziness and vertigo only. Various balance tests have been performed in community-dwelling adults in order to study the risk of imbalance on falls and a meta-analysis reported an overall summary risk ratio of 1.42 (95% confidence interval (CI) 1.08–1.85) and odds ratio 1.98 (1.60–2.46) (34), which was even higher in previous reviews including also institutionalized populations. Among nine measurement scales used,

Table 18.1 Population prevalence and incidence of dizziness and vertigo of moderate/severe intensity in the general adult population

	Population % (95% CI)					
	Women	(95% CI)	Men	(95% CI)	Total	(95% CI)
Dizziness (including vertigo)						
Incidence (1 year)	4.0	(3.2–5.0)	2.3	(1.6–3.1)	3.1	(2.6–3.8)
Prevalence (1 year)	28.9	(26.8–31.1)	16.7	(15.0–18.6)	22.9	(21.5–24.3)
Prevalence (lifetime)	35.9	(33.7–38.3)	22.6	(20.6–24.7)	29.3	(27.8–30.9)
Vestibular vertigo						
Incidence (1 year)	1.9	(1.4–2.7)	0.8	(0.4–1.3)	1.4	(1.0–1.8)
Prevalence (1 year)	7.1	(6.0–8.4)	2.6	(1.9–3.5)	4.9	(4.2–5.7)
Prevalence (lifetime)	10.3	(9.0–11.8)	4.3	(3.4–5.4)	7.4	(6.5–8.3)

Based on data from Neuhauser et al. (20, 26)

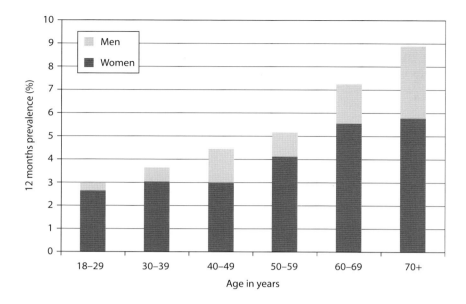

Fig. 18.1 Twelve-month prevalence of vestibular vertigo in adults. From Neuhauser et al. with permission (110).

significant associations for increased fall risk were found for five (tandem stand, tandem walk, one leg stand, Performance Oriented Mobility Assessment, and body sway), and not for Forward Reach Test, Berg Balance Scale, and Timed Up & Go Test. However, the studies did not report prevalences of imbalance. Confusingly, a very high prevalence of 35% of vestibular dysfunction among US adults has been claimed based on data from the National Health and Nutrition Examination Survey (NHANES) (35). The prevalence refers to the failure to stand unassisted for 30 s on a foam-padded surface with eyes closed, a test referred to as the modified Romberg Test of Standing Balance on Firm and Compliant Support Surfaces. This is not a purely vestibular test and documentation of the test validity and reliability as well as on the rationale for the cut-off is not available.

Personal and occupational impact of dizziness and vertigo

Dizziness and vertigo have a considerable personal impact. In the epidemiological study from Germany described earlier, participants with vestibular vertigo and non-vestibular dizziness reported medical consultation (70% and 54%), sick leave (41% and 15%), interruption of daily activities (40% and 12%), and avoidance of leaving the house (19% and 10%).

In addition, age- and sex-adjusted health-related quality of life was lower in individuals with dizziness and vertigo compared with dizziness-free control subjects (Figure 18.2) (19, 20).

Vertigo can trigger or exacerbate psychiatric problems, which do not necessarily correlate with deficits on neuro-otological testing. In a large population-based study more than a quarter of participants with dizziness (28%) reported symptoms of an anxiety disorder and had increased healthcare use and impairment (18). Among current dizziness sufferers 18% had panic disorders, followed by 13% with generalized anxiety disorders, and 9% social phobia (18). In a recent study, patients with vestibular neuritis and persistent vestibular deficits had lower levels of anxiety, depression, and somatization than patients with md or VM (36). Development

of anxiety and depressive disorder *after* the onset of the vestibular disorder was correlated with poor improvement and high persistency of vertigo and dizziness (37).

Little is known about the occupational impact of vertigo. Sick leave due to vestibular vertigo was reported by 41% participants with vestibular vertigo working at the time and by 15% of those with non-vestibular dizziness in a population-based study (20). In employees on long-term sickness leave (more than 8 weeks), dizziness/vertigo was a rather infrequent cause (0.9% of women and 0.7% of men) in a register-based prospective study from Norway (38). This corresponds for women to an annual incidence of long-term sickness leave due to dizziness/vertigo of 7.5/10 000 at risk (vocationally active) and for men 3.2/10 000 at risk. One quarter of these women and men obtained a disability pension. However, most recurrent vertigo is unlikely to cause such long episodes of sickness leave and the occupational impact of repeated short-term absence or more subtle productivity loss is unknown.

Healthcare impact of vertigo

Vertigo and dizziness rank among the ten most common reasons for referral to neurologists both in emergency rooms (39) and in office-based settings (40). The German neuro-otological survey estimated that 1.8% of adults seek medical care annually with the new (first-time) symptom of dizziness or vertigo (0.9% for vestibular vertigo alone) (20). Similarly, a Spanish primary care study reported that 7.6 per 1000 inhabitants (i.e. 0.8%) consulted in primary care over 12 months for incident vertigo and 1.8% for combined incident and recurrent vertigo defined as an illusion of unequivocal rotatory movement (41). This is in line with reports of 3.4% and 8.3% patient records with dizziness diagnoses from adult and geriatric general practice databases (32, 33).

In the German neuro-otological study, the proportion with vestibular vertigo increased with age and varied by medical specialty from 35% among those consulting a general practitioner to 59% of those consulting a neurologist. This shows that vestibular vertigo is frequent in all medical settings. More than half of participants with

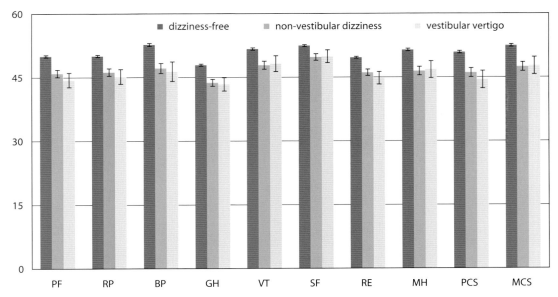

Fig. 18.2 Health-related quality of life in unselected adults with vestibular vertigo, non-vestibular dizziness, and no dizziness/vertigo. SF-8 scores, 95% CI; adjusted for age and sex; higher scores indicate higher health related quality of life. PF, Physical Functioning; RP, Role Physical; BP, Bodily Pain; GH, General Health; VT, Vitality; SF, Social Functioning; RE, Role Emotional; MH, Mental Health; PCS, Physical Component Summary; MCS, Mental Component Summary. From Neuhauser et al. with permission (20)

clear-cut vestibular vertigo were diagnosed with a non-vestibular disorder (20). At least one medical consultation because of dizziness/vertigo at some point in their life was reported by 17% of this representative sample of adults in Germany, but 42% of participants with dizziness/vertigo of at least moderate severity never consulted a physician.

In emergency departments (EDs) in the US, vertigo and dizziness account for an increasing proportion of visits and currently amount to 2–3% of all consultations (42, 43). A median of 3.6 diagnostic tests per patient were performed and 17% of patients had a computed tomography or magnetic resonance imaging scan (42). In primary care, low proportions of specific diagnoses (20% and 60% in studies from Germany and the Netherlands (32) (33) and very low specialist referral rates are reported (4% in the German primary care data base (32) and 3% cited for the Netherlands (11)). Claims that dizziness/vertigo is an non-specific symptom in a high proportion of patients, especially in old age, have been however convincingly contradicted, e.g. by a recent study showing that out of 3400 patients over 70 years of age an accurate diagnosis was possible in more than 75%. In these elderly patients, dizziness often had a multifactorial aetiology and caused age-specific impairment but dizziness caused by age per se was not found (44). In summary, data from primary care and from EDs show that misdiagnosis of vertigo and dizziness is common (21–24, 45) and suggest that appropriate training for these disorders may benefit patients and save costs.

Vertigo as a symptom of stroke/TIA

Identification of central or otherwise serious vertigo is a major concern (43, 46), in particular since isolated vertigo can be the only manifestation of vertebrobasilar ischemia (47). However, stroke was found to be a rare cause of dizziness presentations to the ED in a recent population-based stroke surveillance study: 3.2% of those presenting with any dizziness and only 0.7% of those presenting with *isolated* dizziness had an acute cerebrovascular cause (48).

At the primary care level and even more at the general population level this proportion is likely to be much lower since there are selection mechanisms which drive patients with a higher probability of stroke to present to the ED and those with a lower stroke probability not to. This selection toward a higher stroke probability among ED and hospitalized patients is also one of the caveats of an interesting recent study reporting a three times higher 4-year risk of stroke in patients hospitalized with a principal ICD-9-CM coded diagnosis of a non-central vertiginous syndrome compared to patients hospitalized for appendectomy (49). The reported long-term stroke risk can therefore not be generalized to unselected patients with vertigo but only to patients hospitalized for vertigo, which are likely to be systematically different from those who are not hospitalized. In addition, it is not evident that all patients with these diagnostic codes really had isolated vertigo as suggested by the title of the study since the study was based only on claims, administrative and death record codes and not on medical records. Therefore, the relevant question of the long-term stroke-risk in patients with isolated vertigo of unknown origin (with a normal neurological and preferably also neuro-otological examination) has yet to be answered.

Risk factors for vertigo

Vertigo can be a symptom of a variety of conditions with different aetiologies. Therefore, the potential benefit of investigating risk factors for the *symptom* vertigo is limited and findings must be interpreted cautiously. However, some interesting insights have resulted from such studies, the most prominent being the consistent association of vertigo and migraine (2–4), which has greatly contributed to the recognition of VM as a distinct vestibular syndrome. Migraine is also statistically associated with BPPV (50–52) and MD (53). However, the implications of these associations are not clear yet. Since migraine is more common in women, the association of migraine and specific vestibular disorders may partly explain the marked female preponderance among vertigo sufferers (26) which has also been consistently reported for specific vestibular disorders including BPPV (54), MD (53), and VM (4). Along that line, case series have suggested that premenstrual or drug-related hormonal changes may increase the risk of vestibular disorders (55, 56), but this was not confirmed by two other large studies (26, 57).

There is increasing evidence for an association of vertigo with depression (26, 58, 59) (60). A recent study found that a previous psychiatric disorder is a strong predictor for the development of reactive psychiatric disorders in vestibular patients (61). The same group reported that a history of mental disorders and stressful life events as well as lower scores of protective factors of subjective well-being, i.e. resilience, sense of coherence, and subjective quality of life, were associated with the development of secondary somatoform dizziness and vertigo 1 year after admission for acute vestibular disease (62).

A few studies suggest a link between vertigo and cardiovascular risk factors (for a summary see Neuhauser et al. (26)), but the evidence is insufficient to support an independent association in unselected individuals after taking potential confounders into account. Of note, overt cardiovascular disease was not significantly associated with vertigo after correcting for potential confounders (26).

Epidemiology of benign paroxysmal positional vertigo

BPPV it is not only the most frequent cause of recurrent vertigo but also amenable to successful and inexpensive treatment by liberatory manoeuvres (63). However, the importance of BPPV at the population level is still underestimated due to low recognition rates in primary care (22, 24), and scarce epidemiological data. Two older studies which estimated the incidence of BPPV at 0.01% in Japan (64) and 0.06% in Olmsted County, Minnesota (65) were based on recorded clinical cases and thus likely to considerably underestimate the incidence at the population level. Strikingly higher findings of 9% positive Dix–Hallpike tests in a series of 100 geriatric clinic patients (66) and of 11% and 39% positive Dix–Hallpike tests in unselected dizziness patients in primary care suggested that BPPV may actually be much more common in the community (11, 24). In a population-based postal questionnaire study from Stockholm, 5% of 2547 adults reported dizziness provoked by the movement of lying down in the past year (17), a question with considerable predictive capability for diagnosing BPPV (67). Prevalence and incidence estimates for BPPV have been obtained from the nationally representative neuro-otological survey conducted in Germany (21). Diagnostic criteria for BPPV were at least five attacks of vertigo lasting less than 1 min without concomitant neurological symptoms and invariably provoked by typical changes of head position (i.e. lying down, turning over in the supine position or at least two of the following manoeuvres: reclining the head, rising up from supine position and bending forward). The lifetime prevalence of BPPV was estimated at 2.4%, the 1-year prevalence at 1.6%, and the 1-year incidence at 0.6%. Of note, BPPV diagnoses relied on neuro-otological interviews and not on positioning manoeuvres, but the prevalence estimates are likely to be rather conservative since diagnostic criteria emphasized specificity and not sensitivity (the interviews had a specificity of 92% and a sensitivity of 88% in a concurrent validation study).

BPPV can manifest from childhood to the very old age with a reported peak age of onset in the sixth decade for idiopathic BPPV

and a lower mean age of onset in secondary BPPV (68). The 1-year prevalence of individuals with BPPV attacks (new-onset and recurrent) rises steeply with age: from 0.5% in 18–39-year-olds, to 3.4% in over 60-year-olds (21). The cumulative (lifetime) incidence of BPPV reaches almost 10% by the age of 80 (21). A recent clinical study reported a mean spontaneous remission time of untreated BPPV episodes of 39 days for posterior canal BPPV and 16 days for horizontal canal BPPV (69), a difference which is linked to the anatomical orientation of the canals. In the community, however, untreated episodes appear to be shorter, as suggested by a median episode duration of two weeks among 80 mostly untreated community-sampled individuals with BPPV (this study did not differentiate the affected canals) (21). A recent large case series of 589 BPPV patients from Korea confirmed previous reports of posterior canal BPPV as the most frequent involved canal (over 60%) and showed that frequency of horizontal canal BPPV may be as high as 40% in patients examined within 24 h of symptoms onset, while still accounting for a quarter of cases among those presenting after 7 days of onset (70). A third to a half of patients have recurrences at 3–5 years (71–73) with most recurrences occurring in the first year. A higher recurrence rate has been reported in traumatic BPPV compared to idiopathic BPPV (73, 74) and in women (71, 73), but data on determinants of recurrences are still scarce.

At present, the mechanisms of BPPV may be explained by canalolithiasis and cupulolithiasis. However, the underlying causes which lead to detachment of otoconia from the utricle are still poorly understood in the vast majority of patients. Head trauma and inner ear diseases such as vestibular neuritis and MD, are probably less frequent causes than previously thought, accounting for 6% of unselected BPPV cases (21, 75). More women than men are affected by BPPV (female:male ratio is 1.5:2.2:1) (21, 54, 64) but this seems to be the case only for idiopathic and not for secondary BPPV (76). This female preponderance is still poorly understood pathophysiologically, but may be linked to an equally poorly understood association of BPPV and migraine (50–52). Osteoporosis, which is more frequent in middle-aged and elderly women with BPPV compared to controls (77), may also play a role. Recent studies have found associations of BPPV with diabetes (78), and with hypertension, hyperlipidaemia, and stroke (21), but these observations await replication.

There is also increasingly more evidence of adverse psychosocial consequences of BPPV including reduced health-related quality of life (79), severe subjective impairment in affected individuals (21, 22), and avoidance behaviour in 70% of BPPV sufferers (21). Medical advice is sought by 80% of BPPV sufferers, but specific diagnostic positioning manoeuvres are applied in less than a third of patients seeking medical care (21). The rate of adequate therapy is even lower with only 10–20% of BPPV cases seen by a doctor receiving appropriate positioning manoeuvres (21, 22).

Epidemiology of vestibular migraine

VM is only starting to be perceived as a nosological entity by the medical community although it is the second most common cause of recurrent vertigo after BPPV (4, 80). Various terms, including migrainous vertigo, migraine-associated dizziness, migraine-related vestibulopathy, VM, and benign recurrent vertigo have all been applied to roughly the same patient population. VM accounts for 6–7% of patients in neurological dizziness clinics (4, 80) and has been found in 9% of patients in a migraine clinic case series (4). The term basilar migraine is restricted to patients who fulfil the diagnostic criteria of the International Headache Society (IHS) (81) for basilar migraine which applies to only about 10% of patients with VM (4, 80, 82).

Dizziness before, during and after headache was reported by more than half of headache sufferers in a large population-based study (83), however, various causes other than VM are possible (84). In the general population, migraine headaches and vestibular vertigo concur about three times more often than would be expected by chance. Lifetime prevalences are 14% for migraine (85) and 7% for vestibular vertigo (26). Thus, chance concurrence of the two would be 1%, but the German neuro-otological survey showed it to be 3.2% (23). This survey estimated the prevalence of definite VM in the general adult population based on validated neuro-otological interviews (26) and previously proposed explicit diagnostic criteria (4) that require not only a migraine diagnosis according to the IHS criteria (81) but also that migraine symptoms such as migrainous headache, photophobia, phonophobia or migrainous auras occur concurrently with spontaneous vertigo attacks. The lifetime prevalence of VM was 0.98% (95% CI 0.70–1.37) and the 12-month prevalence 0.89 (95% CI 0.62–1.27) (23). This study did not investigate probable VM, which is a more sensitive but less specific diagnostic category than definite VM, requiring spontaneous vertigo attacks not attributable to another cause, and either a history of migraine *or* concurrence of migraine symptoms during vertigo (4). An even broader term is benign recurrent vertigo (BRV) (86), which describes recurrent spontaneous attacks of vertigo which do not lead to permanent deficits and which cannot be attributed to a specific cause (other than migraine). The population prevalence of probable VM and BRV are not known. A recent large case series of 208 patients with spontaneous episodic vertigo of unknown cause comprised 61% with definite VM, 29% with probable VM and 10% for which only the broadest term of BRV applied (87). These rates confirm expert opinion that VM is a frequent condition both at the population level and in dizziness clinics. Of note, epidemiological studies of VM are prone to misclassification, in particular to high false-positive rates, due to the difficult differentiation of vestibular vertigo versus non-vestibular dizziness in questionnaires and structured interviews and to the differential diagnoses that have to be considered. This may explain recently reported very high VM prevalences (88, 89).

VM may occur at any age (80, 82). The prevalence of recurrent vertigo probably related to migraine is estimated at 2.8% of children between ages 6 and 12 (28). Benign paroxysmal vertigo of childhood, an early manifestation of VM, is the most common diagnosis in children presenting with vertigo, followed by BPPV (90). In adults with VM there is a clear female preponderance with a reported female-to-male ratio between 1.5 and 5 to 1 (4, 80, 82). However, a recent study reported that among unselected VM sufferers there are not significantly more women than among dizziness-free migraineurs (23). In most patients, migraine headaches begin earlier in life than VM (4, 23, 80), but little is known on the determinants of VM. A comparison of patients with VM with dizziness-free migraineurs showed an independent association with coronary heart disease but not with sex, age, migrainous aura, education, stroke, hypertension, hyperlipidaemia, body mass index, or depression (23).

The natural course of VM is not well known, but disease severity has been reported to vary over time (91). However, the impact of VM both at the personal and healthcare level may be considerable, as indicated by lower health-related quality of life scores in VM patients compared to dizziness-free controls (23), higher levels of anxiety and depression in VM patients compared to patients with persistent vestibular deficits (36), and an overall medical consultation rate of almost 70% among VM sufferers (23).

Epidemiology of vestibular neuritis

Epidemiological studies on vestibular neuritis, one of the most severely impairing acute vestibular disorders, are scarce, possibly due to the difficulty of diagnosing it by standardized interviews or questionnaires (67). Vestibular neuritis accounts for 3–10% of diagnoses in specialised dizziness clinics (4, 6, 92) and was reported to be the second most common dizziness diagnosis after BPPV in a British general practice study (93). However, the only published estimation on the frequency of vestibular neuritis in the general population comes from a government report in Japan, stating that vestibular neuritis occurs in 3.5 per 100 000 inhabitants (although this is not further specified, one can assume that this is a 1-year incidence) (94). The methods are not described, but based on the epidemiological data on other vestibular disorders from this report, considerable underestimation of the frequency of vestibular neuritis in the population is likely. Data from the National Hospital Discharge Registry in Germany document 19,828 cases of vestibular neuronitis (ICD 10 H81.2) in 2006, corresponding to 24 per 100,000 inhabitants (personal communication, German National Statistical Office). Also from Japan originates the single largest published series of about 600 patients aged 3–88 years with a peak of age distribution between 30–50. There was no female preponderance as in other vestibular disorders but, on the contrary, a male predominance until the age of 40 (94). A low recurrence rate of 2% was reported in two studies with a follow-up of 5–20 years (95) and 4–6 years (96) respectively. However, the long-term outcome of vestibular neuritis may not be as favourable as previously thought since persisting dizziness has been reported in 30–40% of patients (97, 98) and chronic anxiety in 15% (99). However, complete long-term recovery has been reported in a series of 21 children (100).

Epidemiology of Ménière's disease

MD accounts for 3–11% of diagnoses in dizziness clinics (4, 6, 92), but this reflects selection bias in specialized care settings towards severe, recurrent and difficult to treat vestibulopathies. In the general population, MD is a rare disease, therefore reliable prevalence and incidence estimates are difficult to obtain. Most studies have been based on patient registers and have various methodological restrictions (for a summary see Kotimäki et al. (101)). A thorough re-evaluation of diagnoses of Ménière's from the Mayo clinic's centralized diagnostic index in Rochester according to the previous criteria of the American Academy of Ophthalmology and Otolaryngology (AAOO 1972) resulted in an estimated annual incidence rate of 15/100 000 and a point prevalence of 218/100 000 population, which is higher than previous estimates (102). Since MD is a rare disease, the prevalence is reported per 100 000 population, however for comparison, the estimated 218/100,000 correspond to 0.2%. Furthermore, in the Rochester study, only 65% had classic MD, while 26% had vestibular Ménière's and 9% had cochlear Ménière's, two variants which were included in the 1972

AAOO criteria, but no longer fulfil the 1995 diagnostic criteria for MD of the American Academy of Otolaryngology-Head and Neck Surgery (AAO-HNS) (103). Taking this into account, MD appears to be at least ten times less common than BPPV.

Recently, a prevalence of 513/100,000 was reported from Southern Finland, which is considerably higher than figures from previous studies (25). The study was based on a questionnaire sent to a sample of the general population inquiring about vertigo, hearing loss and tinnitus, and a review of available medical records. The 1995 AAO criteria were used but the published questionnaire suggests that the hearing loss and duration criteria may have been modified. Interestingly, the number of individuals who reported that they suffer from impaired hearing and tinnitus and in addition experienced vertigo at some point in the past was 14 times higher than the number of MD cases. Similarly, a population prevalence of 5% of dizziness in combination with self-reported hearing loss and tinnitus was found in Sweden (17). This illustrates that when a patient presents with the MD triad of symptoms, i.e. vertigo, hearing loss, and tinnitus, possibly without specific information of the temporal association of these symptoms, the probability of MD is rather low and more specific information is required before suspecting MD. In medical practice, MD is overdiagnosed, as suggested by both the Rochester study and a more recent Finish study, which applied the AAOO and AAO-HNS criteria respectively and confirmed only 40% of MD diagnoses suspected in primary care (101, 102).

Generally, MD is regarded as a disease of the middle-aged, which can occasionally occur in children. However, MD is not uncommon after 65 years of age, accounting for 15% of a large case series (104). A female preponderance can be assumed based on the data from Rochester (61% women) (102) and is confirmed by the latest data from Finland (25). More than 10% bilateral involvement within 6 months of onset was present in a recent large case series (105) and a comprehensive review reported up to 35% bilaterality within 10 years and up to 47% within 20 years (106). Hearing loss and reduction of vestibular function appear to take place within 5–10 years, while drop attacks can occur early or late during follow-up.

The debate on the multiple aetiological possibilities of MD is ongoing. An intriguing finding is the increased prevalence of migraine in MD patients (53). In a recent study, MD patients had an earlier onset of symptoms and a greater susceptibility to bilateral hearing loss when they also had migraine (107). However, a frequent occurrence of migrainous symptoms during MD attacks has been found, which may reflect some overlap between the diagnostic criteria for MD and for VM (53) or a shared genetic susceptibility (108). Inhalant and food allergies have been linked with symptoms of MD (109), but the evidence is not conclusive.

Conclusion

The epidemiology of dizziness, vertigo, and imbalance is still an emerging field that can make valuable contributions to patient care and lead to a better understanding of the underlying causes of vestibular disorders. Recent studies have underscored the high frequency and impact of dizziness and vertigo and of underlying conditions such as BPPV and VM as well as of comorbidities such as anxiety and depression at the population level. However, risk factor research is only at its beginning and needs improved study designs. A qualitative leap is only possible if dizziness experts and

epidemiologists work together to improve the validity of study instruments, in particular their content validity, i.e. the extent to which the instruments measure the concepts of interest. This includes further work on classification systems and validation studies including comparisons with gold standards, when available, and cognitive interviewing techniques that investigate the conceptual equivalence between the study participants' and investigators' understanding of a term or question. Epidemiological methods can be used for improvement of patient care in other ways as well, e.g. by improving design, analysis and critical appraisal of randomised controlled treatment trials, or through healthcare research.

References

1. Lurie JD, Sox HC (1999). Principles of medical decision making. *Spine*, 24(5), 493–8.
2. Kuritzky A, Ziegler DK, Hassanein R (1981). Vertigo, motion sickness and migraine. *Headache*, 21(5), 227–31.
3. Kayan A, Hood JD (1984). Neuro-otological manifestations of migraine. *Brain*, 107 (Pt 4), 1123–42.
4. Neuhauser H, Leopold M, von Brevern M, Arnold G, Lempert T (2001). The interrelations of migraine, vertigo, and migrainous vertigo. *Neurology*, 56(4), 436–41.
5. Vukovic V, Plavec D, Galinovic I, Lovrencic-Huzja A, Budisic M, Demarin V (2007). Prevalence of vertigo, dizziness, and migrainous vertigo in patients with migraine. *Headache*, 47(10), 1427–35.
6. Brandt T (2004). A chameleon among the episodic vertigo syndromes: 'migrainous vertigo' or 'vestibular migraine'. *Cephalalgia*, 24(2), 81–2.
7. Guilemany JM, Martinez P, Prades E, Sanudo I, De Espana R, Cuchi A (2004). Clinical and epidemiological study of vertigo at an outpatient clinic. *Acta Otolaryngol*, 124(1), 49–52.
8. Newman-Toker DE, Cannon LM, Stofferahn ME, Rothman RE, Hsieh YH, Zee DS (2007). Imprecision in patient reports of dizziness symptom quality: a cross-sectional study conducted in an acute care setting. *Mayo Clin Proc*, 82(11), 1329–40.
9. Stanton VA, Hsieh YH, Camargo CA, Jr, *et al.* (2007). Overreliance on symptom quality in diagnosing dizziness: results of a multicenter survey of emergency physicians. *Mayo Clin Proc*, 82(11), 1319–28.
10. Sloane P, Blazer D, George LK (1989). Dizziness in a community elderly population. *J Am Geriatr Soc*, 37(2), 101–8.
11. Maarsingh OR, Dros J, Schellevis FG, *et al.* (2010). Causes of persistent dizziness in elderly patients in primary care. *Ann Fam Med*, 8(3), 196–205.
12. Bisdorff A, Von Brevern M, Lempert T, Newman-Toker DE (2009). Classification of vestibular symptoms: towards an international classification of vestibular disorders. *J Vestib Res*, 19(1–2), 1–13.
13. Committee on Hearing and Equilibrium guidelines for the diagnosis and evaluation of therapy in Meniere's disease (1995). American Academy of Otolaryngology-Head and Neck Foundation, Inc. *Otolaryngol Head Neck Surg*, 113(3), 181–5.
14. Kroenke K, Price RK (1993). Symptoms in the community. Prevalence, classification, and psychiatric comorbidity. *Arch Int Med*, 153(21), 2474–80.
15. Yardley L, Owen N, Nazareth I, Luxon L (1998). Prevalence and presentation of dizziness in a general practice community sample of working age people. *Br J Gen Pract*, 48(429), 1131–5.
16. Hannaford PC, Simpson JA, Bisset AF, Davis A, McKerrow W, Mills R (2005). The prevalence of ear, nose and throat problems in the community: results from a national cross-sectional postal survey in Scotland. *Fam Pract*, 22, 227–33.
17. Mendel B, Bergenius J, Langius-Eklof A (2010). Dizziness: A common, troublesome symptom but often treatable. *J Vestib Res*, 20(5), 391–8.
18. Wiltink J, Tschan R, Michal M, *et al.* (2009). Dizziness: anxiety, health care utilization and health behavior – results from a representative German community survey. *J Psychosom Res*, 66(5), 417–24.

19. Gopinath B, McMahon CM, Rochtchina E, Mitchell P (2009). Dizziness and vertigo in an older population: the Blue Mountains prospective cross-sectional study. *Clin Otolaryngol*, 34(6), 552–6.

20. Neuhauser HK, Radtke A, von Brevern M, Lezius F, Feldmann M, Lempert T (2008). Burden of dizziness and vertigo in the community. *Arch Int Med*, 168(19), 2118–24.

21. von Brevern M, Radtke A, Lezius F, *et al.* (2007). Epidemiology of benign paroxysmal positional vertigo. A population-based study. *J Neurol Neurosurg Psychiatry*, 78, 710–5.

22. von Brevern M, Lezius F, Tiel-Wilck K, Radtke A, Lempert T (2004). Benign paroxysmal positional vertigo: Current status of medical management. *Otolaryngol Head Neck Surg*, 130, 381–2.

23. Neuhauser HK, Radtke A, von Brevern M, *et al.* (2006). Migrainous vertigo. Prevalence and impact on quality of life. *Neurology*, 67(6), 1028–33.

24. Ekvall Hansson E, Mansson NO, Hakansson A (2005). Benign paroxysmal positional vertigo among elderly patients in primary health care. *Gerontology*, 51(6), 386–9.

25. Havia M, Kentala E, Pyykkö I (2005). Prevalence of Menière's disease in general population of Southern Finland. *Otolaryngol Head Neck Surg*, 133, 762–8.

26. Neuhauser HK, von Brevern M, Radtke A, *et al.* (2005). Epidemiology of vestibular vertigo: a neurotological survey of the general population. *Neurology*, 65(6), 898–904.

27. Radtke A, Lempert T, von Brevern M, Feldmann M, Lezius F, Neuhauser H (2011). Prevalence and complications of orthostatic dizziness in the general population. *Clin Auton Res*, 21, 161–8.

28. Abu-Arafeh I, Russell G (1995). Paroxysmal vertigo as a migraine equivalent in children: a population-based study. *Cephalalgia*, 15(1), 22–5.

29. Humphriss RL, Hall AJ (2011). Dizziness in 10 year old children: An epidemiological study. *Int J Pediatr Otorhinolaryngol*, 75, 395–400.

30. Niemensivu R, Pyykko I, Wiener-Vacher SR, Kentala E (2006). Vertigo and balance problems in children – an epidemiologic study in Finland. *Int J Pediatr Otorhinolaryngol*, 70(2), 259–65.

31. O'Reilly RC, Morlet T, Nicholas BD, *et al.* (2010). Prevalence of vestibular and balance disorders in children. *Otol Neurotol*, 31(9), 1441–4.

32. Kruschinski C, Kersting M, Breull A, Kochen MM, Koschack J, Hummers-Pradier E (2008). Frequency of dizziness-related diagnoses and prescriptions in a general practice database. *Z Evid Fortbild Qual Gesundhwes*, 102(5), 313–19.

33. Maarsingh OR, Dros J, Schellevis FG, van Weert HC, Bindels PJ, Horst HE (2010). Dizziness reported by elderly patients in family practice: prevalence, incidence, and clinical characteristics. *BMC Fam Pract*, 11, 2.

34. Muir SW, Berg K, Chesworth B, Klar N, Speechley M (2010). Quantifying the magnitude of risk for balance impairment on falls in community-dwelling older adults: a systematic review and meta-analysis. *J Clin Epidemiol*, 63(4), 389–406.

35. Agrawal Y, Carey JP, Della Santina CC, Schubert MC, Minor LB (2009). Disorders of balance and vestibular function in US adults: data from the National Health and Nutrition Examination Survey, 2001–2004. *Arch Intern Med*, 169(10), 938–44.

36. Best C, Eckhardt-Henn A, Diener G, Bense S, Breuer P, Dieterich M (2006). Interaction of somatoform and vestibular disorders. *J Neurol Neurosurg Psychiatry*, 77, 658–64.

37. Best C, Eckhardt-Henn A, Tschan R, Dieterich M (2009). Why do subjective vertigo and dizziness persist over one year after a vestibular vertigo syndrome? *Ann N Y Acad Sci*, 1164, 334–7.

38. Skoien AK, Wilhemsen K, Gjesdal S (2008). Occupational disability caused by dizziness and vertigo: a register-based prospective study. *Br J Gen Pract*, 58(554), 619–23.

39. Moulin T, Sablot D, Vidry E, *et al.* (2003). Impact of emergency room neurologists on patient management and outcome. *Eur Neurol*, 50, 207–14.

40. Schappert SM, Nelson C (1999). National Ambulatory Medical Care Survey, 1995–96 Summary. National Center for Health Statistics. *Vital Health Stat*, 142, 1–122.

41. Garrigues HP, Andres C, Arbaizar A, *et al.* (2008). Epidemiological aspects of vertigo in the general population of the Autonomic Region of Valencia, Spain. *Acta Otolaryngol*, 128(1), 43–7.

42. Kerber KA, Meurer WJ, West BT, Fendrick AM (2008). Dizziness presentations in U.S. emergency departments, 1995–2004. *Acad Emerg Med*, 15(8), 744–50.

43. Newman-Toker DE, Hsieh YH, Camargo CA, Jr, Pelletier AJ, Butchy GT, Edlow JA (2008). Spectrum of dizziness visits to US emergency departments: cross-sectional analysis from a nationally representative sample. *Mayo Clin Proc*, 83(7), 765–75.

44. Katsarkas A (2008). Dizziness in aging: the clinical experience. *Geriatrics*, 63(11), 18–20.

45. Moeller JJ, Kurniawan J, Gubitz GJ, Ross JA, Bhan V (2008). Diagnostic accuracy of neurological problems in the emergency department. *Can J Neurol Sci*, 35(3), 335–41.

46. Eagles D, Stiell IG, Clement CM, *et al.* (2008). International survey of emergency physicians' priorities for clinical decision rules. *Acad Emerg Med*, 15(2), 177–82.

47. Gomez CR, Cruz-Flores S, Malkoff MD, Sauer CM, Burch CM (1996). Isolated vertigo as a manifestation of vertebrobasilar ischemia. *Neurology*, 47(1), 94–7.

48. Kerber KA, Brown DL, Lisabeth LD, Smith MA, Morgenstern LB (2006). Stroke among patients with dizziness, vertigo, and imbalance in the emergency department: a population-based study. *Stroke*, 37(10), 2484–7.

49. Lee CC, Su YC, Ho HC, Hung SK, Lee MS, Chou P, *et al.* (2011). Risk of stroke in patients hospitalized for isolated vertigo: a four-year follow-up study. *Stroke*, 42(1), 48–52.

50. Ishiyama A, Jacobson KM, Baloh RW (2000). Migraine and benign positional vertigo. *Ann Otol Rhinol Laryngol*, 109(4), 377–80.

51. Lempert T, Leopold M, von Brevern M, Neuhauser H (2000). Migraine and benign positional vertigo. *Ann Otol Rhinol Laryngol*, 109(12 Pt 1), 1176.

52. Uneri A (2004). Migraine and benign paroxysmal positional vertigo: an outcome study of 476 patients. *Ear Nose Throat J*, 83, 814–15.

53. Radtke A, Lempert T, Gresty MA, Brookes GB, Bronstein AM, Neuhauser H (2002). Migraine and Meniere's disease: is there a link? *Neurology*, 59(11), 1700–4.

54. Katsarkas A (1999). Benign paroxysmal positional vertigo (BPPV): idiopathic versus post-traumatic. *Acta Otolaryngol*, 119(7), 745–9.

55. Rybak LP (1995). Metabolic disorders of the vestibular system. *Otolaryngol Head Neck Surg*, 112(1), 128–32.

56. Andrews JC, Ator GA, Honrubia V (1992). The exacerbation of symptoms in Meniere's disease during the premenstrual period. *Arch Otolaryngol Head Neck Surg*, 118(1), 74–8.

57. Vessey M, Painter R (2001). Oral contraception and ear disease: findings in a large cohort study. *Contraception*, 63(2), 61–3.

58. Monzani D, Casolari L, Guidetti G, Rigatelli M (2001). Psychological distress and disability in patients with vertigo. *J Psychosom Res*, 50(6), 319–23.

59. Grunfeld EA, Gresty MA, Bronstein AM, Jahanshahi M (2003). Screening for depression among neuro-otology patients with and without identifiable vestibular lesions. *Int J Audiol*, 42(3), 161–5.

60. Ketola S, Havia M, Appelberg B, Kentala E (2007). Depressive symptoms underestimated in vertiginous patients. *Otolaryngol Head Neck Surg*, 137(2), 312–5.

61. Best C, Eckhardt-Henn A, Tschan R, Dieterich M (2009). Psychiatric morbidity and comorbidity in different vestibular vertigo syndromes: Results of a prospective longitudinal study over one year. *J Neurol*, 256(1), 58–65.

62. Tschan R, Best C, Beutel ME, *et al.* (2011). Patients' psychological well-being and resilient coping protect from secondary somatoform vertigo and dizziness (SVD) 1 year after vestibular disease. *J Neurol*, 258(1), 104–12.

63. Bronstein AM (2003). Benign paroxysmal positional vertigo: some recent advances. *Curr Opin Neurol*, 16, 1–3.

64. Mizukoshi K, Watanabe Y, Shojaku H, Okubo J, Watanabe I (1988). Epidemiological studies on benign paroxysmal positional vertigo in Japan. *Acta Otolaryngol Suppl*, 447, 67–72.

65. Froehling DA, Silverstein MD, Mohr DN, Beatty CW, Offord KP, Ballard DJ (1991). Benign positional vertigo: incidence and prognosis in a population-based study in Olmsted County, Minnesota. *Mayo Clin Proc*, 66, 596–601.

66. Oghalai JS, Manolidis S, Barth JL, Stewart MG, Jenkins HA (2000). Unrecognized benign paroxysmal positional vertigo in elderly patients. *Otolaryngol Head Neck Surg*, 122, 630–4.

67. Zhao JG, Piccirillo JF, Spitznagel EL, Jr., Kallogjeri D, Goebel JA (2011). Predictive capability of historical data for diagnosis of dizziness. *Otol Neurotol*, 32(2), 284–90.

68. Baloh RW, Honrubia V, Jacobson K (1987). Benign positional vertigo. Clinical and oculographic features in 240 cases. *Neurology*, 37, 371–8.

69. Imai T, Ito M, Takeda N, *et al.* (2005). Natural course of the remission of vertigo in patients with benign paroxysmal positional vertigo. Neurology, 64, 920–1.

70. Chung KW, Park KN, Ko MH, *et al.* (2009). Incidence of horizontal canal benign paroxysmal positional vertigo as a function of the duration of symptoms. *Otol Neurotol*, 30(2), 202–5.

71. Brandt T, Huppert D, Hecht J, Karch C, Strupp M (2006). Benign paroxysmal positioning vertigo: A long-term follow-up (6–17 years) of 125 patients. *Acta Otolaryngol*, 126, 160–3.

72. Nunez RA, Cass SP, Furman JM (2000). Short- and long-term outcomes of canalith repositioning for benign paroxysmal positional vertigo. *Otolaryngol Head Neck Surg*, 122, 647–52.

73. Kansu L, Avci S, Yilmaz I, Ozluoglu LN (2010). Long-term follow-up of patients with posterior canal benign paroxysmal positional vertigo. *Acta Otolaryngol*, 130(9), 1009–12.

74. Gordon CR, Levite R, Joffe V, Gadoth N (2004). Is posttraumatic benign paroxysmal positional vertigo different from the idiopathic form? *Arch Neurol*, 61, 1590–3.

75. Karlberg M, Hall K, Quickert N, Hinson J, Halmagyi M (2000). What inner ear diseases cause benign paroxysmal positional vertigo? *Acta Otolaryngol*, 120, 380–5.

76. Katsarkas A (1999). Benign paroxysmal positional vertigo (BPPV): Idiopathic versus post-traumatic. *Acta Otolaryngol*, 119, 745–9.

77. Vibert D, Kompis M, Häusler R (2003). Benign paroxysmal positional vertigo in older women may be related to osteoporosis and osteopenia. *Ann Otol Rhinol Laryngol*, 112, 885–9.

78. Cohen HS, Kimball KT, Stewart MG (2004). Benign paroxysmal positional vertigo and comorbid conditions. *ORL J Otorhinolaryngol Relat Spec*, 66(1), 11–5.

79. Lopez-Escamez JA, Gamiz MJ, Fernandez-Perez A, Gomez-Finana M (2005). Long-term outcome and health-related quality of life in benign paroxysmal positional vertigo. *Eur Arch Otorhinolaryngol*, 262, 507–11.

80. Dieterich M, Brandt T (1999). Episodic vertigo related to migraine (90 cases): vestibular migraine? *J Neurol*, 246(10), 883–92.

81. Headache Classification Subcommittee of the International Headache Society (2004). The International Classification of Headache Disorders: 2nd edition. *Cephalalgia*, 24(Suppl), 9–160.

82. Cass SP, Furman JM, Ankerstjerne K, Balaban C, Yetiser S, Aydogan B (1997). Migraine-related vestibulopathy. *Ann Otol Rhinol Laryngol*, 106(3), 182–9.

83. Bisdorff A, Andree C, Vaillant M, Sandor PS (2010). Headache-associated dizziness in a headache population: prevalence and impact. *Cephalalgia*, 30(7), 815–20.

84. Neuhauser H, Lempert T (2004). Vertigo and dizziness related to migraine: a diagnostic challenge. *Cephalalgia*, 24(2), 83–91.

85. Jensen R, Stovner LJ (2008). Epidemiology and comorbidity of headache. *Lancet Neurol*, 7(4), 354–61.

86. Slater R (1979). Benign recurrent vertigo. *J Neurol Neurosurg Psychiatry*, 42(4), 363–7.

87. Cha YH, Lee H, Santell LS, Baloh RW (2009). Association of benign recurrent vertigo and migraine in 208 patients. *Cephalalgia*, 29(5), 550–5.

88. Salhofer S, Lieba-Samal D, Freydl E, Bartl S, Wiest G, Wober C (2010). Migraine and vertigo – a prospective diary study. *Cephalalgia*, 30(7), 821–8.

89. Hsu LC, Wang SJ, Fuh JL (2011). Prevalence and impact of migrainous vertigo in mid-life women: a community-based study. *Cephalalgia*, 31(1), 77–83.

90. Erbek SH, Erbek SS, Yilmaz I, *et al.* (2006). Vertigo in childhood: a clinical experience. *Int J Pediatr Otorhinolaryngol*, 70, 1547–54.

91. Neuhauser H, Radtke A, von Brevern M, Lempert T (2003). Zolmitriptan for treatment of migrainous vertigo: a pilot randomized placebo-controlled trial. *Neurology*, 60(5), 882–3.

92. Guilemany J-M, Martinez P, Prades E, Sanudo I, De Espana R, Cuchi A (2004). Clinical and epidemiological study of vertigo at an outpatient clinic. *Acta Otolaryngol*, 124, 49–52.

93. Hanley K, T OD (2002). Symptoms of vertigo in general practice: a prospective study of diagnosis. *Br J Gen Pract*, 52(483), 809–12.

94. Sekitani T, Imate Y, Noguchi T, Inokuma T (1993). Vestibular neuronitis: epidemiological survey by questionnaire in Japan. *Acta Otolaryngol*, 503, 9–12.

95. Huppert D, Strupp M, Theil D, Glaser M, Brandt T (2006). Low recurrence rate of vestibular neuritis: a long-term follow-up. *Neurology*, 67(10), 1870–1.

96. Mandala M, Santoro GP, Awrey J, Nuti D (2010). Vestibular neuritis: recurrence and incidence of secondary benign paroxysmal positional vertigo. *Acta Otolaryngol*, 130(5), 565–7.

97. Okinaka Y, Sektani T, Okazaki H, Miura M, Tahara T (1993). Progress of caloric response of vestibular neuronitis. *Acta Otolaryngol Suppl*, 503, 18–22.

98. Godemann F, Siefert K, Hantschke-Brüggemann M, Neu P, Seidl R, Ströhle A (2005). What accounts for vertigo one year after neuritis vestibularis – anxiety or a dysfunctional vestibular organ? *J Pychiatr Res*, 39, 529–34.

99. Godemann F, Linden M, Neu P, Heipp E, Dorr P (2004). A prospective study on the course of anxiety after vestibular neuronitis. *J Psychosom Res*, 56(3), 351–4.

100. Taborelli G, Melagrana A, D'Agostino R, Tarantino V, Calevo MG (2000). Vestibular neuronitis in children: study of medium and long term follow-up. *Int J Pediatr Otorhinolaryngol*, 54, 117–21.

101. Kotimäki J, Sorri M, Aantaa E, Nuutinen J (1999). Prevalence of Meniere Disease in Finland. *Laryngoscope*, 109, 748–53.

102. Wladislavosky-Waserman P, Facer GW, Mokri B, Kurland LT (1984). Meniere's disease: a 30-year epidemiologic and clinical study in Rochester, Mn, 1951–1980. *Laryngoscope*, 94, 1098–102.

103. Committee on Hearing and Equilibrium (1995). Committee on Hearing and Equilibrium guidelines for the diagnosis and evaluation of therapy in Meniere's disease. *Otolaryngol Head Neck Surg*, 113, 181–5.

104. Ballester M, Liard P, Vibert D, Häusler R (2002). Menière's disease in the elderly. *Otol Neurotol*, 23, 73–8.

105. Vrabec JT, Simon LM, Coker NJ (2007). Survey of Meniere's disease in a subspecialty referral practice. *Otolaryngol Head Neck Surg*, 137(2), 213–7.

106. Huppert D, Strupp M, Brandt T (2010). Long-term course of Meniere's disease revisited. *Acta Otolaryngol*, 130(6), 644–51.

107. Cha YH, Brodsky J, Ishiyama G, Sabatti C, Baloh RW (2007). The relevance of migraine in patients with Ménière's disease. *Acta Oto-Laryngologica*, 127(12), 1241–5.

108. Cha YH, Kane MJ, Baloh RW (2008). Familial clustering of migraine, episodic vertigo, and Ménière's disease. *Otol Neurotol*, 29, 93–6.

109. Derebery MJ, Berliner KI (2000). Prevalence of allergy in Meniere's disease. *Otolaryngol Head Neck Surg*, 123, 69–75.

110. Neuhauser HK (2007). Epidemiology of vertigo. *Curr Opin Neurol*, 20, 40–6.

CHAPTER 19

Vestibular Neuritis

Michael Strupp and Thomas Brandt

Clinical characteristics: signs and symptoms

Patient history

The main symptoms of acute unilateral vestibular deficit are violent rotatory vertigo, apparent movement of the visual surrounding (oscillopsia), gait and postural imbalance with a tendency to fall toward the side of the affected ear, as well as nausea and vomiting. All of these symptoms have an acute or subacute onset and last for many days or a few weeks. To make the diagnosis, you must first exclude the possibility of hearing disorders or—even more relevant—other neurological deficits, in particular those originating from the brainstem or cerebellum. Therefore, it is important to note that you have to explicitly ask the patient for symptoms that may arise from the inner ear, brainstem, or cerebellum (1). There are no typical antecedent signs or triggers, although some patients have occasional spells of vertigo a few days before (2). Since the patients' complaints are exacerbated by any movements of the head, they intuitively seek peace and quiet.

Clinical signs

Key signs and symptoms of vestibular neuritis are: 1) an acute/subacute onset of sustained rotational vertigo with pathological adjustments of the subjective visual vertical toward the affected ear; 2) peripheral vestibular spontaneous nystagmus with a torsional component toward the non-affected ear, which can be suppressed by visual fixation; 3) a pathological head-impulse test (3); 4) postural imbalance with falls toward the affected ear (positive Romberg test); and 5) nausea and vomiting (Figure 19.1) 4–6). Ocular motor evaluation reveals an incomplete ocular tilt reaction, apparent horizontal saccadic pursuit, and an increase of the intensity of the nystagmus when looking in the direction of the fast phase. All of these symptoms are secondary to the peripheral vestibular spontaneous nystagmus, which indicates a vestibular tone imbalance in the yaw (horizontal) and roll (torsional) planes between the two labyrinths.

Peripheral vestibular spontaneous nystagmus

The nystagmus in vestibular neuritis is horizontal due to the involvement of the horizontal semicircular canal. It has a torsional component due to involvement of the vertical superior canal (beating counterclockwise-left or clockwise-right from the patient's point of view) (7, 8). The three-dimensional features of the spontaneous nystagmus in vestibular neuritis, i.e. the horizontal, vertical, and torsional components as well as the dynamic deficit of the vestibulo-ocular reflex (VOR) of the horizontal, anterior, and posterior semicircular canals (see later), have been measured by means of the scleral-coil technique and analysed by vector analysis (7). These measurements support the earlier view (9) that vestibular neuritis is a partial rather than a complete unilateral vestibular lesion. It affects the superior division of the vestibular nerve (innervating the horizontal and anterior semicircular canals, the maculae of the utricle, and the anterosuperior part of the saccule), which has its own path and ganglion (10, 11). The inferior vestibular nerve (innervating the posterior semicircular canal and the posteroinferior part of the saccule) is spared (7). This has twofold implications: first, with respect to clinical findings, it explains why patients with vestibular neuritis can suffer from benign paroxysmal positioning nystagmus of the posterior canal (9, 12, 13); second, it explains the pathophysiology and aetiology of the disorder (see page 209). It rarely happens that only the inferior division of the vestibular nerve is affected which then causes inferior vestibular neuritis (14–16). In these patients the horizontal semicircular canal (with normal caloric irrigation) and anterior semicircular canal function normally, whereas the posterior canal and the saccule are impaired, as was demonstrated by the three-dimensional head-impulse test (14) and vestibular-evoked potentials (17).

Peripheral vestibular spontaneous nystagmus in vestibular neuritis is typically reduced in amplitude during fixation, because visual fixation suppresses the VOR. The error signal for the suppression is the retinal slip. This visual fixation suppression of the spontaneous nystagmus, however, is only possible if the relevant central structures in the brainstem and cerebellum are intact. On the other hand, the intensity of a peripheral vestibular spontaneous nystagmus is enhanced by eye closure (you can see

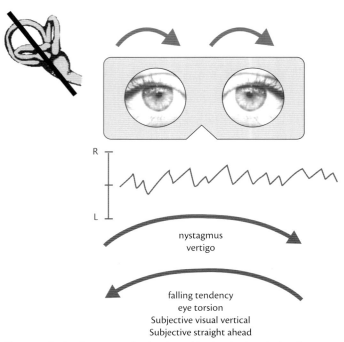

Fig. 19.1 Ocular signs, perception (vertigo, subjective visual vertical, and subjective straight ahead), and posture in the acute stage of right-sided vestibular neuritis. Spontaneous vestibular nystagmus is always horizontal-rotatory away from the side of the lesion (best observed with Frenzel glasses). The initial perception of apparent body motion (vertigo) is also directed away from the side of the lesion, whereas measurable destabilization (Romberg fall) is toward the side of the lesion. The latter is the compensatory vestibulospinal reaction to the apparent tilt.

the nystagmus when looking at the eyelids or even feel it when you touch the eyelids with your fingertips), Frenzel glasses (+16 dioptres), and during convergence. According to Alexander's

law, amplitude and slow-phase velocity are increased with gaze shifts in the direction of the fast phase, and decreased with gaze shifts in the direction of the slow phase of the nystagmus. This may mimic unilateral gaze-evoked nystagmus in a patient with moderate spontaneous nystagmus that is completely suppressed by visual fixation straight ahead, but it is still present when the gaze is directed toward the fast phase.

Head impulse test

A suspected diagnosis of vestibular neuritis is supported by demonstrating a unilateral deficit of the VOR by means of the head impulse test (3, 18–20). When the head is rapidly rotated toward the side with the lesion, the eyes move with the head and the patient has to make a compensatory re-fixation saccade. This indicates a dynamic unilateral high-frequency deficiency of the VOR which persists if the peripheral vestibular function does not recover. Since the diagnosis of a unilateral dynamic deficit of the VOR by the bedside head impulse test is not always reliable, a video head impulse test can be useful (21).

Incomplete ocular tilt reaction and the bucket test

An incomplete ocular tilt reaction with ocular torsion and perceived tilts of the subjective visual vertical occurs in most patients with vestibular neuritis (22). Nowadays a simple bedside device, the so-called bucket test (23), can be used to easily measure the subjective visual vertical, which is the most sensitive parameter for an acute lesion of the vestibular system (Figure 19.2).

Although reported in the older literature (24, 25), patients with vestibular neuritis do not have a skew deviation/vertical divergence. This typically occurs in vestibular pseudoneuritis (19) and can also be found in a complete de-afferentation, which occurs in zoster oticus (26). An ocular tilt reaction indicates a vestibular tone imbalance in the roll plane induced by involvement of the anterior semicircular canal or otolith function, or both.

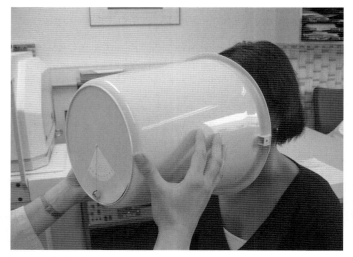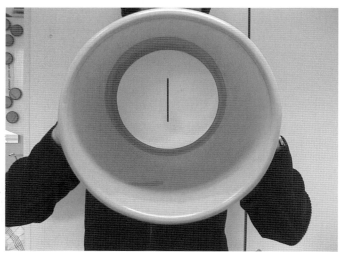

Fig. 19.2 The bucket test. An easy and reliable test to determine the subjective visual vertical. Patients sit upright looking into an opaque plastic bucket so that the bucket rim prevents any gravitational orientation clues. There is a dark, straight, diametric line on the bottom of the bucket, inside. On the bottom of the bucket, outside there is a perpendicular that originates from the centre of a quadrant divided into degrees with the zero line corresponding to the true vertical. To make measurements the examiner rotates the bucket clock- or counterclockwise to an end-position and then slowly rotates it back toward the zero degree position. Patients indicate the position, where they estimate the inside bottom line to be truly vertical by signalling stop. The examiner reads off the degrees on the outside scale. A total of ten repetitions are performed. An eye patch is used for monocular testing. From (23).

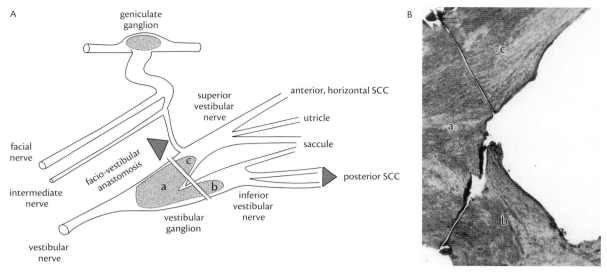

Fig. 19.3 (A) Schematic drawing of the vestibular and facial nerves, the facio-vestibular anastomosis, the geniculate ganglion, and different sections of the vestibular ganglion (a, stem; b, inferior portion; and c, superior portion). (B) Longitudinal cryosection of a human vestibular ganglion, in which the individual portions are separated. Using PCR HSV-1 DNA was found in about 60% of the examined human vestibular ganglia. Moreover, the double innervation of the posterior canal, which led to the preservation of its function during vestibular neuritis, is visible. From (42).

Laboratory examinations

Caloric testing

The principal diagnostic marker of vestibular neuritis is a peripheral vestibular deficit on the affected side. Caloric testing shows a hypo- or unresponsiveness of the tested and affected horizontal canal in vestibular neuritis. Since there is a large intersubject variability of the nystagmus induced by caloric irrigation and a small intraindividual variability of the response of the right and the left labyrinths in healthy subjects, 'Jongkees's formula for vestibular paresis' (27):

$$(((R30° + R44°) − (L30° + L44°))/ (R30° + R44° + L30° + L44°)) \times 100$$

should be used to determine its presence. In this formula, for instance, R30° is the mean peak slow-phase velocity during caloric irrigation with 30°C water. Vestibular paresis is usually defined as greater than 25% asymmetry between the two sides (28). This formula allows a direct comparison of the function of the horizontal semicircular canals of both labyrinths, which is important due to the large interindividual variability of caloric excitability.

Cervical and ocular vestibular-evoked myogenic potentials

In response to loud clicks, cervical vestibular-evoked myogenic potentials (cVEMP) can be recorded from the sternocleidomastoid muscles (29, 30). There is good evidence that cVEMPs originate in the medial (striola) area of the saccular macula (31). Cervical VEMP allow examination of the function of the saccule and, thereby, of the inferior vestibular nerve. VEMPs are preserved in at least two-thirds of the patients with vestibular neuritis (32, 33). This is because the inferior part of the vestibular nerve is spared in most patients (see later), and it supplies the posteroinferior part of the saccule and posterior canal.

Intense air-conducted sound as well as bone-conducted vibration (nowadays preferred with the so-called mini-shaker) can elicit ocular VEMPs (oVEMPs). In ten patients with vestibular neuritis and normal saccular and inferior vestibular nerve function, the oVEMP n10 amplitude was reduced or absent in response to air-conducted sound. This indicates the involvement of utricular receptors and thereby the crossed utriculo-ocular pathway (34).

Aetiology

There is good evidence that vestibular neuritis is caused by a viral inflammation; however, this has not yet been proven (35–37). The following arguments are presented in support of a viral aetiology. First, the vestibular nerve histopathology in cases of vestibular neuritis (38) is similar to that seen in single cases of herpes zoster oticus, when temporal bone histopathology was available. Second, an animal model of vestibular neuritis was developed by inoculating herpes simplex virus 1 (HSV-1) into the auricle of mice (39, 40). Third, HSV-1 DNA was repeatedly detected in about two-thirds of autopsied human vestibular ganglia by polymerase chain reaction (PCR) (41, 42) (Figure 19.3); furthermore, the 'latency associated transcript' was found in about 70% of human vestibular ganglia (43) as well as infiltration of CD8+ T cells (44). All these findings indicate that the vestibular ganglia like other cranial nerve ganglia are latently infected by HSV-1 (45–47). A similar aetiology is also assumed for Bell's palsy and strongly supported by the demonstration of HSV-1 DNA in the endoneural fluid of affected subjects (48).

If HSV-1 is the most likely candidate, it can be assumed to reside in a latent state in the vestibular ganglia, e.g. in the ganglionic nuclei as has been reported in other cranial nerves (19, 45, 49–53). Due to intercurrent factors, the virus suddenly replicates and induces inflammation and oedema, thereby causing secondary cell damage of the vestibular ganglion cells and axons in the bony canals. The canal of the superior vestibular nerve is longer and has more speculae (54), whereas the posterior semicircular canal is innervated by an additional anastomosis (55). This difference may explain why the posterior canal is often spared.

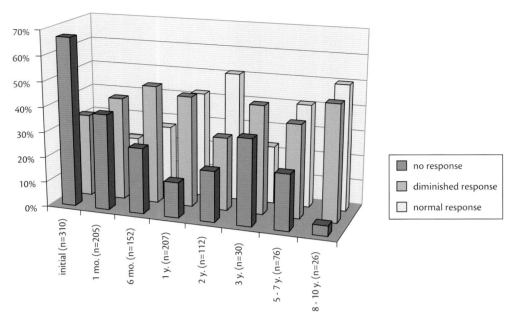

Fig. 19.4 Time course of average recovery of vestibular function after vestibular neuritis as measured by the nystagmus response to caloric irrigation on the basis of ten retrospective or prospective follow-up studies (for references see (69)). There is a tendency for recovery to increase over time. Most of the function that is regained takes place within the first month after onset.

Epidemiology, spontaneous course, recurrences, and complications

Epidemiology

Vestibular neuritis has an incidence of about 3.5 per 100,000 persons (56). It is the third most common cause of peripheral vestibular disorders in our neurological dizziness unit (benign paroxysmal positioning vertigo ranks first, Ménière's disease second). It accounts for about 7% of the patients (57). The usual age of onset is between 30–60 years (58), and age distribution plateaus between 40–50 years (56). There is no significant sexual difference.

Spontaneous recovery

The onset of the disease is usually sudden. Patients feel severely ill and prefer to stay immobilized in bed for about 1–3 days. After 5–7 days spontaneous nystagmus is largely suppressed by fixation in the primary position, although—depending on the severity of the canal palsy—it is still present for 2–3 weeks with Frenzel glasses and during lateral gaze directed away from the lesion. After recovery of peripheral vestibular function, spontaneous nystagmus transiently reverses its direction in some patients (recovery nystagmus), i.e. when the centrally compensated lesion regains function. Recovery nystagmus then reflects a tone imbalance secondary to compensation. Bechterew's phenomenon, a reversal of spontaneous nystagmus that occurs after contralateral labyrinthectomy in animals or humans (59, 60), is produced by a similar mechanism. After 1–6 weeks most of the patients feel symptom free, even during slow body movements, but actual recovery depends on if and how quickly functional restitution of the vestibular nerve occurs during 'central compensation' (61) and possibly on how much physical exercise the patient has done. Rapid head movements, however, may still cause slight oscillopsia of the visual scene and impaired balance for a second in those who do not regain normal

labyrinthine function. This explains why only 34 (57%) of 60 patients with vestibular neuritis reported complete relief from subjective symptoms at long-term follow-up (62), a figure that roughly corresponds to the 50–70% complete recovery rate of labyrinthine function assessed by caloric irrigation (62–64).

Numerous, mostly retrospective rather than prospective, studies have investigated the rate of complete or incomplete recovery of vestibular function as measured by the nystagmus response to caloric irrigation (57, 65). These studies are difficult to compare because of their different study design, the number of patients included, diagnostic criteria, definition of recovery, and duration of follow-up. This explains the great divergence in the numbers of complete or incomplete vestibular recovery following acute vestibular neuritis. The average recovery, which is based on ten studies (Figure 19.4), shows a tendency to functional improvement not only in the first few months but up to 10 years afterwards (57). Tests for ocular torsion, subjective visual vertical, and vestibular-evoked myogenic potentials revealed that otolith function appears to improve more rapidly than canal-related test abnormalities at the short-term follow-up (66).

Recurrence rate

In a long-term follow-up study (5.7–20.5 years, mean 9.8 years) on a total of 103 patients with vestibular neuritis, only two patients (1.9%) had developed a second vestibular neuritis 29–39 months after the first (67). It affected the contralateral ear in both patients and caused less severe, distressing vertigo and postural imbalance. In another study on 131 patients the recurrence was 10.7% (68).

Complications

In 10–15% of patients with vestibular neuritis a typical, benign paroxysmal positioning vertigo develops in the affected ear within a few weeks (9, 13, 68, 69). It is possible that the otoconia loosen

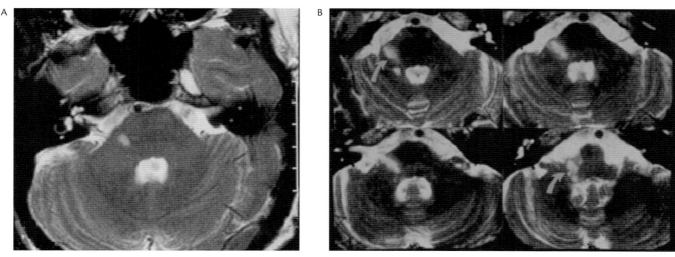

Fig. 19.5 Fascicular and nuclear lesion of the vestibular nerve due to an MS plaque (A) and vascular lesion (B), mimicking vestibular neuritis (T2-weighted MR images).

during the additional inflammation of the labyrinth (HSV-1 DNA was also found in the human labyrinth (70)), and this eventually results in canalolithiasis. Patients should be warned about this possible complication, because there are therapeutic liberatory manoeuvres that can quickly free them of their complaints. The second important complication is that vestibular neuritis can develop into a secondary phobic postural vertigo (71, 72). A recent study shows that the transition from vestibular neuritis to phobic postural vertigo can also be diagnosed by artificial neural network posturography (73). The traumatic experience of a persisting organic rotatory vertigo leads to fearful introspection, resulting in a somatoform, fluctuating, and persistent postural vertigo, which is reinforced in specific situations and culminates in a phobic behaviour of avoidance.

Differential diagnosis and other clinical problems

Topographically, dysfunctions or lesions in the brainstem and/or cerebellum (so-called vestibular pseudoneuritis) as well as other peripheral vestibular disorders may mimic vestibular neuritis. In other words: there is no pathognomonic test or sign for vestibular neuritis as a clinical entity (1, 18, 19, 74). In a strict sense, only an acute unilateral peripheral vestibular hypofunction with horizontal semicircular canal paresis can be diagnosed by the head-impulse test and caloric irrigation.

Central lesions mimicking vestibular neuritis

A lesion that occurs in a small area in the lateral medulla including the root entry zone of the vestibular nerve and the medial and superior vestibular nuclei may be confused with lesions of the peripheral vestibular nerve or labyrinths. We have seen several patients with multiple sclerosis who have pontomedullary plaques or small lacunar ischemia or infarctions in the territory of the anterior inferior cerebellar artery (AICA) (Figure 19.5) (75) at the root entry zone of the VIIIth nerve. This leads to 'fascicular nerve lesion', which mimics vestibular neuritis: 'vestibular pseudoneuritis'. A small lacunar infarction of the vestibular nuclei (76) or the dorsolateral pons (77) may also mimic vestibular neuritis.

The differential diagnosis between central and peripheral causes of unilateral vestibular loss is simple, if the patient has obvious additional brainstem signs. If this is not the case, differential diagnosis is indeed difficult. Therefore, in several studies the clinical signs to differentiate vestibular neuritis from central 'vestibular pseudoneuritis' in the acute situation were correlated, and the final diagnosis was assessed by neuroimaging (18, 19, 78, 79). None of the isolated signs (head impulse test, saccadic pursuit, gaze-evoked nystagmus, subjective visual vertical) is reliable. There are two exceptions: in most studies skew deviation or a normal head impulse test in a patient with acute onset of vertigo and nystagmus was a specific, but non-sensitive sign for vestibular pseudoneuritis (18, 19, 78). A combination of the different clinical signs (skew deviation, head impulse test, gaze-holding function, fixation versus peripheral vestibular spontaneous nystagmus, and smooth pursuit eye movements), however, increased the sensitivity and specificity to more than 90% (18, 19, 78, 79).

Cerebellar infarction may also mimic vestibular neuritis, if it occurs in the territory of the posterior inferior cerebellar artery (PICA; 80–83), especially if it is an isolated nodular infarction (84). It may also cause an incomplete ocular tilt reaction (85), in particular, if the dentate nucleus is involved (86). This could make the differential diagnosis even more difficult. Infarction in the territory of the anterior inferior cerebellar artery (AICA) may also mimic vestibular neuritis, but it is most often associated with AICA unilateral hearing loss (due to cochlear ischemia) and additional brainstem signs (88, 89). All in all, brainstem or cerebellar infarctions may cause isolated vertigo and a pathological Romberg sign, but clinical examination of eye movements and hearing will allow its differentiation from vestibular neuritis and vestibular pseudoneuritis.

Acute attacks of *vestibular migraine* (89, 90) may also mimic vestibular neuritis, because they may be associated with a rotatory vertigo and horizontal-torsional nystagmus. Accompanying symptoms and the course of the disease help to differentiate between the two entities.

Peripheral vestibular lesions

The differential diagnosis of peripheral labyrinthine and vestibular nerve disorders mimicking vestibular neuritis includes numerous

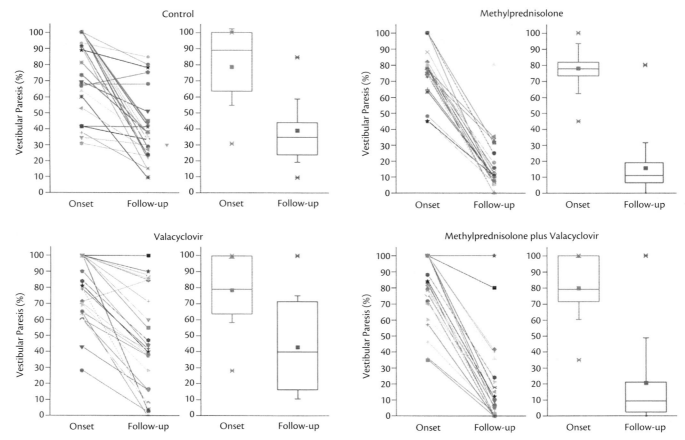

Fig. 19.6 (Also see Colour plate 12.) Unilateral vestibular failure within 3 days after symptom onset and after 12 months. Vestibular function was determined by caloric irrigation, using the 'vestibular paresis formula' (which allows a direct comparison of the function of both labyrinths) for each patient in the placebo (upper left), methylprednisolone (upper right), valacyclovir (lower right), and methylprednisolone plus valacyclovir (lower left) groups. Also shown are box plot charts for each group with the mean (■) ± standard deviation (SD), and 25% and 75% percentile (box plot) as well as the 1% and 99% range (x). A clinically relevant vestibular paresis was defined as greater than 25% asymmetry between the right-sided and the left-sided responses (28). Follow-up examination showed that vestibular function improved in all four groups: in the placebo group from 78.9 ± 24.0 (mean ± SD) to 39.0 ± 19.9, in the methylprednisolone group from 78.7 ± 15.8 to 15.4 ± 16.2, in the valacyclovir group from 78.4 ± 20.0 to 42.7 ± 32.3, and in the methylprednisolone plus valacyclovir group from 78.6 ± 21.1 to 20.4 ± 28.4. Analysis of variance revealed that methylprednisolone and methylprednisolone plus valacyclovir caused significantly more improvement than placebo or valacyclovir alone. The combination of both was not superior to steroid monotherapy. From (96).

rare conditions. Nevertheless, extensive laboratory examinations, lumbar puncture, and computed tomography/magnetic resonance imaging (MRI) are not part of the routine diagnostics of vestibular neuritis for two reasons: 1) the rareness of these disorders and 2) typical additional signs and symptoms indicative of other disorders. An initial monosymptomatic vertigo attack in Ménière's disease or a short attack in *vestibular paroxysmia* (91, 92) can be confused with vestibular neuritis in a patient admitted to the hospital in an acute stage. The shortness of the attack and the patient's rapid recovery, however, allow differentiation. During the course of the disease almost all patients with Ménière's disease develop hypoacusis, tinnitus, or aural fullness in the affected ear, which also allows differentiation. An initially burning pain and blisters as well as hearing disorders and facial paresis are typical for herpes zoster oticus (Ramsay–Hunt syndrome) (in such cases acyclovir or valacyclovir is indicated). It has to be pointed out that there may be a skew deviation in herpes zoster oticus due to the complete unilateral peripheral vestibular deficit, i.e. of the superior and inferior parts of the vestibular nerve (26) and—contrary to vestibular neuritis—a contrast enhancement of the VIIIth cranial nerve. Cogan

syndrome (often overlooked) is a severe autoimmune disease accompanied by interstitial keratitis and audiovestibular symptoms (hearing disorders are very prominent). It occurs most often in young adults and responds, in part only temporarily, to the very early administration of high doses of corticoids (1000 mg per day for 3–5 days, then slowly tapered off) or—like other autoimmune diseases of the inner ear—to a subsequent combination of steroids and cyclophosphamide.

Rare variants of vestibular neuritis have been described, e.g. inferior vestibular neuritis (here there is a selective deficit of the posterior canal combined with sparing of the lateral and anterior canals) (14, 15) and a form in which a dysfunction of the posterior canal is combined with one of the cochlea. The latter probably does not have a viral but rather a vascular aetiology, since both structures have a common area of vascular supply.

Vestibular schwannomas, which arise in the myelin sheaths of the vestibular part of the VIIIth nerve, often cause only vertigo, a tendency to fall, and nystagmus if the pontomedullary brainstem and the flocculus are compressed, and the increasing peripheral tone difference can no longer be neutralized by central compensation.

The main symptom is a slowly progressive unilateral reduction of hearing without any identifiable otological cause. This is combined with a caloric hypoexcitability or non-excitability. There is rarely also a loss of hearing as well as recurrent attacks of vertigo in cases of a purely intracanalicular dilatation, which can be confirmed by MRI and treated early by microsurgery or with the 'gamma knife'.

Management

The management of vestibular neuritis involves: 1) symptomatic treatment with antivertiginous drugs (e.g. dimenhydrinate, scopolamine, or in severe cases benzodiazepines) to attenuate vertigo, dizziness, and nausea/vomiting; 2) 'causal' treatment with corticosteroids to improve recovery of peripheral vestibular function; and 3) physical therapy (vestibular exercises and balance training) to improve central vestibular compensation (93).

Symptomatic treatment

During the first 1–3 days, when nausea is pronounced, vestibular sedatives such as antihistamine dimenhydrinate (50–100 mg every 6 h) or the anticholinergic scopolamine can be administered. Their major side effect is general sedation. Transdermal application of scopolamine hydrobromide avoids some of the side effects of the conventional means of administration. The most probable sites of primary action are the synapses of the vestibular nuclei, which exhibit a reduced discharge and diminished neural reaction to body rotation. These drugs should not be given for more than 3 days, because they evidently prolong the time required to achieve central compensation (94, 95).

Causal treatment

Based on the assumption that vestibular neuritis is caused by the reactivation of a latent HSV-1 infection, a prospective, randomized, double-blind trial was conducted to determine whether steroids, antiviral agents, or a combination of the two might improve outcome in vestibular neuritis (96). This study with a placebo, methylprednisolone, valacyclovir, and methylprednisolone plus valacyclovir groups out of a total 114 patients showed that monotherapy with steroids suffices to significantly improve the peripheral vestibular function of patients with vestibular neuritis; there was no evidence for synergy between methylprednisolone and valacyclovir (Figure 19.6) (96). Glucocorticoids (6-methylprednisolone) should be given within 3 days after symptom onset and for 3 weeks (initially 100 mg/day and then tapered off by 20 mg every 3 days). These findings are supported by a more recent study (97). It must, however, be mentioned that due to the few appropriate studies, treatment with steroids is so far not generally recommended (98). As in Bell's palsy, the benefit of steroids might be due to their anti-inflammatory effects, which reduce the swelling and cause a mechanical compression of the vestibular nerve within the temporal bone.

Physical therapy

A gradual programme of physical exercise under the supervision of a physiotherapist improves the central vestibular compensation of a peripheral deficit. First, static stabilization is concentrated on, and then dynamic exercises are done for balance control and gaze stabilization during eye–head–body movements. It is important that the degree of difficulty of exercises for equilibrium and balance be successively increased above normal levels, both with and without visual stabilization. The efficacy of physiotherapy in improving central vestibulospinal compensation in patients with vestibular neuritis has been proven in a prospective, randomized, and controlled clinical study (99) and confirmed in a meta-analysis (100).

Conclusions

Vestibular neuritis is the third most frequently occurring peripheral vestibular disorder. Its diagnosis is based on the patient history (acute onset of rotatory vertigo) and clinical bedside examination (to exclude any central vestibular, ocular motor, or cerebellar dysfunction) as well as caloric irrigation, which shows a hypo- or unresponsiveness of the affected horizontal canal. The use of three-dimensional recordings of eye movements with a vector analysis of the peripheral vestibular spontaneous nystagmus and head-impulse test in combination with cVEMPs and oVEMPs is helpful for identifying the different parts of the vestibular nerve affected (it is most often the superior vestibular nerve which then affects the horizontal and anterior semicircular canals and utricles). There is good evidence that vestibular neuritis is caused by the reactivation of a latent HSV-1 infection, although further work still has to be done. This is also true for its treatment, because there is only limited evidence so far that the outcome can be improved by the early administration of corticosteroids.

References

1. Mandala M, Nuti D, Broman AT, Zee DS (2008). Effectiveness of careful bedside examination in assessment, diagnosis, and prognosis of vestibular neuritis. *Arch Otolaryngol Head Neck Surg*, 134, 164–9.
2. Lee H, Kim BK, Park HJ, Koo JW, Kim JS (2009). Prodromal dizziness in vestibular neuritis: frequency and clinical implication. *J Neurol Neurosurg Psychiatry*, 80, 355–6.
3. Halmagyi GM, Curthoys IS (1988). A clinical sign of canal paresis. *Arch Neurol*, 45, 737–9.
4. Baloh RW (2003). Clinical practice. Vestibular neuritis. *N Engl J Med*, 348, 1027–32.
5. Strupp M, Brandt T (2009). Vestibular neuritis. *Semin Neurol*, 29, 509–19.
6. Brandt T, Dieterich M, Strupp M (2012). *Vertigo and dizziness—common complaints* (2nd ed). London: Springer.
7. Fetter M, Dichgans J (1996). Vestibular neuritis spares the inferior division of the vestibular nerve. *Brain*, 119, 755–63.
8. Hirvonen TP, Aalto H (2009). Three-dimensional video-oculography in patients with vestibular neuritis. *Acta Otolaryngol*, 129, 1400–3.
9. Büchele W, Brandt T (1988). Vestibular neuritis, a horizontal semicircular canal paresis? *Adv Otorhinolaryngol*, 42, 157–61.
10. Lorente de Nó R (1933). Vestibulo-ocular reflex arc. *Arch Neurol Psychiat*, 30, 245–91.
11. Sando I, Black FO, Hemenway WG (1972). Spatial distribution of vestibular nerve in internal auditory canal. *Ann Otol*, 81, 305–19.
12. Mandala M, Santoro GP, Awrey J, Nuti D (2010). Vestibular neuritis: recurrence and incidence of secondary benign paroxysmal positional vertigo. *Acta Otolaryngol*, 130, 565–7.
13. Lee NH, Ban JH, Lee KC, Kim SM (2010). Benign paroxysmal positional vertigo secondary to inner ear disease. *Otolaryngol Head Neck Surg*, 143, 413–17.
14. Halmagyi GM, Aw ST, Karlberg M, Curthoys IS, Todd MJ (2002). Inferior vestibular neuritis. *Ann N Y Acad Sci*, 956, 306–13.
15. Zhang D, Fan Z, Han Y, Yu G, Wang H (2010). Inferior vestibular neuritis: a novel subtype of vestibular neuritis. *J Laryngol Otol*, 124, 477–81.

16. Monstad P, Okstad S, Mygland A (2006). Inferior vestibular neuritis: 3 cases with clinical features of acute vestibular neuritis, normal calorics but indications of saccular failure. *BMC Neurol*, 6, 45.

17. Lin CM, Young YH (2011). Identifying the affected branches of vestibular nerve in vestibular neuritis. *Acta Otolaryngol*, 131, 921–8.

18. Newman-Toker DE, Kattah JC, Alvernia JE, Wang DZ (2008). Normal head impulse test differentiates acute cerebellar strokes from vestibular neuritis. *Neurology*, 70, 2378–85.

19. Cnyrim CD, Newman-Toker D, Karch C, Brandt T, Strupp M (2008). Bedside differentiation of vestibular neuritis from central 'vestibular pseudoneuritis'. *J Neurol Neurosurg Psychiatry*, 79, 458–60.

20. Chen L, Lee W, Chambers BR, Dewey HM (2011). Diagnostic accuracy of acute vestibular syndrome at the bedside in a stroke unit. *J Neurol*, 258, 855–61.

21. MacDougall HG, Weber KP, McGarvie LA, Halmagyi GM, Curthoys IS (2009). The video head impulse test: diagnostic accuracy in peripheral vestibulopathy. *Neurology*, 73, 1134–41.

22. Böhmer A, Rickenmann J (1995). The subjective visual vertical as a clinical parameter of vestibular function in peripheral vestibular diseases. *J Vestib Res*, 5, 35–45.

23. Zwergal A, Rettinger N, Frenzel C, Frisen L, Brandt T, Strupp M (2009). A bucket of static vestibular function. *Neurology*, 72, 1689–92.

24. Safran AB, Vibert D, Issoua D, Hausler R (1994). Skew deviation after vestibular neuritis. *Am J Ophthalmol*, 118, 238–45.

25. Vibert D, Hausler R, Safran AB, Koerner F (1996). Diplopia from skew deviation in unilateral peripheral vestibular lesions. *Acta Otolaryngol (Stockh)*, 116, 170–6.

26. Arbusow V, Dieterich M, Strupp M, Dreher V, Jäger L, Brandt T (1998). Herpes zoster neuritis involving superior and inferior parts of the vestibular nerve causes ocular tilt reaction. *Neuro-Ophthalmol*, 19, 17–22.

27. Jongkees LB, Maas J, Philipszoon A (1962). Clinical electronystagmography: a detailed study of electronystagmography in 341 patients with vertigo. *Pract Otorhinolaryngol Basel*, 24, 65–93.

28. Honrubia V (1994). Quantitative vestibular function tests and the clinical examination. In Herdman SJ (Ed) *Vestibular rehabilitation*, pp. 113–64. Philadelphia, PA: FA Davis.

29. Murofushi T, Halmagyi GM, Yavor RA, Colebatch JG (1996). Absent vestibular evoked myogenic potentials in vestibular neurolabyrinthitis. An indicator of inferior vestibular nerve involvement? *Arch Otolaryngol Head Neck Surg*, 122, 845–8.

30. Colebatch JG, Halmagyi GM, Skuse NF (2000). Myogenic potentials generated by a click-evoked vestibulocollic reflex. *J Neurol Neurosurg Psychiatry*, 57, 190–7.

31. Murofushi T, Curthoys IS, Topple AN, Colebatch JG, Halmagyi GM (2000). Responses of guinea pig primary vestibular neurons to clicks. *Exp Brain Res*, 103, 174–8.

32. Colebatch JG (2000). Vestibular evoked potentials. *Curr Opin Neurol*, 14, 21–6.

33. Shin BS, Oh SY, Kim JS, *et al.* (2012). Cervical and ocular vestibular-evoked myogenic potentials in acute vestibular neuritis. *Clin Neurophysiol*, 123, 369–75.

34. Curthoys IS, Iwasaki S, Chihara Y, Ushio M, McGarvie LA, Burgess AM (2011). The ocular vestibular-evoked myogenic potential to air-conducted sound; probable superior vestibular nerve origin. *Clin Neurophysiol*, 122, 611–16.

35. Nadol JB, Jr (1995). Vestibular neuritis. *Otolaryngol Head Neck Surg*, 112, 162–72.

36. Brandt T (1999). *Vertigo; Its Multisensory Syndromes* (2nd ed). London: Springer.

37. Baloh RW (2003). Clinical practice. Vestibular neuritis. *N Engl J Med*, 348, 1027–32.

38. Schuknecht HF, Kitamura K (1981). Vestibular neuritis. *Ann Otol*, 90(Suppl. 78), 1–19.

39. Hirata Y, Gyo K, Yanagihara N (1995). Herpetic vestibular neuritis: an experimental study. *Acta Otolaryngol (Stockh) Suppl*, 519, 93–6.

40. Esaki S, Goshima F, Kimura H, *et al.* (2011). Auditory and vestibular defects induced by experimental labyrinthitis following herpes simplex virus in mice. *Acta Otolaryngol*, 131, 684–91.

41. Furuta Y, Takasu T, Fukuda S, Inuyama Y, Sato KC, Nagashima K (1993). Latent herpes simplex virus type 1 in human vestibular ganglia. *Acta Otolaryngol (Stockh) Suppl*, 503, 85–9.

42. Arbusow V, Schulz P, Strupp M, *et al.* (1999). Distribution of herpes simplex virus type 1 in human geniculate and vestibular ganglia: implications for vestibular neuritis. *Ann Neurol*, 46, 416–19.

43. Theil D, Derfuss T, Strupp M, Gilden DH, Arbusow V, Brandt T (2002). Cranial nerve palsies: herpes simplex virus type 1 and varizella-zoster virus latency. *Ann Neurol*, 51, 273–4.

44. Arbusow V, Derfuss T, Held K, *et al.* (2010). Latency of herpes simplex virus type-1 in human geniculate and vestibular ganglia is associated with infiltration of CD8+ T cells. *J Med Virol*, 82, 1917–20.

45. Theil D, Arbusow V, Derfuss T, *et al.* (2001). Prevalence of HSV-1 LAT in human trigeminal, geniculate, and vestibular ganglia and its implication for cranial nerve syndromes. *Brain Pathol*, 11, 408–13.

46. Nahmias AJ, Roizman B (1973). Infection with herpes-simplex viruses 1 and 2. II. *N Engl J Med*, 289, 719–25.

47. Theil D, Derfuss T, Paripovic I, *et al.* (2003). Latent herpesvirus infection in human trigeminal ganglia causes chronic immune response. *Am J Pathol*, 163, 2179–84.

48. Murakami S, Mizobuchi M, Nakashiro Y, Doi T, Hato N, Yanagihara N (1996). Bell palsy and herpes simplex virus: identification of viral DNA in endoneurial fluid and muscle. *Ann Intern Med*, 124, 27–30.

49. Hüfner K, Arbusow V, Himmelein S, *et al.* (2007). The prevalence of human herpesvirus 6 in human sensory ganglia and its co-occurrence with alpha-herpesviruses. *J Neurovirol*, 13, 462–7.

50. Theil D, Horn AK, Derfuss T, Strupp M, Arbusow V, Brandt T (2004). Prevalence and distribution of HSV-1, VZV, and HHV-6 in human cranial nerve nuclei III, IV, VI, VII, and XII. *J Med Virol*, 74, 102–6.

51. Hufner K, Horn A, Derfuss T, *et al.* (2009). Fewer latent herpes simplex virus type 1 and cytotoxic T cells occur in the ophthalmic division than in the maxillary and mandibular divisions of the human trigeminal ganglion and nerve. *J Virol*, 83, 3696–703.

52. Derfuss T, Segerer S, Herberger S, *et al.* (2007). Presence of HSV-1 immediate early genes and clonally expanded t-cells with a memory effector phenotype in human trigeminal ganglia. *Brain Pathol*, 17, 389–98.

53. Hufner K, Derfuss T, Herberger S, *et al.* (2006). Latency of alpha-herpes viruses is accompanied by a chronic inflammation in human trigeminal ganglia but not in dorsal root ganglia. *J Neuropathol Exp Neurol*, 65,1022–30.

54. Gianoli G, Goebel J, Mowry S, Poomipannit P (2005). Anatomic differences in the lateral vestibular nerve channels and their implications in vestibular neuritis. *Otol Neurotol*, 26, 489–94.

55. Arbusow V, Theil D, Schulz P, *et al.* (2003). Distribution of HSV-1 in human geniculate and vestibular ganglia: Implications for vestibular neuritis. *Ann N Y Acad Sci*, 1004, 409–13.

56. Sekitani T, Imate Y, Noguchi T, Inokuma T (1993). Vestibular neuronitis: epidemiological survey by questionnaire in Japan. *Acta Otolaryngol (Stockh) Suppl*, 503, 9–12.

57. Brandt T, Huppert T, Hufner K, Zingler VC, Dieterich M, Strupp M (2010). Long-term course and relapses of vestibular and balance disorders. *Restor Neurol Neurosci*, 28, 69–82.

58. Depondt M (1973). Vestibular neuronitis. Vestibular paralysis with special characteristics. *Acta Otorhinolaryngol Belg*, 27, 323–59.

59. Katsarkas A, Galiana HL (1984). Bechterew's phenomenon in humans. A new explanation. *Acta Otolaryngol Suppl Stockh*, 406, 95–100.

60. Zee DS, Preziosi TJ, Proctor LR (1982). Bechterew's phenomenon in a human patient [letter]. *Ann Neurol*, 12, 495–6.

61. Brandt T, Strupp M, Arbusow V, Dieringer N (1997). Plasticity of the vestibular system: central compensation and sensory substitution for vestibular deficits. *Adv Neurol*, 73, 297–309.

62. Okinaka Y, Sekitani T, Okazaki H, Miura M, Tahara T (1993). Progress of caloric response of vestibular neuronitis. *Acta Otolaryngol (Stockh) Suppl*, 503, 18–22.

63. Meran A, Pfaltz CR (1975). The acute vestibular paralysis. *Arch Otorhinolaryngol*, 209, 229–44.

64. Ohbayashi S, Oda M, Yamamoto M, *et al.* (1993). Recovery of the vestibular function after vestibular neuronitis. *Acta Otolaryngol (Stockh) Suppl*, 503, 31–4.

65. Halmagyi GM, Weber KP, Curthoys IS (2010). Vestibular function after acute vestibular neuritis. *Restor Neurol Neurosci*, 28, 37–46.

66. Kim HA, Hong JH, Lee H, *et al.* (2008). Otolith dysfunction in vestibular neuritis: recovery pattern and a predictor of symptom recovery. *Neurology*, 70, 449–53.

67. Huppert D, Strupp M, Theil D, Glaser M, Brandt T (2006). Low recurrence rate of vestibular neuritis: a long-term follow-up. *Neurology*, 67, 1870–1.

68. Kim YH, Kim KS, Kim KJ, Choi H, Choi JS, Hwang IK (2011). Recurrence of vertigo in patients with vestibular neuritis. *Acta Otolaryngol*, 131, 1172–7.

69. Brandt T, Huppert T, Hüfner K, Zingler VC, Dieterich M, Strupp M (2010). Long-term course and relapses of vestibular and balance disorders. *Restor Neurol Neurosci*, 28, 69–82.

70. Arbusow V, Theil D, Strupp M, Mascolo A, Brandt T (2000). HSV-1 not only in human vestibular ganglia but also in the vestibular labyrinth. *Audiol Neurootol*, 6, 259–62.

71. Brandt T, Dieterich M (1986). Phobischer Attacken-Schwankschwindel, ein neues Syndrom. *M nch Med Wochenschr*, 128, 247–50.

72. Brandt T (1996). Phobic postural vertigo. *Neurology*, 46, 1515–19.

73. Brandt T, Strupp M, Novozhilov S, Krafczyk S (2011). Artificial neural network posturography detects the transition of vestibular neuritis to phobic postural vertigo. *J Neurol*, 259, 182–4.

74. Goddard JC, Fayad JN (2011). Vestibular neuritis. *Otolaryngol Clin North Am*, 44, 361–5.

75. Thomke F, Hopf HC (1999). Pontine lesions mimicking acute peripheral vestibulopathy. *J Neurol Neurosurg Psychiatry*, 66, 340–9.

76. Kim HA, Lee H (2010). Isolated vestibular nucleus infarction mimicking acute peripheral vestibulopathy. *Stroke*, 41, 1558–60.

77. Chang TP, Wu YC (2010). A tiny infarct on the dorsolateral pons mimicking vestibular neuritis. *Laryngoscope*, 120, 2336–8.

78. Kattah JC, Talkad AV, Wang DZ, Hsieh YH, Newman-Toker DE (2009). HINTS to diagnose stroke in the acute vestibular syndrome: three-step bedside oculomotor examination more sensitive than early MRI diffusion-weighted imaging. *Stroke*, 40, 3504–10.

79. Chen L, Lee W, Chambers BR, Dewey HM (2011). Diagnostic accuracy of acute vestibular syndrome at the bedside in a stroke unit. *J Neurol*, 258, 855–61.

80. Duncan GW, Parker SW, Fisher CM (1975). Acute cerebellar infarction in the PICA territory. *Arch Neurol*, 32, 364–8.

81. Huang CY, Yu YL (1985). Small cerebellar strokes may mimic labyrinthine lesions. *J Neurol Neurosurg Psychiatry*, 48, 263–5.

82. Magnusson M, Norrving B (1991). Cerebellar infarctions as the cause of 'vestibular neuritis'. *Acta Otolaryngol (Stockh) Suppl*, 481, 258–9.

83. Magnusson M, Norrving B (1993). Cerebellar infarctions and 'vestibular neuritis'. *Acta Otolaryngol Suppl Stockh*, 503, 64–6.

84. Moon IS, Kim JS, Choi KD, *et al.* (2009). Isolated nodular infarction. *Stroke*, 40, 487–91.

85. Mossman S, Halmagyi GM (2000). Partial ocular tilt reaction due to unilateral cerebellar lesion. *Neurology*, 49, 491–3.

86. Baier B, Bense S, Dieterich M (2008). Are signs of ocular tilt reaction in patients with cerebellar lesions mediated by the dentate nucleus? *Brain*, 131, 1445–54.

87. Lee H, Sohn SI, Jung DK, *et al.* (2002). Sudden deafness and anterior inferior cerebellar artery infarction. *Stroke*, 33, 2807–12.

88. Lee H, Sohn SI, Cho YW, *et al.* (2006). Cerebellar infarction presenting isolated vertigo: frequency and vascular topographical patterns. *Neurology*, 67, 1178–83.

89. Strupp M, Versino M, Brandt T (2010). Vestibular migraine. *Handb Clin Neurol*, 97, 755–71.

90. Dieterich M, Brandt T (1999). Episodic vertigo related to migraine (90 cases): vestibular migraine? *J Neurol*, 246, 883–92.

91. Hufner K, Barresi D, Glaser M, *et al.* (2008). Vestibular paroxysmia: diagnostic features and medical treatment. *Neurology*, 71, 1006–14.

92. Brandt T, Dieterich M (1994). VIIIth nerve vascular compression syndrome: vestibular paroxysmia. *Baillieres Clin Neurol*, 3, 565–75.

93. Walker MF (2009). Treatment of vestibular neuritis. *Curr Treat Options Neurol*, 11, 41–5.

94. Zee DS (1985). Perspectives on the pharmacotherapy of vertigo. *Arch Otolaryngol*, 111, 609–12.

95. Curthoys IS, Halmagyi GM (2000). Vestibular compensation: A review of the oculomotor, neural, and clinical consequences of unilateral vestibular loss. *J Vest Res Equilib Orientat*, 5, 67–107.

96. Strupp M, Zingler VC, Arbusow V, *et al.* (2004). Methylprednisolone, valacyclovir, or the combination for vestibular neuritis. *N Engl J Med*, 351, 354–61.

97. Karlberg ML, Magnusson M (2011). Treatment of acute vestibular neuronitis with glucocorticoids. *Otol Neurotol*, 32;1140–43.

98. Fishman JM, Burgess C, Waddell A (2011). Corticosteroids for the treatment of idiopathic acute vestibular dysfunction (vestibular neuritis). *Cochrane Database Syst Rev*, CD008607.

99. Strupp M, Arbusow V, Maag KP, Gall C, Brandt T (1998). Vestibular exercises improve central vestibulospinal compensation after vestibular neuritis. *Neurology*, 51, 838–44.

100. Hillier SL, McDonnell M (2011). Vestibular rehabilitation for unilateral peripheral vestibular dysfunction. *Cochrane Database Syst Rev*, 2, CD005397.

CHAPTER 20

Positional Vertigo and Benign Paroxysmal Positional Vertigo

Daniele Nuti and David S. Zee

Benign paroxysmal positional vertigo (BPPV) is caused by the unwanted stimulation of the vestibular receptors within the semicircular canals. In 1969, H. F. Schucknecht (1) proposed the term 'cupulolithiasis', and hypothesized that the disease was caused by otoconia that had become detached from the utricular macula and then migrated to and became fixed upon the cupula of the posterior semicircular canal (PC). The cupulolithiasis hypothesis is still tenable for some patients with BPPV, but in most canalolithiasis, in which the dislodged otoconia are free floating within the posterior semicircular canals, is the better explanation (2). Both the posterior and the lateral canal (LC) can cause BPPV, with a predominance of the former. BPPV arising from the anterior canal (AC) may also be possible, but it is harder to envision how otoconia get into or stay in the canal because of its vertical and superior orientation within the labyrinth.

Paroxysmal positional nystagmus (PPN) is the pathognomonic sign of BPPV. In most cases its features are easily explained by an excitation/inhibition of the vestibular receptors in the ampulla following an inappropriate flow of endolymph related to the aberrant otoconia within the semicircular canal.

The therapy of the most common causes of BPPV, canalolithiasis of the PC and of the LC, is a physical manoeuvre that moves (repositions) the otoconia out of the canals. Results are generally satisfactory for both the patient and the doctor. Cupulolithiasis and atypical forms, such as downbeat positional nystagmus, are more refractory to physical therapy treatment.

Despite the growing understanding of the disease, many unresolved points remain. For example, why are some patients particularly prone to recurrences? Why are women more frequently affected than men? Why is the right PC more affected than the left one? How often is downbeat positional nystagmus of peripheral origin due to involvement of the AC?

Epidemiology

The incidence and prevalence of BPPV are underestimated due to lack of recognition by primary care physicians though well-conducted epidemiological studies are lacking (3). This lack of knowledge among general practitioners converts what should be a 'low-cost' easily diagnosed and treatable condition into an expensive evaluation with unnecessary laboratory testing, imaging, and medications. In 2007 von Brevern et al. published epidemiological data based upon a German representative neuro-otological survey (4). The lifetime prevalence was estimated as 2.4% and the incidence 0.6% per year. This means that in Germany about one million people are affected by BPPV every year. The 1-year prevalence of BPPV in patients older than 60 years is almost seven times higher than patients under 40. In this survey the diagnosis was based on the neuro-otological interview, not on diagnostic manoeuvres, but the estimates were conservative since the diagnostic criteria were based mainly on specificity rather than sensitivity. BPPV is the most common cause of vertigo seen in neuro-otological clinics (5, 6), accounting for about 20–30% of diagnoses. Women are more affected than men by about 2:1 (7), which could also be related to the higher incidence of migraine in women as there is an association between migraine and BPPV (8). The PC is usually responsible for BPPV. In a large group of patients, more than 70% presented with the typical clinical features of unilateral PC-BPPV. The right canal is more often involved than the left, with a ratio of 1.5:1, perhaps related to the habit of most people sleeping on the right side (9). Bilateral involvement of the posterior canal affects 7.5% of patients, and almost 90% of these are post-traumatic. LC-BPPV accounts for about 17% of all BPPV patients, with no difference in gender or on which side is involved. About 80% of patient with lateral canal BPPV present with the geotropic form (beating toward the ground) and 20% with the apogeotropic form (beating away from the ground). In about 5% of patients, PPN is atypical (7). Once diseases of the central nervous system are excluded, atypical forms suggest an unusual location of the canaliths in the labyrinth (common crus, anterior canal), simultaneous involvement of the posterior and lateral canals, or cupulolithiasis, in which the otoliths adhere to the cupula.

Aetiology and pathogenesis

While we understand the basic pathogenesis of the symptoms and signs of BPPV, little is known about the primary (underlying) causes of the disease in most patients.

Particles of different sizes have been observed inside the PCs during surgery for patients affected by BPPV (10, 11). The particles are calcium carbonate crystals, similar to the normal otoliths attached to the utricular macula. There is also evidence that dislodged otoconia are common in all the semicircular canals, both within the lumen and on the cupulae, in asymptomatic patients (12). It is likely that otoconial debris enters the semicircular canals and, once inside, they move in the endolymph when the attitude of the head is changed relative to gravity. But only when a critical mass is reached do they alter the endolymphatic pressure enough to displace the cupula. According to the canalolithiasis theory, the debris can fall towards or away from the ampulla, creating ampullopetal or ampullofugal deflection of the cupula by a pump or suction mechanism, or by hydrodynamic drag. Otoconial particles may also adhere to the cupula rendering it sensitive to gravitational forces (cupulolithiasis). It is not possible to know if otoconia are attached to the cupula on the side of the vestibule or on the side of the long arm of the canal. Probably both locations are possible. In this regard a 'chronic' canalolithiasis within the short arm of the PC (utricular side) has been proposed for positional vertigo without positional nystagmus (13). When detached from the otolithic membrane, otoconia should eventually dissolve in the endolymphatic fluid and the concentration of calcium of the endolymph may be important in this clearing action (14).

As previously mentioned, everyone probably has free-floating otoconia in the utricular endolymph, especially in older people. The syndrome is triggered when the head of the patient is positioned such that the debris can enter the semicircular canals. The posterior canal is by far the most commonly affected because of its anatomical position. When the patient is lying supine the common crus is lower than the utricle, and free otoconia can enter the non-ampulla orifice of the PC. Once in the canal, the otolithic debris moves under the force of gravity, tending to settle at the bottom. This is why the first symptoms generally occur in bed or on getting up. Quantitative recordings of eye movements in BPPV by Aw and colleagues (15) and Yagi and colleagues (16) indicate that involvement of a single canal does not always explain the patterns of nystagmus. Furthermore, natural variability in the orientation of the semicircular canals within the skull might also contribute to different patterns of nystagmus among patients (e.g. more torsional in some, more vertical in others).

In about 15% of cases, the otoconia become detached because of trauma, sometimes minor, since the symptoms begin after head trauma, whiplash injury, high-impact exercises, scuba diving, or following surgery on the head in which a drill is used (nasal, dental).

Why do otoconia detach from the utricular maculae spontaneously? Is it a consequence of aging, since the disease is rare in childhood and frequent in the elderly? (4, 17). Is it a disorder of calcium metabolism (18)? Hormonal effects and migraine may underlie the higher incidence of BPPV in females. Vasospasm of the inner ear, leading to release of otoconia from the macula was postulated as a mechanism (8). In some patients a viral cause seems likely, as the disease begins during or after a flu-like episode. BPPV may be a delayed effect of labyrinthine injury, of viral or vascular origin, as in the Lindsay–Hemenway syndrome (19) in which only the vestibular structures innervated by the superior division of the vestibular nerve and perfused by the anterior vestibular artery are affected leading to detachment of otoconia and then entry into an intact PC. Sometimes BPPV begins after a long confinement to bed, or after holding certain positions at the hairdresser, dentist or even after general surgery with prolonged positioning with the head back. Ménière's disease

also seems to predispose to BPPV (20). Associations of BPPV with diabetes (21), hypertension, hyperlipidaemia, and stroke (4) have been suggested, but need to be confirmed.

Symptoms

In most patients with BPPV, the symptoms are so typical that the diagnosis can be made over the phone. 'Do you get vertigo when you lie down or when you turn in bed?' is the key question. If yes, there are very few alternatives to BPPV, and in this way we also exclude orthostatic dizziness.

When the vertical canals are involved, vertigo is also triggered by movement in the *pitch* plane, such as lying down and getting up, looking at or reaching for things above the head, bending forward or tying one's shoe. The vertiginous sensation is often one of rotation, since it arises from the semicircular canals, and generally lasts for many seconds. Some patients are also able to describe the direction of rotation, i.e. clockwise or counterclockwise, and also that it occurs in the same way every time a critical head position is assumed. The episodes of vertigo are generally intense when the condition begins and then decrease with each passing day. Especially at the beginning, the vertigo is often accompanied by nausea or vomiting and patients may overestimate the duration of single attacks. In patients with LC-BPPV the attacks of vertigo are provoked mainly by rolling onto a side while lying down. In this case the symptoms are generally much more intense, forcing the patient to lie immobile in a supine position, so it can be difficult to know whether it is a positional vertigo or not.

If not treated, the symptomatic period lasts for days, weeks, or, rarely, months. This period is also known as the active phase of BPPV. BPPV is often self-limited and it is not uncommon to see the patients after they have become asymptomatic. However, recurrences of active phases are frequent. Some patients have closely spaced active phases; in others, the asymptomatic period lasts for years. Chronic forms with a persistent active phase cause intractable BPPV. Typically, patients with BPPV have no problems while standing up and can safely drive a car. However, some complain of a feeling of floating and postural instability.

BPPV is, by definition, not associated with hearing or neurological symptoms, unless secondary to other diseases. Vertigo is often a stressful, terrifying event that can easily lead to anxiety, phobic behaviour, and a reduction of the quality of life (22). There are patients who, despite being symptom free, sleep in semi-sitting position or avoid turning in bed. This can give rise to neck discomfort that is often incorrectly considered the cause of vertigo.

Diagnosis and pathophysiology

The diagnosis is based on the finding of PPN induced by diagnostic manoeuvres that move the head in planes parallel to the individual semicircular canals. The features of the nystagmus often allow one to identify which semicircular canal is involved and also in which part of the semicircular canal the otoconial debris are located. PPN is usually seen well even without Frenzel glasses, though the exact pattern of nystagmus is best appreciated when fixation is eliminated.

Posterior canal

Diagnostic manoeuvre

The Dix–Hallpike manoeuvre, originally described by Dix and Hallpike in 1952 (23) is still the most efficient technique to

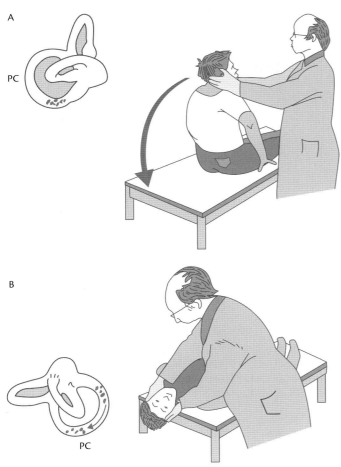

A

PC

B

PC

Fig. 20.1 Dix–Hallpike test for right PC-BPPV. (A) The head is turned 45° to the right and then (B) the patient is quickly brought into the right head hanging position. It is advisable to keep this position for at least 30 seconds since positional nystagmus may appear after a long latency. The patient is next returned to the sitting position with the head facing forward, observing again for nystagmus. The procedure is then repeated for the left posterior canal. The position and movement of particles inside the PC are shown on the left side of the figure (for details, see text).

are free-floating as in canalolithiasis. A pillow under the shoulders of the patient, or a bed with an adjustable headrest can be used so that at the end of the manoeuvre the patient's head is lower than the horizontal plane and rotated to one side. When the cause of the BPPV is cupulolithiasis a 'half Hallpike', in which the patient lies flat, may produce a stronger nystagmus because the *cupula* is now in the position to be maximally stimulated by the pull of gravity (24). From the head-hanging position, the patient is then returned to the sitting position with the head facing forward. The manoeuvre is then repeated on the other side. The positions should be held for at least 20–30 seconds, since there may be a delay before the nystagmus appears. It is always necessary to test both sides not to miss the diagnosis in bilateral forms, beginning from the left side because the right side is more frequently involved. In patients in whom you strongly suspect BPPV but elicit no nystagmus on the first Dix–Hallpike manoeuvre it may be worth repeating it after you have performed manoeuvres looking for a LC-BPPV (25).

An alternative to the Dix–Hallpike test is the Semont diagnostic manoeuvre, also called 'side-lying' test (26, 27). The manoeuvre corresponds to the first step of the Semont therapeutic manoeuvre (see later). It is particularly useful when the examiner already knows the pathological side and wants to check if the positional nystagmus is gone after the treatment. If the treatment was not effective the patient is already in the correct position for retreatment

Paroxysmal positional nystagmus

The characteristic features of the PPN evoked by the Dix–Hallpike test are illustrated in Table 20.1. These features are as predicted when canalolithiasis of the PC is the presumed cause (see also later in chapter). The *latency* is the delay between reaching the diagnostic Dix–Hallpike position and the onset of nystagmus. It is generally shorter in the early stages of the disease. The *direction* and *plane* of the nystagmus are the most important features. Nystagmus is mixed torsional and vertical. If the *right* PC is involved, the right Dix–Hallpike manoeuvre provokes a nystagmus in which the fast phases of the vertical component beat toward the forehead (up) and the fast phases of the torsional component beat toward the right ear (top pole beating to the right ear), i.e. beating clockwise *with respect to the patient's view*. With involvement of the left PC, the nystagmus in the left Dix–Hallpike position is also upbeating, but fast phases of the torsional component beat toward the left ear (top pole beating to the left ear), i.e. counterclockwise *with respect to the patient's view*. The torsional component may appear more prominent if the patient looks toward the lowermost ear, and the vertical component more prominent if the patient looks toward the uppermost ear. PPN is *paroxysmal*, with a rapid increase followed by a slower decrease in intensity. The frequency

diagnose involvement of the PC (Figure 20.1). The patient sits on an examination table and the head is rotated 45° in the direction of the examiner. The patient is then rapidly moved into the supine position with the head hyperextended. In this position the undermost. PC is aligned with the plane of movement and the long arm nearly vertical so that it is maximally stimulated when the otoconia

Table 20.1 Features of paroxysmal positional nystagmus in posterior canal canalolithiasis. Note the directions of the nystagmus are named from the patient's view

Latency	1–20 seconds
Direction and plane	Torsional and vertical. Counterclockwise (patient reference) quick phases for left PC-BPPV and clockwise for right PC. Always upbeating
Temporal profile	Intensity increases rapidly and then declines more slowly
Duration	Usually <30–40 seconds
Direction change	Reverses direction on returning to the sitting position
Fatigability	Reduction in intensity by repeating the manoeuvres

Table 20.2 Typical features of paroxysmal positional nystagmus due to lateral canal canalolithiasis

Latency	0–10 seconds
Direction and plane	Horizontal. Geotropic (beating toward the ground) or apogeotropic (beating away from the ground)
Temporal profile	Increases rapidly in intensity and then declines more slowly
Duration	<60 seconds
Direction change	Reverses direction when rolling the head to the either side
Fatigability	Absent? (but difficult to assess)

may be as high as three beats per second. It is *transient*, usually ending in 10–40 seconds, though it may last only a few seconds. When the patient returns to the sitting position, the nystagmus reverses direction, i.e. becoming downbeating and beating clockwise if it were previously counterclockwise. It is less intense and shorter in duration than the previous one. It is often characterized by fatigability, which is a reduction of intensity on repeating the diagnostic manoeuvres. Some patients show a spontaneous reversal of the nystagmus direction without any change in head position, especially if the paroxysm was intense. Known as secondary nystagmus, it begins a few seconds after the end of the previous paroxysmal nystagmus.

Bilateral BPPV also occurs, especially after head trauma. In these patients PPN is up and clockwise beating on the right and up and counterclockwise beating on the left side. Finally, some patients do not show the typical features of canalolithiasis. Their positional nystagmus is long lasting and stationary (not paroxysmal) and more resistant to physical treatment, suggesting cupulolithiasis.

Pathophysiology

In a patient with BPPV of the right PC, the right Dix–Hallpike manoeuvre brings the ampulla to a higher position with respect to the canal, so that the particles fall in an ampullofugal direction and, with a plunger effect in the narrow canal, cause an endolymphatic flow that displaces the cupula away from the utricle (Figure 20.1). This is an excitatory stimulus that provokes a mixed upbeating torsional (top pole beating toward the affected lower ear) paroxysmal nystagmus consistent with the excitatory connections of the right PC to the vertical extraocular muscles (right superior oblique muscle and left inferior rectus muscle) (28).

Bringing the patient to the sitting position, the particles fall in the opposite direction and, acting as a plunger, produce an ampullopetal displacement of the cupula with an inhibitory response from the PC. The resulting nystagmus is less intense and in the opposite direction, i.e. downbeating with the torsional component now directed such that the top pole of the eyes beat away from the previously downward (affected) ear. A delay in the movement of the otoconia accounts for the latency between the positioning and the onset of the positional nystagmus. The short duration of positional vertigo and nystagmus is due to the elasticity of the cupula that allows it to return to its primary position with its time constant once the otoconial debris has reached its lowest position in the canal. Fatigability is explained by dispersion of the debris, making it less effective as a plunger (29), but this hypothesis has been questioned on the basis of a mathematical model of BPPV (30).

The features of the PPN just described are typical for canalolithiasis of the posterior canal, which is the cause in about 80% of patients with BPPV. In some patients the nystagmus is more persistent and

not paroxysmal. This may reflect adherence of some of the otolithic debris to the cupula (cupulolithiasis). Animal experiments suggest that cupulolithiasis of the PC should have a shorter latency and longer duration of the PPN (31). On the other hand it may not be possible to distinguish canalolithiasis from cupulolithiasis only on the basis of the parameters of PPN since they may coexist (32). The diagnostic key to distinguish canalo- from cupulolithiasis may be the response to the therapeutic manoeuvres designed to expel the debris from the canals (see later in chapter). In fact we can deduce that the otoconia have moved into the vestibule by the appearance of the so called 'liberatory nystagmus', which indicates ampullofugal displacement of the cupula. If instead the patient does not respond to repeated treatments and/or the therapeutic manoeuvre causes a nystagmus suggesting ampullopetal displacement of the cupula, a cupulolithiasis is suspected.

Lateral canal

Diagnostic manoeuvre

If the history suggests involvement of the LC, we must first look for spontaneous nystagmus, with the patient seated. In some patients affected by LC-BPPV, horizontal 'spontaneous' nystagmus can also be evoked by a gentle shaking of the head. If spontaneous nystagmus is present, it is necessary to look for changes of direction, disappearance, or increase of its intensity by bending the head about 30° and 60° forward and then 60° backward. Next bring the patient to the supine position; with the head straight (nose upward) and bent 30° forward to bring the lateral canal in the vertical plane. An adjustable head rest or a pillow can be useful. In this position check for the appearance of positional nystagmus or for a change in the intensity or direction of the spontaneous nystagmus that was seen in the upright position (33). Continue with the McClure–Pagnini test (supine roll test), which acts in a plane parallel to that of the lateral canal, by rolling the patient's head 90° to one side. The head is then rotated 180° to the other side, looking for changes of direction and intensity of nystagmus (34, 35). In patients who cannot easily turn their head on their torso, for example, the elderly, the whole body can be rotated. Sometimes one must repeat the diagnostic manoeuvres, because the first rotation may not evoke the positional nystagmus. Horizontal PPN from the lateral canal may also be provoked by the Dix–Hallpike manoeuvre.

Paroxysmal positional nystagmus

Positional nystagmus due to lateral canal canalolithiasis differs from that of the PC (Table 20.2). The most important diagnostic finding is a *horizontal* and *direction-changing* positional nystagmus provoked by the supine head roll test. Its *latency* is usually shorter;

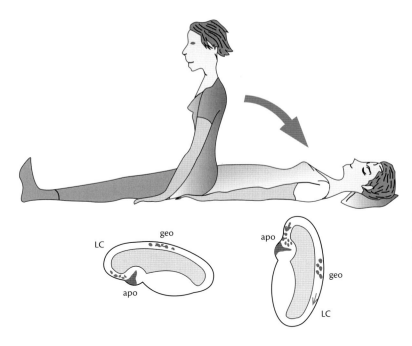

Fig. 20.2 Sitting-supine positioning test in LC-BPPV. The patient is rapidly moved from the sitting to the supine position with the head straight. In the geotropic type (geo), the manoeuvre causes otoconial particles to gravitate away from the ampulla, to the most dependent part of the canal, provoking an ampullofugal flow and mild positional nystagmus beating away from the affected side (apogeotropic type, apo). If located close to the ampulla, particles can move towards the cupula, provoking an ampullopetal flow and nystagmus beating towards the affected side.

sometimes no latency is appreciable. Generally it is more intense and longer lasting, but again *transient*. Rotation of the head towards the pathological side causes an intense horizontal positional nystagmus beating towards the lower ear. Since it beats towards the ground it is named *geotropic*. Rotation of the head to the other side reverses the direction of the nystagmus, i.e. beating towards the opposite ear (but again geotropic). This is less intense and sometimes longer lasting. The inversion of the direction of the nystagmus, caused by two different head positions, is comparable to the inversion of direction that occurs when the patient with PC-BPPV is brought from the Dix–Hallpike position to the sitting position. The more intense positional nystagmus is often followed by a secondary reversal nystagmus, where the direction changes without any further change in head position. This secondary nystagmus is usually less intense but longer lasting. Sometimes the nystagmus reverses on both sides (36).

In about 20% of patients, LC-BPPV presents with an *apogeotropic* nystagmus, i.e. it beats toward the uppermost ear. It is again more intense on one side than on the other. The affected side is indicated by the direction of the fast phase of the strongest nystagmus. In both variants, geotropic and apogeotropic, it is sometimes difficult to identify the pathological side because the intensity of the nystagmus on the two sides is similar (37).

Lateral canal PPN is often associated with severe autonomic symptoms, and it may not be possible to continue testing to determine whether the nystagmus is fatigable. In many patients with apogeotropic nystagmus there may be a transformation into the geotropic form spontaneously or after therapeutic manoeuvres. The converse is also possible, especially if the therapeutic manoeuvres are incorrectly performed, confirming that otoconia are free to move inside the endolymph of the canals. Physical manoeuvres can also cause a lateral canal BPPV to become a posterior canal BPPV, and occasionally vice versa. In a few patients, the profile of nystagmus suggests that both the lateral and posterior canals are affected.

The features so far described are typical of canalolithiasis of the lateral canal. Similar to the posterior canal, there are patients with apogeotropic nystagmus with features that suggest a cupulolithiasis.

PPN appears less intense, long lasting and not paroxysmal, reflecting adherence of some otolithic debris to the cupula.

Patients with LC-BPPV may also have a 'spontaneous' horizontal nystagmus while in the sitting position (34, 38). It is called pseudo-spontaneous nystagmus and is modulated by head position and movement. In patients with the geotropic form, the direction of the fast phase of pseudo-spontaneous nystagmus is towards the healthy side with the apogeotropic form beating towards the affected side. Generally of low intensity, it increases by bending the head 30° backward, stops with the head bent 30° forward, and reverses direction if the head is further bent forward to 60°. These manoeuvres are known as the 'bow and lean test' (39) or 'head pitch test' (40). The finding of spontaneous nystagmus in LC-BPPV may be more common when patients are observed in darkness using recordings rather than when using Frenzel glasses to eliminate fixation which is imperfect.

In some patients positional nystagmus in LC-BPPV is also evoked by quickly bringing the patient from the sitting position to the supine position, with the nose up. Often a mild, low intensity, horizontal nystagmus appears. It beats towards the healthy ear in the geotropic form and towards the affected side in the apogeotropic form (36). Central causes of positional nystagmus will be considered further later in the chapter.

Pathophysiology

Otoconia can also enter the long arm of the LC, since its entrance is close to the exit of the common crus into the utricle. Once inside, they move under the force of gravity, tending to settle at the bottom of the canal, far from the cupula. Taking the example of a patient with BPPV of the *right* LC, the rapid change from sitting to supine position, causes the debris to settle in the most dependent portion of the LC, in an ampullofugal direction. This could cause an ampullofugal flow, which is inhibitory, and a mild horizontal positional nystagmus beating towards the left, normal ear (Figure 20.2). Less frequently, in cases where otoconial debris is located near to the ampulla, or is attached to the cupula, nystagmus beats towards the affected side.

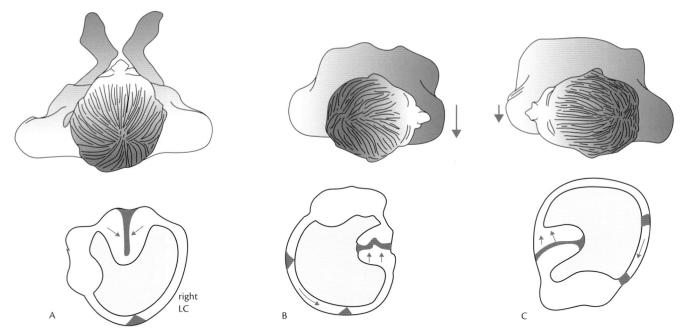

Fig. 20.3 Supine head roll test (Mc Clure–Pagnini test) in right LC-BPPV (geotropic form). (A) Patient in the supine position and the head straight: particles are located in the most dependent part of the lateral canal. (B) Rotating the head 90° to the right side causes particles to fall towards the ampulla, producing an ampullopetal flow and intense horizontal nystagmus beating to the right, affected, ear (geotropic). (C) Rolling the head 180° to the left side causes particles to move in the opposite direction, producing ampullofugal flow and left-beating horizontal nystagmus (again geotropic) that is less intense than in B.

Rolling the head to the right side, by the supine head roll test, causes these particles to fall towards the ampulla and induces ampullopetal (excitatory) endolymphatic flow. This provokes a right-beating (geotropic) paroxysmal horizontal nystagmus consistent with the excitatory connections of the right LC to the horizontal extraocular muscles (right medial rectus and left lateral rectus). When the head is then rolled to the other side (to the left), the particles fall in the opposite direction and cause a flow of endolymph away from the utricle. This provokes a left beating nystagmus, again geotropic, which is less intense because it is caused by an inhibitory stimulus which has a smaller effect (Ewald's second law). (Figure 20.3)

The different direction of the apogeotropic variant of LC-BPPV is probably due to the different initial position of the particles in the LC. If debris is close to the ampulla of the right LC, rotation of the head to the right side would cause the otoconia to fall away from the ampulla, producing an inhibitory apogeotropic nystagmus beating towards the left (upper) ear. When the head is rotated to the left, otoconia fall towards the ampulla, causing an apogeotropic nystagmus toward the affected right ear, which is uppermost. In this case, excitatory ampullopetal flow occurs and produces the strongest nystagmus with the affected ear up (Figure 20.4).

The excitatory nystagmus of the LC is stronger and lasts longer compared to PC-BPPV. This is probably due to a greater central action of the velocity storage mechanism (which perseverates peripheral nystagmus) of the horizontal more than the vertical vestibulo-ocular reflex (41).

The apogeotropic form may convert to the geotropic form in patients who are treated by being asked to lie on the pathological side for a period of time (see later). The transformation of the apogeotropic form into the geotropic form, or vice versa, after diagnostic or therapeutic manoeuvres, is further support for the canalolithiasis hypothesis, as the reversal is linked to a change in

position of the debris in the LC. The cupulolithiasis theory, however, probably better explains persistent direction changing apogeotropic nystagmus. When the affected ear is down, the mass located on the cupula causes it to deviate away from the utricle, inhibiting the ampullary nerve and causing nystagmus beating away from the undermost affected ear. The opposite occurs when the patient turns on the side of the normal ear. In this position the mass causes the cupula to deviate toward the utricle, again producing nystagmus beating away from the ground (42). Cupulolithiasis is also expected to cause a weaker nystagmus than canalolithiasis (30).

The 'spontaneous' nystagmus that has been reported in lateral canal BPPV is explained by the angle between the plane of the lateral canal and the horizontal plane of the head (Figure 20.5). When the head is erect the lateral canal is tilted about 30° from the horizontal plane, with the ampulla *higher* than the canal. Gravity and head movements, even if minimal, could cause debris that is floating inside the canal to move away from the ampulla, provoking nystagmus beating away from the affected ear. Or, if the debris were attached to the cupula or close to the ampulla, the cupula would deviate toward the utricle and produce nystagmus beating towards the affected right ear (40). The spontaneous nystagmus usually disappears if the head is bent 30° forward, because the LC assumes a horizontal position and particles inside the canal or the heavy cupula are not influenced by the gravity vector. By bending the head farther forward to about 60°, gravity causes the debris to move toward the ampulla with a resulting nystagmus beating toward the affected ear, i.e. in the opposite direction observed with the head erect. On the contrary, if otoconia are located near the ampulla or if the cupula is heavy, the deflection of the cupula and nystagmus will be in the opposite direction. Finally, bending the head backwards will cause an increase in the spontaneous nystagmus because the

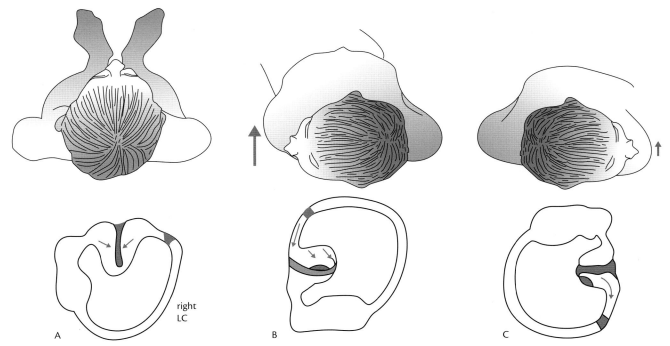

Fig. 20.4 Supine head roll test in right LC-BPPV with apogeotropic positional nystagmus. (A) Patient in the supine position and the head straight: particles are located close to the ampulla. (B) Rotating the head 90° to the left side causes particles to fall towards the cupula, provoking an intense horizontal right-beating nystagmus (apogeotropic) due to the excitatory stimulus. (C) Rolling the head 180° to the right side causes particles to move in the opposite direction, producing less intense left-beating horizontal nystagmus (apogeotropic).

canal will be approximately vertical, similar to when the patient is lying supine and the head is bent 30° forward.

Anterior canal

Diagnostic manoeuvre
Since the ACs are roughly coplanar to the PCs of the opposite side, when we test the right posterior canal we also stimulate in the plane of the left AC.

Therefore BPPV of the AC should be detected with both Dix–Hallpike positions but also with straight head hanging, by bringing the patient supine and the head 30° below the earth-horizontal (43, 44).

Paroxysmal positional nystagmus
Positional nystagmus due to canalolithiasis or cupulolithiasis of the AC should be mixed torsional and vertical. If the *right* AC is involved, the *left* Dix–Hallpike manoeuvre should provoke a PPN in which the fast phase of the vertical component is down-beating and the fast phase of the torsional component beats with the top pole toward the right ear, i.e. clockwise with respect to the patient's view. However, the torsional component is often not detectable and positional nystagmus attributed to the anterior canal is usually better seen with straight head hanging (43). Furthermore it is often relatively sustained and of low intensity. The latency of the nystagmus varies from zero to a few seconds and the duration of nystagmus is less than one minute. The nystagmus fatigues in most patients. When the patient is returned to the sitting position, the nystagmus may not reverse, even if the patient still has dizziness. In many patients this type of positional vertigo and nystagmus lasts for weeks or months, even after various treatments attempts.

Pathophysiology
The existence of canalolithiasis of the anterior canal is still debated. The anterior canal is located in the top of the labyrinth and it is unlikely that particles enter normally unless the patient is upside down. Even if this were the case, the condition should be short-lived because of gravity, since the posterior arm of the AC descends directly into the common crus when the patient is upright. Nevertheless the incidence of the anterior canal variant of BPPV is reported to be from 2–20% (45, 46). Regardless, in an otherwise normal patient, when the Dix–Hallpike manoeuvre provokes a positional nystagmus with a downbeating component, the anterior canal variant should be considered. For example, the right Dix–Hallpike test provokes a backwards rotation of the left AC, and otoconial debris located in the ampullar region would fall in the ampullofugal direction, thus provoking an excitatory stimulus. The resulting nystagmus is mixed downbeat and torsional with the top pole of the eyes beating toward the left upper ear, consistent with the primary excitatory connections of the left AC to the ipsilateral superior rectus and contralateral inferior oblique muscles.

As already mentioned, AC-BPPV remains poorly understood, Why would there be positional nystagmus evoked with both Dix–Hallpike manoeuvres and with straight head-hanging? This is explained by the vertical upward orientation of the ampullary segment of the AC in the normal upright head position. Such an orientation should reduce the right–left specificity of the Dix–Hallpike manoeuvre for AC compared to PC-BPPV. Why is the nystagmus mainly vertical? Presumably, this is related to the more upright orientation of the ACs (43). Furthermore, why is the positional nystagmus rarely paroxysmal and does not reverse direction when the patient is returned to the sitting position?

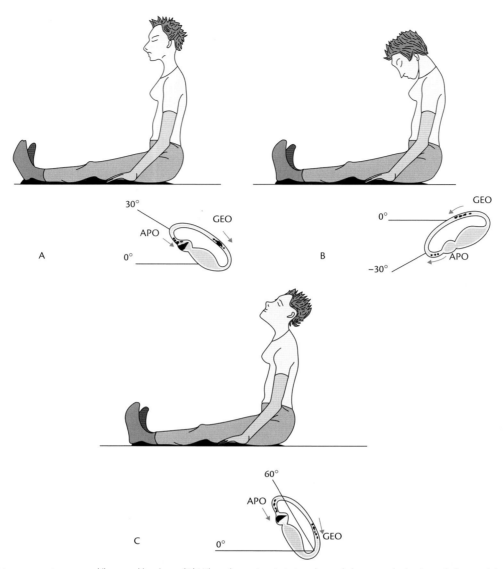

Fig. 20.5 Pseudo-spontaneous nystagmus and 'bow and lean' test. (A) When the patient is sitting, the angle between the horizontal plane and the plane of the lateral canal could cause particles to move inside the canal. If far from the ampulla, debris move in an ampullofugal direction, provoking a nystagmus beating away from the affected side (GEO tropic). If debris are attached to the cupula or located close to the ampulla, the cupula will be deflected towards the utricle with nystagmus towards the affected side (APO geotropic). (B) Bending the head about 60° forward, gravity causes debris to move towards (GEO) or away (APO) from the ampulla (APO), producing a reversal of direction of the 'spontaneous' nystagmus. (C) By bending the head backwards, the pseudo spontaneous nystagmus may increase its intensity because the canal is in the vertical plane, favouring the fall of particles towards or away from the ampulla.

In conclusion, downbeat positional nystagmus of peripheral origin is likely more common than previously reported, but its precise relationship to canalo- or cupulolithiasis of the anterior canal is not settled. One possibility is that the positional downbeating nystagmus may actually arise from the PC. If the otoconial debris does not reach the bottom of the canal and, for any reason, is held in the distal portion with respect to the ampulla (perhaps due to the amount of the debris and its relationship to the size of the lumen or the structure of the walls of the canal), the Dix–Hallpike manoeuvre could cause the debris to move in the ampullopetal direction, so provoking an inhibitory nystagmus, that is downbeating. In other words it is possible that, by analogy with LC involvement, BPPV of the posterior canal could lead to a geotropic or apogeotropic positional nystagmus.

Central causes of positional nystagmus

Differentiating peripheral from central causes of positional vertigo and nystagmus is usually straightforward: the symptoms and signs are relatively stereotyped and the neurological symptoms or signs pointing toward more central lesions are absent. In particular the most common form of BPPV, due to PC involvement, is almost never confused with other lesions. There are, however, rare reports of PC-like positional nystagmus presenting as a sign of a central lesion though careful reading of the clinical descriptions of both symptoms and signs almost always reveals a 'red flag' pointing to a more central process. Likewise posterior canal BPPV can sometimes seem purely torsional and other times purely vertical. If fixation is not eliminated the vertical component may be suppressed leaving the torsional component alone. BPPV arising from the lateral canals may be more difficult to distinguish from more central lesions and the putative AC-BPPV can look just like the downbeat positional nystagmus associated with cerebellar lesions and cranial-junction anomalies. The most common mimics of peripheral positional nystagmus are demyelinating lesions, small tumours in the cerebellum or in the structures around the fourth ventricle, and small ischaemic lesions, involving the vestibulocerebellum and especially the nodulus, the cerebellar peduncles or the brainstem structures close to the fourth ventricle (47). Features that point to a central cause of paroxysmal positional vertigo are lack of a latency and lack of fatigability with respective testing; an unusual direction of the nystagmus, sometimes with a changing direction over time; and a pure vertical or a pure torsional nystagmus. A careful examination of eye movements including provocative vestibulo-ocular manoeuvres such as head shaking, mastoid vibration, Valsalva, and hyperventilation, will usually reveal 'atypical features' prompting further investigations. Positional downbeat nystagmus, however, always mandates careful imaging of the posterior fossa, looking especially for small lesions in the nodulus (48).

Treatment

The development of simple treatment procedures for the most common cause of vertigo is probably 'the most important (therapeutic) breakthrough in the field of neuro-otology in the past 25 years' (49). The aim of physical therapy is to eliminate the episodes of positional vertigo by dislodging the otoconial debris from the semicircular canals. Special movements and positions of the head and body are used to trigger a series of clinical events that are consistent with the canalolithiasis hypothesis. Therapies for PC- and LC-BPPV have been validated. On the other hand, specific diagnostic criteria and effective treatment for the anterior canal variant of BPPV are still elusive. Surgery and medications play a minor role in BPPV.

Physical treatment of posterior canal BPPV

PC-BPPV is treated effectively by Epley's canalith repositioning procedure (CRP) or Semont's liberatory manoeuvre. The aim of the manoeuvres is to allow the particles to fall out of the canal using gravity. With Semont's manoeuvre the movement of the particles is also affected by the acceleration of the head. A recent evidence-based review of the American Academy of Neurology considers CRP as effective and safe therapy that should be offered to patients of all ages with PC-BPPV. Semont's manoeuvre is classified as 'possibly effective' since Class I and II studies were lacking (50) though a recent class I study has been performed (51). The efficacy of the two treatments is probably similar (52, 53).

The canalith repositioning procedure

The manoeuvre was designed to allow free canaliths to migrate by gravity out of the PC through the common crus (54). The treatment

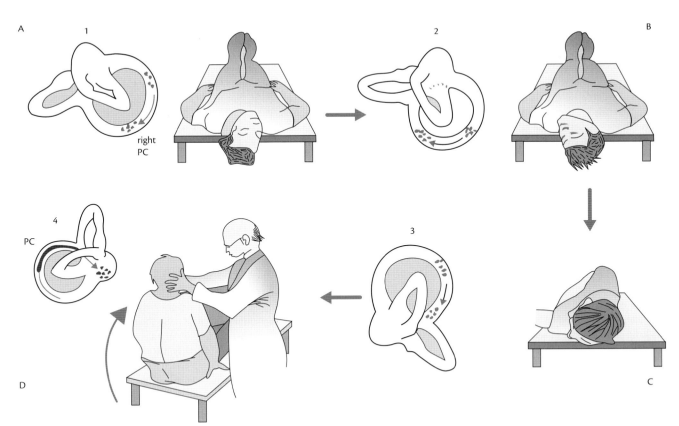

Fig. 20. 6 Canalith repositioning procedure (Epley manoeuvre) for right PC-BPPV. (A) The patient is moved into the right Dix–Hallpike position (head hyperextended and rotated 45° to the right). In this position particles gravitate towards the centre of the PC (1). (B) After about 30 seconds the head is rotated 90° leftward, maintaining the hyperextension. This movement provokes a progression of debris towards the common crus (2). (C) The head and the shoulders are rotated leftward another 90° until the head is face down. With this movement particles should cross the common crus (3). (D) The patient is returned to the sitting position and the head still turned to the left. In this way debris should enter the utricle (4). At the end the head is turned forward and tilted about 20° down.

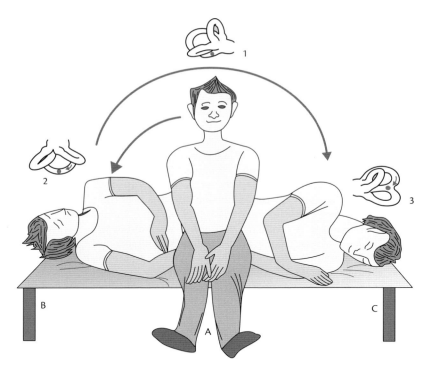

Fig. 20.7 Semont's liberatory manoeuvre for right posterior canal BPPV. (A) Patient in the sitting position and debris located in the most dependent part of the PC (1). The head is first turned 45° to the left and then (B) the patient is brought in the right side-lying position with the back of the head resting on the bed. With this 'provoking manoeuvre' particles move away from the ampulla (2). After about 2 minutes the patient is rapidly moved to the opposite side (C), without changing the head position relative to shoulders. At the end of the manoeuvre the patient lies on his left shoulder with the cheek-bone and nose in contact with the bed (liberatory position). With the liberatory manoeuvre debris should be expelled through the common crus into the utricle (3). After 2 minutes the patient is slowly returned to the sitting position, with the head bent slightly forward.

consists of a series of five movements to different positions beginning with the examiner standing in front of the patient who is seated on the bed. With the first movement the patient is brought into the Dix–Hallpike provoking position on the affected side. For right BPPV, the head is rotated 45° to the right and the body moved supine with the head over the end of the table. This position would cause canaliths to gravitate towards the centre of the posterior canal. The head is then rotated 90° leftward, while maintaining neck hyperextension, until the head reaches a 45° left position. In this way the canaliths should approach the common crus. The head and body are further rotated leftward 90° so the patient is lying on their left side with his head at 135° with respect to the supine position (almost looking at the floor). This third position would cause the canaliths to cross the common crus. The patient is then brought up to the sitting position with their head kept turned to the left, so that the canaliths enter the utricle. Finally, the head is turned forward with the chin down at 20° (Figure 20.6). The five-position cycle should provoke a nystagmus that reflects the direction in which the canaliths move (in this case excitatory for the PC). Every position is held until the nystagmus subsides, which typically takes up to about 15 seconds in each position. The cycle is repeated until no nystagmus is observed. A vibrator can be applied to the ipsilateral mastoid area during at least one positioning cycle to dislodge canaliths that might be adherent to the canal wall. Various modifications have been proposed to simplify the Epley's original method, obtaining similar results in most cases (55, 56).

The Semont liberatory manoeuvre

The original manoeuvre suggested by Semont et al. (26) is currently applied in a simplified version. After identifying the pathological ear with the Dix–Hallpike test, the examiner stands in front of the patient who is seated on the side of the examining table. If, for example, the right side is affected, the patient's head is rotated 45° to

the left, and then the patient is brought so as to lie on his right side, with the back of the head resting on the table, that is in a position similar to the right Dix–Hallpike diagnostic test. The movement must be quick and continuous. The manoeuvre provokes a paroxysmal vertical torsional nystagmus caused by movement of otoconia away from the ampulla. The patient is kept in this position for about 2 minutes and is then quickly rolled 180° onto the opposite side (a cartwheel), maintaining the head in the same position relative to the shoulders (Figure 20.7). This movement, called the liberatory manoeuvre, provokes acceleration in the plane of the right PC and should bring the head of the patient in a position that allows the debris to fall into the utricle. At the end the patient is in the liberatory position, i.e. lying on his left shoulder with the cheekbone and nose in contact with the bed. The liberatory manoeuvre must be rapid and continuous. If too slow, the debris might fall back in the wrong direction. The acceleration acting on the canal is important so that the duration of the swing must not exceed 1.5 seconds (57).

The expected response to the liberatory manoeuvre is another episode of intense vertigo and paroxysmal nystagmus with the same direction of rotation as in the provoking right Dix–Hallpike position. In the example of a right BPPV, it is again mixed vertical upbeating-torsional clockwise, due to excitation of the right posterior semicircular canal. This is called the liberatory nystagmus. The latency of appearance of the liberatory nystagmus varies considerably, from a few seconds up to 20–30 seconds. Liberatory nystagmus is due to the progressive movement of otoconial debris in the ampullofugal direction, until it is expelled through the common crus into the utricle, where it no longer affects endolymph dynamics. The presence of the liberatory nystagmus is therefore a good prognostic sign (58, 59); its absence does not necessarily mean that the manoeuvre has been unsuccessful (51, 59). In contrast, after the Epley manoeuvre, the absence of a liberatory nystagmus or even reversal (downbeating) of nystagmus when the patient finally sits up does not automatically exclude a successful outcome. The patient is held in the liberatory position for 2 minutes and then slowly returned to the sitting position with the head bent slightly forward. In this final position, neither nystagmus nor vertigo should appear. If the liberatory manoeuvre did not lead to liberatory nystagmus the vertigo and nystagmus may recur when the patient is returned to the sitting position. The direction of nystagmus will be in the opposite direction to that seen in the provoking position and is to be considered a 'reversal' nystagmus due to ampullopetal movement of otoconia back into the canal.

After the treatment with either the CRP or Semont manoeuvre, patients are often advised to keep their heads erect for several days, to sleep in the sitting position or to wear a cervical collar. These precautions are probably unnecessary because once the otoconial debris has left the canals, it is unlikely to re-enter them (50, 52, 58). Patients are advised, however, to avoid bending up or down or to the side in the immediate 20–30 minutes after completion of the treatment manoeuvres, and are warned they could loss their balance and even fall in the minutes to hours after the treatment.

If the treatment is not effective, it can be repeated several times. In the few patients with intractable BPPV, they can perform self-treatment with the purpose of facilitating the dispersion of canaliths and of promoting habituation. Another option is Brandt–Daroff exercises (60), since they allow patients to better tolerate positional vertigo. The patient is instructed to sit on the edge of their bed and then to quickly move to one lateral position, with the head turned approximately 45° up; to stay in this position until the vertigo subsides, or for 30 seconds; then to sit up for 30 seconds before assuming the lateral, down position on the opposite side for an additional 30 seconds. The positional changes are repeated three to five times in each session, and the sessions are repeated three times a day until the vertigo no longer occurs.

Physical treatment of lateral canal BPPV

Lateral canal BPPV is also treated with physical manoeuvres that allow the otoconial debris to exit the lateral canal by centrifugal inertia and/or gravity.

Many physical treatments have been proposed, beginning with barbecue rotation by Lempert in 1994 (61). According to the review of the American Academy of Neurology, all the studies belong to the Class IV level of evidence studies, corresponding to uncontrolled trials or derived from case reports or from expert opinion (50). According to our empirical experience, the most effective treatments for LC-BPPV are the forced prolonged position, Gufoni's manoeuvre, or a combination of the two.

The forced prolonged position

The so-called 'forced prolonged position', by Vannucchi et al. (62), is simple and well tolerated, with a remission rate of about 75–90% (63–65) in patients with the geotropic form of LC-BPPV. Having identified the pathological side, the patient is instructed to lie supine, then to turn on the side of the healthy ear and to stay in this position as long as possible, *all night if possible*. In this way otoconial debris exit the canal by gravity. It is particularly useful in those patients with severe autonomic symptoms.

Gufoni's manoeuvre

The manoeuvre proposed by Gufoni et al. in 1998 (66) is a liberatory manoeuvre developed to clear the LC immediately in the geotropic form of LC-BPPV. Starting from the sitting position with the

head looking forward, the patient is rapidly brought down onto the healthy side, and then the head is rotated about 45° down, in order to put the nose in contact with the bed. The head must decelerate rapidly as it makes contact with the bed (Figure 20.8). After about 2 minutes in this position, the patient is returned to the upright position. The manoeuvre should allow the particles to exit the canal due to the centrifugal force created by rapid deceleration and by gravity, when the head is maintained with the nose down for 2 minutes. The manoeuvre can be repeated two or three times sequentially. The Gufoni treatment is a good option when the patient is moderately tolerant of vertigo. Several studies have reported success using this manoeuvre, with remission rates of 80–90% (64, 65).

Treating apogeotropic lateral canal BPPV

In patients affected by the apogeotropic form paroxysmal positional nystagmus of the LC-BPPV, either the Gufoni manoeuvre or the forced prolonged position may also be used to convert the positional nystagmus into the more treatable geotropic form. In the example of a right apogeotropic LC-BPPV, the stronger positional nystagmus beats toward the right ear when uppermost. In this example it is necessary to perform the Gufoni manoeuvre onto the right side, the affected one. In this way particles should migrate away from the ampulla, towards the posterior part of the lateral canal. The outcome of the manoeuvre should be verified after 10–15 minutes by repeating the supine head roll test. If positional nystagmus changed its direction, becoming geotropic and more intense with the right ear down, the manoeuvre will be repeated onto the left, healthy, side.

The success of the therapeutic manoeuvre for LC-BPPV depends on the correct identification of the pathological side, whatever the treatment option. A wrong diagnosis can cause the otoconia to move in the wrong direction, transforming a geotropic into an apogeotropic nystagmus. Identification of the affected side is sometimes more difficult than in PC-BPPV because there may be no clear difference in the nystagmus intensity between the two sides. The patient may sometimes help by reporting which side provokes more intense vertigo. Caloric testing may be also helpful since a reversible caloric deficit is often present in the pathological ear (35). The caloric paresis is due to a functional plugging of the canal and disappears when the patient is cured (67). The presence of pseudo-spontaneous nystagmus and the head pitch test may be also useful in identifying the affected side, once we know if positional nystagmus is geotropic or apogeotropic. The most useful method is probably to check for horizontal positional nystagmus by quickly bringing the patient from the sitting position to the supine position, with the nose up: if beating to the left it indicates a right canalolithiasis if the form is geotropic or a left canalo-cupulolithiasis if the form is apogeotropic (36, 68, 69).

Treatment of anterior canal BPPV

In the last decade many physical procedures have been proposed for the treatment of AC-BPPV, each of them with the aim of dislodging canaliths from the *canal*. Since one AC is roughly coplanar to the PC of the opposite side, a 'reverse' Epley's manoeuvre, starting from the healthy side, seems to be logical (70). Excellent results were also reported with Epley's manoeuvre starting from the affected side (46). Hamid (71) reported that patients undergoing repeated Dix–Hallpike manoeuvres, performed to check fatigability of positional nystagmus, were improved. The manoeuvre

997608997

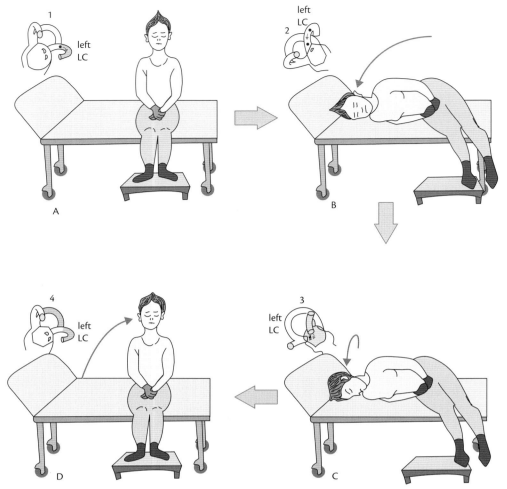

Fig. 20.8 Gufoni's manoeuvre for left lateral canal BPPV (geotropic form). (A) Patient in the sitting position and debris located in the middle of the LC (1). (B) The patient is moved to the healthy side, without changing the head position relative to shoulders. The manoeuvre must be rapid and with deceleration as the head makes contact with the bed. With this movement debris should move away from the ampulla (2). (C) After a few second the head is rotated about 45° down. In this way particle should exit the canal, by gravitation (3). (D) After 2 minutes the patient is returned in the sitting position.

proposed by Yacovino et al. (72), which followed the suggestion of Crevits (73), has the advantage of not requiring the identification of the affected side. It consists of four steps with 30-second intervals: the patient is brought from the sitting to the supine position with the head extended 30° backwards; then the head is tilted forward so that the chin is in contact with the chest; finally the patient returns to the sitting position. The efficacy of this kind of treatment has been recently confirmed (44). Other physical treatments of AC-BPPV have been proposed (for review see (74)) but at present no controlled studies are available, and, in our experience their effectiveness is questionable. Home treatment with manoeuvres similar to the Brandt–Daroff exercises is another option for these patients. The purpose is to facilitate dispersion of otoconia and to promote habituation.

References

1. Schuknecht HF (1969). Cupulolithiasis. *Arch Otolaryngol*, 90, 765–78.
2. Hall SF, Ruby RRF, McClure JA (1979). The mechanics of benign paroxysmal vertigo, *J Otolaryngol*, 8, 151–8.
3. Neuhauser HK (2007). Epidemiology of vertigo. *Curr Opin Neurol*, 20, 40–6.
4. Von Brevern M, Radtke A, Lezius F, et al. (2007). Epidemiology of benign paroxysmal positional vertigo: a population based study. *J Neurol Neurosurg Psychiatry*, 78, 710–15.
5. Neuhauser HK, Leopold M, von Brevern M, et al. (2001). The interrelations of migraine, vertigo and migrainous vertigo. *Neurology*, 56, 436–41.
6. Brandt T (2003). *Vertigo. Its multisensory syndromes* (2nd ed). London: Springer.
7. Caruso G, Nuti D (2005). Epidemiological data from 2270 PPV patients. *Audiological Med*, 3, 7–11
8. Ishiyama A, Jacobson KM, Baloh RW (2000). Migraine and benign positional vertigo. *Ann Otol Rhinol Laryngol*, 109, 377–80.
9. von Brevern M, Seelig T, Neuhauser H, et al. (2004). Benign paroxysmal positional vertigo predominantly affects the right labyrinth. *J Neurol Neurosurg Psychiatry*, 75, 1487–8.
10. Parnes LS, McClure JA (1992). Free-floating endolymph particles: a new operative finding during posterior semicircular canal occlusion. *Laryngoscope*, 102, 988–92.
11. Welling DB, Parnes LS, O'Brien B Bakalletz LO, Brackmann DE, Hinojosa R (1997). Particulate matter in the posterior semicircular canal. *Laryngoscope*, 107, 90–4.
12. Kveton JF, Kashgarian M (1994). Particular matter within the membranous labyrinth: pathologic or normal? *Am J Otol*, 15, 173–6.

13. Buki B, Simon L, Garab S, Lundberg YW, Straumann D (2011). Sitting-up vertigo and trunk retropulsion in patients with positional vertigo but without positional nystagmus. *J Neurol Neurosurg Psychiatry*, 82, 98–104.

14. Zucca G, Valli S, Valli P, Perrin P, Mira E (1998). Why do benign positional vertigo episodes recover spontaneously? *J Vestib Res*, 8, 325–9.

15. Aw ST, Todd MJ, Aw GE, et al. (2005). Benign positional nystagmus: a study of its three-dimensional spatio-temporal characteristics. *Neurology*, 64, 1897–905.

16. Yagi T, Koizumi Y, Kimura M, Aoyagi M (2006). Pathological localization of so-called posterior canal BPPV. *Auris Nasus Larynx*, 33, 391–5.

17. Baloh RW (2005). Clinical features and pathophysiology of posterior canal benign positional vertigo. *Audiological Med*, 3, 12–15.

18. Vibert D, Kompis M, Hausler R (2003). Benign paroxysmal positional vertigo in older women may be related to osteoporosis and osteopenia. *Ann Otol Rhinol Laryngol*, 112, 885–9.

19. Lindsay JR, Hemenway WG (1952). Postural vertigo due to unilateral sudden partial loss of vestibular function. *Ann Otol Rhinol Laryngol*, 65, 692–707.

20. Gross EM. Ress BD, Viirre ES, Nelson JR, Harris JP (2000). Intractable benign paroxysmal positional vertigo in patients with Ménière's disease. *Laryngoscope*, 110, 655–9.

21. Cohen HS, Kimball KT (2005). Effectiveness of treatments for benign paroxysmal positional vertigo of the posterior canal. *Otol Neurotol*, 26, 1034–40.

22. Lopez-Escamez JA, Gamiz MJ, Fernandez-Perez A, et al. (2005). Long term outcome and health-related quality of life in benign paroxysmal positional vertigo. *Eur Arch Otorhinolaryngol*, 262, 507–11.

23. Dix MR, Hallpike CS (1952). The pathology, symptomatology and diagnosis of certain common diseases of vestibular system. *Proc R Soc Med*, 78, 987–1016.

24. Epley JM (2001). Human experience with canalith repositioning procedure. *Ann N Y Acad Sci*, 942, 179–91.

25. Viirre E, Purcell I, Baloh RW (2005). The Dix Hallpike test and the canalith repositioning maneuver. *Laryngoscope*, 115, 184–7.

26. Semont A, Freyss G, Vitte E (1988). Curing the BPPV with a liberatory maneuver. *Adv Oto-Rhino-Laryng*, 42, 290–3.

27. Cohen HS (2004). Side-lying as an alternative to the Dix-Hallpike test of the posterior canal. *Otol Neurotol*, 25, 130–4.

28. Baloh RW, Honrubia V, Jacobson K (1987). Benign positional vertigo: clinical and oculographic features in 240 cases. *Neurology*, 37, 371–9.

29. Brandt T, Steddin S, Daroff RB (1994). Therapy for benign paroxysmal positioning vertigo. *Neurology*, 44, 254–61.

30. Hain TC, Squires TM, Stone HA (2005). Clinical implications of a mathematical model of benign paroxysmal positional vertigo. *Ann N Y Acad Sci*, 1039, 384–94.

31. Otsuka K, Suzuki M, Furuya M (2003). Model experiment of benign paroxysmal positional vertigo mechanism using the whole membranous labyrinth. *Acta Otolaryngol*, 123, 515–18.

32. Cohen HS, Sangi-Haghpeykar H (2010). Nystagmus parameters and subtypes of benign paroxysmal positional vertigo. *Acta Otolaryngol*, 130, 1019–23.

33. Nuti D, Mandalà M, Salerni L (2009). Lateral canal paroxysmal positional vertigo revisited. *Ann N Y Acad Sci*, 1164, 316–23.

34. McClure J (1985). Horizontal canal BPV. *J Otolaryngol*, 14, 30–5.

35. Pagnini P, Nuti D, Vannucchi P (1989). Benign paroxysmal vertigo of the horizontal canal. *ORL J Otorhinolaryngol Relat Spec*, 51, 161–70.

36. Nuti D, Vannucchi P, Pagnini P (1996). Benign paroxysmal positional vertigo of the horizontal canal: a form of canalolithiasis with variable clinical features. *J Vestib Res*, 6, 173–84.

37. Nuti D, Vannucchi P, Pagnini P (2005). Lateral canal BPPV: which is the affected side? *Audiological Med*, 3, 16–20.

38. Bisdorff AR, Debatisse D (2001). Localizing signs in positional vertigo due to lateral canal cupulolithiasis. *Neurology*, 57, 1085–8.

39. Choung YH, Shin YR, Kahng H, Park K, Choi SJ (2006). 'Bow and lean test' to determine the affected ear of horizontal canal benign paroxysmal positional vertigo. *Laryngoscope*, 116, 1776–81.

40. Asprella Libonati G (2008). Pseudo-spontaneous nystagmus: a new sign to diagnose the affected side in lateral semicircular canal benign paroxysmal positional vertigo. *Acta Otorhinolaryngol Ital*, 28, 73–8.

41. Baloh RW, Jacobson KJ, Honrubia V (1993). Horizontal semicircular canal variant of benign paroxysmal positional vertigo. *Neurology*, 43, 2542–9.

42. Baloh, R.W, Yue Q, Jacobson KM, et al. (1995). Persistent direction-changing positional nystagmus: another variant of benign positional nystagmus? *Neurology*, 45, 1297–301.

43. Bertholon P, Bronstein AM, Davies RA, Rudge P, Thilo KV (2002). Positional down beating nystagmus in 50 patients: cerebellar disorders and possible anterior semicircular canalithiasis. *J Neurol Neurosurg Psychiatry*, 72, 366–72.

44. Casani AP, Cerchiai N, Dallan I, Sellari-Franceschini S (2011). Anterior canal lithiasis: diagnosis and treatment. *Otolaryngol Head Neck Surg*, 144, 412–18.

45. Korres S, Balatsouras DG, Kaberos A, Kandiloros D, Ferekidis E (2002). Occurrence of semicircular canal involvement in benign paroxysmal positional vertigo. *Otol Neurotol*, 23, 926–32.

46. Jackson L, Morgan B, Fletcher J, Krueger WW (2007). Anterior canal benign paroxysmal vertigo: an underappreciated entity. *Otol Neurotol*, 28, 218–22.

47. Lee, S-H, Kim JS (2010). Benign paroxysmal positional vertigo. *J Clin Neurol*, 6, 51–63.

48. Fernandez C, Alzate R, Lindsay JR (1960). Experimental observations on postural nystagmus. Lesions of the nodulus. *Ann Otol Rhinol Laryngol*, 69, 94–114.

49. Baloh RW (2005). Preface. *Audiological Med*, 3, 2–3.

50. Fife TD, Iverson DJ, Lempert T, et al. (2008). Practice parameter: therapies for benign paroxysmal positional vertigo (an evidence-based review): report of the Quality Standards Subcommittee of the American Academy of Neurology. *Neurology*, 70, 2067–74.

51. Mandalà M, Santoro GP, Asprella Libonati G, et al. (2012). Double-blind randomized trial on short-term efficacy of Semont maneuver for treatment of posterior canal benign paroxysmal positional vertigo. *J Neurol*, 259, 882–5.

52. Massoud E, Ireland DJ (1996). Post treatment instructions in the nonsurgical management of benign paroxysmal positional vertigo. *J Otolaryngol*, 25, 121–5.

53. Cohen HS, Kimball KT (2005). Effectiveness of treatments for benign paroxysmal positional vertigo of the posterior canal. *Otol Neurotol*, 26, 1034–40.

54. Epley J (1992). The canalith repositioning procedure: For treatment of benign paroxysmal positional vertigo. *Otolaryngol Head Neck Surg*, 107, 399–404.

55. Herdman SJ, Tusa RJ, Zee DS, Proctor LR, Mattox DE (1993). Single treatment approach to benign paroxysmal positional vertigo. *Arch Otolaryngol Head Neck Surg*, 119, 450–4.

56. Harvey SA, Hain TC, Adamiec LC (1994). Modified liberatory manoeuvre: effective treatment for benign paroxysmal positional vertigo. *Laryngoscope*, 104, 1206–12.

57. Faldon ME, Bronstein AM (2008). Head accelerations during particle repositioning manoeuvres. *Audiol Neurotol*, 13, 345–56.

58. Nuti D, Nati C, Passali D (2000). Treatment of benign paroxysmal positional vertigo: no need for postmaneuver restrictions. *Otolaryngol Head Neck Surg*, 122, 440–4.

59. Soto-Varela A, Rossi-Izquierdo M, Santos-Pérez S (2011). Can we predict the efficacy of the Semont maneuver in the treatment of benign paroxysmal positional vertigo of the posterior semicircular canal? *Otol Neurotol*, 32, 1008–11.

60. Brandt T, Daroff Rb (1980). Physical therapy for benign paroxysmal positional vertigo. *Arch Otolaryngol*, 106, 484–5.

61. Lempert T (1994). Horizontal benign positional vertigo. *Neurology*, 44, 2213–14.
62. Vannucchi P, Giannoni B, Pagnini P (1997). Treatment of horizontal semicircular canal benign paroxysmal positional vertigo. *J Vestib Res*, 7, 1–6.
63. Nuti D, Agus G, Barbieri MT, Passali D (1998). The management of horizontal-canal paroxysmal positional vertigo. *Acta Otolaryngol (Stockh)*, 118, 445–60.
64. Casani AP, Vannucci G, Fattori B, Berrettini S (2002). The treatment of horizontal canal positional vertigo: our experience in 66 cases. *Laryngoscope*, 112, 172–8.
65. Vannucchi P, Asprella Libonati G, Gufoni M (2005). The physical treatment of lateral semicircular canal canalolithiasis. *Audiological Med*, 3, 52–6.
66. Gufoni M, Mastrosimone L, Di Nasso F (1998). Repositioning maneuver in benign paroxysmal vertigo of horizontal semicircular canal. *Acta Otorhinolaryngol Ital*, 18, 363–7.
67. Strupp M, Brandt T, Steddin S (1995). Horizontal canal benign paroxysmal positioning vertigo: reversible ipsilateral caloric hypoexcitability caused by canalolithiasis? *Neurology*, 45, 2072–6.
68. Asprella Libonati G (2005). Diagnostic and treatment strategy of the lateral semicircular canal canalolithiasis. *Acta Otorhinolaryngol Ital*, 25, 277–83.
69. Han BI, Oh HJ, Kim JS (2006). Nystagmus while recumbent in horizontal canal benign paroxysmal positional vertigo. *Neurology*, 66, 706–10.
70. Honrubia V, Baloh R, Harris M, Jacobson K (1999). Paroxysmal positional vertigo syndrome. *Am J Otol*, 20, 465–70.
71. Hamid M (2001). The manoeuvres for benign positional vertigo. *Oper Tech Otolaryngol Head Neck Surg*, 12, 148–50.
72. Yacovino DA, Hain TC, Gualtieri F (2009). New therapeutic manoeuvre for anterior canal benign paroxysmal positional vertigo. *J Neurol*, 256, 1851–5.
73. Crevits L. (2004). Treatment of anterior canal benign paroxysmal positional vertigo by a prolonged forced position procedure. *J Neurol Neurosurg Psychiatry*, 75, 779–81.
74. Korres S, Riga M, Sandris V, Danielides V, Sismanis A (2010). Canalithiasis of the anterior semicircular canal (ASC): Treatment options based on the possible underlying pathogenetic mechanisms. *Int J Audiol*, 49, 606–12.

CHAPTER 21

Migraine and Other Episodic Vestibular Disorders

Michael von Brevern

Epidemiological association of vertigo and migraine

Given the high prevalence of vertigo and migraine in the general population it is not surprising that many patients suffer from both symptoms. Nonetheless, in the last decade epidemiological arguments have progressively accumulated to strengthen the hypothesis that vertigo is linked to migraine beyond a chance concurrence. All case–control studies published to date indicate a more than chance association of migraine with vertigo. The prevalence of migraine was 1.6 times higher in 200 dizziness clinic patients than in 200 age and sex-matched controls (1). Conversely, in migraineurs, the prevalence of vertigo is higher as compared to non-migraineurs. In a seminal study, 27% of unselected migraine patients reported vertigo, compared with 8% of patients with tension headache (2). Similarly, two other case–control studies found an increased prevalence of vertigo and dizziness in migraineurs (3, 4).

Even more striking is the preponderance of migraine in patients with recurrent vertigo of unknown cause, not fulfilling diagnostic criteria for Ménière's disease. Cha et al. found that 87% of 208 patients with recurrent vertigo of unknown cause met the criteria for migraine and that 70% of these fulfilled the diagnostic criteria for definite vestibular migraine (5). In a similar group of 72 patients, the prevalence of migraine was six times higher as compared to an age and sex-matched control group (6). Likewise, in patients with recurrent vertigo of unknown cause a prevalence of migraine of 81% has been found, as compared to 22% in patients with Ménière's disease (7).

Only recently, the intersection of vertigo and migraine has been examined on the population level. Assuming a lifetime prevalence of migraine of 14% (8) and a lifetime prevalence of vertigo of 7.4% (9), we can calculate a chance coincidence of 1%. Notably, a large epidemiological general population study found that about three times more adults have a history of both vertigo and migraine than would be expected by chance alone, namely 3.2% (9). Recently, the link between migraine and vertigo has been confirmed by another population-based study showing that individuals with migraine are much more likely to have vertigo and vertigo with accompanying headache (odds ratio 3.8 and 8, respectively) than non-migraineurs (10).

Besides clinical experience, this epidemiological data is the scientific basis for vestibular migraine as a syndrome that causally links migraine to vestibular symptoms. Of note, two other vestibular diseases, namely benign paroxysmal positional vertigo (BPPV; 11, 12) and Ménière's disease (13), are epidemiologically linked to—but not caused by—migraine. Furthermore, the interrelation between migraine and vertigo is complicated by the observation that migraine can be triggered by vestibular stimulation (14).

Vestibular migraine

Vestibular migraine is an episodic vertigo syndrome that has been shaped during the last three decades, gaining increasingly recognition but being still debated as an entity. To date, most dizziness clinic experts consider vestibular migraine as one of the most common causes for episodic vertigo. Numerous synonyms have been used including benign recurrent vertigo, migrainous vertigo, migraine associated vertigo, and migraine-related vestibulopathy.

Diagnostic criteria

At first, the diagnosis of vestibular migraine requires the recognition of migraine according to universally accepted diagnostic criteria (Table 21.1). Similar to migraine itself, the diagnosis of vestibular migraine is made on the basis of the history and the exclusion of other causes. So far, there are no internationally approved diagnostic criteria for vestibular migraine. The International Classification of Headache Disorders (ICHD) of the International Headache Society includes vertigo as a migrainous symptom in adults only in the setting of basilar-type migraine. For this diagnosis, the ICHD requires at least two aura symptoms originating from the brainstem and/or both hemispheres, lasting 5–60 minutes, and followed by migraine headaches. Only a minority of less than 10% of patients fulfil these criteria (1, 5, 15). As a consequence, most patients with vestibular migraine cannot be classified according to the current ICHD. Neuhauser and co-workers (1) have proposed operational clinical criteria that are in wide use nowadays and are currently revised by the Classification Committee of the Bàràny Society (Table 21.2). These criteria have a high positive predictive value. A re-evaluation of 75 patients 105 ± 16 months after the initial diagnosis of

Table 21.1 Diagnostic criteria for migraine

A	At least 5 attacks fulfilling criteria B–D
B	Headache attacks lasting 4–72 hours
C	Headache has at least two of the following characteristics: 1. Unilateral localization 2. Pulsating quality 3. Moderate or severe pain intensity 4. Aggravation by or causing avoidance of routine physical activity
D	During headache at least one of the following: 1. Nausea and/or vomiting 2. Photophobia and phonophobia
E	Not attributable to another disorder

From International Headache Society Classification Subcommittee (64).

vestibular migraine confirmed vestibular migraine in 84% whereas a competing diagnosis was considered in 16% (16).

Demographic aspects of vestibular migraine

Vestibular migraine is the second most common cause of recurrent vertigo after BPPV with a lifetime prevalence of about 1% (17). In neurological dizziness clinics, vestibular migraine accounts for 6–7% of diagnoses (1, 18). The onset may be at any age, most commonly between the third and sixth decade. Usually, migraine headaches begin earlier in life than vestibular migraine (18). Similar to migraine there is a clear female preponderance with a female-to-male ratio of around 3:1.

Clinical features

Vestibular migraine can present with spontaneous vertigo, positional vertigo, or head-motion dizziness (19) in isolation or in

Table 21.2 Diagnostic criteria for vestibular migraine

Definite vestibular migraine	
A	Recurrent vertigo of moderate or severe intensity
B	Current or previous history of migraine according to the criteria of the International Classification of Headache Disorders
C	One or more of the following migraine symptoms during at least 50% of the vertigo attacks: migraine headache, photophobia, phonophobia, aura
D	Not attributed to another disorder
Probable vestibular migraine	
A	Recurrent vertigo of moderate or severe intensity
B	One of the following: Current or previous history of migraine according to the ICHD criteria Migraine symptoms during at least 50% of the vertigo attacks Menstrual precipitation of at least 50% of the vertigo attacks
C	Not attributed to another disorder

Adapted from Neuhauser et al. (1).

any combination (Table 21.3). Most patients complain of episodic spontaneous vertigo. In addition, about half of patients experience positional vertigo in the course of the disorder, but not necessarily with every attack (20, 21). Rarely, vestibular migraine presents with isolated episodes of positional vertigo (22) mimicking BPPV. Head-motion dizziness, a distorted sensation of spatial orientation during self-motion, is a frequent additional symptom (15). A transition from spontaneous to positional and finally to head-motion dizziness is often reported. Vertigo and dizziness can be additionally triggered by complex visual, large field, or moving visual stimuli: visually-induced dizziness (15). Autonomic symptoms with nausea and vomiting are frequent but unspecific accompaniments of acute vestibular migraine (20, 21).

The duration of symptomatic episodes ranges from seconds (about 10%) and minutes (30%) to hours (30%) and several days (30%), sometimes even in the same patient (1, 2, 18, 23). Although the core attack with objective clinical signs rarely exceeds 72 hours, for some patients it may take weeks to fully recover from an episode. Only 10–30% of patients experience vertigo with the typical duration of a migraine aura, i.e. 5–60 min (1, 18).

The temporal relationship of vestibular symptoms to migraine headache is highly variable: vertigo can precede headache, may begin with headache, or appear late in the headache phase. Many patients experience attacks both with and without headache (1, 23). The intensity of headache accompanying vertigo is attenuated in most patients as compared to migraine episodes without vestibular symptoms. Often patients develop vestibular migraine after the intensity of their migraine headaches has declined during lifetime.

Table 21.3 Symptoms during acute vestibular migraine (n = 20)

Symptom	%
Vestibular[1]	
Spontaneous vertigo	30
Positional vertigo	40
Head induced dizziness	30
Cochlear	
Aural pressure	20
Hearing loss	0
Tinnitus	0
Autonomic	
Nausea	95
Vomiting	50
Diarrhoea	10
Polyuria	5
Visual	
External vertigo (oszillopsia)	50
Migrainous	
Photophobia	70
Headache	65
Osmophobia	15
Phonophobia	10
Aura	10

[1] Leading vestibular symptom.

From von Brevern et al. (20).

Thus, the dominating clinical feature of vestibular migraine is usually vertigo, not headache. In up to 30% of patients, vestibular symptoms and headache never occur together (1, 5, 23). In these patients, diagnosis can be based on migrainous symptoms other than headache during the attack, i.e. photophobia, phonophobia, osmophobia, and aura symptoms (see Table 21.2). Patients need to be specifically asked about these symptoms since they usually do not volunteer them. A dizziness diary is useful for prospective recording of associated symptoms.

Cochlear symptoms may occur but are not prominent in vestibular migraine. In a prospective study of 20 patients with acute vestibular migraine examined during the attack, none reported hearing loss and four had bilateral aural pressure at the beginning of the episode (20).

In women, vestibular migraine can be precipitated by hormonal changes, appearing just before the menses, similar to migraine headaches. Migraine patients often also report other precipitants such as lack of sleep, stress, sunlight, red wine, which are, however, not specific enough to support a diagnosis of vestibular migraine.

Pathophysiology

The vestibular origin of vestibular migraine has been ascertained by the observation of pathological nystagmus in the acute phase, indicating central vestibular dysfunction in most cases (20, 21). However, it remains unclear how migraine affects the vestibular system. Various hypothesis have been proposed, all of which are derived from the presumed pathophysiology of migraine. Heterogeneous findings during acute episodes indicate that more than one mechanism may be involved in vestibular migraine.

A vasospasm of the internal auditory artery could explain: 1) peripheral vestibular and auditory symptoms during the attack, 2) persisting vestibular deficits und hearing loss in migraine, and 3) the association of migraine with BPPV and Ménière's disease. A spreading depression of the neuronal cortex is likely to be the mechanism of a migraine aura and a spreading depression of brainstem structures could account for short-lasting episodes of vestibular migraine (18). During a migraine attack, various neuropeptides such as calcitonin gene-related peptide are released, which are also involved in peripheral and central vestibular structures and may lead to distorted signal processing (23, 24). Peripheral vestibular and cochlear signs and symptoms could also be explained by activation of the trigeminovascular system during migraine, which can lead to plasma extravasation in the inner ear in animal experiments (25). In line with this finding it is interesting that painful trigeminal stimulation can evoke nystagmus in migraineurs (26). Finally, a deficit of ion channels could account for peripheral and central vestibular dysfunction. This last hypothesis is the only one systematically tested and appears to be promising as other paroxysmal disorders presenting with migraine and vertigo such as episodic ataxia type 2 (EA2) and familial hemiplegic migraine have been found to result from a channelopathy. However, searching for mutations in various candidate genes was negative in patients with vestibular migraine (27, 28).

Investigations

Vestibular migraine is diagnosed primarily on the basis of the history and there is no specific testing abnormality. However, laboratory testing can be useful to reassure that there is no severe vestibular damage such as a complete canal paresis, which would rather suggest another disorder. On the other hand, minor findings on vestibular testing are not uncommon in patients with vestibular migraine. In most patients, the clinical neuro-otological examination is normal in the symptom-free period (23) or shows only subtle ocular motor abnormalities such as impaired smooth pursuit (18, 29).

A unilaterally reduced caloric response is the most often reported finding with a prevalence of about 20% in several case series (29, 30). Usually, unilateral vestibular hypofunction is only mild and the head thrust test is almost always normal. Interestingly, patients with vestibular migraine are four times more likely to have an emetic response to caloric stimulation than migraine patients without vertigo (31).

In rotatory chair testing, an isolated directional preponderance has been found in about 20% of patients (15, 18). A reduced gain of the horizontal vestibulo-ocular reflex during rotatory testing has been reported by some authors (32, 33), but occurred only rarely in a large patient series (15).

Assessment of vestibular-evoked myogenic potentials (VEMPs) has yielded reduced amplitudes in around two-thirds of patients with vestibular migraine indicating saccule dysfunction. Unfortunately, this method does not seem to be helpful for the differentiation from Ménière's disease, where similar results can be found (34).

Audiometry revealed sensorineural hearing loss not attributable to any cause in up to 20% of patients (35). A review on audiometric findings in vestibular migraine summarized results of nine studies and found an average prevalence of unexplained hearing loss of 7.5% (36). Thus, hearing loss is rather unusual, and low-frequency, progressive, or fluctuating hearing loss, typical for Ménière's disease, is a rare finding in vestibular migraine.

Findings during an episode

Examination during an episode of vestibular migraine usually yields pathological nystagmus, indicating central vestibular dysfunction in most patients. A prospective neuro-otolneuro-otological study of 20 patients during the acute phase of vestibular migraine recorded pathological nystagmus in 70% of patients by means of three-dimensional video-oculography (20). A peripheral type of spontaneous nystagmus with a unilateral deficit of the horizontal vestibulo-ocular reflex was observed in three patients, a central type of spontaneous nystagmus in three, a central positional nystagmus in five, and a combined central spontaneous and positional nystagmus in three (Figure 21.1; Video 21.1). Hearing was not affected in any patient during the episode. Saccadic pursuit was only noted in two patients during the attack. Overall, findings pointed to central vestibular dysfunction in 10 patients (50%), to peripheral vestibular dysfunction in three patients (15%), and were inconclusive with regard to the involved structure in 35%. On follow-up vestibular and ocular motor abnormalities had disappeared in almost all patients. Various patterns of spontaneous and positional nystagmus, almost exclusively of a central type, have also been observed by other authors (18, 21).

Differential diagnosis

Due to its lack of characteristic clinical features (except for a temporal association with migrainous symptoms) vestibular migraine has been designated a chameleon (37) that can mimic peripheral vestibular disorder (e.g. Ménière's disease, BPPV),

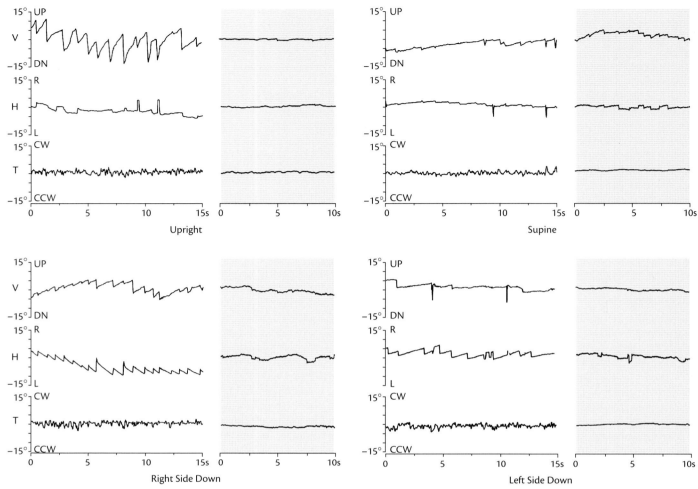

Fig. 21.1 Video-oculography recording of spontaneous and persistent positional nystagmus in a patient with acute vestibular migraine and during the symptom-free interval (grey shading). Vertical (V), horizontal (H), and torsional (T) eye movement components are shown. Note the downbeating nystagmus in the upright position, which ceases in the supine position. In the lateral positions a predominantly horizontal, geotropic nystagmus appears. From von Brevern et al. (20), by permission of Oxford University Press.

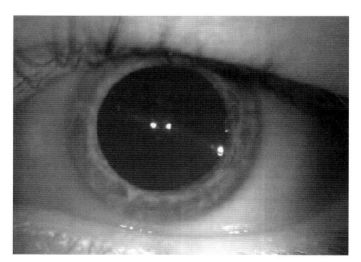

Video 21.1 Video-oculography recording of two patients during acute vestibular migraine: patient 3 shows spontaneous and persistent positional nystagmus indicating central vestibular dysfunction and patient 11 has spontaneous horizontal nystagmus and a positive head thrust test (not shown) pointing to peripheral vestibular dysfunction.

central vestibular disorders (e.g. vertebrobasilar ischaemia), and non-vestibular psychiatric disorders presenting with dizziness and vertigo. Furthermore, the interrelation between migraine and vestibular dysfunction is complicated by the fact that vertigo can trigger migraine headaches in susceptible individuals, similar to lack of sleep and menstrual cycling (14). Therefore, disorders causing episodic vertigo have to be prudently excluded even in those patients presenting concurrently with both migraine and vertigo.

The most challenging differential diagnosis of vestibular migraine is Ménière's disease, particularly in the early course when permanent hearing loss may not yet be detectable in the latter. Both disorders present similar in terms of severity and duration of vertigo episodes (38). Usually, the distinction can be made based on hearing loss being only occasional and mild in vestibular migraine, while it is a regular and disabling accompaniment in Ménière's disease. Furthermore, when hearing loss develops in vestibular migraine, it is often bilateral (16, 36) whereas involvement of both ears from the onset has been described in only 2% of Ménière's patients (39). Tinnitus and aural fullness may also occur during vertigo attacks in vestibular migraine. Again, in comparison with Ménière's disease, these symptoms are rarely unilateral and more often bilateral (15, 38). Nonetheless, there is a diagnostic overlap between vestibular migraine and Ménière's disease, not only in the early stage. After a mean follow-up of 9 years in 75 patients with the initial diagnosis of vestibular migraine, 10% of patients fulfilled both diagnostic criteria for Ménière's disease and vestibular migraine. Yet, these patients had clinical features atypical of classical Ménière's disease such as symmetrical and mostly mild hearing loss and long duration of vertigo episodes, raising doubts that Ménière's disease is the correct diagnosis (16). These findings can be interpreted in two ways: either current diagnostic criteria for Ménière's disease and vestibular migraine are not sufficiently discriminative or both disorders share an underlying mechanism. A genetic link between both disorders would be supported by familial clustering of migraine, episodic vertigo, and Ménière's disease but this constellation is rather rare (40, 41). To complicate matters further, migrainous symptoms such as headache and photophobia are also frequent accompaniments in attacks of Ménière's disease (13, 38). For practical purposes, when patients present with prominent and initially unilateral hearing loss and vertigo attacks lasting at least 20 minutes, Ménière's disease should be diagnosed, even when migraine symptoms occur during vertigo episodes. In those patients with only minor hearing symptoms and a history compatible with both vestibular migraine and Ménière's disease, medical treatment with a trial of migraine prophylaxis is advisable. Failure of this approach should prompt consideration of the alternative management but invasive procedures for Ménière's disease should be avoided.

Occasionally, vestibular migraine can mimic BPPV when presenting with isolated positional vertigo. Several factors help to distinguish vestibular migraine from BPPV: short symptomatic episodes of one to few days (versus weeks to months in BPPV), manifestation early in life, frequent recurrences of episodes, and atypical positional nystagmus (22).

Vestibular migraine shares some clinical features with EA2. In both disorders, a history of migraine and a positive family history for episodic vertigo are often present. EA2 is a rare autosomal dominant, inherited paroxysmal disorder of early onset characterized by episodes of incoordination and truncal ataxia. Manifestation after the age of 20 is exceptional. The attacks are commonly triggered by physical and emotional stress and last typically hours. In about half of the patients at least one of the following can be found: vestibular symptoms with vertigo, nausea and vomiting during attacks, generalized weakness during attacks, gradual progressive baseline ataxia, and a history of migraine (42). Between attacks, the vast majority of patients present with gaze-evoked nystagmus and a third with spontaneous or positional downbeat nystagmus (43). These interictal ocular motor signs are an important key to differentiate vestibular migraine from EA2 as they are no more than subtle in the former and prominent in the latter. Other features that may help to distinguish vestibular migraine from EA2 are the age at onset, triggers and response to treatment with acetazolamide (Table 21.4). Genetic testing is commercially available for EA2 and identifies a mutation in the CACNA1A gene in about 60% of patients.

There is a complex interrelation between vertigo and dizziness, migraine, and some psychiatric disorders. Both panic disorders and major depression are bidirectionally associated with migraine (44, 45). With regard to all vestibular disorders, patients with vestibular migraine seem to be at highest risk to develop comorbid psychiatric disorders, particularly anxiety and depression disorders (46). Hence, besides vestibular episodes, patients with vestibular migraine may exhibit episodic or constant psychogenic dizziness in the course of the disease. Episodes of psychogenic dizziness usually can be identified on the basis of the history as they are often triggered by specific environments and are not accompanied by severe nausea, vomiting, external vertigo, and falls (see Chapter 29). However, in individual patients with co-occurrence of vestibular migraine and psychogenic dizziness, the differentiation between both syndromes can be problematic.

Table 21.4 Comparison between episodic ataxia type 2 and vestibular migraine

	EA2	Vestibular migraine
Episodic ataxia	+	−
Episodic vertigo	50%	Almost 100%
History of migraine	50%	100%
History of epilepsy	7%	Risk not increased
Age of onset	2–20	Predominantly in adulthood
Duration of attack	Hours	Minutes to hours, rarely seconds
Trigger	Exertion Emotional stress	Menstruation Emotional stress?
Interictal findings	90% gaze-evoked nystagmus 30% downbeat nystagmus 50% mild ataxia	Mild central ocular motor abnormalities may occur
Family history	Usually	Occasionally
Gene	CACN1A1	Unknown
Treatment	Acetazolamide 4-Aminopyridine	Migraine prophylaxis

Adapted from Baloh and Jen (63).

Table 21.5 Pharmacological treatment of vestibular migraine

Drug and dose	Common side effects	Contraindications/precautions
Acute attacks		
Dimenhydrinate 50–100 mg PO or 150 mg supp every 8 h	Sedation, dry mouth	Glaucoma, asthma, urinary retention
Sumatriptan 50–100 mg PO, 25 mg supp, 6 mg SC	Chest pain, palpitations, paraesthesia	Hypertension, coronary artery disease, basilar-type migraine
Zolmitriptan 2.5 mg PO, 5 mg IN	Same as above	Same as above
Prophylaxis		
Metoprolol 50–200 mg/day PO	Hypotension, sedation, bronchospasm, bradycardia, impotence	Asthma, bradycardia, heart block, heart insufficiency, diabetes, orthostatic hypotension, depression
Propranolol 40–240 mg/day PO	Same as above	Same as above
Topiramate 50–100 mg/day PO	Sedation, paraesthesia, cognitive impairment, weight loss, paraesthesia, renal stone formation	Renal insufficiency, psychosis, glaucoma
Valproic acid 500–600 mg/day PO	Sedation, weight gain	Liver disease, pregnancy
Amitriptyline 50–100 mg/day PO	Sedation, orthostatic hypotension, dry mouth	Glaucoma, urinary retention
Acetazolamide 500–750 mg/day PO	Paraesthesia, hypokalaemia	Severe kidney or liver disease, hypokalaemia

IN, intranasally; PO, by mouth; SC, subcutaneously; supp, suppository.

Adapted from Bronstein AM, Lempert T (2007). *Dizziness. A practical approach to diagnosis and management*. Cambridge: Cambridge University Press.

Treatment

A thorough explanation of the migrainous origin of the episodes is essential to relieve unnecessary fears of a serious disorder and prepares the ground for adherence to lifestyle changes and medications. At first, many patients are surprised when the diagnosis is explained to them, particularly when the presenting symptom is vertigo and not headache. Non-pharmaceutical approaches in the prophylactic treatment of vestibular migraine should not be neglected and can be as effective as drugs. Avoidance of identified triggers, regular sleep and meals, and physical exercise has a firm place in migraine prophylaxis. In migraine headaches, relaxation methods and biofeedback are as effective as pharmacological prophylaxis (47).

Symptomatic treatment during episodes of vestibular migraine lasting longer than 1 hour can be achieved with vestibular suppressants such as dimenhydrinate (Table 21.5). There is anecdotal evidence that triptans may be effective for vestibular migraine. The only controlled trial on the efficacy of triptans in vestibular migraine remained inconclusive due to its limited power (48). A retrospective study found that the effect of triptans on vertigo was related to its effect on headache (49). Interestingly, triptans seem also to reduce motion-sickness in migraineurs, possibly by influencing serotonergic vestibulo-autonomic projections (50). As nausea is often present during an attack, acute medication should be administered non-orally.

In many patients, episodes of vestibular migraine are severe, long, and frequent enough to warrant prophylactic medication. Unfortunately, there is a lack of solid data derived from placebo-controlled trials. Several retrospective and observational analysis have reported a reduction of intensity and frequency of attacks of vestibular migraine with prophylactic migraine drugs such as metoprolol, propranolol, flunarizine, topiramate, lamotrigine, valproate, and amitriptyline (51). Furthermore, response to the carbonic anhydrase inhibitor acetazolamide, which is usually not used for migraine prophylaxis, has been reported (52). These reports have to be regarded with caution as the clinical course is variable and spontaneous remissions often occur (48). However, most experts agree that prophylactic drug treatment can be effective in vestibular migraine. In the absence of evidence for the most effective medication, comorbid conditions and side effects must be taken into consideration for the choice of drug. In patients with hypertension, a beta-blocker is usually the first choice. The use of several drugs can be limited by weight-gaining side effects (flunarizine, valproate, amitriptyline). Sedation and other side effects can be greatly reduced with slow titration of dosage. Patients should keep a diary of events and treatment efficacy should be evaluated after 3 months. A reduction in attack frequency of about 50–70% is a realistic goal.

In patients with constant dizziness and unsteadiness in addition to episodes of vertigo migraine, vestibular rehabilitation can be effective (53). Psychiatric illness often significantly adds to reduction of life quality and patients with coexisting anxiety disorders or depression should be treated with antidepressants and psychotherapy.

Benign paroxysmal vertigo of childhood

Benign paroxysmal vertigo of childhood is recognized by the International Headache Society as a precursor of migraine (Table 21.6) and can be regarded as an early variant of vestibular migraine manifesting before puberty. It has been estimated that 2.6% of children aged 6–12 years are affected by benign paroxysmal vertigo of childhood (54) and that vertigo is due to a migraine mechanism in about a third of children suffering from dizziness and vertigo (55).

Benign paroxysmal vertigo of childhood is characterized by sudden brief attacks of vertigo with imbalance, occurring without warning and lasting minutes, rarely hours, in otherwise healthy children (56). The attacks may be accompanied with nausea, vomiting, pallor, sweating, and nystagmus, but headache is lacking. The ictal oculomotor findings of benign paroxysmal vertigo of

Table 21.6 Diagnostic criteria for benign paroxysmal vertigo of childhood

A	At least 5 attacks fulfilling criterion B
B	Multiple episodes of severe vertigo, occurring without warning and resolving spontaneously after minutes to hours
C	Normal neurological examination, audiometric and vestibular functions between attacks
D	Normal electroencephalogram

From International Headache Society Classification Subcommittee (64).

childhood have not been well documented. Usually the condition ceases spontaneously after few years. Many of these children have a family history of migraine and later develop migraine headache, often years after vertigo attacks have ceased (57).

Benign recurrent vertigo

The term 'benign recurrent vertigo' was coined in 1979 by Slater for patients with recurrent attacks of spontaneous vertigo that cannot be explained by other known peripheral or central vestibular disorders and in the absence of cochlear signs. Other authors have used 'recurrent vestibulopathy' as a synonym (58). To date, this syndrome is ill defined as some authors include patients with vestibular migraine (5) whereas others exclude patients with a migraine history (59).

There is a large overlap between benign recurrent vertigo and vestibular migraine and Slater has speculated on benign recurrent vertigo as a migraine equivalent. Several large case series endorse the association between benign recurrent vertigo and migraine (5, 6, 38). Besides the strikingly increased prevalence of migraine there are several clinical similarities between benign recurrent vertigo and vestibular migraine: 1) female preponderance (5), 2) family occurrence suggestive of an autosomal dominant inheritance with reduced penetrance in some patients (60), 3) precipitation by lack of sleep and emotional stress (61), and 4) transition from spontaneous to positional vertigo during an episode (61). In conclusion, the majority of patients with benign recurrent vertigo can be classified as definite or probable vestibular migraine. However, the term benign recurrent vertigo (or recurrent vestibulopathy) is not dispensable but should be restricted to patients with episodic spontaneous vertigo of unknown cause and without a history of migraine. Only a few authors have reported on benign recurrent vertigo in this stricter sense (5, 59).

The clinical presentation of benign recurrent vertigo is similar to vestibular migraine and Ménière's disease with respect to duration, severity, and triggers (38). Cochlear symptoms during episodes of vertigo are not rare. The incidence of bilateral hearing impairment, tinnitus, or aural fullness during vertigo episodes is not different from patients with Ménière's disease. In contrast, unilateral cochlear symptoms occurring with at least half of the vertigo attacks have been reported by 81% of Ménière's patients versus only 32% of patients with benign recurrent vertigo (38). The age at onset peaks in the middle of life and women are affected twice as often as men (59). The most common duration of episodes is 1 hour to 1 day but attacks of shorter and longer duration may also occur (5). Nausea is often an accompaniment. The mean frequency of episodes was five per year in a group of 105 patients (59).

The natural course of this syndrome is benign with about 60% of patients reporting a spontaneous remission after few years (59, 62). The rate of conversion to Ménière's disease 3 years after initial diagnosis ranges between 1% (59) and 7% (58).

Benign recurrent vertigo remains a diagnosis of exclusion and a provisional diagnosis. Several other disorders that can cause episodic vertigo should be ruled out, in particular vestibular migraine, Ménière's disease, vertebrobasilar insufficiency, and panic disorder. Laboratory testing is useful to exclude other vestibular disorders but provides unspecific results in patients with benign recurrent vertigo. Similar to vestibular migraine, unilateral caloric hyporesponsiveness has been found in about 10–20% of patients with benign recurrent vertigo (59, 62).

The pathophysiology of benign recurrent vertigo in the stricter sense (without migraine history) is unclear. A migraine mechanism is conceivable even in the absence of a history of migraine headaches, just as an isolated migraine aura may occur in patients who have never had a migraine headache. This hypothesis is supported by the female preponderance of benign recurrent vertigo.

For treatment of acute episodes patients should be provided with vestibular sedatives. There is a lack of reports on prophylactic treatment of benign recurrent vertigo without a history of migraine in the literature.

Conclusion

The association between migraine and vestibular symptoms has been well ascertained by epidemiological studies. There is a complex interrelation between vestibular disorders and migraine: 1) vestibular migraine is conceptualized as an episodic vestibular disorder that is caused by a not yet identified migraine pathomechanism, 2) benign paroxysmal positional vertigo and Ménière's disease are vestibular disorders epidemiologically associated with migraine, and 3) migraine headache can be triggered by vestibular activation. Vestibular migraine has emerged during the last three decades as a new syndrome that accounts for up to 10% of diagnosis in dizziness clinics. As vestibular migraine can mimic other vestibular disorders, it is worthwhile taking a migraine history in all patients presenting with vertigo. At the beginning of the medical history, diagnostic ambiguity between vestibular migraine and Ménière's disease may be problematic, but later cochlear deficits discriminate both disorders in most patients. Given the frequency of vestibular migraine, more research into the mechanisms of how migraine can affect the vestibular system and well-designed treatment trials are needed. The integration of vestibular migraine as a subcategory of migraine in the International Classification of Headache Disorders would help to promote these goals.

References

1. Neuhauser H, Leopold M, von Brevern M, Arnold G, Lempert T (2001). The interrelations of migraine, vertigo, and migrainous vertigo. *Neurology*, 56, 436–41.
2. Kayan A, Hood JD (1984). Neuro-otological manifestations of migraine. *Brain*, 107, 1123–42.
3. Kuritzky A, Ziegler DK, Hassanein R (1981). Vertigo, motion sickness and migraine. *Headache*, 21, 227–31.
4. Vuković V, Plavec D, Galinivic I, Lovrencic-Huzja A, Budisic M, Demarin V (2007). Prevalence of vertigo, dizziness, and migrainous vertigo in patients with migraine. *Headache*, 47, 1427–35.

5. Cha YH, Santell LS, Baloh RW (2009). Association of benign recurrent vertigo and migraine in 208 patients. *Cephalalgia*, 29, 550–5.

6. Lee H, Sohn SI, Jung DK, *et al.* (2002). Migraine and isolated recurrent vertigo of unknown cause. *Neurol Res*, 24, 663–5.

7. Rassekh CH, Harker LA (1992). The prevalence of migraine in Ménière's disease. *Laryngoscope*, 102, 135–8.

8. Jensen R, Stovner LJ (2008). Epidemiology and comorbidity of headache. *Lancet Neurol*, 7, 354–61.

9. Neuhauser HK, von Brevern M, Radtke A, *et al.* (2005). Epidemiology of vestibular vertigo. A neurotologic survey of the general population. *Neurology*, 65, 898–904.

10. Neuhauser HK, von Brevern M, Radtke A, Lempert T (2008). Population-based epidemiological evidence for the link between dizziness and migraine. 25th Barany Society Meeting 2008, Kyoto, Abstract 177.

11. Ishiyama A, Jacobson KM, Baloh RW (2000). Migraine and benign paroxysmal vertigo. *Ann Otol Rhinol Laryngol*, 109, 377–80.

12. von Brevern M, Radtke A, Lezius F, Feldmann M, Lempert T, Neuhauser H (2007). Epidemiology of benign paroxysmal positional vertigo: a population based study. *J Neurol Neurosurg Psychiatry*, 78, 710–5.

13. Radtke A, Lempert T, Gresty MA, Brookes GB, Bronstein AM, Neuhauser H (2002). Migraine and Ménière's disease. Is there a link? *Neurology*, 59, 1700–4.

14. Murdin L, Davies RA, Bronstein AM (2009). Vertigo as a migraine trigger. *Neurology*, 7, 638–42.

15. Cass SP, Ankerstjerne JKP, Yetiser S, Furman J, Balaban C, Aydogan B (1997). Migraine-related vestibulopathy. *Ann Otol Rhinol Laryngol*, 106, 182–9.

16. Radtke A, Neuhauser H, von Brevern M, Hottenrott T, Lempert T (2011). Vestibular migraine—validity of clinical diagnostic criteria. *Cephalalgia*, 31, 906–13.

17. Neuhauser HK, Radtke A, von Brevern M, *et al.* (2006). Migrainous vertigo: prevalence and impact on quality of life. *Neurology*, 67, 1028–33.

18. Dieterich M, Brandt T (1999). Episodic vertigo related to migraine (90 cases): vestibular migraine? *J Neurol*, 246, 883–92.

19. Bisdorff A, von Brevern M, Lempert T, Newman-Toker DE (2009). Classification of vestibular symptoms: towards an international classification of vestibular disorders. *J Vest Res*, 19, 1–13.

20. von Brevern M, Zeise D, Neuhauser H, Clarke A, Lempert T (2005). Acute migrainous vertigo: clinical and oculographic findings. *Brain*, 128, 365–74.

21. Polensek SH, Tusa RJ (2010). Nystagmus during attacks of vestibular migraine: an aid in diagnosis. *Audiol Neurootol*, 15, 241–46.

22. von Brevern M, Radtke A, Clarke AH, Lempert T (2004). Migrainous vertigo presenting as episodic positional vertigo. *Neurology*, 62, 469–72.

23. Cutrer FM, Baloh RW (1992). Migraine-associated dizziness. *Headache*, 32, 300–4.

24. Furman JM, Marcus DA, Balaban CD (2003). Migrainous vertigo: development of a pathogenetic model and structured diagnostic interview. *Curr Opin Neurol*, 16, 5–13.

25. Koo JW, Balaban CD (2006). Serotonin-induced plasma extravasation in the murine inner ear: possible mechanism of migraine-associated inner ear dysfunction. *Cephalalgia*, 26, 1310–19.

26. Marano E, Marcelli V, Di Stasio E, *et al.* (2005). Trigeminal stimulation elicits a peripheral vestibular imbalance in migraine patients. *Headache*, 45, 325–31.

27. Kim JS, Yue Q, Jen JC, Nelson SF, Baloh RW (1998). Familial migraine with vertigo: no mutation found in CACNA1A. *Am J Med Gen*, 79, 148–51.

28. von Brevern M, Ta N, Shankar A, *et al.* (2006). Migrainous vertigo: mutation analysis of the candidate genes CACNA1A, ATP1A2, SCN1A, and CACNB4. *Headache*, 46, 1136–41.

29. Çelebisoy N, Gökçay F, Şirin H, Biçak N (2007). Migrainous vertigo: clinical, oculographic and posturographic findings. *Cephalalgia*, 28, 72–7.

30. Teggi R, Colombo B, Bernasconi L, Bellini C, Comi G, Bussi M (2009). Migrainous vertigo: results of caloric testing and stabilometric findings. *Headache*, 49, 435–44.

31. Vitkovic J, Paine M, Rance G (2008). Neuro-otological findings in patients with migraine- and nonmigraine-related dizziness. *Audiol Neurotol*, 13, 113–22.

32. Dimitri PS, Wall C, Oas JG, Rauch SD (2001). Application of multivariate statistics to vestibular testing: discrimination between Ménière's disease and migraine associated dizziness. *J Vest Res*, 11, 53–65.

33. Furman JM, Sparto PJ, Soso M, Marcus D (2005). Vestibular function in migraine-related dizziness: a pilot study. *J Vest Res*, 15, 327–32.

34. Baier B, Dieterich M (2009). Vestibular-evoked myogenic potentials in 'vestibular migraine' and Ménière's disease. A sign of electrophysiological link? *Ann N Y Acad Sci*, 1164, 324–7.

35. Maione A (2006). Migraine-related vertigo: diagnostic criteria and prophylactic treatment. *Laryngoscope*, 116, 1782–6.

36. Battista RA (2004). Audiometric findings of patients with migraine-associated dizziness. *Otol Neurotol*, 25, 987–92.

37. Brandt T (2004). A chameleon among the episodic vertigo syndromes: 'migrainous vertigo' or 'vestibular migraine'. *Cephalalgia*, 24, 81–2.

38. Brantberg K, Baloh RW (2011). Similarity of vertigo attacks due to Meniere's disease and benign recurrent vertigo, both with and without migraine. *Acta Otolaryngol*, 131, 722–7.

39. Huppert D, Strupp M, Brandt T (2010). Long-term course of Ménière's disease revisited. *Acta Otolaryngol*, 130, 644–651.

40. Cha YH, Kane KJ, Baloh RW (2007). Familial clustering of migraine, episodic vertigo and Ménière's disease. *Otol Neurotol*, 29, 93–6.

41. Hietikko E, Kotimäki J, Kentala E, Klockars T, Sorri M, Männikkö M (2011). Finnish familial Meniere disease is not linked to chromosome 12p12.3, and anticipation and consegration with migraine are not common findings. *Genet Med*, 13, 415–20.

42. Jen J, Kim GW, Baloh RW (2004). Clinical spectrum of episodic ataxia type 2. *Neurology*, 62, 17–22.

43. Jen JC, Graves TD, Hess EJ, Hanna MG, Griggs RC, Baloh RW and the CINCH investigators (2007). Primary episodic ataxias: diagnosis, pathogenesis, and treatment. *Brain*, 130, 2484–493.

44. Breslau N, Schulz LR, Steward WF, Lipton RB, Lucia VC, Welch KM (2000). Headache and major depression: is the association specific for migraine? *Neurology*, 54, 308–13.

45. Breslau N, Schulz LR, Steward WF, Lipton RB, Welch KM (2001). Headache types and panic disorders: directionally and specificity. *Neurology*, 56, 350–54.

46. Eckhardt-Henn A, Best C, Bense S, Breuer P, Diener G, Tschan R, Dieterich M (2008). Psychiatric comorbidity in different organic vertigo syndromes. *J Neurol*, 255, 420–8.

47. Holroyd KA, Penzien DB (1990). Pharmacological versus non-pharmacological prophylaxis of recurrent migraine headaches: a meta-analytic review of clinical trials. *Pain*, 42, 1–13.

48. Neuhauser H, Radtke A, von Brevern M, Lempert T (2003). Zolmitriptan for treatment of migrainous vertigo: a pilot randomized placebo-controlled trial. *Neurology*, 60, 882–3.

49. Bikhazi P, Jackson C, Ruckenstein MJ (1997). Efficacy of antimigrainous therapy in the treatment of migraine-associated dizziness. *Am J Otol*, 18(3), 350–4.

50. Furman JM, Marcus DA, Balaban CD (2011). Rizatriptan reduces vestibular-induced motion sickness in migraineurs. *J Headache Pain*, 12, 81–88.

51. Fotuhi M, Glaun B, Quan SY, Sofare T (2009). Vestibular migraine: a critical review of treatment trials. *J Neurol*, 256, 711–16.

52. Baloh RW, Foster CA, Yue Q, Nelson SF (1996). Familial migraine with vertigo and essential tremor. *Neurology*, 46, 458–60.

53. Whitney SL, Wrisley DM, Brown KE, Furman JM (2000). Physical therapy for migraine-related vestibulopathy and vestibular dysfunction with history of migraine. *Laryngoscope*, 110, 1528–34.

54. Abu-Arafeh I, Russel G (1995). Paroxysmal vertigo as a migraine equivalent in children: a population-based study. *Cephalalgia*, 15, 22–5.

55. Riina N, Ilmari P, Kentala E (2005). Vertigo and imbalance in children. A retrospective study in a Helsinki university otolaryngology clinic. *Arch Otolaryngol Head Neck Surg*, 131, 996–1000.

56. Basser LS (1964). Benign paroxysmal vertigo of childhood. *Brain*, 87, 141–52.

57. Krams B, Echenne B, Leydet J, Rivier F, Roubertie A (2011). Benign paroxysmal vertigo of childhood: long-term outcome. *Cephalalgia*, 31, 439–43.

58. Leliever WC, Barber HO (1981). Recurrent vestibulopathy. *Laryngoscope*, 91, 1–6.

59. van Leeuwen RB, Bruintjes TD (2010). Recurrent vestibulopathy: natural course and prognostic factors. *J Laryngol Otol*, 124, 19–22.

60. Lee H, Jen JC, Wang H, *et al.* (2006). A genome-wide linkage scan of familial benign recurrent vertigo: linkage to 22q12 with evidence of heterogeneity. *Hum Mol Gen*, 15, 251–8.

61. Slater R (1979). Benign recurrent vertigo. *J Neurol Neurosurg Psychiatry*, 42, 363–7.

62. Kentala E, Pyykkö I (1997). Benign recurrent vertigo—true or artificial diagnosis? *Acta Otolaryngol Suppl* 529, 101–103.

63. Baloh RW, Jen JC (2002). Genetics of familial episodic vertigo and ataxia. *N Y Acad Sci*, 956, 338–45.

64. International Headache Society Classification Subcommittee (2004). International classification of headache disorders. 2nd edition. *Cephalgia*, 24(Suppl 1), 1–160.

CHAPTER 22

Ménière's Disease and Other Causes of Episodic Vertigo

Yuri Agrawal and Lloyd B. Minor

Introduction

Ménière's syndrome is an inner ear disorder characterized by spontaneous attacks of vertigo, fluctuating low-frequency sensorineural hearing loss, aural fullness, and tinnitus. When the syndrome is idiopathic and cannot be attributed to any other cause (e.g. syphilis, immune-mediated inner ear disease, surgical trauma), it is referred to as Ménière's disease (1). Ménière's syndrome exhibits a relapsing–remitting pattern, with episodic attacks terminated by periods of restitution to normal auditory and vestibular function. Additionally, the natural history of Ménière's syndrome is such that auditory and vestibular function typically decline over time (2).

Prosper Ménière first described this constellation of symptoms in 1861, and given the co-occurrence of auditory and vestibular phenomena he proposed that the pathological locus was the labyrinth (3). Subsequent investigations have corroborated his hypothesis: postmortem temporal bone analyses of individuals with Ménière's syndrome demonstrated histopathological abnormalities in the labyrinth. Additionally, physiological tests of labyrinthine function were also found to be abnormal in these patients.

In this chapter we will review the clinical and pathophysiological features of Ménière's disease that distinguish it from other disease processes in the differential diagnosis of vertigo and imbalance. We will begin by describing some key clinical characteristics of Ménière's disease. We will then outline the central pathological hypothesis behind Ménière's disease—endolymphatic hydrops—insofar as this informs our understanding of physiological and radiographic tests as well as management strategies in Ménière's disease. We will explore the physiological effects of Ménière's disease on vestibular function, as measured by caloric, head impulse, and vestibular-evoked myogenic potential (VEMP) testing. Finally, we will review management strategies for the treatment of Ménière's disease.

Ménière's disease: clinical features

The prevalence of Ménière's disease has been reported to range from 3.5 per 100,000 persons in Japan,(4) 157 per 100,000 persons in the United Kingdom (5), 190 per 100,000 in the United States (6), to 513 per 100,000 in Finland (7). Disease onset typically occurs in the fourth to sixth decade of life, with a 1.3–1.9:1 female predominance (6, 8). Ménière's disease tends to be unilateral and involves the contralateral ear in 30% of cases (9). The diagnosis of Ménière's disease is largely clinical at this time; there are no pathognomonic tests that confirm this diagnosis. The most widely-used guidelines to establish a diagnosis of Ménière's disease were published by the American Academy of Otolaryngology-Head and Neck Surgery (AAO-HNS), which termed 'definite' Ménière's disease as two or more spontaneous episodes of vertigo each lasting 20 minutes or longer, hearing loss documented by audiograms on at least one occasion, tinnitus or aural fullness in the affected ear, and other causes excluded (typically with gadolinium-enhanced magnetic resonance imaging (MRI) of the cranial base) (10). The staging system established by the AAO-HNS is based on audiometric criteria, with four-frequency pure-tone averages at 0.5, 1, 2, and 3 kHz of <25, 26–40, 41–70 and >70 corresponding to Stages 1, 2, 3, and 4 respectively.

The presentation of Ménière's disease typically includes recurring attacks of vertigo (96.2%), with tinnitus (91.1%) and ipsilateral hearing loss (87.7%) (11). The clinical course of Ménière's disease varies considerably between patients, from long periods of remission punctuated by episodic attacks to intervals of unrelenting recurring attacks. Longitudinal studies suggest that vertigo ceases spontaneously in 57% of cases at 2 years and 71% after 8.3 years (12). Patients classically present with a low-frequency sensorineural hearing loss that is fluctuating and progressive. With long-standing disease (>10 years), the audiometric pattern flattens and the hearing loss stabilizes at a pure-tone average of 50 dB and a speech discrimination score of 50% (13). Profound sensorineural hearing loss occurs in 1–2% of patients (14); if the losses are bilateral patients may benefit from cochlear implantation. Interestingly, some patients with Ménière's disease who undergo cochlear implantation continue to experience fluctuation in hearing in their implanted ear (15). Ménière's disease has been shown to have significant adverse effects on quality of life, as measured by the Quality of Well-Being Scale (16). Poor physical and mental functioning scores as well as increased levels of depression were also noted in patients with Ménière's disease (16).

Endolymphatic hydrops

Endolymphatic hydrops has long been held to be the pathological basis for Ménière's disease (17–19). Endolymph, the potassium-enriched fluid in the inner ear, may be either excessively synthesized or inadequately resorbed, resulting in expansion of the endolymphatic space (19, 20). Surgical ablation of the endolymphatic sac in experimental animals has reproduced the histopathological finding of endolymphatic hydrops seen in temporal bone specimens of individuals with Ménière's disease, although these animals do not seem to experience the classic signs and symptoms associated with Ménière's disease in humans (21, 22).

Endolymphatic hydrops typically involves the pars inferior of the labyrinth (comprising the saccule and cochlea) (18, 23). Saccular hydrops may range from mild to severe, based on the degree of membrane distension towards the stapes footplate (24). Cochlear hydrops is typified by bowing of Reissner's membrane into the scala vestibuli; severity of cochlear hydrops also varies according to the degree of convexity towards the scalar wall of the modiolus (25). The pars superior (utricle and semicircular canals) may also be involved in endolymphatic hydrops, although changes tend to be less dramatic and occur less frequently.

Several mechanisms have been suggested to explain how endolymphatic hydrops may produce the spontaneous attacks of vertigo characteristic of Ménière's disease. The most prominent theory holds that hydropic distension of the endolymphatic duct causes rupture of the distended membranes, a phenomenon that has been observed throughout the labyrinth (26). Membrane rupture allows the potassium-rich endolymph to leak into the perilymphatic space and contact the basal surface of the hair cells as well as the VIIIth cranial nerve. Initial excitation then subsequent inhibition of the hair cells manifests as a direction-changing nystagmus and may underlie the clinical phenotype of episodic vertigo.

Long-term declines in auditory and vestibular function may be the result of repeated exposure of the vestibular hair cells to toxic levels of potassium-enriched perilymph (27). The increased susceptibility of type II relative to type I hair cells in Ménière's disease supports the hypothesis that chronic perilymph toxicity may cause neurosensory dysfunction (28). The vestibular neuroepithelium consists of type I and type II hair cells as well as supporting cells. Both hair cell types have cuticular plates and stereociliary bundles, reflecting their role in mechanosensory signal transduction. However, the two hair cell types can be distinguished based on other morphological characteristics: type I hair cells are flask-shaped, have a round nucleus and are enveloped on their basal surface by an afferent nerve chalice. In contrast, type II hair cells are cylindrically-shaped, have oval nuclei, and small bouton-type nerve terminals from afferent and efferent nerve endings (29). The sparse nerve endings on the basal surface of type II hair cells may provide decreased protection against harmful ionic changes in the perilymph (28). The physiological and functional implications of the selective depletion of type II hair cells in Ménière's disease are still poorly understood.

Alternatively it has been postulated that hydrops itself may occur in an episodic manner, as a result of sudden increases in the secretory function of the stria vascularis or of spontaneous obstruction of the endolymphatic sac (30). Hydropic distension may then cause a mechanical deflection of the macula and crista of the otoliths and semicircular canals respectively and thus vestibular hair cell depolarization, leading to the sensation of vertigo (30). Long-term changes to the neurosensory function of the vestibular apparatus may be the consequence of increased hydrodynamic pressure causing increased vascular resistance, compromised blood flow, and chronic ischaemic injury (31, 32).

Several lines of evidence challenge the primacy of endolymphatic hydrops in the pathophysiology of Ménière's disease. As mentioned previously, experimentally-induced endolymphatic hydrops in animal models does not produce the clinical phenotype of Ménière's disease in these animals. Moreover, a double-blind study of temporal bone specimens and associated clinical histories demonstrated that all individuals with Ménière's syndrome diagnosed during life had evidence of endolymphatic hydrops on postmortem examination of their temporal bones; however, not all individuals with histopathological evidence of endolymphatic hydrops had clinical histories consistent with Ménière's disease (33). If endolymphatic hydrops was central to the development of Ménière's disease, one would expect the correlation between the clinical manifestations of Ménière's disease and endolymphatic hydrops to be absolute.

Alternatively, studies are increasingly suggesting that endolymphatic hydrops may be a marker of some other pathological process that causes Ménière's disease, such as disordered cochlear homeostasis (34). Emerging evidence implicates the fibrocytes of the spiral ligament which play a crucial role in maintaining cochlear fluid homeostasis: dysregulation of these cells appears to precede the development of hydrops (35). Genetic studies may generate additional insights into the pathological basis of Ménière's disease. A familial genetic predisposition has been reported in 2–14% of cases (36), following an autosomal dominant inheritance pattern (37). Recent genome-wide association studies have identified polymorphisms in a potassium ion transporter and a protein also linked to hypertension in individuals with Ménière's disease (38). Auto-immune mechanisms may also play a role, as evidenced by associations between specific human leukocyte antigens such as Cw7 and Ménière's disease (39). This molecular genetic line of inquiry shows promise for yielding the true pathological basis for Ménière's disease.

Based on endolymphatic hydrops as a presumed pathological correlate of Ménière's disease, various electrophysiological and radiographic tests have been explored as providing supportive evidence for a diagnosis of Ménière's disease. Electrocochleography measures electrical potentials generated by the cochlea in response to repeated sound stimulation. The cochlear response typically consists of a cochlear microphonic and summating potential (SP), both of which represent cochlear outer hair cell function, and the compound action potential (AP), which reflects auditory nerve activity and corresponds to wave I of the auditory brainstem reflex. The SP has been observed to be larger and more negative in patients with Ménière's disease, leading to an elevated SP/AP ratio (>0.4). This is thought to reflect hydropic distension of the basilar membrane into the scala tympani causing an increase in the normal asymmetry of its vibration. The sensitivity of the SP/AP ratio has been reported to be 50–70% (40), and efforts to augment the sensitivity have included combining the SP/AP ratio with SP amplitude, AP latency, and audiometric parameters (41).

The pursuit of a diagnostic test for Ménière's disease has also motivated research into imaging of endolymphatic hydrops. MRI scanning with the intravenous and intratympanic delivery of gadolinium has allowed for the visualization of the labyrinthine fluid

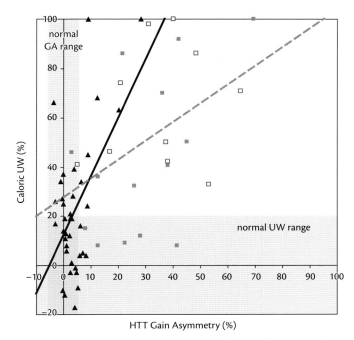

Fig. 22.1 Head thrust test gain asymmetry (HTT GA) is plotted versus the caloric unilateral weakness (UW) in subjects with Ménière's disease (filled triangles), and the regression line (solid line) fitting Ménière's disease is also plotted. For comparison, data from Schmid-Priscoveanu et al. (85) for subjects with acute (open rectangles) and chronic (filled rectangles) vestibular neuritis (VN) are also plotted, along with the regression line (broken line) for both groups of VN subjects. Shaded regions indicate normal HTT GA (−5.8% to +5.8%) and normal caloric UW values (−20% to +20%). Figure reproduced with permission (46).

spaces *in vivo*, and endolymphatic hydrops has been observed in many cases of clinically-diagnosed Ménière's disease (42). As technological refinements continue to augment the power of MRI, the ability of MRI to resolve endolymphatic hydrops should concomitantly rise. It should be noted that studies of the predictive value of various tests for Ménière's disease inherently suffer from the lack of an objective gold standard diagnosis for Ménière's disease.

Caloric and head impulse testing in Ménière's disease

Caloric and head impulse testing are both tests of semicircular canal function. In caloric testing, bithermal irrigation is applied to the external auditory canals, which causes a convective movement of endolymph within the ipsilateral horizontal semicircular canal (43). The movement of fluid within the horizontal canal results in excitatory or inhibitory deflection of the cupula (depending upon the direction of endolymph flow). Motion of the cupula then leads to hair-cell excitation or inhibition with a corresponding change in the discharge rate of vestibular-nerve afferents. Compensatory eye movements are thereby elicited (corresponding to the slow phases of nystagmus), followed by a rapid corrective saccades (corresponding to the fast phase of nystagmus). The maximum velocities of the slow phases of nystagmus are compared bilaterally and used to compute unilateral weakness or caloric asymmetry. A caloric asymmetry of 20% or greater is usually considered indicative of unilateral peripheral vestibular hypofunction.

Head impulse (or head thrust) testing assesses the integrity of the three-dimensional angular vestibulo-ocular reflex (AVOR). Head and eye movements are recorded during high-velocity, high-acceleration rotary head impulses in the plane excitatory for each of the six semicircular canals. Normal subjects are able to maintain visual fixation on a target during rapid head movement and thus have gain values (computed as the ratio of eye velocity to head velocity) close to 1.0 (44).

A significant reduction in the caloric response of affected ears has been observed in 42–79% of individuals with unilateral Ménière's disease, and caloric asymmetries of 100% (i.e. absent caloric response in the affected ear) have been noted in 6–11% of patients (45–51). In contrast, abnormalities of the AVOR in Ménière's disease are much less prevalent. A study comparing caloric and head impulse testing in individuals with Ménière's disease observed caloric testing abnormalities in 42% of subjects but AVOR abnormalities in only 13% of patients, although a significant linear correlation was noted between head impulse test gain asymmetry and caloric unilateral weakness percentage (Figure 22.1) (46).

The results of caloric and head impulse testing in Ménière's disease are informative. First, although caloric testing is abnormal, the normal AVOR gains in Ménière's disease suggest that there is substantial preservation of semicircular canal function in these patients (52). Additionally, although both caloric and head impulse testing are measures of semicircular canal function they appear to be capturing distinct phenomena. Caloric irrigation causes a slow convective flow of endolymph and provides a low-frequency stimulus to the vestibular system. In contrast, high-velocity rotary head thrusts cause rapid endolymph movement and generate a high-frequency input to vestibular afferents. It is possible that Ménière's disease preferentially impairs the ability of the vestibular apparatus to process low-frequency signals. It should be noted that the low-frequency caloric stimulus is a non-physiological input, whereas the high-frequency head thrust approximates commonly-occurring stimulus frequencies to the vestibular apparatus. Thus it is also possible that mechanisms of central adaptation can only be established for physiological stimuli (leading to normal responses to head impulse testing) but not for inputs outside the normal range (i.e. caloric stimuli).

A similar dissociation between caloric and head impulse testing was observed in a study of semicircular canal function during acute attacks and quiescent periods (53). The authors found that in patients with early-stage unilateral Ménière's disease, there was no asymmetry in caloric testing or AVOR gain during quiescent intervals. During acute vertigo attacks, these patients demonstrated ipsilateral caloric weakness and an increase in VOR gain with rotations towards the ipsilesional side (53). The hydropic ear may function as a high-pass filter: it dampens sensitivity to low-frequency stimulation and enhances sensitivity to high frequency stimulation.

VEMP testing in Ménière's disease

Vestibular-evoked myogenic potentials are thought to reflect otolith function. The cervical VEMP (cVEMP) appears to be generated by a sacculocollic reflex. In the afferent limb of this reflex pathway, acoustically-sensitive cells in the saccule respond to brief, loud, monaural sound stimuli and transmit an electrical signal centrally via the inferior vestibular nerve. The efferent limb of this

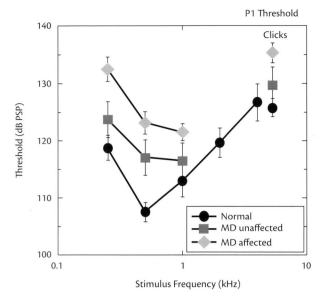

Fig. 22.2 Mean ± standard error of the mean vestibular-evoked myogenic potential thresholds for tone-burst and click stimuli in normal subjects' ears (n = 14) and affected and unaffected ears of subjects with unilateral Ménière's disease (n = 34). Figure reproduced with permission (63).

reflex arc sends an inhibitory impulse to the fibres of the ipsilateral sternocleidomastoid muscle; electromyographic recordings from this muscle in response to a sound input thus reflect saccular function (54, 55). Typical cVEMP testing paradigms elicit responses to broadband clicks and frequency-specific tonebursts. In normal subjects, click-evoked cVEMP responses can be elicited 98% of the time and short toneburst-evoked cVEMP responses occur 88% of the time (56).

Ocular VEMPs (oVEMP) are a newer vestibular-evoked potential to air-conducted sound or bone-conducted vibrational (BCV) stimuli. Responses are crossed and are excitatory to the contralateral inferior oblique muscle. One study found that the oVEMP in response to BCV is abolished in the setting of superior vestibular neuritis, suggesting that the vibration-evoked oVEMP may be a measure of utricular function (57). Studies of otolith function and Ménière's disease have largely focused on the cVEMP; these studies will be reviewed in this section. More recent investigations into the diagnostic utility of the oVEMP will be discussed at the end of this section.

Individuals with normal saccular function exhibit frequency tuning of their cVEMP responses, such that sound thresholds required to elicit a cVEMP response are lowest when the sound stimuli are delivered at particular frequencies (58). The greatest sensitivity of the sacculocollic reflex appears to occur over the 200–1000-Hz frequency range (59, 60). Frequency tuning appears to be a function of both the testing apparatus as well as resonance properties of the saccule (which in part reflects the size of the saccule).

Given that Ménière's disease is associated with cochleosaccular hydrops, and that cVEMP responses reflect saccular mechanics, it is logical that cVEMP testing would be altered in individuals with Ménière's disease. Indeed, cVEMP responses to click stimuli were observed to be delayed or absent in 51–54% of patients with Ménière's disease (61, 62) compared to the normal click-evoked response rates of 98% discussed previously. Additionally, cVEMP responses in

individuals with Ménière's disease exhibit altered frequency tuning, such that the greatest sensitivity of the sacculocollic reflex appears to occur at higher frequencies and across broader frequency ranges compared to normal subjects (Figure 22.2) (63). Changes in saccular resonance characteristics in the setting of hydrops are thought to underlie the abnormalities in cVEMP testing.

Further evidence that cVEMP responses are indicative of saccular dysfunction in Ménière's disease comes from the observation of 'dose–response' relationships. Individuals with severe saccular dysfunction who experience drop attacks—otherwise known as otolithic crises of Tumarkin (64, 65)—have the greatest blunting and frequency shift of their cVEMP tuning curves (66). Additionally, 27% of individuals with unilateral Ménière's disease were found to have cVEMP response abnormalities in their unaffected ear; the cVEMP tuning curves in these asymptomatic ears were noted to be intermediate in phenotype between affected and normal ears (67).

Cervical VEMP testing appears to be a powerful tool in the diagnosis of Ménière's disease, likely because it specifically measures saccular function which is impaired in Ménière's disease. Indeed, a study evaluating the relative ability of various vestibular physiologic tests to predict the side of lesion in individuals with unilateral Ménière's disease found that cVEMP testing using a toneburst stimulus at 250 Hz correctly assigned the side of lesion in 80% of cases (68). This test performance was second only the 85% correct assignment seen with caloric testing where caloric asymmetry was defined as greater than 5% interaural difference (as opposed to the more conventional 20–30%). Another study evaluated differences in cVEMP thresholds between affected and unaffected ears in patients with unilateral Ménière's disease as a measure of disease severity (69). The authors found a significant correlation between interaural cVEMP amplitude differences and Ménière's disease stage based on AAO-HNS 1995 clinical criteria (69). Cervical VEMP testing shows particular promise as a measure of Ménière's disease severity and in its ability to prognosticate bilateral disease.

Emerging evidence suggests that oVEMPs to air-conducted sounds demonstrate similar sensitivity to sound-evoked cVEMPs in the diagnosis of Ménière's disease. Both the oVEMP and cVEMP in response to air-conducted sounds are thought to reflect saccular function, and in one study the sound-evoked oVEMP had a higher correlation with other measures of cochleovestibular function in Ménière's disease—including caloric testing and hearing loss—than the sound-evoked cVEMP (70). Alterations in frequency tuning of the sound-evoked oVEMP in patients with Ménière's disease have also been observed (71). Changes in otolith function during acute attacks and periods of remission have been explored using oVEMPs, and an increase in utricular function as measured by the vibration-evoked oVEMP and a decrease in saccular function as measured by the vibration-evoked cVEMP during acute attacks have been reported (72). The proliferation and specification of tests of otolith function will likely be of diagnostic utility and also shed light on the pathophysiology of Ménière's disease.

Treatment

Given that the pathological basis of Ménière's disease remains elusive, it follows that a curative treatment remains to be elucidated. Current therapies are directed at mitigating symptoms, particularly vertigo. First-line medical regimens include salt restriction and

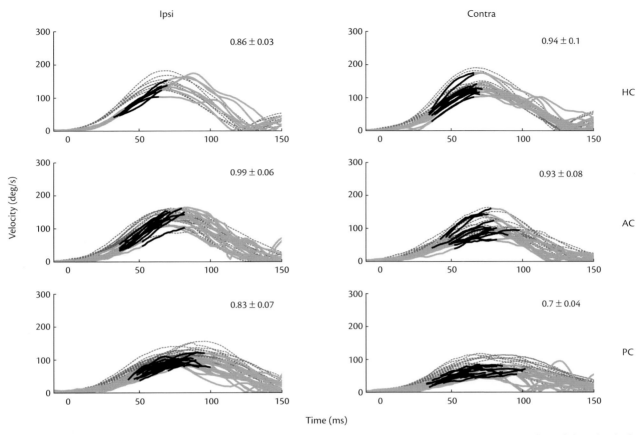

Fig. 22.3 Responses to head impulse testing in a patient with Ménière's disease measured before intratympanic gentamicin injection. Each panel shows head velocity (light grey dashed) and eye velocity (dark grey and black) for rotations in the excitatory direction for each canal. Data from 8–12 stimulus repetitions are shown for each canal. Head velocity has been inverted to permit a direct comparison of the stimulus and the response. The interval over which gain was analysed (30 ms prior to peak head velocity) is shown in black for each trace. The eye velocity before and after this analysis interval is shown in dark grey. A gain value was calculated as eye/head velocity for every point in time during the analysis interval. The response gain for each stimulus repetition was defined as the maximum gain value during the interval of analysis. The response gain (mean ± standard deviation for all stimulus repetitions) is given in each panel's upper right corner. Figure reproduced with permission (52).

diuretics, aimed at alleviating endolymphatic hydrops. Betahistine, an H1-histamine receptor antagonist that increases inner ear blood flow, has been shown to reduce the frequency and severity of vertigo episodes. Betahistine is widely used in Europe in the treatment of Ménière's disease although its use is limited in the United States given insufficient evidence for its efficacy (73). Increasing evidence is supporting the use of corticosteroids, particularly delivered intratympanically, in the treatment of Ménière's disease. One large retrospective study found that control of vertigo symptoms was achieved in 91% of patients treated with intratympanic dexamethasone, allowing them to defer or avoid ablative therapies (74).

Medical therapy is insufficient to control vertigo symptoms in 10% of cases (75). Options for patients with refractory Ménière's disease include surgical decompression of the endolymphatic system, and surgical or chemical ablation of vestibular function. In endolymphatic sac surgery, a transmastoid approach is used to decompress the sac with or without placement of a shunt to drain endolymph. Studies demonstrate positive outcomes from endolymphatic shunt surgery in terms of hearing preservation and vertigo control (76), although a recent meta-analysis found that there is insufficient evidence showing efficacy of this procedure relative to placebo (77). Selective vestibular neurectomy via middle fossa or posterior fossa approach has been shown to relieve vertigo symptoms in over 90%

of cases, although potential complications of these procedures, including hearing loss, facial nerve weakness, cerebrospinal fluid leak, speech and language deficits (from temporal lobe retraction in the middle fossa approach), and headaches (from the posterior fossa approach) must be considered. Surgical labyrinthectomy achieves excellent vertigo control rates, although hearing in the operated ear is abolished. A new area of investigation involves the use of a vestibular neurostimulator in the treatment of Ménière's disease. Using cochlear implant technology, an implantable device that delivers a fixed electrical signal during acute attacks to suppress the symptoms of vertigo has been tested in animal models and is being adapted for human use (78). The ongoing development of a multichannel vestibular prosthesis may also find use in patients with bilateral Ménière's disease and bilateral vestibular hypofunction (79).

Surgical procedures are increasingly being supplanted by chemical ablation of the peripheral vestibular apparatus using intratympanic gentamicin. Gentamicin is a selective vestibulotoxic aminoglycoside antibiotic that is preferentially taken up by type I hair cells of the vestibular neuroepithelium (80). The use of low-dose intratympanic gentamicin has been shown to yield 70–90% vertigo control rates (81), and is associated with hearing loss in only 17% of cases (82). One study examined AVOR gain before and after intratympanic gentamicin administration (52). As noted

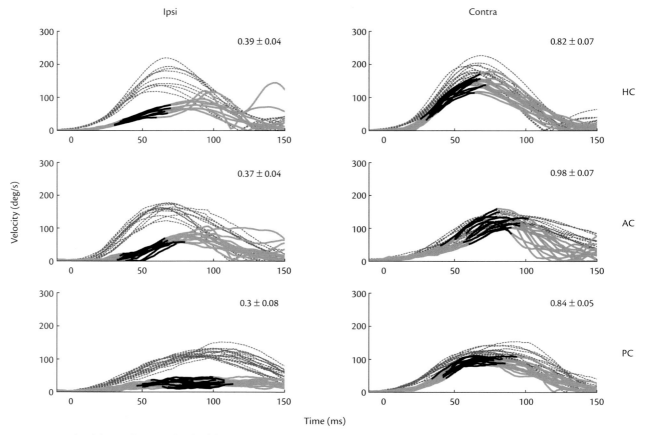

Fig. 22.4 Responses to head thrusts that excited each of the six semicircular canals in a patient with Ménière's disease (same as in Figure 22.1) measured 49 days after a single intratympanic injection of gentamicin. Panels, traces, and gain values are as described for Figure 22.1. Figure reproduced with permission (52).

previously, gain values in patients with Ménière's disease were close to unity, although caloric responses were diminished in the majority of patients. Figure 22.3 depicts representative head (light grey dashed) and eye (dark grey and black) velocity traces for a 38-year-old woman with a 3-year history of episodic vertigo and right fluctuating sensorineural hearing loss and tinnitus before intratympanic gentamicin (52). Caloric testing showed a 23% right unilateral weakness. Each trace shows the patient's head and eye velocities for head impulses that excited the indicated canal; ipsilateral impulses were directed toward the affected ear and contralateral impulses were in the direction of the intact ear. Figure 22.4 shows the head and eye velocity traces from the same woman obtained 49 days after a single intratympanic gentamicin injection to the right ear (52). She reported no further vertigo episodes after treatment. Her caloric testing revealed a 92% right unilateral caloric weakness, and her AVOR data showed marked reductions in the gain for rotations to the ipsilesional side.

Studies suggest that control of vertigo symptoms occurs with successful and enduring ablation of vestibular function: patients who sustained decreases in AVOR gain and increases in caloric weakness following intratympanic gentamicin were found to have fewer episodes of post-treatment vertigo and were less likely to require repeat therapy (83, 84). However, the correlation between the loss of semicircular canal function and symptom control is not absolute (84). It is possible that the natural history of Ménière's disease—typified by a high spontaneous remission rate—may obscure an association between decreased vestibular function and relief from vertigo symptoms. Alternatively, recurrent vertigo may in part reflect otolith function which is not captured by caloric or head impulse testing.

Superior semicircular canal dehiscence syndrome and vestibular paroxysmia

Other vestibular disorders may present similarly to Ménière's disease and should be included in the differential diagnosis. Superior semicircular canal dehiscence syndrome (SCDS) and vestibular paroxysmia will be discussed here; the reader is referred to the following chapters for a discussion of vestibular migraine (Chapter 21), vascular etiologies (Chapter 23) and recurrent BPPV (Chapter 9). In 1998, Minor et al. described that dehiscence of bone overlying the superior semicircular canal can result in a clinical syndrome with symptoms and signs related to vestibular and auditory dysfunction.[86] These patients may exhibit a Tullio phenomenon (eye movements induced by loud noises) or Hennebert's sign (eye movements induced by pressure in the external auditory canal). Chronic disequilibrium may also be present, and the auditory manifestations include autophony and pulsatile tinnitus.

The pathophysiology of superior canal dehiscence can be understood in terms of the effects of the dehiscence in creating a 'third mobile window' into the inner ear, thereby allowing the superior canal to respond to sound and pressure stimuli.[86] The finding that eye movements evoked by sound or by pressure stimuli are in the same plane as the superior canal of the affected ear was important in focusing attention on the superior canal as the cause

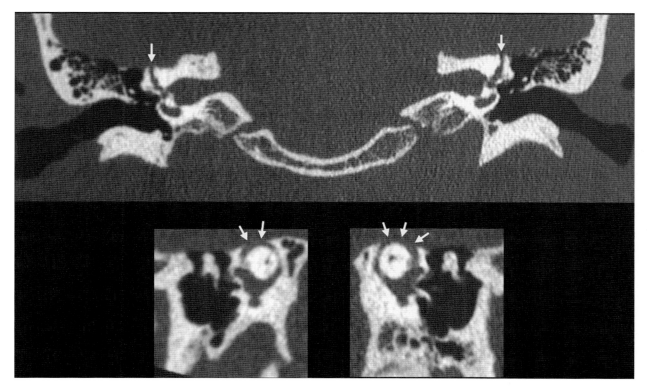

Fig. 22.5 CT scan of a patient with bilateral superior canal dehiscences. Top panel is a coronal image, bottom panels are reformatted in the plane of the superior canals on the right (left panel) and left (right panel) sides.

of these abnormalities.[86,87] Typical physiologic findings in patients with SCDS include an air-bone gap on audiometry accompanied by supra-normalbone conduction thresholds ('conductive hyperacusis'),[88,89] and a lowered threshold for eliciting a cervical and ocular VEMP response in the affected ear.[90,91] The diagnosis of SCDS is established with a high-resolution temporal bone CT scan showing a dehiscence of the bone overlying the superior canal (Figure 22.5).

Treatment in symptomatic patients includessurgical repair of SCD performed through the middle cranial fossa approach,[86] although a transmastoid approach has also been described.[92] The dehiscent superior canal is plugged with fascia and bone thereby obliterating the canal lumen, and the bony middle fossa plate is resurfaced with bone cement. Plugging the superior canal has been shown to result in resolution of symptoms, closure of the air-bone gap, and normalization of VEMP responses.[93,94]

Vestibular paroxysmia is a syndrome of episodic vertigo associated with neurovascular compression of the VIIIth cranial nerve, leading to nerve demyelination and ephaptic transmission of action potentials.[95] A recent study established diagnostic criteria for definite and probable vestibular paroxysmia.[96] Definite vestibular paroxysmia is characterized by: (a) at least five attacks of vertigo spells lasting seconds to minutes, (b) attacks associated with specificprovocative factors (e.g. head turn), and (c) attacks accompanied by tinnitus, hearing loss, aural fullness, or gait disturbance. Additionally, (d) certain objective criteria must be met, including neurovascular compression demonstrated on MRI (CISS sequence), hyperventilation-induced nystagmus as measured by electronystagmography (ENG), progression of vestibular deficit

based on repeated ENG, or treatment response to antiepileptics. Moreover, (e) the symptoms cannot be explained by another disease. Probable vestibular paroxysmia has been defined as at least five attacks fulfilling criterion (a), and at least three of the criteria B–E.[96] Treatment of vestibular paroxysmia typically includes antiepileptics(e.g. carbamazepine), and in selected symptomatic patients, microvascular decompression has been shown to be effective at reducing symptoms and improving quality of life in 80–85% of patients.[97,98]

Summary

Prosper Ménière first described the symptom complex of episodic vertigo, fluctuating hearing loss, aural fullness, and tinnitus 150 years ago. Despite the significant disability and diminished quality of life associated with this disease, a definitive understanding of the pathophysiological basis as well as curative treatment remain elusive. Fortunately, progress is being made on numerous fronts, specifically with respect to the molecular genetic basis of Ménière's disease, enhanced imaging of endolymphatic hydrops, a heightened understanding of otolith dysfunction in Ménière's disease, the increased use of otolith tests, and the development and refinement of therapeutics including intratympanic gentamicin and vestibular stimulators and prostheses. Hopefully definitive diagnosis and cure now lie within reach.

References

1. Paparella MM, Sajjadi H (1987). Endolymphatic sac enhancement. Principles of diagnosis and treatment. *Am J Otol*, 8(4), 294–300.

2. Minor LB, Schessel DA, Carey JP (2004). Meniere's disease. *Curr Opin Neurol*, 17(1), 9–16.

3. Ménière P (1861). Sur une forme de surdite grave dependant d'une lesion de l'oreille interne. *Gaz Med de Paris*, 16, 29.

4. Nakae K, Nitta H, Hattori Y, *et al.* (1980). The prevalence of Ménière's disease in Japan (in Japanese). *Prac Otol (Kyoto)*, 73, 1023–29.

5. Cawthorne T, Hewlett AB (1954). Ménière's disease. *Proc R Soc Med*, 47(8), 663–70.

6. Harris JP, Alexander TH (2010). Current-day prevalence of Meniere's syndrome. *Audiol Neurootol*, 15(5), 318–22.

7. Havia M, Kentala E, Pyykko I (2005). Prevalence of Meniere's disease in general population of Southern Finland. *Otolaryngol Head Neck Surg*, 133(5), 762–8.

8. Shojaku H, Watanabe Y, Fujisaka M, *et al.* (2005). Epidemiologic characteristics of definite Meniere's disease in Japan. A long-term survey of Toyama and Niigata prefectures. *ORL J Otorhinolaryngol Relat Spec*, 67(5), 305–9.

9. Thomas K, Harrison MS (1971). Long-term follow up of 610 cases of Meniere's disease. *Proc R Soc Med*, 64(8), 853–7.

10. American Academy of Otolaryngology-Head and Neck Foundation, Inc. (1995). Committee on Hearing and Equilibrium guidelines for the diagnosis and evaluation of therapy in Meniere's disease. *Otolaryngol Head Neck Surg*, 113(3), 181–5.

11. Paparella MM, Mancini F (1985). Vestibular Meniere's disease. *Otolaryngol Head Neck Surg*, 93(2), 148–51.

12. Silverstein H, Smouha E, Jones R (1989). Natural history vs. surgery for Meniere's disease. *Otolaryngol Head Neck Surg*, 100(1), 6–16.

13. Friberg U, Stahle J, Svedberg A (1984). The natural course of Meniere's disease. *Acta Otolaryngol Suppl*, 406, 72–7.

14. Stahle J (1976). Advanced Meniere's disease. A study of 356 severely disabled patients. *Acta Otolaryngol*, 81(1–2), 113–19.

15. Lustig LR, Yeagle J, Niparko JK, Minor LB (2003). Cochlear implantation in patients with bilateral Meniere's syndrome. *Otol Neurotol*, 24(3), 397–403.

16. Anderson JP, Harris JP (2001). Impact of Meniere's disease on quality of life. *Otol Neurotol*, 22(6), 888–94.

17. Hallpike CS, Cairns H (1938). Observations on the pathology of Meniere's syndrome. *J Laryngol Otol*, 53, 625–55.

18. Schuknecht HF, Igarashi M (1986). Pathophysiology of Meniere's disease. In Pfaltz CR (Ed) *Controversial aspects of Meniere's disease*, pp. 46–54. New York: Georg Thieme Verlag Stuttgart.

19. Anatoli-Candela F (1976). The histopathology of Meniere's disease. *Acta Otolaryngol Suppl (Stockh)*, 340, 5–42.

20. Paparella MM (1985). The cause (multifactorial inheritance) and pathogenesis (endolymphatic malabsorption) of Meniere's disease and its symptoms (mechanical and chemical). *Acta Otolaryngol*, 99(3–4), 445–51.

21. Fukuda S, Keithley EM, Harris JP (1988). The development of endolymphatic hydrops following CMV inoculation of the endolymphatic sac. *Laryngoscope*, 98(4), 439–43.

22. Kimura RS (1967). Experimental blockage of the endolymphatic duct and sac and its effect on the inner ear of the guinea pig: a study of endolymphatic hydrops. *Ann Otol Rhinol Laryngol*, 76, 664–87.

23. Schuknecht HF (1986). Endolymphatic hydrops: can it be controlled? *Ann Otol Rhinol Laryngol*, 95(1 Pt 1), 36–9.

24. Horner KC (1993). Review: morphological changes associated with endolymphatic hydrops. *Scanning Microsc*, 7(1), 223–38.

25. Schuknecht HF (1974). *Pathology of the ear*. Cambridge, MA: Harvard University.

26. Schuknecht HF (1963). Meniere's disease: a correlation of symptomatology and pathology. *Laryngoscope*, 73, 651–65.

27. Thomsen J, Bretlau P (1986). General conclusions. In Pfaltz CR (Ed) *Controversial aspects of Meniere's disease*, pp. 120–36. New York: Georg Thieme Verlag Stuttgart.

28. Tsuji K, Velazquez-Villasenor L, Rauch SD, Glynn RJ, Wall C, 3rd, Merchant SN (2000). Temporal bone studies of the human peripheral vestibular system. Meniere's disease. *Ann Otol Rhinol Laryngol Suppl*, 181, 26–31.

29. Merchant SN, Velazquez-Villasenor L, Tsuji K, Glynn RJ, Wall C, 3rd, Rauch SD (2000). Temporal bone studies of the human peripheral vestibular system. Normative vestibular hair cell data. *Ann Otol Rhinol Laryngol Suppl*, 181, 3–13.

30. Honrubia V (1999). Pathophysiology of Meniere's disease: Vestibular system. In Harris JP (Ed) *Ménière's Disease*, pp. 231–60. The Hague: Kugler Publications.

31. Nakashima T, Ito A (1981). Effect of increased perilymphatic pressure on endocochlear potential. *Ann Otol Rhinol Laryngol*, 90(3 Pt 1), 264–6.

32. Andrews JC, Honrubia V (1988). Vestibular function in experimental endolymphatic hydrops. *Laryngoscope*, 98(5), 479–85.

33. Rauch SD, Merchant SN, Thedinger BA (1989). Meniere's syndrome and endolymphatic hydrops. Double-blind temporal bone study. *Ann Otol Rhinol Laryngol*, 98(11), 873–83.

34. Merchant SN, Adams JC, Nadol JB, Jr (2005). Pathophysiology of Meniere's syndrome: are symptoms caused by endolymphatic hydrops? *Otol Neurotol*, 26(1), 74–81.

35. Shinomori Y, Kimura RS, Adams JC (2001). Changes in immunostaining for Na+, K+, 2Cl-cotransporter 1, taurine and c-Jun N-terminal kinase in experimentally induced endolymphatic hydrops. *ARO Abstr*, 24, 134.

36. Birgerson L, Gustavson KH, Stahle J (1987). Familial Meniere's disease: a genetic investigation. *Am J Otol*, 8(4), 323–6.

37. Morrison AW, Bailey ME, Morrison GA (2009). Familial Meniere's disease: clinical and genetic aspects. *J Laryngol Otol*, 123(1), 29–37.

38. Vrabec JT (2010). Genetic investigations of Meniere's disease. *Otolaryngol Clin North Am*, 43(5), 1121–32.

39. Xenellis J, Morrison AW, McClowskey D, Festenstein H (1986). HLA antigens in the pathogenesis of Meniere's disease. *J Laryngol Otol*, 100(1), 21–4.

40. Adams ME, Heidenreich KD, Kileny PR (2010). Audiovestibular testing in patients with Meniere's disease. *Otolaryngol Clin North Am*, 43(5), 995–1009.

41. Claes GM, De Valck CF, Van de Heyning P, Wuyts FL (2011). The Meniere's Disease Index: An objective correlate of Meniere's disease, based on audiometric and electrocochleographic Data. *Otol Neurotol*, 32, 887–92.

42. Nakashima T, Naganawa S, Pyykko I, *et al.* (2009). Grading of endolymphatic hydrops using magnetic resonance imaging. *Acta Otolaryngol Suppl*, 560, 5–8.

43. Proctor L, Dix R, Hughes D, Rentea R (1975). Stimulation of the vestibular receptor by means of step temperature changes during continuous aural irrigation. *Acta Otolaryngol*, 79(5–6), 425–35.

44. Aw ST, Haslwanter T, Halmagyi GM, Curthoys IS, Yavor RA, Todd MJ (1996). Three-dimensional vector analysis of the human vestibuloocular reflex in response to high-acceleration head rotations. I. Responses in normal subjects. *J Neurophysiol*, 76(6), 4009–20.

45. Stahle J, Klockhoff I (1986). Diagnostic procedures, differential diagnosis and general conclusions. In Pfaltz CR (Ed) *Controversial aspects of Ménière's disease*, pp. 71–86. New York: Georg Thieme Verlag Stuttgart.

46. Park HJ, Migliaccio AA, Della Santina CC, Minor LB, Carey JP (2005). Search-coil head-thrust and caloric tests in Meniere's disease. *Acta Otolaryngol*, 125(8), 852–7.

47. Black FO, Kitch R (1980). A review of vestibular test results in Meniere's disease. *Otolaryngol Clin North Am*, 13(4), 631–42.

48. Oosterveld WJ (1980). Meniere's disease, signs and symptoms. *J Laryngol Otol*, 94(8), 885–92.

49. Martin E, Perez N (2003). Hearing loss after intratympanic gentamicin therapy for unilateral Meniere's disease. *Otol Neurotol*, 24(5), 800–6.

50. Enander A, Stahle J (1969). Hearing loss and caloric response in Meniere's disease. A comparative study. *Acta Otolaryngol*, 67(1), 57–68.

51. Hone SW, Nedzelski J, Chen J (2000). Does intratympanic gentamicin treatment for Meniere's disease cause complete vestibular ablation? *J Otolaryngol*, 29(2), 83–7.

52. Carey JP, Minor LB, Peng GC, Della Santina CC, Cremer PD, Haslwanter T (2002). Changes in the three-dimensional angular vestibulo-ocular reflex following intratympanic gentamicin for Meniere's disease. *J Assoc Res Otolaryngol*, 3(4), 430–43.

53. Maire R, van Melle G (2008). Vestibulo-ocular reflex characteristics in patients with unilateral Meniere's disease. *Otol Neurotol*, 29(5), 693–8.

54. McCue MP, Guinan JJ, Jr (1994). Acoustically responsive fibers in the vestibular nerve of the cat. *J Neurosci*, 14(10), 6058–70.

55. Colebatch JG, Halmagyi GM (1992). Vestibular evoked potentials in human neck muscles before and after unilateral vestibular deafferentation. *Neurology*, 42(8), 1635–6.

56. Cheng PW, Huang TW, Young YH (2003). The influence of clicks versus short tone bursts on the vestibular evoked myogenic potentials. *Ear Hear*, 24(3), 195–7.

57. Iwasaki S, Chihara Y, Smulders YE, et al. (2009). The role of the superior vestibular nerve in generating ocular vestibular-evoked myogenic potentials to bone conducted vibration at Fz. *Clin Neurophysiol*, 120(3), 588–93.

58. Cheng PW, Murofushi T (2001). The effects of plateau time on vestibular-evoked myogenic potentials triggered by tone bursts. *Acta Otolaryngol*, 121(8), 935–8.

59. Todd NP, Cody FW, Banks JR (2000). A saccular origin of frequency tuning in myogenic vestibular evoked potentials?: implications for human responses to loud sounds. *Hear Res*, 141(1–2), 180–8.

60. Welgampola MS, Colebatch JG (2001). Characteristics of tone burst-evoked myogenic potentials in the sternocleidomastoid muscles. *Otol Neurotol*, 22(6), 796–802.

61. de Waele C, Huy PT, Diard JP, Freyss G, Vidal PP (1999). Saccular dysfunction in Meniere's disease. *Am J Otol*, 20(2), 223–32.

62. Murofushi T, Shimizu K, Takegoshi H, Cheng PW (2001). Diagnostic value of prolonged latencies in the vestibular evoked myogenic potential. *Arch Otolaryngol Head Neck Surg*, 127(9), 1069–72.

63. Rauch SD, Zhou G, Kujawa SG, Guinan JJ, Herrmann BS (2004). Vestibular evoked myogenic potentials show altered tuning in patients with Meniere's disease. *Otol Neurotol*, 25(3), 333–8.

64. Tumarkin A (1936). The otolithic catastrophe: a new syndrome. *BMJ*, 2, 175–7.

65. Baloh RW, Jacobson K, Winder T (1990). Drop attacks with Meniere's syndrome. *Ann Neurol*, 28(3), 384–7.

66. Timmer FC, Zhou G, Guinan JJ, Kujawa SG, Herrmann BS, Rauch SD (2006). Vestibular evoked myogenic potential (VEMP) in patients with Meniere's disease with drop attacks. *Laryngoscope*, 116(5), 776–9.

67. Lin MY, Timmer FC, Oriel BS, et al. (2006). Vestibular evoked myogenic potentials (VEMP) can detect asymptomatic saccular hydrops. *Laryngoscope*, 116(6), 987–92.

68. Rauch SD, Silveira MB, Zhou G, et al. (2004). Vestibular evoked myogenic potentials versus vestibular test battery in patients with Meniere's disease. *Otol Neurotol*, 25(6), 981–6.

69. Young YH, Huang TW, Cheng PW (2003). Assessing the stage of Meniere's disease using vestibular evoked myogenic potentials. *Arch Otolaryngol Head Neck Surg*, 129(8), 815–18.

70. Taylor RL, Wijewardene AA, Gibson WP, Black DA, Halmagyi GM, Welgampola MS (2011). The vestibular evoked-potential profile of Meniere's disease. *Clin Neurophysiol*, 122, 1256–63.

71. Winters SM, Berg IT, Grolman W, Klis SF (2012). Ocular vestibular evoked myogenic potentials: Frequency tuning to air-conducted acoustic stimuli in healthy subjects and Meniere's disease. *Audiol Neurootol*, 17(1), 12–19.

72. Manzari L, Tedesco AR, Burgess AM, Curthoys IS (2010). Ocular and cervical vestibular-evoked myogenic potentials to bone conducted vibration in Meniere's disease during quiescence vs during acute attacks. *Clin Neurophysiol*, 121(7), 1092–101.

73. James AL, Burton MJ (2001). Betahistine for Meniere's disease or syndrome. *Cochrane Database Syst Rev*, 1, CD001873.

74. Boleas-Aguirre MS, Lin FR, Della Santina CC, Minor LB, Carey JP (2008). Longitudinal results with intratympanic dexamethasone in the treatment of Meniere's disease. *Otol Neurotol*, 29(1), 33–8.

75. Glasscock ME, 3rd, Gulya AJ, Pensak ML, Black JN, Jr (1984). Medical and surgical management of Meniere's disease. *Am J Otol*, 5(6), 536–42.

76. Derebery MJ, Fisher LM, Berliner K, Chung J, Green K (2010. Outcomes of endolymphatic shunt surgery for Meniere's disease: comparison with intratympanic gentamicin on vertigo control and hearing loss. *Otol Neurotol*, 31(4), 649–55.

77. Pullens B, Giard JL, Verschuur HP, van Benthem PP (2010). Surgery for Meniere's disease. *Cochrane Database Syst Rev*, 1, CD005395.

78. Rubinstein JT, Nie K, Bierer S, Ling L, Phillips JO (2010). Signal processing for a vestibular neurostimulator. *Conf Proc IEEE Eng Med Biol Soc*, 6247.

79. Davidovics NS, Fridman GY, Chiang B, Della Santina CC (2011). Effects of biphasic current pulse frequency, amplitude, duration, and interphase gap on eye movement responses to prosthetic electrical stimulation of the vestibular nerve. *IEEE Trans Neural Syst Rehabil Eng*, 19(1), 84–94.

80. Lyford-Pike S, Vogelheim C, Chu E, Della Santina CC, Carey JP (2007). Gentamicin is primarily localized in vestibular type I hair cells after intratympanic administration. *J Assoc Res Otolaryngol*, 8(4), 497–508.

81. Chia SH, Gamst AC, Anderson JP, Harris JP (2004). Intratympanic gentamicin therapy for Meniere's disease: a meta-analysis. *Otol Neurotol*, 25(4), 544–52.

82. Wu IC, Minor LB (2003). Long-term hearing outcome in patients receiving intratympanic gentamicin for Meniere's disease. *Laryngoscope*, 113(5), 815–20.

83. Lin FR, Migliaccio AA, Haslwanter T, Minor LB, Carey JP (2005). Angular vestibulo-ocular reflex gains correlate with vertigo control after intratympanic gentamicin treatment for Meniere's disease. *Ann Otol Rhinol Laryngol*, 114(10), 777–85.

84. Nguyen KD, Minor LB, Della Santina CC, Carey JP (2009). Vestibular function and vertigo control after intratympanic gentamicin for Meniere's disease. *Audiol Neurootol*, 14(6), 361–72.

85. Schmid-Priscoveanu A, Bohmer A, Obzina H, Straumann D (2001). Caloric and search-coil head-impulse testing in patients after vestibular neuritis. *J Assoc Res Otolaryngol*, 2(1), 72–8.

86. Minor LB, Solomon D, Zinreich JS, Zee DS (1998). Sound- and/or pressure-induced vertigo due to bone dehiscence of the superior semicircular canal. *Arch Otolaryngol Head Neck Surg*, 124(3), 249–58.

87. Cremer PD, Minor LB, Carey JP, Della Santina CC (2000). Eye movements in patients with superior canal dehiscence syndrome align with the abnormal canal. *Neurology*, 55(12), 1833–41.

88. Minor LB, Carey JP, Cremer PD, Lustig LR, Streubel SO, Ruckenstein MJ (2003). Dehiscence of bone overlying the superior canal as a cause of apparent conductive hearing loss. *Otol Neurotol*, 24(2), 270–8.

89. Mikulec AA, McKenna MJ, Ramsey MJ, et al. (2004). Superior semicircular canal dehiscence presenting as conductive hearing loss without vertigo. *Otol Neurotol*, 25(2), 121–9.

90. Brantberg K, Bergenius J, Tribukait A (1999). Vestibular-evoked myogenic potentials in patients with dehiscence of the superior semicircular canal. *Acta Otolaryngol*, 119(6), 633–40.

91. Streubel SO, Cremer PD, Carey JP, Weg N, Minor LB (2001). Vestibular-evoked myogenic potentials in the diagnosis of superior canal dehiscence syndrome. *Acta Otolaryngol Suppl*, 545, 41–9.

92. Deschenes GR, Hsu DP, Megerian CA (2009). Outpatient repair of superior semicircular canal dehiscence via the transmastoid approach. *Laryngoscope*, 119(9), 1765–69.

93. Welgampola MS, Myrie OA, Minor LB, Carey JP (2008). Vestibular-evoked myogenic potential thresholds normalize on plugging superior canal dehiscence. *Neurology*, 70(6), 464–72.

94. Limb CJ, Carey JP, Srireddy S, Minor LB (2006). Auditory function in patients with surgically treated superior semicircular canal dehiscence. *Otol Neurotol*, 27(7), 969–80.

95. Brandt T, Dieterich M (1994). Vestibular paroxysmia: vascular compression of the eighth nerve? *Lancet*, 343(8900), 798–9.

96. Hufner K, Barresi D, Glaser M, *et al.* (2008). Vestibular paroxysmia: diagnostic features and medical treatment. *Neurology*, 71(13), 1006–14.

97. Brackmann DE, Kesser BW, Day JD (2001). Microvascular decompression of the vestibulocochlear nerve for disabling positional vertigo: the House Ear Clinic experience. *Otol Neurotol*, 22(6), 882–7.

98. Moller MB, Moller AR, Jannetta PJ, Jho HD, Sekhar LN (1993). Microvascular decompression of the eighth nerve in patients with disabling positional vertigo: selection criteria and operative results in 207 patients. *Acta neurochirurgica*, 125(1–4), 75–82.

CHAPTER 23

Posterior Circulation Stroke and Vestibular Syndromes

Ji Soo Kim and Hyung Lee

Introduction

Approximately 20% of ischaemic events involve tissue supplied by the posterior (vertebrobasilar) circulation territory (1). The symptoms of posterior circulation stroke can be devastating, and some forms have high rates of death (1). Vertigo/dizziness is considered as a most common symptom of posterior circulation stroke and episodic vertigo frequently occurs in patients with suffering from ischaemia in the distribution of the posterior circulation (2–4). It may occur in isolation, without other symptoms of posterior circulation ischaemia or with persisting symptoms and signs of the infarction of the brainstem and/or cerebellum (2–4). When other symptoms and signs are present, the diagnosis is usually obvious, whereas, when vertigo occurs in isolation it can be difficult to differentiate from benign disorders involving the inner ear (2–4). The stroke involving the brainstem or cerebellum may produce a wide spectrum of isolated or combined eye movement disorders, in addition to vertigo. We summarize the clinical symptoms and signs of acute vestibular syndromes associated with stroke in the posterior circulation.

Isolated episodic vertigo of a vascular cause

Transient ischaemia within the vertebrobasilar circulation (i.e. vertebrobasilar insufficiency) is a common cause of episodic vertigo in elderly patients. The vertigo is usually accompanied by other neurological symptoms or signs. It is typically abrupt in onset, and usually lasting several minutes (2). Earlier reports (5, 6) emphasized that isolated vertigo, when present for more than several weeks, is rarely due to vascular events. However, recent studies (2–4) reported contradictory findings. Grad and Baloh (2) reported that of patients with vertigo due to vertebrobasilar insufficiency, 62% had at least one isolated episode of vertigo, and in 19% vertigo was the initial symptom. Moreover, 26% had canal paresis to caloric stimulation, indicating permanent damage to the peripheral vestibular system involving the inner ear or vestibular nerve. Subsequent studies (4, 7) also reported similar results: of 29 patients with vertebrobasilar insufficiency, 21% had episodic vertigo for at least 4 weeks as the only presenting symptom (4). Cho and Hyung recently reported

three patients with anterior inferior cerebellar artery (AICA) infarction who experienced isolated episode of recurrent vertigo, fluctuating hearing loss, and/or tinnitus (similar to Ménière's disease) as initial symptoms 1–10 days prior to the infarction (7). All of these data suggested that isolated episodic vertigo with or without auditory symptoms can be the only manifestation of transient ischaemia within the vertebrobasilar circulation. Isolated vertigo can occur particularly when there is a stenosis of the caudal or middle portion of the basilar artery (presumably close to the AICA origin) or widespread slow vertebrobasilar flow on magnetic resonance angiography (MRA; 3, 7). However, it is still unclear whether isolated episodic vertigo originates from the brain or the inner ear. When isolated vertigo occurs in transient ischaemia of the peripheral vestibular labyrinth, the superior part of the vestibular labyrinth may selectively be vulnerable to ischaemia, possibly due to the small calibre of the anterior vestibular artery (AVA) and little collateralization (2, 8). Patients with AVA infarction may subsequently develop typical episodes of benign paroxysmal positional vertigo; these have been ascribed to ischaemic necrosis of the utricular macule and release of otoconia into the posterior canal. Since the posterior canal is supplied by the posterior vestibular artery, a branch of the common cochlear artery, it may be spared in AVA infarction (8, 9). Although isolated episodic vertigo can occur as a manifestation of vertebrobasilar insufficiency, long-lasting (>6 months) recurrent episodes of vertigo without other symptoms are almost never caused by vertebrobasilar disease.

Brainstem stroke

Medullary stroke

Lateral medullary infarction (Wallenberg syndrome)

Infarction in the dorsolateral medulla (Wallenberg syndrome) commonly involves the inferior and medial vestibular nuclei and usually manifests with nausea/vomiting, vertigo, and imbalance. Commonly associated signs are ipsilateral Horner's syndrome, decreased pain and temperature sensation in the ipsilateral face and contralateral body and extremities, dysphagia, ataxia, and hoarseness. Lateral medullary infarction (LMI) is commonly caused by thrombosis of the ipsilateral vertebral artery just proximal to the

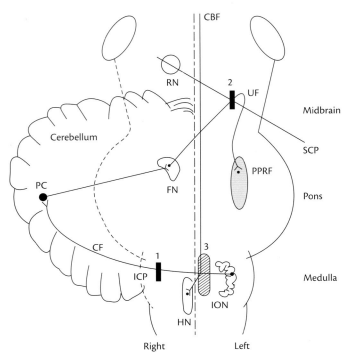

Fig. 23.1 Schematic representation of the pathways involved in ocular lateropulsion. Ocular lateropulsion may occur in lesions involving neural pathways connecting the inferior olivary nucleus (ION), cerebellar Purkinje cells (PC), fastigial nucleus (FN), and paramedian pontine reticular formation (PPRF). Ocular ipsipulsion in Wallenberg syndrome may be ascribed to damaging the climbing fibres (CF) from the contralesional ION to the PC of dorsal vermis after decussation [1] while ocular contrapulsion in superior cerebellar artery infarction occurs due to damage to the fibres from the contralesional FN to the ipsilesional PPRF near the uncinate fasciculus [2]. In medial medullary infarction, disruption of the CF before decussation [3] gives rise to ocular contrapulsion. CBF, corticobulbar fibers to the contralateral hypoglossal nucleus; HN, hypoglossal nucleus; ICP, inferior cerebellar peduncle; RN, red nucleus; SCP, superior cerebellar peduncle; UF, uncinate fasciculus.

origin of PICA (10). In younger patients, especially in patients with a history of head trauma or neck manipulation (11) or with posterior neck pain or occipital headache, traumatic dissection of the distal vertebral artery should be considered (12).

Spontaneous nystagmus in LMI varies considerably. Typically, horizontal nystagmus beats away from the lesion side (13–15). The vertical component is usually upbeating, and torsional nystagmus may be ipsi- or contralesional (13–15). In monkeys, spontaneous nystagmus beat contralesionally for unilateral lesions of the vestibular nerve root and caudal lateral parts of the vestibular nuclei (16). In contrast, the nystagmus was ipsilesional when the superior vestibular nucleus or the rostral portion of the medial vestibular nucleus was lesioned (16). Later, the spontaneous nystagmus may change directions (15). Gaze-evoked nystagmus is observed in almost all the patients, which is mostly horizontal (17). Positional nystagmus is rare and usually torsional (17).

In Wallenberg syndrome, head-shaking nystagmus (HSN) is frequently observed, and the horizontal component of HSN is ipsilesional in most patients (15). Even in patients with contralesional spontaneous nystagmus, horizontal head shaking reverses the direction of spontaneous horizontal nystagmus (15). HSN may also be unusually strong or perverted, i.e. the nystagmus develops in the

plane other than that being stimulated (downbeat or upbeat after horizontal head oscillation) (15). Since visual fixation markedly suppressed HSN even in patients with vigorous HSN, removal of visual fixation (e.g. Frenzel goggles) is required for proper observation of HSN.

The ocular tilt reaction (OTR), which consists of head tilt, ocular torsion, and skew deviation, is commonly observed during the acute phase and is ipsilesional, i.e. the head is tilted to the lesion side, the upper poles of the eyes rotate toward the ipsilesional shoulder, and the ipsilesional eye lies lower than the contralesional one (17). OTR is mostly associated with ipsilesional tilt of the subjective visual vertical (SVV) (17). The OTR and SVV tilt are explained by interruption of the otolith-ocular pathways at the level of the vestibular nucleus (17).

Patients also show an ocular motor bias toward the lesion side without limitation of eye motion (ipsipulsion), which is comprised of a steady-state ocular deviation, hypermetric saccades to the side of the lesion and hypometric saccades opposite the lesion, and oblique misdirection of vertical saccades (18). Ocular lateropulsion may occur in lesions involving neural pathways connecting the inferior olivary nucleus (ION), cerebellar Purkinje cells, fastigial nucleus, and paramedian pontine reticular formation (PPRF) (19). Ocular ipsipulsion in Wallenberg syndrome has been ascribed to damage to the climbing fibres from the contralesional inferior olivary nucleus to the dorsal vermis (19). Increased Purkinje cell activity following damage to the climbing fibres in the lateral medulla after decussation would inhibit the ipsilateral fastigial nucleus and create a bias toward ipsilateral saccades (Figure 23.1).

Wallenberg syndrome may disrupt descending vestibulospinal tracts and cause prominent imbalance with falling to the ipsilesional side as if being pulled by a strong external force. Leaning, veering, falling, or toppling to the lesion side when the patient is placed in an erect or sitting position is invariable (18). Posturography demonstrated an increased diagonal sway in Wallenberg syndrome. Truncal lateropulsion is correlated with SVV tilt, i.e. the more pronounced the lateropulsion, the greater the SVV tilt (17). Diplopia due to skew deviation and oscillopsia from the spontaneous nystagmus also contribute to disequilibrium. Cervical vestibular-evoked myogenic potentials (cVEMPs) can be abnormal if the sacculocollic reflex pathways are damaged at the level of the vestibular nucleus (Figure 23.2) (20).

Medial medullary infarction

Medial medullary infarction (MMI) is characterized by a triad of contralesional hemiparesis, ipsilesional tongue paralysis, and decreased position and vibration sensation in the contralateral side of the body. MMI is usually caused by thrombosis of the anterior spinal artery or distal intracranial vertebral artery and is frequently bilateral (21). The anteromedial arteries irrigate several structures: the ascending efferent fibres from the vestibular nuclei, the medial longitudinal fasciculus (MLF), the perihypoglossal nuclear complex, the climbing fibres emanating from the inferior olive, and the cell groups of the paramedian tracts (PMTs), which probably function in gaze-holding.

MMI generates distinct patterns of ocular motor abnormalities (22–24) especially when lesions extend into the tegmentum in the rostral medulla. Whereas the horizontal nystagmus is typically contralesional in LMI, it beats ipsilesionally in patients with MMI probably by involving the nucleus prepositus hypoglossi (NPH)

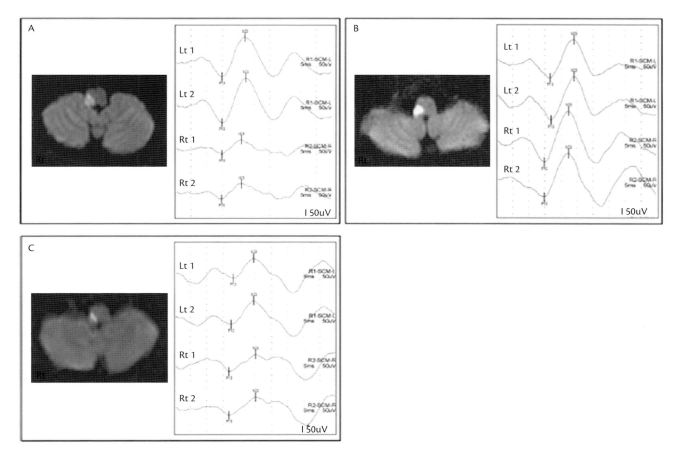

Fig. 23.2 Abnormal cervical vestibular-evoked myogenic potentials (cVEMP) and diffusion-weighted magnetic resonance images (DWI). A patient with right lateral medullary infarction (LMI) shows decreased amplitude on cVEMP in the ipsilesional side (A) while another patient with right LMI exhibits delayed p13 responses in the contralesional side (B). The other patient with right LMI shows delayed p13 responses and decreased amplitude in the ipsi- and contralesional side (C).

(23, 24). Gaze-evoked nystagmus is usually more intense on looking ipsilesionally (23). Upbeat nystagmus occasionally occurs in MMI has been ascribed to the involvement of the perihypoglossal nuclei, which consist of NPH, nucleus of Roller, and nucleus intercalatus (25). However, the evolution of upbeat into hemi-seesaw nystagmus with the resolution of a unilateral lesion in a patient with bilateral MMI suggests an involvement of the vestibulo-ocular reflex (VOR) pathways from both anterior semicircular canals as a mechanism of upbeat nystagmus (26). Since the MLF is a midline structures that carries signals from the vestibular to the ocular motor nuclei, upbeat nystagmus in unilateral lesions may be explained by concurrent damage to decussating fibres from both anterior semicircular canals at the rostral medulla (26). In the caudal medullary lesions, the nucleus of Roller and the caudal subgroup of the PMT cell, which are involved in processing of vertical eye position through their projections to the cerebellar flocculus, may be another neural substrates for upbeat nystagmus (25, 27). OTR with isolated MMI is contralesional (22–24, 26). The contralesional OTR in MMI indicates a unilateral lesion of the graviceptive brainstem pathways from the vestibular nuclei after decussation, which occurs at the pontomedullary junction. In MMI, damage to the climbing fibres before decussation also causes ocular contrapulsion (Figure 23.1) (22, 23). About half of the patients with MMI show abnormal cVEMP in the lesion side, especially when the lesions are extended to the dorsal tegmentum

(Figure 23.3) (24). The abnormal cVEMP in MMI involving the tegmentum supports that VEMP is mediated by the medial vestibulospinal tract descending within the MLF (24).

Pontine stroke

Pontine infarction

Neurotological and neuro-ophthalmological findings are most frequently observed in infarctions of the pontine tegmentum that is mainly supplied by anterior medial pontine arteries, AICA (lower pons), and superior cerebellar artery (SCA) (upper pons). Pontine tegmental infarction may occur in isolation or in association with paramedian (anteromedial and anterolateral) or lateral pontine infarction.

Nystagmus and saccadic intrusions/oscillations

Upbeat nystagmus may occur in tegmental infarction by disrupting upward VOR pathways from both anterior semicircular canals, which lie in the MLFs (27). Since the MLF carries excitatory fibres originating in the contralateral anterior and posterior canals and projecting to the ocular motor nuclei, various patterns of dissociated torsional-vertical nystagmus may occur in MLF lesions, depending on the patterns involving the pathways from contralateral vertical semicircular canals (28). Upbeat nystagmus was also reported in a focal infarction between the basis pontis and tegmentum slightly above the midpons level and was ascribed to damaging

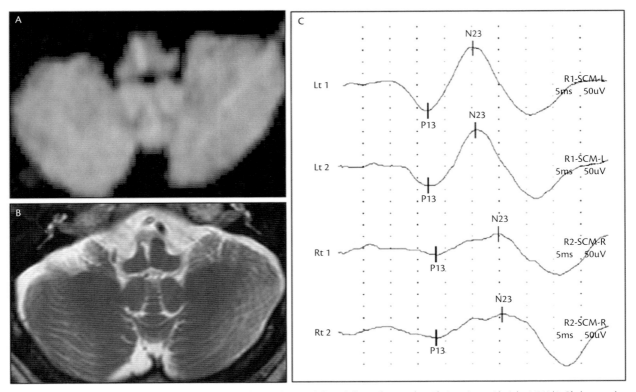

Fig. 23.3 Abnormal cervical vestibular evoked myogenic potential (cVEMP) in medial medullary infarction (MMI). A patient with right MMI (A, B) shows a decreased amplitude of cVEMP in the lesion side.

the decussating ventral tegmental tracts, which is also believed to transmit upward VOR (25). Ocular bobbing, intermittent downward jerks of the eyes followed by slow return to the primary position, can be observed in extensive infarction of the pontine base and tegmentum.

Horizontal gaze palsy
Since several neural structures involved in horizontal gaze are located in the pontine tegmentum, tegmental infarction may give rise to varied combinations of horizontal gaze palsy from isolated abducens palsy to total horizontal gaze palsy (29).

Internuclear ophthalmoplegia
Internuclear ophthalmoplegia (INO) is caused by a lesion in the MLF, which contains fibres connecting the abducens interneurons and contralateral medial rectus subnucleus (Figure 23.4). INO is characterized by an impairment of adduction in the ipsilesional eye and dissociated abducting nystagmus of the contralateral eye on attempted contralesional gaze (Figure 23.5). Convergence may be normal or impaired. Since the MLF also carries the fibres involved in the vertical VOR and the fibres from the utricle to the interstitial nucleus of Cajal (INC), INO is usually accompanied by vertical, torsional or dissociated vertical-torsional nystagmus (28), OTR (Figure 23.5). (18, 30), and impaired vertical VOR (31). Selective impairment of vertical VOR originating from the contralateral posterior semicircular canal may be demonstrated in INO by the head impulse test (32). The preserved anterior canal function suggests an extra-route for the ascending VOR pathway from the anterior canal, possibly the ventral tegmental tract. Exotropia of the contralesional eye or both eyes is common

in unilateral (wall-eyed monocular INO, WEMINO) or bilateral (wall-eye bilateral INO, WEBINO) INO. In bilateral INO, vertical smooth pursuit, vertical optokinetic nystagmus and after-nystagmus, and vertical gaze-holding are also impaired (31). INO may occur as an isolated or predominant symptom of dorsal brainstem infarction and has an excellent prognosis (33).

Conjugate horizontal gaze palsy
The PPRF contains burst neurons for ipsilateral horizontal saccades. Burst neurons in PPRF receive input from the contralateral frontal eye field and projects to the ipsilateral abducens nucleus. Selective damage to the pontine burst neurons results in isolated ipsilesional saccadic palsy with contralesional conjugate deviation of the eyes (34). In contrast, damage to the abducens nucleus produces ipsilesional palsy of saccades, smooth pursuit, and VOR. A nuclear lesion gives rise to an ipsilesional conjugate gaze palsy rather than a unilateral abduction deficit since the nucleus includes the lateral rectus motor neurons as well as interneurons that project to the contralateral medial rectus subnucleus via the MLF (29). However, lesions restricted to the abducens nucleus rarely occur, and nuclear lesions usually involve adjacent tegmental structures, especially the MLF, PPRF, and genu of the facial nerve fascicle.

One-and-a-half syndrome
This syndrome refers to a combination of unilateral conjugate gaze palsy (one) and INO on the same side (a half) (35). Consequently, the only remaining eye movement is abduction of the contralateral eye (a half). The one-and-a-half syndrome is caused by combined damage to the PPRF/abducens nucleus and the MLF. The term paralytic pontine exotropia was coined

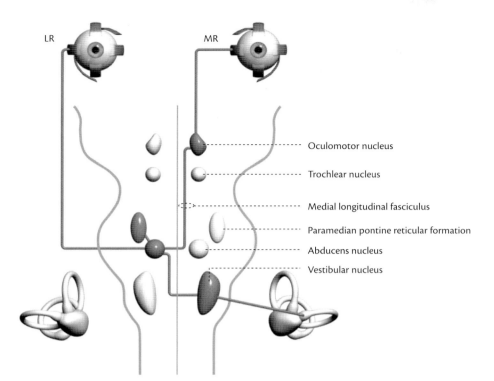

Fig. 23.4 Schematic illustrations of neural structures involved in the horizontal gaze. LR, lateral rectus, MR, medial rectus.

for patients who had an exotropia of the contralesional eye with the one-and-a-half syndrome (36).

Abducens palsy

Intra-axial abducens palsy is mostly caused by disruption of the abducens fascicle. Fascicular abducens nerve palsy may be isolated (37) but is usually accompanied by contralateral hemiplegia (Raymond's syndrome) and ipsilateral facial weakness

(Millard–Gubler syndrome) since the abducens nerve fascicle courses through the medial pons and passes next to the pyramidal tract.

Other findings

A focal pontine tegmental infarction may generate perverted HSN (38). The dorsolateral pontine nuclei (DLPN) and the nucleus reticularis tegmenti pontis (NRTP) are involved in the control of

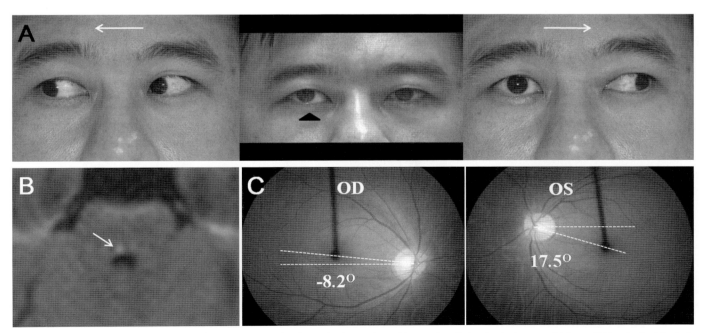

Fig. 23.5 Internuclear ophthalmoplegia (A) and contraversive ocular tilt reaction in a patient with a restricted infarction in the area of right medial longitudinal fasciculus (B, arrow). The patient shows diminished adduction of the right eye on attempted leftward gaze (A), and contraversive skew (A, right hypertropia, arrowhead) and ocular torsion (C).

smooth pursuit eye movements. Damage to DLPN impairs ipsilesional smooth pursuit (39), and NRTP lesions cause impairment of vertical smooth pursuit (40) and vergence eye movements (41). Lateral pontine infarction may be due to occlusion of the AICA or the SCA. However, isolated infarction of the posterior lateral tegmentum is extremely rare and is usually associated with involvement of the cerebellum (42). Small infarction in the tegmental area just ventral to the fourth ventricle causes body lateropulsion as a presenting symptom that probably results from damage to the graviceptive pathway ascending through the paramedian pontine tegmentum (43).

Pontine haemorrhage

The pons is a common site of intracerebral haemorrhage. Pontine haemorrhage usually causes a rapid onset of coma, pinpoint but reactive pupils, ocular bobbing, horizontal gaze palsy, and quadriplegia. Inferior olivary pseudohypertrophy and oculopalatal tremor may develop as delayed complications (44–46).

Midbrain stroke

The midbrain is irrigated by branches arising from the posterior cerebral artery, upper basilar artery, and the SCA. Pure midbrain infarction frequently causes gait ataxia and ocular motor abnormalities including third cranial nerve palsy, INO, and vertical gaze palsy, especially when the anteromedial portion is involved (47, 48).

Top of the basilar syndrome

Occlusion of the rostral tip of the basilar artery gives rise to a characteristic combination of ocular motor abnormalities by damaging the pretectum that contains the rostral interstitial nucleus of the medial longitudinal fasciculus (riMLF), the INC, the rostral portion of the mesencephalic reticular formation (MRF), and the posterior commissure, which are involved in the premotor control of vertical and torsional eye movements (pretectal syndrome) (49). The riMLF lies in the prerubral area near the midline and contains medium lead burst neurons that generate vertical and ipsiversive (top pole toward the side) torsional saccades (50). Each riMLF projects bilaterally to motoneurons for the elevator muscles (superior rectus and inferior oblique) but ipsilaterally to motoneurons for the depressor muscles (inferior rectus and superior oblique) (51, 52). Unilateral lesions of the riMLF result in contralesional ocular torsion, contralesional torsional nystagmus, and loss of ipsitorsional quick phases and vertical gaze (53). Bilateral lesions of the riMLF cause loss either of downward saccades or of all vertical saccades (53). The INC, together with the vestibular nuclei, is an element of the neural integrator for vertical and torsional eye motion, which transforms vertical eye velocity signals to position signals (54). It sends eye-position, saccade, and pursuit-related signals, combined in variable proportions on each axon, to extraocular motoneurons (55). The INC is separated from the riMLF by the fasciculus retroflexus, but fibres from the riMLF pass through the INC, providing axon collaterals to the INC (51, 52). Unilateral lesions of INC produce contralesional OTR and ipsitorsional nystagmus while bilateral lesions reduce the range of all vertical eye movements without saccadic slowing (56). The OTR may be paroxysmal due to intermittent irritation of partially damaged riMLF or INC mostly by mesodiencephalic haemorrhage (57). Unilateral inactivation of the rostral MRF produces slowed and hypometric upward and downward saccades without postsaccadic drift (58). Pretectal syndrome

may cause various ocular motor disorders related to vergence, which include convergence insufficiency, convergence spasm, and convergence nystagmus (59). The pretectal syndrome is also associated with bilateral ptosis or lid retraction (Collier's sign) (59).

Other ocular motor abnormalities

Third cranial nerve palsy

Varied combinations of signs of an oculomotor palsy may occur which are related to the spatial organization of the oculomotor nuclei and fascicles in the midbrain (60). Isolated palsy of individual extraocular muscle may occur due to nuclear or fascicular lesions (61, 62). Fascicular third nerve palsy may accompany crossed hemiplegia (Weber's syndrome), cerebellar signs (Claude's syndrome), or involuntary movements (Benedikt's syndrome).

Trochlear palsy

Ipsilateral trochlear palsy, Horner's syndrome, and contralateral ataxia may be observed in an infarction in the SCA territory since the SCA supplies the posterior aspect of the caudal midbrain and the superior cerebellum. However, midbrain involvement is rare in SCA infarction, and the classic syndrome of SCA infarction (ipsilateral trochlear palsy, Horner's syndrome, and contralateral ataxia) is rarely encountered (21). The trochlear nucleus is located in the central grey matter of the midbrain, close to the midline, near the MLF and the decussating fibres of the superior cerebellar peduncle. Fibres emerging from the trochlear nucleus pass laterally and posteriorly round the central grey matter, decussate in the superior medullary velum, and leave the midbrain below the inferior colliculus. Hence the innervation of the superior oblique muscle is crossed. The trochlear nucleus is supplied by paramedian branches at the basilar artery bifurcation. Trochlear palsy alone or with tinnitus and upbeat nystagmus may occur in brainstem stroke involving the trochlear nucleus or fascicle (63, 64).

Internuclear ophthalmoplegia

INO alone or in association with the cerebellar syndrome (limb and gait ataxia) may occur in restricted caudal paramedian midbrain infarction, which damages the decussation of the brachium conjunctivum and the MLF (65).

Three cerebellar ischaemic stroke syndromes

There are three major cerebellar arteries: the posterior inferior cerebellar artery (PICA), the AICA, and the SCA. After supplying branches to the brainstem, each of these arteries supplies the part of the cerebellum indicated by its name.

Acute vestibular syndrome due to AICA territory cerebellar infarction

Labyrinthine infarction as an important sign for the diagnosis of AICA territory infarction

Internal auditory artery (IAA) infarction mostly occurs due to thrombotic narrowing of either the AICA itself, or of the basilar artery at the orifice of the AICA (66). Occlusion of the IAA causes a sudden loss of both auditory and vestibular functions, resulting in acute onset of hearing loss and vertigo, so-called labyrinthine (inner ear) infarction. When a labyrinthine infarction occurs, infarction of the brainstem and/or cerebellum in the territory of the AICA is usually associated.

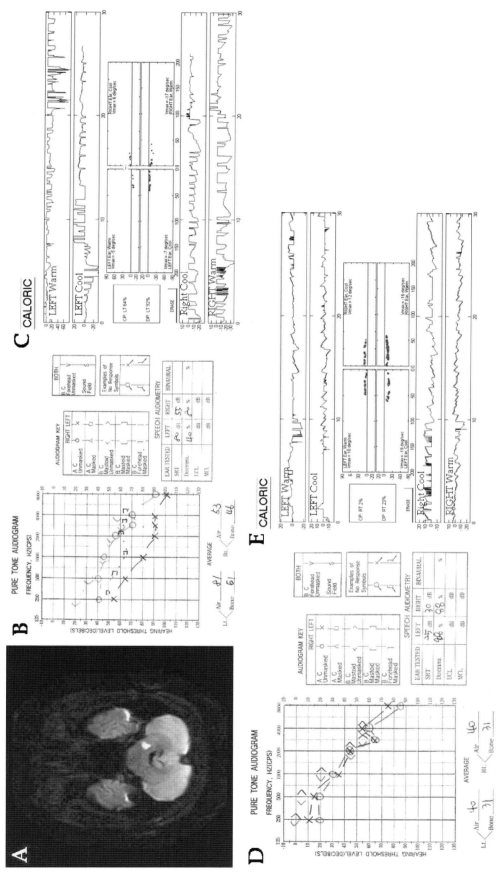

Fig. 23.6 MRI and progress of audiovestibular dysfunction in a patient with AICA territory infarction who had severe hearing loss initially, but showed normal hearing level on the last follow-up. (A) Axial diffusion-weighted MRI demonstrates acute infarcts involving the right middle cerebellar peduncle. (B) Initial pure tone audiogram reveals severe hearing loss (80 dB) with 40% speech discrimination in the right ear. Hearing levels in decibels (dB) (American National Standards Institute, 1989) are plotted against stimulus frequency on a logarithmic scale. (C) Initial video-oculographic recordings of bithermal caloric tests disclose the left CP (84%). (D) Follow-up testing performed 4 years after the onset of symptoms showed a complete recovery of hearing loss in the right ear. (E) Follow-up caloric test performed 4 years after the onset of symptoms also showed normal caloric response on the left side. AICA, anterior inferior cerebellar artery; CP, canal paresis; Vmax, maximal velocity of slow phase of nystagmus.

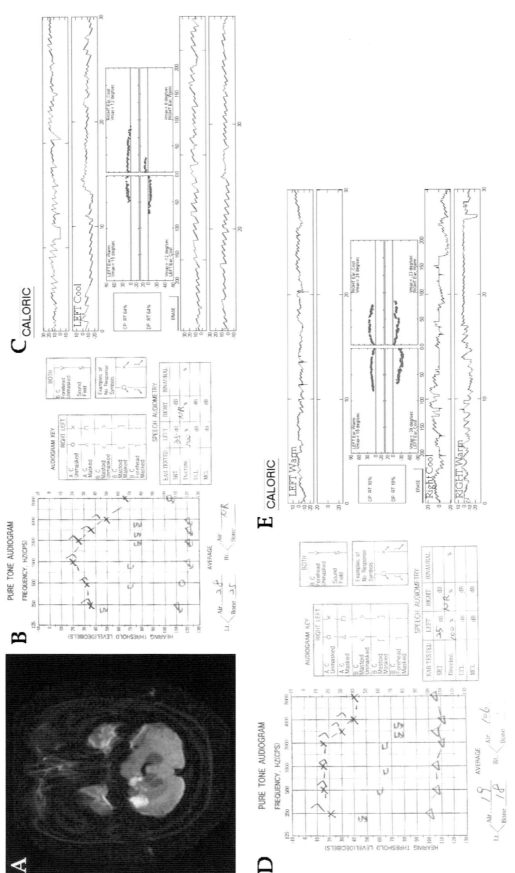

Fig. 23.7 (Also see Colour plate 13.) MRI and progress of audiovestibular dysfunction in a patient with AICA territory infarction who had profound hearing loss at initial and last follow-up. (A) Axial diffusion-weighted MRI demonstrates acute infarcts involving the right middle cerebellar peduncle and right anterior cerebellar hemisphere. (B) Initial pure tone audiogram reveals profound hearing loss on the right side. Hearing levels in decibels (dB) (American National Standards Institute, 1989) are plotted against stimulus frequency on a logarithmic scale. (C) Initial video-oculographic recordings of bithermal caloric tests showed a right CP (64%). (D) Follow-up testing performed 6 years after the onset of symptoms showed persistent hearing loss with no interval change. (E) Follow-up caloric test performed 6 years after the onset of symptoms showed normal caloric responses on the right side. AICA, anterior inferior cerebellar artery; CP, canal paresis; Vmax, maximal velocity of slow phase of nystagmus.

However, AICA infarction rarely causes sudden hearing loss and vertigo without brainstem or cerebellar signs (i.e. isolated labyrinthine infarction), in which case an acute infarct may still be seen on brain magnetic resonance imaging (MRI) (67). Hearing loss is a less widely appreciated and has been traditionally considered as a less common sign of AICA territory infarction. This may be explained by two facts. First, patients may not be aware of their hearing loss during an attack of vertigo and vomiting when the unilateral hearing loss is mild or the associated vertigo is severe. Second, neurologists do not included the audiogram as a routine diagnostic tool for the evaluation of AICA infarction. However, a recent report (68) showed that 11 out of 12 patients (92%) with AICA infarction showed labyrinthine infarction, which is clinically diagnosed by sudden sensorineural hearing loss on pure tone audiogram (PTA) and canal paresis to standardized bithermal caloric tests. Subsequently there have been other reports (69–71) emphasizing that AICA infarction commonly accompanied inner ear involvement and labyrinthine infarction is an important sign for the diagnosis of AICA infarction. Hearing loss is usually permanent, but dizziness and imbalance gradually improve with central compensation. However, a recent report (72) showed that most patients with labyrinthine infarction who were followed for at least 1 year (17/21, 81%) follow show improved hearing loss partially or completely. Another recent paper (73) showed that caloric response is also normalized in 20 (67%) of 30 patients with canal paresis associated with posterior circulation ischaemic stroke who were followed for at least 1 year. These findings suggested that audiovestibular loss associated with posterior circulation ischaemic stroke often has a good long-term outcome. Illustrative cases with good outcome with complete recovery of both hearing loss and canal paresis and with poor outcome with no recovery of hearing loss associated with AICA territory infarction are shown in Figures.23.6 and 23.7, respectively.

Isolated labyrinthine infarction as a harbinger of incoming AICA territory infarction

Since the blood supply to the inner ear arises from the IAA, partial ischaemia in the AICA territory could lead to an isolated acute audiovestibular loss. Several case reports (74–76) have shown that labyrinthine infarction may be served as an impending sign of incoming AICA territory infarction. A recent study (77) reported that approximately 9% (4/43) of patients with documented AICA territory infarction on brain MRI experienced an isolated audiovestibular disturbance (i.e. sudden onset of vertigo and hearing loss) with an initially normal MRI, and subsequently suffered from other neurological symptoms or signs indicative of AICA territory infarction. All of these studies suggest that the clinician should keep in mind the differential diagnosis of a posterior circulation stroke when caring for patients with acute peripheral-type audiovestibular syndrome, especially in patients with vascular risk factors and vertebrobasilar compromise on brain MRA, even though the classic brainstem or cerebellar signs are absent and MRI does not demonstrates acute infarction in the brain. Since the inner ear is not well visualized on routine MRI, a definite diagnosis of labyrinthine infarction is not possible unless a pathological study is done. It should be keep in mind that clinicians should consider all of the clinical evidence when attempting to determine the aetiology of the acute audio-vestibular syndrome rather than emphasizing that MRI is the best way to distinguish a viral (i.e. labyrinthitis) from a vascular (i.e. labyrinthine infarction) aetiology (78).

Characteristic pattern of vestibular dysfunction in AICA territory infarction

The most common pattern of vestibular dysfunction in AICA territory infarction was a combination of peripheral (i.e. unilateral canal paresis), and central ocular motor or vestibular signs (i.e. asymmetrically impaired smooth pursuit, bidirectional gaze-evoked nystagmus, or impaired modulation of the vestibular responses using visual input). These findings can be explained by the fact that AICA constantly supplied the peripheral vestibular structures such as the inner ear and vestibulocochlear nerve, in addition to the central vestibular structures (66). As a result, in contrast to other cerebellar artery territory infarction, complete AICA infarction usually results in combined peripheral and central vestibular damages in addition to hearing loss, facial weakness, limb and facial sensory loss, gait ataxia, and cerebellar dysmetria (66, 68). Since ischaemia of any structures supplied by AICA can lead to vertigo, determining the responsible site(s) for the prolonged vertigo seems difficult in individual patient with AICA infarction. However, as noted earlier, most patients with AICA infarction had a unilateral weakness to caloric stimulation, suggesting that the vertigo was from the dysfunction of the peripheral vestibular structure at least in part. On the other hand, some patients showed normal caloric response, indicating that in these patients vertigo may have resulted from ischaemia to the central vestibular structures. Overall, prolonged vertigo in AICA infarction mostly results from ischaemia to both the peripheral and central vestibular structures.

Spectrum of audiovestibuar loss in AICA territory infarction

It is well known that acute audiovestibular loss commonly occurs in acute ischaemic stroke in the distribution of the AICA, but the detailed spectrum of audiovestibular dysfunction has not been systematically studied in AICA infarction. Two dizziness clinics from South Korea investigated the pattern of audiovestibuar loss in AICA infarction (79). Eighty-two consecutive patients with AICA infarction diagnosed by MRI completed a standardized audiovestibular questionnaire and underwent a neuro-otological evaluation including bithermal caloric tests and PTA (79). All but two (80/82: 98%) patients had acute prolonged (lasting more than 24 hours) vertigo and vestibular dysfunction of peripheral, central, or combined origin. The most common pattern of audiovestibular dysfunctions was the combined loss of auditory and vestibular function (60%); selective loss of vestibular (5%) or cochlear (4%) function was rarely observed (79). We could classify AICA infarction into seven subgroups according to the patterns of neurotological presentations: 1) acute prolonged vertigo with audiovestibular loss (n = 35), 2) acute prolonged vertigo with audiovestibular loss preceded by an episode(s) of transient vertigo/auditory disturbance within 1 month before the infarction (n = 13), 3) acute prolonged vertigo and isolated auditory loss without vestibular loss (n = 3), 4) acute prolonged vertigo and isolated vestibular loss without auditory loss (n = 4), 5) acute prolonged vertigo, but without documented audiovestibular loss (n = 24), 6) acute prolonged vertigo and isolated audiovestibular loss without any other neurological symptoms/signs (n = 1), 7) nonvestibular symptoms with normal audiovestibular function (n = 2) (79). These findings suggested that infarction in the AICA territory mostly present with vertigo with a broad spectrum of audiovestibular dysfunctions. Considering the low incidence of selective cochlear or vestibular involvement in AICA infarction, vascular compromise

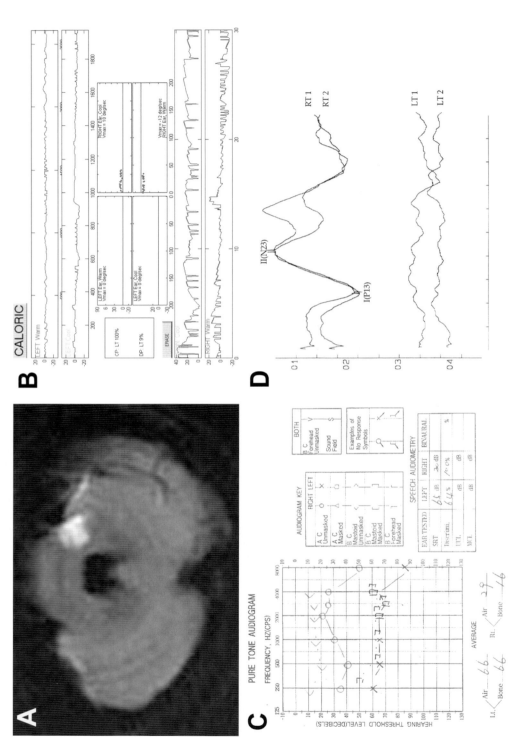

Fig. 23.8 (Also see Colour plate 14.) MRI, audiovestibular function tests, and cervical VEMP in a patient (patient 2) with AICA territory infarction. (A) Axial diffusion-weighted MRI demonstrates acute infarcts involving the left middle cerebellar peduncle. (B) Video-oculographic recordings of bithermal caloric tests disclose the left CP of 100%. (C) PTA reveals severe degree of hearing loss of 66 dB with 64% speech discrimination in the left ear. Hearing levels in decibels (dB) (American National Standards Institute, 1989) are plotted against stimulus frequency on a logarithmic scale. (D) Recording of cervical VEMP shows no wave formation in the ipsilesional side. AICA, anterior inferior cerebellar artery; CP, canal paresis; PTA, pure tone audiogram; VEMP, vestibular evoked myogenic potential; Vmax, maximal velocity of slow phase of nystagmus.

appears to give rise to combined loss of auditory and vestibular functions while viral illness commonly presents as an isolated vestibular (i.e. vestibular neuritis) or cochlear loss (i.e. sudden deafness) (79).

Otolith dysfunction in AICA territory infarction

OTR, a sign of vestibular dysfunction in the roll plane, is characterized by the triad of conjugate ocular torsion, skew deviation, and head tilt. It is typically caused by damage to the brainstem tegmentum (80). AICA infarction can cause the OTR (i.e. ipsilateral head tilt, skew deviation, and conjugate ocular torsion with upper pole of the eye rotated toward the side of the lesion) associated with a deviation of the SVV in the direction of the head tilt (81, 82). Since AICA infarction with normal caloric response produce contralateral ocular torsion only, the peripheral vestibular structure with inner ear probably plays a crucial role in determining the direction of ocular torsion associated with AICA territory infarction (82). Another recent report focused on acute cerebellar stroke emphasized that the dentate nucleus is a critical anatomical structure within the cerebellum, belonging to a network involved in vestibular processing such as the perception of verticality (83). Like ocular torsion, the peripheral vestibular structure with the inner ear may have a crucial role in producing abnormal VEMP response associated with AICA territory infarction since abnormal VEMP response is almost occurred in patients with canal paresis and acute hearing loss, which is usually ascribed to damage to the peripheral audiovestibular structure with inner ear (Figure 23.8). Further study is needed to clarify the issue on which structure(s) is a critical for production of otolith dysfunction in AICA territory infarction.

Acute vestibular syndrome due to PICA territory cerebellar infarction

Pseudo-acute peripheral vestibulopathy (APV associated with medial PICA territory cerebellar infarction)

The classic medial PICA cerebellar ischaemic stroke syndrome is characterized by severe vertigo, vomiting, prominent axial (body) lateropulsion, dysarthria, and limb dysmetria. The key structure responsible for vertigo is the nodulus, which is strongly connected to the ipsilateral vestibular nucleus and receives direct projections from the labyrinth (84, 85). Functionally, nodulovestibular Purkinje fibres have an inhibitory effect on the ipsilateral vestibular nucleus (85, 86). Since extremity ataxia can be minimal or absent with mPICA cerebellar infarction particularly if the infarcts is small (87, 88), the clinical pattern of cerebellar infarction in the territory of the medial PICA can mimic APV. As many as 25 % of patients with vascular risk factors who presented to an emergency medical setting with isolated severe vertigo, nystagmus and postural instability have a cerebellar infarction in the territory of the medial PICA (89). Recent case reports (90, 91) also described a unique clinical presentation of a vascular vestibular syndrome that is characterized by severe vertigo, ipsilesional spontaneous nystagmus, and contralesional axial lateropulsion due to the medial PICA cerebellar infarction, in which the clinical symptoms were similar to those of APV contralateral to the side of lesion on brain MRI. All of these reports suggest that patients with vertigo associated with medial PICA territory cerebellar infarction are often misdiagnosed with APV.

A report on clinical findings of 240 patients with isolated cerebellar infarction showed that approximately 11% (25/240) of patients with isolated cerebellar infarction had isolated vertigo only, and most (24/25: 96%) had an infarct in the medial PICA territory including the nodulus (92). The key findings differentiating isolated vertigo associated with medial PICA infarction from APV were the normal head impulse and caloric test results in cerebellar infarction. Since the head impulse test can be performed at the bedside without special equipment, it is invaluable for separating pseudo-APV due to cerebellar infarction. Physicians who evaluate stroke patients should be trained to perform and interpret the results of the head impulse test. The prominent cerebellar signs, particularly severe axial instability and direction changing gaze-evoked nystagmus (occurred in 71% and 54%, respectively in the aforementioned series) can also help in the differential, but these findings are less reliable and the findings in some patients with central vertigo are similar to those with peripheral vertigo (92). The significance of head impulse test for differentiating cerebellar stroke from APV has been confirmed by another paper (93) that showed that a negative head impulse test (i.e. normal VOR) is strongly suggestive of a central lesion with a pseudo-APV presentation.

For patients with spontaneous prolonged vertigo, in addition to the obvious cases with associated neurological symptoms or signs, MRI to rule out medial PICA territory cerebellar infarction should be considered in: 1) older patients presenting with isolated spontaneous prolonged vertigo, in 2) any patient with vascular risk factors and isolated spontaneous prolonged vertigo who has a normal head impulse test, and in 3) any patient with isolated spontaneous prolonged vertigo who has a direction-changing gaze- evoked nystagmus or severe gait ataxia with falling in the upright posture (92, 94).

Although small PICA territory cerebellar infarction generally has a benign prognosis, isolated PICA territory cerebellar infarction usually results from emboli originating from the heart or great vessels (95), and recurrent emboli require appropriate treatments. Cerebellar infarction causes brain swelling in up to 25% of cases; PICA territory infarcts are more likely to produce a mass effect than SCA territory infarcts (96, 97). Large PICA territory cerebellar infarction can cause brainstem compression, hydrocephalus, cardiorespiratory complications, coma, and death (98).

Otolith dysfunction in PICA territory cerebellar infarction

Although OTR and its components such as head tilt, ocular torsion, and skew deviation, as well as tilts of the perceived SVV are usually considered as a sign of brainstem dysfunction (80), recent studies (83, 99, 100) have shown that cerebellar dysfunction can also cause partial (incomplete) OTR. One case report (99) described two patients with isolated medial PICA territory cerebellar stroke who showed a contraversive partial OTR (i.e. skew torsion without head tilt) with a contraversive deviation of the SVV. Isolated PICA territory cerebellar infarction usually produces two distinct patterns of otolith dysfunction: Ipsilesional SVV tilt and falling without accompanying OT or skew deviation if the nodulus is spared, and contralesional SVV tilt and falling with OT and skew deviation if nodulus is infracted (100). The authors speculated that interruption of nodular inhibitory projections to graviceptive neurons in the ipsilesional vestibular nuclei caused the contraversive conjugate ocular torsion. Lesion of the dentate nucleus can also lead to tilts of the SVV in the contraversive direction (i.e. a vestibular tone imbalance to the contralateral side), whereas cerebellar lesions excluding the dentate nucleus can induce a tone imbalance to the ipsilesional side (83).

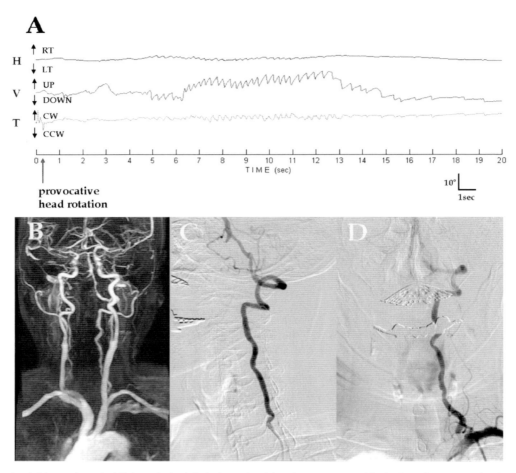

Fig. 23.9 Three-dimensional video-oculography (A) showed mixed clockwise torsional downbeat nystagmus with a horizontal component beating toward the left side with a latency of about 5 s during her neck rotated to the right side. MRA showed the left vertebral artery is dominant and the distal segment (V4) of the right vertebral artery is non-visualized (B). Cerebral angiography shows a patent left vertebral artery (C), but dynamic angiography discloses near complete occlusion of the left vertebral artery at the just distal to the C 2 level with rightward head rotation (D). H, horizontal, V, vertical, T, torsional, RT, right, LT, left, CW, clockwise, CCW, counterclockwise.

Acute hearing loss associated with non-AICA (mostly PICA) territory cerebellar infarction

Rarely, PICA territory cerebellar infarction can cause acute hearing loss because internal auditory artery sometimes originates from the PICA or directly from the basilar artery (101). A recent report showed that 7 (1%) of 685 patients with posterior circulation infarction had acute unilateral hearing loss associated with PICA territory cerebellar infarction (n = 5) or brainstem infarction (n = 2) (102). Although the site of injury responsible for hearing loss in these patients can not be confirmed without pathological examination, a detailed auditory function testing indicates a cochlear site of injury (102). Acute hearing loss associated with non-AICA territory posterior circulation ischaemic stroke is probably attributable to damage to the peripheral auditory system with the inner ear that is supplied by the IAA mostly originated from the PICA (102).

Acute vestibular syndrome due to SCA territory cerebellar infarction

Body lateropulsion as a presenting symptom of medial SCA territory cerebellar infarction

Since the superior cerebellum supplied by the SCA does not have significant vestibular connections, cerebellar infarction in the SCA rarely causes vertigo (103, 104). The vestibulo-ocular portion of the cerebellum is located primarily in the flocculonodular lobes, which are supplied by branches of the AICA and PICA. The low incidence of vertigo in SCA distribution may be a useful clinical distinction from PICA or AICA cerebellar infarction in patients with acute vertigo and limb ataxia (103, 104). Among the broad spectrum of clinical manifestations of SCA territory infarction, infarction in the territory of the lateral SCA is the most common, representing about a half of the cases (103–105). Lateral SCA territory cerebellar infarction is characterized by dizziness, nausea, unsteadiness, mild truncal ataxia, and severe limb ataxia (103–105). One study suggested that the most prominent clinical presentation in the medial SCA territory cerebellar infarction is severe gait ataxia with a sudden fall or severe veering, observed in 11 (76%) of 14 patients with isolated medial SCA territory cerebellar infarction (106). Prominent body lateropulsion in isolated medial SCA territory cerebellar infarction may be explained by involvement of rostral vermis that is related predominantly to gait, muscle tone, and postural control (107). The high incidence of sudden falling with body lateropulsion in the medial SCA cerebellar infarction may be a useful clinical distinction from the lateral SCA cerebellar infarction in patients with acute dizziness and postural instability.

Acute vestibular syndromes due to cerebellar haemorrhage

Cerebellar haemorrhage is also a common cause of vertigo in older patients, especially in those with hypertension. The initial symptoms of acute cerebellar haemorrhage are vertigo, nausea, vomiting, headache, and prominent body lateropulsion with falling to lesion side. The clinical features are similar to those of acute cerebellar infarction and might be confused with an APV. Patients with cerebellar haemorrhage usually complain of more severe occipital headache and nuchal rigidity than in cerebellar infarction. Approximately 50% of patients lose consciousness within 24 h of the initial symptoms, and 75% become comatose within 1 week of the onset (108). The condition is often fatal unless surgical decompression is performed. A widely accepted neurosurgical adage is to evacuate a cerebellar haemorrhage that is more than 3 cm in cross-sectional diameter by computed tomography scan (109).

Vascular compression syndromes

Vertebrobasilar dolichoectasia

Dolichoectasia refers to an enlargement and elongation of the artery. Vertebrobasilar dolichoectasia may generate neurotological manifestations by compression of the brainstem or VIIIth cranial nerves (110) or by ischaemia in the vertebrobasilar territory (111).

Vestibular paroxysmia

Paroxysmal vertigo or tinnitus may occur due to compression of the VIIIth cranial nerve by a vascular loop in the cerebellopontine angle. This syndrome has been described as 'disabling positional vertigo' (112) or 'vestibular paroxysmia' (113). Microvascular decompression or antiepileptic medication may be effective in ameliorating the symptoms.

Rotational vertebral artery syndrome

Paroxysmal vertigo induced by head rotation occurs in patients with rotational vertebral artery syndrome (RVAS), which is characterized by recurrent attacks of vertigo, nystagmus, and ataxia that are mainly induced by head rotation or tilt (114–119). In this very rare syndrome, patients usually have one hypoplastic or stenotic vertebral artery, and a contralateral dominant vertebral artery that is compressed or occluded at the atlantoaxial junction during head rotation to the contralateral side (116). Oculographic analyses of nystagmus revealed various patterns of nystagmus during the attack (115, 116). The initial nystagmus is mostly downbeat, with the horizontal and torsional components beating either towards the compressed vertebral artery side (Figure 23.9) or directed away. Some patients show spontaneous reversal of the nystagmus and no or markedly diminished responses on immediate retrial of head rotation (habituation) (116). Tinnitus develops several seconds after the onset of vertigo and nystagmus, which suggests that the vestibular system is more sensitive to ischaemia than the cochlear system (116). The different patterns of nystagmus suggest that RVAS may result from various mechanisms (115–117). Surgical interventions (decompression or fusion) should be considered, especially in younger patients with frequent attacks and severe vertebral artery compression during attacks (116).

Conclusion

Since posterior circulation stroke can produce unique symptoms and signs, recognizing the characteristic patterns of each individual posterior circulation stroke syndrome is a key to the efficient diagnosis and treatment of this group of patients. The head impulse test is a useful bedside tool for differentiating acute cerebellar infarction from more benign disorders involving the inner ear.

References

1. Savitz SI, Caplan LR (2005). Vertebrobasilar disease. *N Engl J Med*, 352(25), 2618–26.
2. Grad A, Baloh RW (1989). Vertigo of vascular origin: clinical and electronystagmographic features in 84 cases. *Arch Neurol*, 46(3), 281–4.
3. Fife TD, Baloh RW, Duckwiler GR (1994). Isolated dizziness in vertebrobasilar insufficiency: Clinical features, angiography, and follow-up. *J Stroke Cerebrovasc Dis*, 4(1), 4–12.
4. Gomez CR, Cruz-Flores S, Malkoff MD, Sauer CM, Burch CM (1996). Isolated vertigo as a manifestation of vertebrobasilar ischemia. *Neurology*, 47(1), 94–7.
5. Fisher CM (1967). Vertigo in cerebrovascular disease. *Arch Otolaryngol*, 85(5), 529–34.
6. Troost BT (1980). Dizziness and vertigo in vertebrobasilar disease. *Stroke*, 11(4), 413–15.
7. Lee H, Cho YW (2003). Auditory disturbance as a prodrome of anterior inferior cerebellar artery infarction. *J Neurol Neurosurg Psychiatry*, 74(12), 1644–8.
8. Kim JS, Lopez I, DiPatre PL, Liu F, Ishiyama A, Baloh RW (1999). Internal auditory artery infarction: Clinical-pathologic correlation. *Neurology*, 52(1), 40–4.
9. Lindsay JR, Hemenway WG (1956). Postural vertigo due to unilateral sudden partial loss of vestibular function. *Ann Otol Rhinol Laryngo*, 65(3), 696–706.
10. Fisher CM, Karnes WE, Kubik CS (1961). Lateral medullary infarction-the pattern of vascular occlusion. *J Neuropath Exp Neurol*, 20, 323–79.
11. Frumkin LR, Baloh RW (1990). Wallenberg's syndrome following neck manipulation. *Neurology*, 40(4), 611–15.
12. Silbert PL, Mokri B, Schievink WI (1995). Headache and neck pain in spontaneous internal carotid and vertebral artery dissections. *Neurology*, 45(8), 1517–22.
13. Morrow MJ, Sharpe JA (1988). Torsional nystagmus in the lateral medullary syndrome. *Ann Neurol*, 24(3), 390–8.
14. Rambold H, Helmchen C (2005). Spontaneous nystagmus in dorsolateral medullary infarction indicates vestibular semicircular canal imbalance. *J Neurol Neurosurg Psychiatry*, 76(1), 88–94.
15. Choi KD, Oh SY, Park SH, Kim JH, Kim JS, Koo JW (2007). Head-shaking nystagmus in lateral medullary infarction: Patterns and possible mechanism. *Neurology*, 68(17), 1337–44.
16. Uemura T, Cohen B (1973). Effects of vestibular nuclei lesions on vestibulo-ocular reflexes and posture in monkeys. *Acta Otolaryngol Suppl*, 315, 1–71.
17. Dieterich M, Brandt T (1992). Wallenberg's syndrome: Lateropulsion, cyclorotation, and subjective visual vertical in thirty-six patients. *Ann Neurol*, 31(4), 399–408.
18. Kim JS, Moon SY, Park SH, Yoon BW, Roh JK (2004). Ocular lateropulsion in Wallenberg syndrome. *Neurology*, 62(12), 2287.
19. Helmchen C, Straube A, Büttner U (1994). Saccadic lateropulsion in Wallenberg's syndrome may be caused by a functional lesion of the fastigial nucleus. *J Neurol*, 241(7), 421–6.
20. Kim S, Kim HJ, Kim JS (2011). Impaired sacculocollic reflex in lateral medullary infarction. *Front Neur*, 2, 8.
21. Mohr JP, Caplan LR (2004). Vertebrobasilar disease. In: Mohr JP, Choi DW, Grotta JC, Weir B, Wolf PA (Eds) *Stroke: pathophysiology, diagnosis, and management* (4th ed), pp. 207–74. Philadelphia, PA: Churchill Livingstone.

22. Kim JS, Moon SY, Kim KY, *et al.* (2004). Ocular contrapulsion in rostral medial medullary infarction. *Neurology*, 63(7), 1325–7.

23. Kim JS, Choi KD, Oh SY, *et al.* (2005). Medial medullary infarction: Abnormal ocular motor findings. *Neurology*, 65(8), 1294–8.

24. Kim S, Lee HS, Kim JS (2010). Medial vestibulospinal tract lesions impair the sacculocollic reflex . *J Neurol*, 257(5), 825–32.

25. Pierrot-Deseilligny C, Milea D (2005). Vertical nystagmus: clinical facts and hypotheses. *Brain*, 128(Pt 6), 1237–46.

26. Choi KD, Jung DS, Park KP, Koo JW, Kim JS (2004). Bowtie and upbeat nystagmus evolving into hemi-seesaw nystagmus in medial medullary infarction: possible anatomic mechanisms. *Neurology*, 62(4), 663–5.

27. Kim JS, Yoon BW, Choi KD, Oh SY, Park SH, Kim BK (2006). Upbeat nystagmus: Clinico-anatomical correlations in 15 patients. *J Clin Neurol*, 2(1), 58–65.

28. Oh K, Chang JH, Park KW, Lee DH, Choi KD, Kim JS (2005). Jerky see-saw nystagmus in isolated internuclear ophthalmoplegia from focal pontine lesion. *Neurology*, 64(7), 1313–14.

29. Leigh RJ, Zee DS (2006). *The neurology of eye movements* (4th ed), pp. 261–314. New York: Oxford University Press.

30. Zwergal A, Cnyrim C, Arbusow V, *et al.* (2008). Unilateral INO is associated with ocular tilt reaction in pontomesencephalic lesions. INO plus. *Neurology*, 71(8), 590–3.

31. Ranalli PJ, Sharpe JA (1988). Vertical vestibulo-ocular reflex, smooth pursuit and eye-head tracking dysfunction in internuclear ophthalmoplegia. *Brain*, 111(Pt 6), 1299–317.

32. Cremer PD, Migliaccio AA, Halmagyi GM, Curthoys IS (1999). Vestibulo-ocular reflex pathways in internuclear ophthalmoplegia. *Ann Neurol*, 45(4), 529–33.

33. Kim JS (2004). Internuclear ophthalmoplegia as an isolated or predominant symptom of brainstem infarction. *Neurology*, 62(9), 1491–6.

34. Johnston JL, Sharpe JA, Morrow MJ (1992). Paresis of contralateral smooth pursuit and normal vestibular smooth eye movements after unilateral brainstem lesion. *Ann Neurol*, 31(5), 495–502.

35. Fisher CM (1967). Some neuro-ophthalmological observations. *J Neurol Neurosurg Psychiatry*, 30(5), 383–92.

36. Sharpe JA, Rosenberg M, Hoyt W, Daroff RB (1974). Paralytic pontine exotropia. *Neurology*, 24(11), 1076–81.

37. Paik JW, Kang SY, Sohn YH (2004). Isolated abducens nerve palsy due to anterolateral pontine infarction. *Eur Neurol*, 52(4), 254–6.

38. Kim HA, Kim JS, Lee H (2011). Perverted head-shaking nystagmus in focal dorsal pontine infarction. *J Neurol Sci*, 301(1–2), 93–5.

39. Ahn BY, Choi KD, Kim JS, *et al.* (2007). Impaired ipsilateral smooth pursuit and gaze-evoked nystagmus in paramedian pontine lesion. *Neurology*, 68(17), 1436.

40. Suzuki DA, Yamada T, Hoedema R, Yee RD (1999). Smooth-pursuit eye movement deficits with chemical lesions in macaque nucleus reticularis tegmenti pontis. *J Neurophysiol*, 82(3), 1178–86.

41. Rambold H, Neumann G, Helmchen C (2004). Vergence deficits in pontine lesions. *Neurology*, 62(10), 1850–3.

42. Kumral E, Bayulkem G, Evyapan D (2002). Clinical spectrum of pontine infarction: Clinical-MRI correlations. *J Neurol*, 249(12), 1659–70.

43. Yi HA, Lim HA, Lee H, Baloh RW (2007). Body lateropulsion as an isolated or predominant symptom of a pontine infarction. *J Neurol Neurosurg Psychiatry*, 78(4), 372–4.

44. Moon SY, Park SH, Hwang JM, Kim JS (2003). Oculopalatal tremor after pontine hemorrhage. *Neurology*, 61(11), 1621.

45. Kim JS, Moon SY, Choi KD, Kim JH, Sharpe JA (2007). Patterns of ocular oscillation in oculopalatal tremor: Imaging correlations. *Neurology*, 68(14), 1128–35.

46. Shaikh AG, Hong S, Liao K, *et al.* (2010). Oculopalatal tremor explained by a model of inferior olivary hypertrophy and cerebellar plasticity. *Brain*, 133(3), 923–40.

47. Sharpe JA, Kim JS (2002). Midbrain disorders of vertical gaze: A quantitative re-evaluation. *Ann N Y Acad Sci*, 956, 143–54.

48. Kim JS (2005). Pure midbrain infarction. Clinical, radiologic, and pathophysiologic findings. *Neurology*, 64(7), 1227–32.

49. Wall M, Slamovits TL, Weisberg LA, Trufant SA (1986). Vertical gaze ophthalmoplegia from infarction in the area of the posterior thalamo-subthalamic paramedian artery. *Stroke*, 17(3), 546–55.

50. Suzuki Y, Bütner-Ennever JA, Straumann D, Hepp K, Hess BJM, Henn V (1995) Deficits in torsional and vertical rapid eye movements and shift of Listing's plane after uni- and bilateral lesions of the rostral interstitial nucleus of the medial longitudinal fasciculus (riMLF). *Exp Brain Res*, 106(2), 215–32.

51. Moschovakis AK, Scudder CA, Highstein SM (1991). Structure of the primate oculomotor burst generator. I. Medium-lead burst neurons with upward on-directions. *J Neurophysiol*, 65(2), 203–17.

52. Moschovakis AK, Scudder CA, Highstein SM, Warren JD (1991). Structure of the primate oculomotor burst generator. II. Medium-lead burst neurons with downward on-directions. *J Neurophysiol*, 65(2), 218–29.

53. Leigh RJ, Zee DS (2006). *The neurology of eye movements* (4th ed), pp. 598–718. New York: Oxford University Press.

54. Fukushima K, Fukushima J, Harada C, Ohashi T, Kase M (1990). Neuronal activity related to vertical eye movement in the region of the interstitial nucleus of Cajal in alert cats. *Exp Brain Res*, 79(1), 43–64.

55. Dalezios Y, Scudder CA, Highstein SM, Moschovakis AK (1998). Anatomy and physiology of the primate interstitial nucleus of Cajal. II. Discharge pattern of single efferent fibers. *J Neurophysiol*, 80(6), 3100–11.

56. Helmchen C, Rambold H, Fuhry L, Büttner U (1998). Deficits in vertical and torsional eye movements after uni- and bilateral muscimol inactivation of the interstitial nucleus of Cajal of the alert monkey. *Exp Brain Res*, 119(4), 436–52.

57. Oh SY, Choi KD, Shin BS, Seo MW, Kim YH, Kim JS (2009). Paroxysmal ocular tilt reactions after mesodiencephalic lesions: Report of two cases and review of the literature. *J Neurol Sci*, 277(1–2), 98–102.

58. Waitzman DM, Silakov VL, DePalma-Bowles S, Ayers AS (2000). Effects of reversible inactivation of the primate mesencephalic reticular formation. II. Hypometric vertical saccades. *J Neurophysiol*, 83(4), 2285–99.

59. Keane JR (1990). The pretectal syndrome. *Neurology*, 40(4), 684–90.

60. Ksiazek SM, Slamovits TL, Rosen CE, Burde RM, Parisi F (1994). Fascicular arrangement in partial oculomotor paresis. *Am J Ophthalmol*, 118(1), 97–103.

61. Lee DK, Kim JS (2006). Isolated inferior rectus palsy due to midbrain infarction detected by diffusion-weighted MRI. *Neurology*, 66(12), 1956–7.

62. Lee HS, Yang TI, Choi KD, Kim JS (2008). Teaching Video NeuroImmage: Isolated medial rectus palsy in midbrain infarction. *Neurology*, 71(21), e64.

63. Lee SH, Park SW, Kim BC, Kim MK, Cho KH, Kim JS (2010). Isolated trochlear palsy due to midbrain stroke. *Clin Neurol Neurosurg*, 112(1), 68–71.

64. Choi SY, Song JJ, Hwang JM, Kim JS (2010). Tinnitus in superior oblique palsy: An indicator for intra-axial lesion. *J Neuro-Ophthalmol*, 30(4), 325–7.

65. Mossuto-Agatiello L (2006). Caudal paramedian midbrain syndrome. *Neurology* 2006, 66(11), 1668–71.

66. Amarenco P, Hauw JJ (1990). Cerebellar infarction in the territory of the anterior and inferior cerebellar artery. *Brain*, 113(1), 139–55.

67. Lee H, Ahn BH, Baloh RW (2004). Sudden deafness with vertigo as a sole manifestation of anterior inferior cerebellar infarction. *J Neurol Sci*, 222(1–2), 105–7.

68. Lee H, Sohn SI, Jung DK, *et al.* (2002). Sudden deafness and anterior inferior cerebellar artery infarction. *Stroke*, 33(12), 2807–12.

69. Rajesh R, Rafeequ M, Girija AS (2004). Anterior inferior cerebellar artery infarct with unilateral deafness. *J Assoc Physicians India*, 52, 333–4.

70. Patzak MJ, Demuth K, Kehl R, Lindner A (2005). Sudden hearing loss as the leading symptom of an infarction of the left anterior inferior cerebellar artery. *HNO*, 53(9), 797–9.

71. Son EJ, Bang JH, Kang JG (2007). Anterior inferior cerebellar artery infarction presenting with sudden hearing loss and vertigo. *Laryngoscope*, 117(3), 556–8.

72. Lee H, Baloh RW (2005). Sudden Deafness in vertebrobasilar Ischemia: clinical features, vascular topographical patterns, and long-term outcome. *J Neuro Sci*, 228(1), 99–104.

73. Lee H, Yi HA, Chung IS, Lee SR (2011). Long-term outcome of canal paresis of a vascular cause. *J Neurol Neurosurg Psychiatry*, 82(1), 105–9.

74. Lee H, Whitman GT, Lim JG, Lee SD, Park YC (2001). Bilateral sudden deafness as a prodrome of anterior inferior cerebellar artery infarction. *Arch Neurol*, 58(8), 1287–9.

75. Yi HA, Lee SR, Lee H, Ahn BH, Park BY, Whitman GT (2005). Sudden deafness as a sign of stroke with normal diffusion-weighted brain MRI. *Acta Otolaryngol*, 125(10), 1119–21.

76. Lee H, Kim HJ, Koo JW, Kim JS (2009). Progression of acute cochleovestibulopathy into anterior inferior cerebellar artery infarction. *J Neurol Sci*, 278(1–2), 119–22.

77. Kim JS, Cho KH, Lee H (2009). Isolated labyrinthine infarction as a harbinger of anterior inferior cerebellar artery territory infarction with normal diffusion-weighted brain MRI. *J Neurol Sci*, 278(1–2), 82–4.

78. Kim HA, Lee SR, Lee H (2007). Acute peripheral vestibular syndrome of a vascular cause. *J Neurol Sci*, 254(1–2), 99–101.

79. Lee H, Kim JS, Chung EJ, et al. (2009). Infarction in the territory of anterior inferior cerebellar artery: spectrum of audiovestibular loss. *Stroke*, 40(12), 3745–51.

80. Dieterich M, Brandt T (1993). Ocular torsion and tilt of subjective visual vertical are sensitive brainstem signs. *Ann Neurol*, 33(3), 292–9.

81. Lee H, Lee SY, Lee SR, Park BR, Baloh RW (2005). Ocular tilt reaction and anterior inferior cerebellar artery syndrome. *J Neurol Neurosurg Psychiatry*, 76(12), 1742–3.

82. Lee H, Yi HA, Lee SR, Lee SY, Park BR (2008). Ocular torsion associated with infarction in the territory of the anterior inferior cerebellar artery: frequency, pattern, and a major determinant. *J Neurol Sci*, 269(1–2), 18–23.

83. Baier B, Bense S, Dieterich M (2008). Are signs of ocular tilt reaction in patients with cerebellar lesions mediated by the dentate nucleus? *Brain*, 131(Pt 6), 1445–54.

84. Barth A, Bogousslavsky J, Regli F (1994). Infarcts in the territory of the lateral branch of the posterior inferior cerebellar artery. *J Neurol Neurosurg Psychiatry*, 57(9), 1073–6.

85. Voogd JAN, Gerrts NM, Ruigrok TH (1996). Organization of the vestibulocerebellum. *Ann N Y Acad Sci*, 781, 553–79.

86. Fushiki H, Barmack NH (1997). Topography and reciprocal activity of cerebellar purkinje cells in the uvula-nodulus modulated by vestibular stimulation. *J Neurophysiol*, 78(6), 3083–94.

87. Duncan GW, Parker SW, Fisher CM (1975). Acute cerebellar infarction in the PICA territory. *Arch Neurol*, 32(6), 364–8.

88. Huang CY, Yu YL (1985). Small cerebellar stroke may mimic labyrinthine lesions. *J Neurol Neurosurg Psychiatry*, 48(3), 263–5.

89. Norrving B, Magnusson M, Holtas S (1995). Isolated acute vertigo in the elderly; vestibular or vascular disease? *Acta Neurol Scand*, 91(1), 43–8.

90. Lee H, Yi HA, Cho YW, et al. (2003). Nodulus infarction mimicking acute peripheral vestibulopathy. *Neurology*, 60(10), 1700–2.

91. Lee H, Cho YW (2004). A case of isolated nodulus infarction presenting as a vestibular neuritis. *J Neuro Sci*, 221(1–2), 117–19.

92. Lee H, Sohn SI, Cho YW, et al. (2006). Cerebellar infarction presenting isolated vertigo: frequency and vascular topographical patterns. *Neurology*, 67(7), 1178–83.

93. Newman-Toker DE, Kattah JC, Alvernia JE, Wang DZ (2008). Normal head impulse test differentiates acute cerebellar strokes from vestibular neuritis. *Neurology*, 70(24 Pt2), 2378–85

94. Hotson JR, Baloh RW (1998). Acute vestibular syndrome. *N Eng J Med*, 339(10), 680–5.

95. Amarenco P, Levy C, Cohen A, Touboul PJ, Roullet E, Bousser MG (1994). Causes and mechanisms of territorial and nonterritorial cerebellar infarcts in 115 consecutive patients. *Stroke*, 25(1), 105–12.

96. Macdonell RA, Kalnins RM, Donnan GA (1987). Cerebellar infarction: natural history, prognosis, and pathology. *Stroke*, 18(5), 849–55.

97. Kase CS, Norrving B, Levine SR, et al. (1993). Cerebellar infarction: clinical and anatomic observations in 66 cases. *Stroke*, 24(1), 76–83.

98. Koh MG, Phan TG, Atkinson KL, Wijdicks EF (2001). Neuroimaging in deteriorating patients with cerebellar infarcts and mass effect. *Stroke*, 31(9), 2062–7.

99. Mossman S, Halmagyi M (1997). Partial ocular tilt reaction due to unilateral cerebellar lesion. *Neurology*, 49(2), 491–3.

100. Kim HA, Lee H, Yi HA, Lee SR, Lee SY, Baloh RW (2009). Pattern of otolith dysfunction in posterior inferior cerebellar artery territory cerebellar infarction. *J Neurol Sci*, 280(1–2), 65–70.

101. Sunderland S (1945). The arterial relations of the internal auditory meatus. *Brain*, 68, 23–7.

102. Lee H (2008). Sudden deafness related to posterior circulation infarction in the territory of the nonanterior inferior cerebellar artery: frequency, origin, and vascular topographical pattern. *Eur Neurol*, 59(6), 302–6.

103. Kase CS, White JL, Joslyn JN, Williams JP, Mohr JP (1985). Cerebellar infarction in the superior cerebellar artery distribution. *Neurology*, 35(5), 705–11.

104. Amarenco P, Hauw JJ (1990). Cerebellar infarction in the territory of the superior cerebellar artery: a clinicopathologic study of 33 cases. *Neurology*, 40(9), 1383–90.

105. Chaves CJ, Caplan LR, Chung CS, et al. (1994). Cerebellar infarcts in the New England Medical Center Posterior Circulation Stroke Registry. *Neurology*, 44(8), 1385–90.

106. Sohn SI, Lee H, Lee SR, Baloh RW (2006). Cerebellar infarction in the territory of the medial branch of the superior cerebellar artery. *Neurology*, 66(1), 115–17.

107. Nitschke MF, Kleinschmidt A, Wessel K, Frahm J (1996). Somatotopic motor representation in the human anterior cerebellum. A high-resolution functional MRI study. *Brain*, 119(3), 1023–9.

108. Brennen RW, Bergland RM (1977). Acuet cerebellar hemorrhage. Analysis of clinical findings and outcome in 12 cases. *Neurology*, 27(6), 527–32.

109. Jensen MB, St Louis EK (2005). Management of acute cerebellar stroke. *Arch Neurol*, 62(4), 537–44.

110. Passero S, Filosomi G (1998). Posterior circulation infarcts in patients with vertebrobasilar dolichoectasia. *Stroke*, 29(3), 653–9.

111. Besson G, Bogousslavsky J, Moulin T, Hommel M (1995). Vertebrobasilar infarcts in patients with dolichoectatic basilar artery. *Acta Neurol Scand*, 91(1), 37–42.

112. Jannetta PJ, Moller MB, Moller AR (1984). Disabling positional vertigo. *New Engl J Med*, 310(26), 1700–5.

113. Brandt T, Dieterich M (1994). VIIIth nerve vascular compression syndrome: vestibular paroxysmia. *Baillieres Clin Neurol*, 3(3), 565–75.

114. Tatlow W, Bammer H (1957). Syndromes of vertebral artery compression. *Neurology*, 7(5), 331–40.

115. Strupp M, Planck JH, Arbusow V, Steiger HJ, Bruckmann H, Brandt T (2000). Rotational vertebral artery occlusion syndrome with vertigo due to 'labyrinthine excitation'. *Neurology*, 54(6), 1376–9.

116. Choi KD, Shin HY, Kim JS, et al (2005). Rotational vertebral artery syndrome: oculographic analysis of nystagmus. *Neurology*, 65(8), 1287–90.

117. Marti S, Hegemann S, von Büdingen HC, Baumgartner RW, Straumann D (2008). Rotational vertebral artery syndrome. 3D kinematics of nystagmus suggest bilateral labyrinthine dysfunction. *J Neurol*, 255(5), 663–7.

118. Noh Y, Kwon OK, Kim JS (2011). Rotational vertebral artery syndrome due to compression of nondominant vertebral artery terminating in posterior inferior cerebellar artery. *J Neurol*, 258, 1775–80.

119. Choi JH, Kim MJ, Lee TH, Moon IS, Choi KD, Kim JS (2011). Dominant vertebral artery occlusion during ipsilateral head tilt. *Neurology*, 76, 1679.

CHAPTER 24

Gait and Disequilibrium

P. D. Thompson and T. E. Kimber

In this chapter, equilibrium refers to a stable upright posture of the body in which the trunk is balanced on the legs during quiet standing and locomotion. The precise organization of equilibrium is complex and poorly understood. Body motion and truncal sway is controlled by the interplay of mechanical (musculoskeletal) and neural mechanisms. Whilst it is convenient to think of these as separate, mechanical and neural factors may be inter-related in controlling body motion (1). For example, widening the stance width reduces lateral motion of the trunk and to a lesser extent anteroposterior sway (1). Mechanical coupling of the ankles and hips with a wide stance base alters the intersegmental motion between legs and trunk and neural (vestibular, proprioceptive) responses (1). During quiet standing the control of truncal position is largely mechanical with relatively little contraction of 'posturally active' muscles. Several factors bring neural mechanisms into play. These include dynamic equilibrium during walking, upper limb movements, and postural adjustments in response to external perturbations. The neural control of equilibrium involves postural responses generated in networks connecting the frontal and parietal lobes, basal ganglia, thalamus, brainstem and cerebellum, and motor efferents to proximal and axial muscles. In humans the control of posture occurs 'automatically' without conscious thought while maintaining bipedal stance, walking, or concentrating on the planning of movement, intent, direction, obstacles, and terrain. This process is orchestrated at the highest levels of the motor system. As will be discussed in this chapter, disequilibrium has a profound influence on gait and in many circumstances an altered gait pattern dominates the clinical picture, obscuring the presence of disequilibrium. For this reason, disequilibrium has been considered one manifestation of a higher-level gait disorder (2), most commonly encountered in the elderly but also in other age groups where there is diffuse cerebral pathology.

Postural responses

Postural responses can be summarized as: 1) righting reactions that bring the head and body into an upright position and an erect posture, 2) supporting reactions maintaining antigravity muscle contraction to maintain an upright position, and 3) postural reactions that control body sway during movement or in response to external perturbations (2). Postural reactions consist of a hierarchy ranging from: 1) automatic anticipatory postural reflexes programmed in advance of movement to stabilize the trunk, 2) reactive postural responses employing long latency stretch reflexes during movement,

and finally 3) rescue and protective reactions that are partly under voluntary control and determined by the circumstances threatening balance and an impending fall.

Some of these responses are 'feedforward' signals incorporated into the planned movement to control body position, truncal motion, and stabilize the trunk in advance of limb movement (3). Other responses utilize feedback from multiple sensory inputs including vestibular, proprioceptive, tactile, graviceptive, and visual afferents to shape motor control body motion and balance during movement.

The obvious though neglected corollary to the role of multisensory inputs are the motor efferent systems that convey information driving postural reactions and responses information. These efferent motor pathways innervate motor neurons of axial and proximal muscles. In monkeys, bilateral ventromedial pathways descending from brainstem locomotor regions control the axial and proximal limb movements necessary for standing (4, 5). In humans, the axial and proximal limb musculature is innervated bilaterally from direct corticospinal and descending brainstem (reticulospinal) pathways (6). The latter receive bilateral projections from the premotor cortex which plays an important role in governing truncal and proximal limb movement (6, 7).

Disequilibrium

Disequilibrium is regarded as the inability to balance the trunk on the legs to stand or walk and may be caused by any process that interferes with the control of truncal motion while standing or walking. A number of acute clinical disequilibrium syndromes are associated with well-defined lateralized lesions (Table 24.1). However, these causes of disequilibrium are rare. Disequilibrium usually presents in an elderly patient with a slowly evolving history of instability, unsteadiness, or related subjective complaints and falls. Typically the symptoms cannot be explained by ataxia, weakness, sensory loss, or vestibular failure. Indeed the problem is often not readily explained by the clinical findings (8). After excluding medication effects and non-neurological (e.g. musculoskeletal) causes of instability and falls in the elderly, the commonest finding is of multiple peripheral and central nervous system lesions (Table 24.2). This has given rise to the concept that disequilibrium might be caused by combinations of peripheral sensory deficits depriving the central nervous system of proprioceptive, vestibular, or visual signals (9, 10). It is also apparent that disequilibrium is

Table 24.1 Well-defined lesions that interfere with control of truncal position and produce disequilibrium

Anatomy of lesion	Physiology	Clinical signs
Lateral medullary syndrome (28)	Acute vestibular asymmetry	Lateropulsion eyes Trunk Deviation to affected side Active pushing Ipsilateral limb ataxia
Posterolateral thalamic lesions, 'thalamic astasia' (29)	Disorder integration truncal position, posture	Acute truncal instability Fall away from the side of lesion Fall backwards standing or sitting Arms used to correct the posture Minimal or no hemiparesis
Putamen, globus pallidus lesions, 'thalamic astasia' (30)	Disorder integration truncal position, posture	Slow tilt may be unaware fall without corrective movements minimal or no hemiparesis
Posterolateral thalamic lesions, 'pusher syndrome' (31, 32)	Disruption trunk graviceptive sensory relays Disruption subjective visual vertical	Unaffected limbs actively push trunk towards affected side Sensation of falling, need to correct perceived tilt of trunk to unaffected side Unaffected limbs resist attempts to correct the posture during rehabilitation Hemiparesis, sensory loss and neglect
Cerebellar syndrome Flocculonodular lobe (33)	Impairment of axial muscle tone	Severe imbalance, Disequilibrium Falls backwards
Anterior lobe (34)	Abnormal postural reflexes increased extensor tone	AP truncal oscillations (tremor)

associated with multiple dispersed lesions in the central nervous system (Table 24.2) notably subcortical, periventricular vascular lesions of the cerebral hemispheric white matter (11, 12).

Clinical manifestations of disequilibrium

In the earliest stages of disequilibrium, the deficit may be subtle and limited to a perceived increase in body sway. This may be accompanied by slight widening of the stance base and hesitation when shifting weight onto one leg to start walking or turning. Steps are short especially when starting to walk or turning corners in contrast to the irregular dysmetric steps of cerebellar ataxia and the catastrophic deviations in acute vestibulopathy. This combination of start hesitation, short shuffling steps, and slow walking speeds may be misinterpreted as parkinsonian though unsteadiness and falls are not characteristic of early Parkinson's disease. Stepping may improve with external support suggesting shuffling is compensatory for imbalance caused by poor truncal control, increased body sway, and the threat of falling.

Table 24.2 Multiple lesions associated with disequilibrium

Multiple peripheral sensory deficits	Central nervous system
Proprioception	Cerebrovascular disease
Vestibular failure	(periventricular white matter)
Impaired vision	Hydrocephalus
	Frontal lesions
	Frontal lesions

As disequilibrium progresses, the stance base widens and stepping becomes shallower and shorter (shuffling). Upper body motion is guarded and appears awkward or stiff. The arms are held away from the body when walking as if to provide extra balance. The trunk is extended (in contrast to the flexed posture of Parkinson's disease) with flexion of the hips and knees. Eventually, standing may not be possible without support and assistance may be necessary to rise from a sitting position. Truncal movements when lying down or standing up become increasingly difficult, are often ineffective, and attempted with inappropriate postural strategies. This is evident in the patient who tilts backwards when standing. This may be accompanied by active pushing backwards that threatens balance and prevents standing.

Falls are commonly the presenting feature of disequilibrium. Patients often are unable to explain why falls occur. Further inquiry reveals that falls occur during postural adjustments when standing from a seated position (or vice versa), turning, leaning, bending over, following minor perturbations, or performing multiple tasks at once such as when walking while carrying objects or opening doors ('multitasking'). Falls also may follow a distracting stimulus that diverts attention away from walking and maintaining balance. Falls are typically backwards but toppling to either side can occur.

Stepping and the cautious gait

The initiation of walking requires a postural adjustment tilting the trunk to one side, supporting body weight and balancing the trunk on one leg while the opposite (leading) leg swings forward to initiate stepping. The same regulation of truncal motion sway is necessary during rhythmic stepping when walking. If truncal motion cannot be stabilized on one leg for that short period of time, balance will be threatened. Widening the stance width reduces motion in the mediolateral and, to a lesser extent, the anteroposterior planes and augments the sensitivity of neural compensation controlling truncal motion (1).

The cautious gait pattern (2) reflects the stabilizing effect of widening the stance base, short shallow steps (shuffling) and reducing upper body motion. These voluntary manoeuvres to compensate for the uncertainty of truncal control are readily appreciated when walking on a slippery or unstable surface or if balance is threatened for any reason. Accordingly, poor balance or disequilibrium alone can lead to an alteration in stepping patterns to minimize truncal motion and imbalance.

Measurement of stepping in elderly gait disturbances reveals a wide stance base, slow short steps, shuffling when turning, a stooped posture, and general loss of axial mobility, regardless of the cause (13). These changes are considered 'non-specific stride-dependent compensation' (14). Studies of stepping patterns in gait disorders associated with deep white matter cerebrovascular disease (subcortical arteriosclerotic encephalopathy) indicate that step generation is preserved (14). Body sway is increased in all directions and steps are short, slow, and variable in timing and amplitude (ataxic) possibly compensatory for disequilibrium (16). Control of the initial postural adjustments before stepping is abnormal, leading to false steps to control the direction and extent of body sway and delay in initiation of walking (14). This suggests that impaired control of truncal motion or disequilibrium is a major determinant of the initial stepping abnormality. It follows that compensatory manoeuvres for disequilibrium will be superimposed on the stepping pattern during each subsequent step cycle.

Trunk motion

The control of truncal motion during stepping has received scant examination and is not generally emphasized in the traditional neurological examination. The control of truncal movement can be examined by asking the patient to stand up, sit down, start to walk then stop, during turning, standing on one leg, hopping, and when lying down and rolling over. Loss of truncal mobility during any of these manoeuvres points towards a disturbance of truncal axial muscle control. Such findings are common in disequilibrium. In the majority of reports of disequilibrium associated with frontal lobe disease, attention has focused on the initiation of gait, stepping and the striking discrepancy between the inability to step while standing, and preservation of stepping movements while seated or lying down leading to the concept of 'gait apraxia' (17) or 'apraxia of gait and of trunk movements' (18). In many of these case descriptions truncal movements were impaired, suggesting poor truncal control and resulting disequilibrium might have been responsible for the gait disturbance, consistent with the observed improvement in walking with support.

Disequilibrium and degenerative diseases of the brainstem and frontal lobes

Falls due to disequilibrium are an early and significant problem in more than 80% of patients with Steele–Richardson–Olszewski (SRO) syndrome (progressive supranuclear palsy) (19). The falls

are often dramatic without corrective postural adjustments or protective rescue reactions leading to head injuries and fractures. The propensity to fall coupled with the characteristic impulsivity of frontal executive dysfunction results in reckless lurching postural movements and falls. This was referred to as an 'apraxia for truncal or turning movements' in the original description (20). The widespread pathology in SRO, affecting frontal lobe, midbrain, and thalamus makes it difficult to ascribe the deficits to one site. Medial frontal lobe degeneration (21), frontal lobe infarction, deep white matter small-vessel cerebrovascular disease (Binswanger disease), chronic subdural haematoma, callosal glioma, and hydrocephalus all may present with disequilibrium, falls, and a progressive higher-level gait disorder (2).

Disequilibrium and hemispheric subcortical white matter disease

Cerebral white matter lesions in the ambulatory elderly are correlated with disequilibrium, falls, increased body sway, and cognitive decline (22–24). Single leg stance time was negatively correlated with the extent of white matter changes on magnetic resonance brain imaging and was significantly reduced in those who had fallen in the previous year (12). Disequilibrium and falls were particularly associated with frontal and prefrontal periventricular deep white matter disease (12). The findings in this cohort presumably represent the precursor, or a mild form, of subcortical arteriosclerotic encephalopathy in which the increased body sway is accompanied by abnormal stepping patterns as described earlier (16, 25).

The frontal and prefrontal periventricular distribution of white matter disease, interrupting parietal-frontal and frontal-subcortical connections to basal ganglia and brainstem, is placed to interrupt the cerebral hemisphere processing of both afferent and efferent arms of postural reflexes and truncal control. Interruption of premotor cortical–brainstem linkages innervating truncal muscles provides one explanation for the poor truncal mobility that is commonly encountered in bilateral, diffuse frontal white matter pathology. Since the innervation is bilateral, clinical deficits only appear with diffuse bilateral pathology. After unilateral lesions any deficits in truncal control will be subtle or compensated for by the intact premotor cortical inputs (6).

Unexplained falls and disequilibrium

'Unexplained' falls in the elderly are frequently attributed to impaired postural reflexes (26). Impaired postural reflexes are likely to be responsible for the increase in body sway that occurs with aging and body sway is greater in those whose falls are attributed to loss of balance (27). Increased body sway particularly in the mediolateral plane is associated with falls (9). People who fall have variable stride width and increased lateral sway when standing on a narrow base but the extent of sway was not significantly changed by eye closure or deprivation of proprioception (9). These findings from static measures of body motion may greatly underestimate the impact of excessive truncal motion and disequilibrium during the dynamic process of walking when the complexities of controlling truncal motion in all directions are much greater. External perturbations and other distractions (for example, multitasking) will further interfere with compensatory manoeuvres for disequilibrium and lead to 'unexplained' falls.

Concluding remarks

A common theme in disequilibrium is the presence of inappropriate postural synergies, impaired postural reflexes, and absent rescue reactions that interfere with walking and the initiation of walking (15). Impairment of these postural mechanisms leads to loss of 'automatic' control of truncal motion when walking and demands extra attention and conscious effort to control truncal motion, maintain balance, and stepping strategies. Distraction, unexpected obstacles, and multitasking precipitate falls by reducing the conscious attention available to maintain truncal control.

The presence of multiple dispersed hemispheric and brainstem networks governing equilibrium explains why anatomical correlation with subtle signs of disequilibrium is imprecise. Multiple bilateral lesions may be necessary to disconnect these networks and produce clinical symptoms or signs of disequilibrium. The processes that gradually disrupt the fine control of equilibrium will simultaneously interfere with compensatory mechanisms driven by postural responses and voluntary control of truncal motion.

Variation in the extent and location of disconnection along with the degree to which compensatory manoeuvres are affected accounts for the wide range of clinical presentations of disequilibrium, further confounding attempts to identify anatomical correlations. Compensation will continue as long as there is redundancy in the system to cope with the deficits. Ultimately a critical level is reached beyond which compensation to maintain equilibrium is inadequate. Falls then occur and locomotion becomes increasingly difficult if not impossible. The onset of falls often creates the impression of a sudden deterioration though subtle multifocal disconnections will have been underway for some time by the time compensation fails and falls occur. Disequilibrium, particularly after a fall, leads to additional factors such as a fear of falling, a dislike of open spaces and moving objects, adding further complexity to the clinical picture.

References

1. Day BL, Steiger MJ, Thompson PD, Marsden CD. (1993). Effect of vision and stance width on human body motion when standing: implications for afferent control of body sway. *J Physiol*, 469, 479–99.
2. Nutt JG, Marsden CD, Thompson PD. (1993). Human walking and higher level gait disorders, particularly in the elderly. *Neurology*, 43, 268–79.
3. Marsden CD, Merton PM, Morton HB. (1981). Human postural responses. *Brain*, 104, 513–34.
4. Lawrence DG, Kuypers HGJM. (1968). The functional organisation of the motor system in the monkey II. The effects of lesions of descending brainstem pathways. *Brain*, 91, 15–36.
5. Takakusaki K. (2008). Forebrain control of locomotor behaviors. *Brain Res Rev*, 57(1), 192–8.
6. Freund HJ, Hummelsheim H. (1985). Lesions of premotor cortex in man. *Brain*, 108, 697–733.
7. Wise SP, Boussaoud D, Johnson PB, Caminiti R. (1997). Premotor and parietal cortex: corticocortical connectivity and combinatorial computations. *Annu Rev Neurosci*, 20, 25–42.
8. Sudarsky L. (1997). Clinical approach to gait disorders of aging: an overview. In Masdeu JC, Sudarsky L, Wolfson L (Eds) *Gait Disorders of Aging*, pp. 147–57. Philadelphia, PA: Lippincott-Raven.
9. Lord SR, Rogers MW, Howland A, Fitzpatrick R. (1999). Lateral stability, sensorimotor function and falls in older people. *J Am Geriatr Soc*, 47, 1077–81.
10. Fife TD, Baloh RW. (1993). Disequilibrium of unknown cause in older people. *Ann Neurol*, 34, 694–702.
11. Whitman GT, Tang T, Lin A, Baloh RW. (2001). A prospective study of cerebral white matter abnormalities in older people with gait dysfunction. *Neurology*, 57, 990–4.
12. Blahak C, Baezner H, Pantoni L, et al. (2009). Deep frontal and periventricular age related white matter changes but not basal ganglia and infratentorial hyperintensities are associated with falls: cross sectional results from the LADIS study. *J Neurol, Neurosurg Psychiatry*, 80, 608–13.
13. Elble RJ, Higgins C, Hughes L. (1991). The syndrome of senile gait. *J Neurol*, 230, 71–5.
14. Elble RJ, Cousins R, Leffler K, Hughes L. (1996). Gait initiation by patients with lower half parkinsonism. *Brain*, 119, 1705–16.
15. Elble RJ. (2007). Gait and dementia: moving beyond the notion of gait apraxia. *J Neural Transm*, 114, 1253–8.
16. Ebersbach G, Sojer M, Valdeoriola F, et al. (1999). Comparative analysis of gait in Parkinson's disease, cerebellar ataxia and subcortical arteriosclerotic encephalopathy. *Brain*, 122, 1349–55.
17. Meyer JS, Barron DW. (1960). Apraxia of gait: a clinicophysiological study. *Brain*, 83, 261–84.
18. Petrovici K. (1968). Apraxia of gait and of trunk movements. *J Neurol Sci*, 7, 229–43.
19. Williams DR, de Silva R, Paviour DC, et al. (2005). Characteristics of two distinct clinical phenotypes in pathologically proven progressive supranuclear palsy: Richardson's syndrome and PSP-parkinsonism. *Brain*, 128, 1247–58.
20. Steele JC, Richardson JC, Olszewski J. (1964). Progressive supranuclear palsy. A heterogenous degeneration involving the brainstem, basal ganglia and cerebellum with vertical supranuclear gaze and pseudobulbar palsy, nuchal dystonia and dementia. *Arch Neurol*, 10, 333–59.
21. Rossor MN, Tyrell PJ, Warrington EK, Thompson PD, Marsden CD, Lantos P. (1999). Progressive gait disturbance with atypical Alzheimer's disease and corticobasal degeneration. *J Neurol Neurosurg Psychiatry*, 67, 345–52.
22. Masdeu JC, Wolfson L, Lantos G. (1989). Brain white matter changes in the elderly prone to falling. *Arch Neurol*, 46, 1292–6.
23. Baloh RW, Yue Q, Socotch TM, Jacobson KM. (1995). White matter lesions and disequilibrium in older people. I. Case control comparison. *Arch Neurol*, 52, 970–4.
24. Tell GS, Lekfowitz DS, Diehr P, Elster AD. (1998). Relationship between balance and abnormalities in cerebral magnetic resonance imaging in older adults. *Arch Neurol*, 55, 73–9.
25. Thompson PD, Marsden CD. (1987). Gait disorder of subcortical arteriosclerotic encephalopathy: Binswanger's disease. *Movement Disord*, 2, 1–8.
26. Weiner WJ, Nora LM, Glantz RH. (1984). Elderly inpatients: postural reflex impairment. *Neurology*, 34, 945–7.
27. Overstall RW, Exton-Smith AN, Imms FJ, Johnson AZ. (1977). Falls in the elderly related to postural imbalance. *BMJ*, 1, 261–4.
28. Dieterich M, Brandt T. (1992). Wallenberg's syndrome: lateropulsion, cyclorotation and subjective visual vertical in thirty six patients. *Ann Neurol*, 31, 399–408.
29. Masdeu JC, Gorelick PB. (1988). Thalamic astasia: Inability to stand after unilateral thalamic lesions. *Annals of Neurol*, 23, 596–603.
30. Labadie EL, Awerbuch GI, Hamilton RH, Rapesak SZ. (1989). Falling and postural deficits due to acute unilateral basal ganglia lesions. *Arch Neurol* 45, 492–6.
31. Karnath HO, Johannsen L, Broets D, Kuker W. (2005). Posterior thalamic haemorrhage induces 'pusher syndrome'. *Neurology*, 64, 1014–19.
32. Saj A, Honore J, Coello Y, Rousseaux M. (2005). The visual vertical in the pusher syndrome: influence of hemispace and body position. *J Neurol*, 252, 885–91.
33. Fulton JF. (1949). *Physiology of the Nervous System* (3rd ed), pp. 528–36. New York: Oxford University Press.
34. Mauritz KH, Dichgans J, Hufschmidt A. (1979). Quantitative analysis of stance in late cortical cerebellar atrophy of the anterior lobe and other forms of cerebellar ataxia. *Brain*, 102, 461–82.

CHAPTER 25

Progressive Vestibulocerebellar Syndromes

Tracey D. Graves and Joanna C. Jen

Introduction

Vestibulocerebellar syndromes broadly encompass neurological disorders affecting the vestibulocerebellum to cause dizziness and imbalance. A detailed history helps distinguish these syndromes from other common causes of dizziness, including near-faint (presyncopal) dizziness and recurrent vertigo variably associated with migraine without neurological symptoms or signs. Careful physical examination may uncover focal neurological deficits referable to the cerebellum to distinguish the vestibulocerebellar syndromes from diseases affecting the peripheral vestibular apparatus, such as vestibular neuritis, Ménière's disease, and benign paroxysmal positional vertigo.

The cerebellum plays an important role in the motor control of eye movement, speech, and swallowing, truncal stability and gait, as well as appendicular coordination. Although patients with peripheral vestibulopathy can also present with nystagmus, there are important differences in the associated clinical features and the characteristics of the nystagmus to set apart peripheral and central causes of dizziness and imbalance (see Table 25.1). Because the cerebellum exerts critical control on the speed, consistency, and precision of eye movement, patients who suffer from diseases of the cerebellum frequently demonstrate persistent eye movement abnormalities. These patients commonly present with gaze-evoked nystagmus, saccadic dysmetria, and impairment in smooth pursuit and optokinetic response, which are not observed in peripheral vestibulopathy. Slurring of speech, truncal instability, and clumsiness in the setting of dizziness and imbalance are strongly suggestive of cerebellar disease.

Not only are the vestibulocerebellar syndrome heterogeneous in their clinical features, they are also heterogeneous regarding the underlying causes. Only those with nystagmus may complain of vertigo, while most are bothered by a sense of disequilibrium. A wide range of acquired infectious, inflammatory, metabolic, neoplastic, and vascular neurological and systemic disease processes can damage the cerebellum to present with an acute onset of vertigo and ataxia. Yet, an insidious onset with progressive vestibulocerebellar deficits is most commonly caused by neurodegeneration, either inherited or idiopathic. In this chapter, we discuss the diagnostic approach to common acquired causes as well as review recent advances in the elucidation of genetic bases of a growing number of autosomal dominant, autosomal recessive, as well as X-linked disorders presenting with abnormal eye movement control and imbalance, with an emphasis on the episodic ataxias. The chapter concludes with current treatment options and ongoing research.

Acquired causes

Common acquired causes of a progressive vestibulocerebellar syndrome are listed in Table 25.2.

Table 25.1 Comparison between central and peripheral vestibular disorders

Symptoms and signs	Peripheral vestibulopathy	Central disorders
Hearing loss	Common	Rare
Nausea & vomiting	Severe	Variable
Imbalance	Mild to moderate	Severe
Neurological symptoms	Rare	Common
Nystagmus	Unidirectional, never pure vertical or torsional Suppressed by fixation	Gaze-evoked, direction-changing can be downbeat, upbeat, or pure torsional Not inhibited by fixation
VOR	May be absent	Normal
Compensation	Rapid	Slow

Table 25.2 Acquired causes of progressive vestibulocerebellar syndromes

Disease process	Disease	Clinical pointers
Immune	Primary/secondary progressive multiple sclerosis Opsoclonus-myoclonus syndrome Paraneoplastic/autoimmune cerebellar degeneration	Other neurological symptoms and signs Oscillopsia Possible malignancy, no other neurological symptoms or signs
Mass lesion	Metastasis Primary neoplasm Vascular malformation Sarcoidosis	Evidence of malignancy Possible symptoms of hydrocephalus Previous haemorrhage or stroke Extraneurological manifestations
Endocrine	Hypothyroidism Hypoparathyroidism	Signs of hypothyroidism Carpopedal spasm
Gastrointestinal disease	Whipple's disease Coeliac disease Vitamin E deficiency (hereditary)	GI symptoms, lymphadenopathy Weight loss Head tremor
Toxic	Ethanol Drugs (phenytoin, lithium, amiodarone, ciclosporin, isoniazid, metronidazole, platins) Toxins	Other neurological markers (peripheral neuropathy, memory decline), signs of chronic liver disease or neglect History Occupational exposure
Degenerative	Multiple system atrophy Creutzfeldt–Jakob disease Spinocerebellar ataxia	Signs of Parkinsonism, autonomic neuropathy Myoclonus, dementia, mutism (See Table 25.4)
Vascular	Stroke Superficial siderosis of the nervous system	Sudden onset of symptoms Deafness, pyramidal signs

Inherited causes

Autosomal dominant: progressive

The spinocerebellar ataxias (SCAs) are a large group of cerebellar degenerations and are the commonest cause of dominant adult-onset ataxia. There are some SCAs which have distinctive phenotypes (usually extracerebellar features) which may be diagnostic, however, they all have ataxia and dysarthria and can be difficult to distinguish on clinical grounds. They are therefore divided by the gene or locus first found in large families, as the same phenotype can be caused by multiple genes. The commonest and first to be identified are the trinucleotide expansion polyglutamine disorders. These show anticipation and the phenotype is largely related to repeat size. Although many genes have now been identified, genetic testing is often restricted to the commonest conditions. Others are only available on a research basis, whilst some have only been seen in individual pedigrees. On the whole, the clinical classification put forward by Harding in 1982 (1) still stands (see Table 25.3).

A comparison of the genetic, ocular motor, and other clinical features of the autosomal dominant SCAs is summarized in Table 25.4.

Autosomal dominant: episodic

The episodic ataxias (EAs) are early-onset autosomal dominant disorders. All the EA genes identified to date are cell-membrane bound ion channels or transporters important in regulating neuronal excitability. Patients experience paroxysmal attacks of dizziness, unsteadiness, nausea with other associated features in response to various triggers such as sudden movement, emotion, or intercurrent infection. These last minutes to days and in between attacks, patients can be completely well, although interictal myokymia is common in EA1 (27–30) and interictal nystagmus is common in EA2 (31) (see Table 25.5). These are reviewed in detail in (32) and compared in Table 25.6.

Episodic ataxia type 1 (EA1)

Patients with EA1 have frequent, brief attacks of imbalance, dizziness and dysarthria. They may occasionally describe true vertigo or they may have a more non-specific light headedness. All patients tend to experience a profound sense of imbalance or dysequilibrium during an attack and want to sit or lay down. Attacks can be precipitated by sudden movement, emotion, or intercurrent infection. Patients have continuous peripheral nerve excitability, known as myokymia, even between attacks. This is manifest as continuous

Table 25.3 Harding's classification of autosomal dominant cerebellar ataxia (1)

Autosomal dominant cerebellar ataxia type	Clinical phenotype	Diseases
ADCA I	Cerebellar syndrome plus other CNS manifestations (pyramidal, extrapyramidal, ophthalmoplegia, dementia)	SCA1, SCA2, SCA3, SCA4, SCA8, SCA9, SCA12, SCA17, SCA27, SCA28, SCA32, SCA35, SCA36
ADCA II	Cerebellar syndrome and pigmentary maculopathy	SCA7
ADCA III	Pure cerebellar syndrome	SCA5, SCA6, SCA10, SCA11, SCA14, SCA15, SCA22, SCA26, SCA30, SCA31

Table 25.4 Comparison of the ocular motor features of the SCAs

Disease	Gene	Trinucleotide repeat	Ocular motor features	Additional clinical features	Reference
SCA1	*Ataxin-1*	Yes	Gaze paresis, slow/absent saccades ± nystagmus	Extrapyramidal, spasticity, bulbar, polyneuropathy, MCI	(2)
SCA2	*Ataxin-2*	Yes	Slow saccades, gaze paresis	Extrapyramidal, sphincter disturbance, polyneuropathy	(3)
SCA3	*Ataxin-3*	Yes	Impaired VOR gain, square wave jerks	Extrapyramidal, spasticity, polyneuropathy	(4)
SCA5	*β-III Spectrin*	No	Downbeat nystagmus, not suppressed by fixation, impaired smooth pursuit	Facial myokymia	(5)
SCA6	*CACNA1A*	Yes	Nystagmus: downbeating, gaze-evoked (all directions) & rebound. Impaired: VOR, OKN, smooth pursuit	Extrapyramidal (rare, late feature)	(6)
SCA8	*ATXN8/ ATXN8OS*	Yes	Impaired smooth pursuit, horizontal nystagmus	Sensory neuropathy	(7)
SCA10	*ATXN10*	Pentanucleotide	Gaze-evoked nystagmus, fragmented pursuit	Epilepsy	(8)
SCA11	*TTBK2*	No	Nystagmus (horizontal > vertical), saccadic pursuit	Hyper-reflexia	(9)
SCA12	*PPP2R2B*	Yes	Slow saccades, broken pursuit, nystagmus	Extrapyramidal, polyneuropathy, facial myokymia, hyper-reflexia, dementia	(10)
SCA13	*KCNC3*	No	Horizontal nystagmus	Hyper-reflexia, mental retardation	(11)
SCA15/16	*ITPR1*	No	Gaze-evoked nystagmus, dysmetric saccades		(12, 13)
SCA17	*TBP*	No	Nystagmus: gaze-evoked, downbeat & rebound, hypometric saccades, impaired smooth pursuit initiation & maintenance	Extrapyramidal, psychiatric, hyper-reflexia, dementia, epilepsy	(14)
SCA19/22	*KCNC3*	No	Intermittent microsaccadic pursuits, gaze-directed horizontal nystagmus	Bulbar, hyporeflexia	(15) (16)
SCA23	*PDYN*	No	Slow saccades, ocular dysmetria	Sensory loss, hyper-reflexia	(17)
SCA25	Linkage to 2p15–p21	N/A	Slow eye movement speed, nystagmus: some patients	Sensory neuropathy	(18)
SCA26	Linkage to 19p13	N/A	Irregular vertical & horizontal visual pursuit movements, nystagmus: some patients		(19)
SCA28	*AFG3L2*	No	Gaze-evoked nystagmus, ophthalmoparesis (late), ptosis: later in disease course, slow saccades	Spasticity, myoclonic epilepsy	(20)
Ataxia with spasmodic cough	unknown	No	Downbeat nystagmus, diplopia	Cough occurs in bursts, hyper-reflexia	(21)
SCA30	Linkage to 4q34.3–q35.1	Unknown	Hypermetric saccades, gaze evoked nystagmus		(22)
SCA31	Intronic complex pentanucleotide expansion 16q22.1	No	Saccadic pursuits		(23)
SCA32	Linkage to 7q32–q33	Unknown		Cognitive impairment, infertility in males	(24)
SCA35	*TGM6*	No	Slow saccades without nystagmus in some patients	Upper motor neuron signs, spasmodic torticollis	(25)
SCA36	Intronic hexanucleotide repeat in *NOP56*	No	Not described	Motor neuron degeneration with skeletal muscle and tongue atrophy	(26)

fine muscular twitching movements which often flit from place to place and may involve the craniofacial and/or limb musculature. Sometimes this may be exacerbated during an attack and patients may describe this as a 'tremor'. There is often a delay in diagnosis as patients do not seek medical attention or are misdiagnosed with epilepsy or psychological disorders. EA1 is due to mutations in the potassium channel *KCNA1* (33). Carbamazepine can be useful in treating both the ataxia and the myokymia (34). Acetazolamide has been used for the ataxia (35), but is less effective than in EA2 (34). There is an increased relative risk of seizures in patients with EA1 (34, 36). These include partial and generalized seizures, with varying response to anticonvulsant medications (27, 28, 34).

Table 25.5 The known episodic ataxias (EAs)

	EA1	EA2	EA3	PATX/EA4	EA5	EA6	EA7	Late-onset EA	Other EAs
OMIM	160120	108500	606554	606552	601949	600111	611907	Unassigned	Unassigned
Attack duration	Secs–min	Hours	1 min–6 h	Brief	Hours	Hours–days	Hours–days	Minutes	Hours–days
Age of onset	<20	<20	1–42	23–60	<20	5	<20	40–64	After 30
Myokymia	Usual	No	Usual	No	No	No	No	No	No
Nystagmus	No	Usual	Occasional	Usual	Usual	No	No	Yes	Usual
Epilepsy	Occasional	Infrequent	Occasional	Occasional	Usual	Yes	No	No	No
Tinnitus	Infrequent	No	Usual	Occasional	No	No	No	No	No
Vertigo	No	Yes	Yes	Yes	Yes	No	Yes	Yes	Yes
Acetazolamide	Occasional	Usual	Usual	No	Transient	No	No	No	Occasional
Inheritance	AD	AD	AD	AD	AD	Sporadic	AD	AD/AR	Multiple
Chromosomal locus	12q13	19p13	1q42	Unknown	2q22–q23	5p13	19q13	13p12–p13	Unknown
Mutated gene	KCNA1	CACNA1A	Unknown	Unknown	CACNB4	SLC1A3	Unknown	Unknown	Unknown
Mutant protein	Kv1.1	Ca$_v$2.1	Unknown	Unknown	Ca$_v$2.1	EAAT1	Unknown	Unknown	Unknown

Episodic ataxia type 2 (EA2)

Episodes of ataxia often manifest once walking is attempted i.e. between the ages of 1 and 2 years, where it is observed that an affected child has intermittent problems with balance. Parents may also notice triggers or precipitating factors, such as tiredness, stress or emotion. Some parents describe the child becoming generally 'floppy' or hypotonic during an attack. Attacks typically consist of ataxia, vertigo, and dysarthria lasting between 10 minutes to many hours. There may be associated dizziness, headache, diplopia, tinnitus, or dystonia. EA2 is due to mutations in *CACNA1A* (37). Patients often display interictal nystagmus, classically in the downbeat direction. Other clinical signs include hypometric saccades (38), impaired vestibulo-ocular reflex (VOR) (39) and loss of VOR suppression (40). Patients may develop a progressive cerebellar syndrome (41) in addition to paroxysmal ataxia. Approximately 50% of patients complain of headaches indistinguishable from migraine attacks (40). Acetazolamide is the mainstay of therapy and may completely ameliorate attacks in selected patients (42). Patients unresponsive to acetazolamide may respond to 4-aminopyridine (43). Anecdotal evidence suggests that dichlorphenamide is also effective.

Episodic ataxia type 3 (EA3)

One Canadian pedigree has been reported where patients had the sensation of vertigo and tinnitus not usually seen in EA1 and they lacked the interictal nystagmus characteristic of EA2. The age of onset was considered too late for either EA1 or EA2 and the duration of attacks was intermediate between EA1 and EA2. Initially myokymia was reported clinically in 46% of affected individuals but this was not confirmed by subsequent EMG studies. Patients also responded to acetazolamide, as can be seen in both EA1 and EA2 (44). Recently, a genome-wide screen of this pedigree showed linkage to chromosome 1q42, with a maximum two-point LOD score of 4.12. As the only ion channel in the region, the most promising candidate gene was the potassium channel *KCNK1*, however no mutations were identified (45).

Table 25.6 Comparison between episodic ataxia type 1 (EA1) and type 2 (EA2)

	Episodic ataxia type 1	Episodic ataxia type 2
Mode of inheritance	Autosomal dominant	Autosomal dominant
Age of onset	Early childhood	Before age 20
Features	Ataxia Dizziness often without vertigo Visual blurring No nystagmus	Ataxia, truncal instability which may persist between attacks, dysarthria, nystagmus May be associated with vertigo, nausea, vomiting & headache Weakness may occur during spells and can precede onset of episodic ataxia
Precipitating factors	Abrupt postural change, emotion, startle, vestibular stimulation, intercurrent infection	Physical or emotional stress e.g. intercurrent infection
Duration	Brief, attacks last minutes	Attacks often last 30 min to hours
Frequency	Many per day	Variable, less frequent. Not usually more than one in a day
Additional features	Neuromyotonia on electromyography (continuous spontaneous muscle fibre activity) myokymia seen clinically during & between episodes of ataxia. Seizures may occur	Downbeating gaze-evoked nystagmus in all directions between episodes. Impaired VOR, OKN, and smooth pursuits. Some patients develop progressive cerebellar atrophy. Dystonia rarely described. Seizures may occur
Treatment	Phenytoin, carbamazepine	Acetazolamide
Gene	KCNA1	CACNA1A, allelic with FHM and SCA6

Episodic ataxia type 4 (EA4)

Periodic vestibulocerebellar ataxia (PATX) was initially described in two North Carolina families (46) exhibiting autosomal dominant inheritance. The age of onset ranged from the third to the sixth decade and symptoms included episodic attacks of horizontal diplopia, oscillopsia, ataxia, nausea, vertigo, and tinnitus, which escalate over time to become constant. Attacks were precipitated by sudden movement of the head, fatigue or by observing movement in the peripheral vision. Symptoms were alleviated by lying down with eyes closed and acetazolamide was ineffective. Eye movement abnormalities included gaze-evoked nystagmus, abnormal smooth pursuits, reduced optokinetic nystagmus, failure of VOR suppression and strabismus. Linkage was excluded to the known autosomal dominant cerebellar ataxias, including chromosomes 12 (EA1) and 19 (EA2) (47). EA3 patients differ from this syndrome also as they did not display eye movement abnormalities (44).

Episodic ataxia type 5 (EA5)

The apparent genetic heterogeneity in EA2 has led the search for other candidate genes, primarily focused on auxiliary calcium channel subunits. The β4-subunit, encoded by *CACNB4* is the most abundant in cerebellum and is mutated in the mouse model, lethargic, which displays both ataxia and epilepsy (48). It has a crucial role in membrane trafficking and function of $Ca_v2.1$ in neurons. A *CACNB4* mutation was identified (C104F) in six affected members of a French-Canadian family with an EA2 phenotype, but with no mutations in the coding region of *CACNA1A*. The same mutation was seen in a small German family (two affected individuals) with idiopathic generalized epilepsy. A nonsense mutation (R482X) was also found, in a small family with juvenile myoclonic epilepsy (49). Further mutations have not been identified, suggesting that these may be rare polymorphisms or a very rare cause of an EA2-like phenotype.

Episodic ataxia type 6 (EA6)

A patient with a complicated phenotype of episodic ataxia, hemiplegic migraine and seizures was the index case of EA6. The proband had episodes of ataxia lasting days provoked by febrile illness. He later developed hemiplegic migraine and coma. A magnetic resonance image (MRI) scan during an episode of coma showed mild cerebellar atrophy and cortical hyperintensity contralateral to the hemiparesis. An EEG showed a left frontotemporal epileptiform focus, he later developed complex partial seizures. On examination he had truncal ataxia, generalized hyper-reflexia but with flexor plantar responses. Interestingly there was no nystagmus; however, the eye movements were abnormal with reduced smooth pursuits, optokinetic nystagmus and failure of fixation-suppression of the VOR. A novel *de novo* mutation in *SLC1A3* which encodes the excitatory amino acid transporter type 1 (EAAT1) was identified (50). Excitatory amino acid transporters are the sole means of removing glutamate from the extracellular fluid and are therefore critical to the control of neurotransmission. The mutation, leads to the substitution of arginine at a highly conserved proline residue in the fifth transmembrane segment (P290R). This is likely to change the conformation of the protein within the membrane as proline residues allow kinking of peptides and this is the sole proline present in that segment. Functional analysis using a glutamate uptake assay showed reduced uptake via mutant transporters and a dominant negative effect on wild-type cell surface expression. The mutation therefore causes disease by both reduced level of protein

function and expression, leading to reduced glutamate reuptake (50). These findings highlight the role of glutamate in the related channelopathies, EA2, and both familial hemiplegic migraine type 1 (FHM1) and FHM2. Glutamate release is dependent on calcium entry via P/Q-type calcium channels (dysfunctional in EA2/FHM1). Glutamate uptake from the synaptic cleft into astrocytes is via EAAT1, which requires a sodium gradient across the cell membrane to function which is provided by a Na^+/K^+ exchanger ATP1A2, itself dysfunctional in FHM2 (51). This raises interesting questions regarding the possible interrelationship between EAAT1, P/Q-type calcium channels and ATP1A2, in causing similar clinical phenotypes via the same common pathway of glutamate excess.

Episodic ataxia type 7 (EA7)

A new EA phenotype has recently been identified. Six affected members of a US pedigree experienced episodes of ataxia, dysarthria, and weakness, lasting hours to days, which were triggered by exercise or excitement. The phenotype is similar to that of EA2; however, no interictal nystagmus or ataxia were found on examination. Two patients had vertigo as part of their attacks. Linkage analysis showed a LOD score of 2.95 to a 10-cM region at 19q13. Although two ion channel genes lie within the linked region, *KCNC3*, a potassium channel and *SLC17A7*, a solute transporter, no pathogenic mutations were identified in these (52).

Late-onset episodic ataxia

A late-onset syndrome of vertical oscillopsia and slowly progressive gait ataxia was recently described. Attacks were intermediate in length between EA1 and EA2, lasting from 5–60 minutes. In common with EA2, attacks were triggered by exertion, alcohol, and caffeine; however, treatment with acetazolamide was ineffective and no pathogenic mutations were found in *CACNA1A*. Patients all had downbeat nystagmus and most had abnormal smooth pursuit eye movements. All probands had normal MRI brain scans. Four families were investigated by identity-by-descent mapping and linkage was demonstrated to a 14.2-Mb region on chromosome 13q12–13, with a LOD score of higher than 2.7. The initial three candidate genes in the region have yielded no pathogenic mutations and further sequencing is ongoing (53).

Autosomal recessive

Although rare, Friedreich's ataxia is the most common form of hereditary ataxia worldwide, with an estimated carrier frequency of 1 in 120 and a prevalence of 1 in 50,000. Biallelic intronic GAA repeat expansions in the *frataxin* (*FXN*) gene are found in the majority of patients with Friedreich's ataxia and markedly diminish the level of the *frataxin* transcript (54). *Frataxin* is a mitochondrial protein with iron-binding capacity. The multiorgan involvement in Friedreich ataxia has been attributed to systemic mitochondrial dysfunction and oxidative stress. Several other autosomal recessive ataxias are caused by mutations in genes important in DNA repair. Commonly observed eye movement abnormalities are summarized in Table 25.7.

X-linked ataxias

The X-linked ataxias are relatively rare, with the exception of fragile X tremor-ataxia syndrome (FXTAS). FXTAS is due to smaller repeat expansions in *FMR1* than those which cause fragile X syndrome. This is a multisystem disorder with tremor and ataxia with nystagmus as prominent symptoms. Patients may also have

Table 25.7 The autosomal recessive ataxias and their ocular motor features

Disease	Gene	Ocular motor features	Additional features	Reference
Friedreich's ataxia	FXN	Saccadic intrusions with ocular flutter	Areflexia, cardiomyopathy, diabetes, scoliosis, hearing loss, visual loss	(54)
Ataxia telangiectasia	ATM	Poor ocular pursuit, ocular apraxia	Malignancies, immunodeficiencies	(55)
Autosomal recessive spastic ataxia of Charlevoix–Saguenay (ARSACS)	SACS	Nystagmus, poor ocular pursuit	Spasticity, amyotrophy, myelinated retinal nerve fibres, mitral valve prolapse	(56)
Cayman ataxia	ATCAY	Nystagmus	Non-progressive cerebellar syndrome, psychomotor retardation	(57)
Ataxia with oculomotor apraxia type 1 (AOA1)	APTX	Oculomotor apraxia	Axonal motor neuropathy	(58)
Ataxia with oculomotor apraxia type 2 (AOA2)	SETX	Disordered smooth pursuit, absent OKN, slow saccades	Peripheral neuropathy, extrapyramidal, oculomotor apraxia, extensor plantar responses	(59)
Spinocerebellar ataxia with saccadic intrusions (SCAR4)	Linked to 1p36	Macrosaccadic oscillations horizontal, large saccades have increased speed, induced with each gaze shift, intersaccadic intervals present	Hyper-reflexia, myoclonus, fasciculations	(60)
Spinocerebellar ataxia recessive type 8 (SCAR8)	SYNE1	Gaze-evoked nystagmus, abnormal saccades, slow/jerky pursuit	Onset mean 30 years (range 17–46), hyper-reflexia	(61)
Ataxia and motor neuropathy type 1	PEX10	Impaired smooth pursuit	Early onset, distal amyotrophy	(62)
Ataxia and motor neuropathy type 2	ANO10	Hypermetric saccades, nystagmus	Late onset, proximal amyotrophy, tortuous conjunctival vessels, hyper-reflexia	(63)
Cerebellar ataxia and hypergonadotropic hypogonadism	Unknown	Nystagmus or mild saccade disorders	Sensory neuropathy, hypogonadism, sensorineural hearing loss, vestibular hypofunction, mental retardation	(64)
Late-onset Tay–Sachs disease	HEXA	Nystagmus	Cramps/fasciculations, proximal weakness, peripheral neuropathy, dementia, Friedreich's ataxiaphenocopy	(65, 66)

dementia, psychiatric disturbance, sensory and autonomic neuropathy, hyper-reflexia, and Parkinsonism (67).

Combined cerebellar ataxia and bilateral vestibulopathy

Patients with cerebellar ataxia combined with bilateral vestibulopathy and normal hearing were first described in 1991 (68). In a large case series on patients with downbeat nystagmus, which is the most common form of acquired involuntary eye movement, the investigators found bilateral vestibulopathy to be a common comorbidity (based on caloric irrigation and head thrust test) (69). The distinctive clinical presentation of impaired visually enhanced vestibulo-ocular reflex, which reflected impairment in VOR, optokinetic nystagmus (OKN), and smooth pursuit as a result of combined damage to the cerebellum and the peripheral vestibular apparatus) was described in detail in four unrelated patients (70). Subsequently, a follow-up report of 23 additional subjects focused on a newly designated cerebellar ataxia, neuropathy, vestibular areflexia syndrome (CANVAS) (71). The mean age of onset was 60 years, ranging from 33–71. Patients often presented with slowly progressive imbalance and oscillopsia. Physical findings are notable for gaze-evoked nystagmus, dysarthria, appendicular ataxia, and truncal instability with gait difficulties. In the majority of these patients, there was evidence on MRI of anterior and dorsal cerebellar vermian atrophy. The observation of CANVAS in two sib-pairs raised the possibility that this condition may be autosomal recessive but does not rule out other possibilities in the majority of the patients without a positive family history.

Non-progressive congenital cerebellar ataxia

There is a separate clinical entity of congenital cerebellar ataxia that is not associated with progressive clinical deterioration with both genetic and acquired causes (72). Patients typically present with developmental delay and truncal ataxia with evidence of cerebellar hypoplasia on MRI. Different modes of inheritance have been proposed in hereditary non-progressive congenital cerebellar ataxia, including autosomal recessive, autosomal dominant and X-linked. A homozygous mutation in a DNA-binding zinc finger gene, ZNF592, was recently identified in an inbred family with CAMOS (cerebellar ataxia with mental retardation, optic atrophy and skin abnormalities), which is a rare non-progressive ataxia syndrome (73). Two separate genetic loci have been identified in two families with X-linked non-progressive ataxia (74, 75). In one large family with autosomal dominant disease, the disease locus was mapped to chromosome 3p overlapping the SCA15 locus (76). In another family with autosomal dominant non-progressive cerebellar ataxia, the chromosome 3p locus was ruled out, suggesting genetic heterogeneity (77). The symptomatic subjects in this family complained of intermittent oscillopsia, with persistent imbalance and clumsiness. Their examination is notable for upbeat nystagmus in the primary position, with gaze-evoked nystagmus.

Idiopathic

Even with rigorous investigation, about 30% of patients with sporadic adult onset progressive ataxia remain without a firm clinical diagnosis and are labelled as idiopathic late-onset cerebellar ataxia (ILOCA). Family history is usually difficult to ascertain, since these patients present late in life, when their parents are no longer alive, and their children may be too young to manifest symptoms. Despite the genetic advances, the proportion of ILOCA has not really fallen over time and suggests that there are multiple causes which have henceforth not been identified. Patients in this category are heterogeneous but usually have a slowly progressive clinical course.

Downbeat nystagmus is a common presentation and can precede other symptoms of ataxia in patients with idiopathic cerebellar ataxia. An important differential diagnosis is Arnold–Chiari malformation and other pathologies at the foramen magnum, phenytoin toxicity and lesions in the cerebellum (such as strokes and MS). Downbeat nystagmus is a central nystagmus present in the primary position, accentuated by downward gaze and horizontal gaze, and exacerbated by head down position. Acquired downbeat nystagmus leads to oscillopsia, often interfering with reading, playing golf, and walking down stairs. The mechanism is unclear but is thought to be due to asymmetry of the smooth pursuit pathways.

Diagnosis

A careful history (including family history) and physical examination (with particular attention to eye movement abnormalities) may facilitate the recognition and diagnosis of vestibulocerebellar syndromes. Once the symptoms are localized to the cerebellum, MRI of the brain should be obtained to identify structural abnormalities in the posterior fossa. The main purpose of performing neuroimaging in patients with progressive ataxia is to exclude a space occupying lesion, cerebellar/brainstem infarct or haemorrhage, multiple sclerosis or superficial siderosis of the nervous system. This may also show cerebellar atophy in hereditary or longstanding acquired cases. There are specific changes related to different conditions which may be seen, i.e. multiple system atrophy (hot cross bun sign) or Creutzfeldt–Jakob disease (cortical ribboning on diffusion-weighted imaging and fluid-attenuated inversion recovery (FLAIR)). Basic laboratory tests for treatable causes, including hepatic/metabolic abnormalities and nutritional deficiencies, should be performed. First-round screening blood tests are aimed at confirming or excluding common and reversible causes of ataxia. These should include a full blood count, urea and electrolytes, thyroid function, vitamin B12, and vitamin E. The presentation of acute ataxia without obvious neuroimaging findings may be consistent with infection or an immune-mediated process, which dictates a thorough evaluation of cerebrospinal fluid and peripheral blood to identify pathogens and immunological biomarkers. Profound ataxia suspicious for a paraneoplastic syndrome should be further investigated to identify autoantibodies and to search for occult malignancy by positron emission tomography/computed tomography of the chest, abdomen, and pelvis. Quantitative eye movement testing can help clarify subtle bedside physical findings to examine the cerebellar, brainstem, and cortical control of eye movement.

The hereditary vestibulocerebellar syndromes can present early in life and the progression is usually gradual. Differential diagnosis of hereditary vestibulocerebellar syndromes includes a consideration of acquired and non-hereditary degenerative disorders. An acute or subacute onset of symptoms and rapid decline may suggest toxic/metabolic (alcohol, drugs, etc.) causes, vitamin deficiencies, infections, or immune-mediated (e.g. paraneoplastic, gluten allergy)

processes, or superficial siderosis. Although early on multiple system atrophy may mimic cerebellar ataxia, relatively rapid clinical deterioration and dysautonomia are clinically distinctive features. It is not unusual for patients to present with isolated downbeat nystagmus and a vague sense of imbalance with normal structures in the posterior fossa on neuroimaging studies.

At present, exhaustive genetic testing for all the known hereditary vestibulocerebellar syndromes can be prohibitively costly, and the yield can be low depending on the presentation and the clinical course. We are hopeful that with rapid advances in molecular genetic techniques we may soon be able to broadly survey the exome or genome efficiently and economically.

Treatment

Principles of therapy are similar whether the condition is acquired or inherited. Specific conditions will have specific treatments, which ideally should either be curative or may slow the disease process. Immune-mediated diseases can be treated with immunomodulation, such as intravenous (IV) corticosteroids, IV immunoglobulin, and plasmapheresis. In paraneoplastic cases, treatment of the underlying malignancy can halt neurological decline but rarely results in symptomatic benefit. Avoiding alcohol can prevent further decline, but this can be difficult to achieve in those who are dependent upon it. Withdrawal of drugs leading to vestibulocerebellar toxicity may reverse symptoms but not in all cases. There may be no alternative medications for some patients, leading to a delicate balance between the wanted and unwanted effects of the drug. Correction of endocrinopathy can reverse symptoms and signs. The link between celiac disease and neurological symptoms is controversial; however, adherence to a strict gluten-free diet has shown symptomatic benefit in individual cases. Whipple's disease is a rare but treatable condition, which requires prolonged courses of IV antibiotics. Patients with stroke may have very variable outcomes and should undergo investigations into the underlying cause, and start secondary prevention and rehabilitation as any stroke patient would do. Identifying the source of bleeding and treating this can prevent progression in superficial siderosis of the nervous system, but this does not address the damage caused by previous haemorrhage. Trials of chelating agents have been disappointing. There are no available treatments for the degenerative causes of vestibulocerebellar disease, but this is an active field of research and clinical trials are underway.

There is intense effort to identify effective drugs that may lessen the symptoms and halt the progression of Friedreich's ataxia and other hereditary ataxia syndromes. For those with a constant sense of disequilibrium, it is best to avoid meclizine and benzodiazepines that are sedating and can further impair patient gait stability and coordination. Some patients with vertical nystagmus have responded to 3,4-diaminopyridine (78) and 4-aminopyridine (79).

Patients are strongly encouraged to stay active physically and mentally to prevent deconditioning and to improve function. Patients will benefit from physical therapy with gait training and general strengthening exercises. Occupational therapy should be arranged to assist patients with activities of daily living as well as home safety inspections to prevent falls. A speech therapist can assist patients with exercises to improve clarity in enunciation and help assess swallowing if indicated. Patient support groups such as the National Ataxia Foundation and Ataxia UK can provide valuable information and support for patients.

Future directions

There is ongoing effort to improve the diagnosis, unravel the pathomechanisms, and develop treatment for vestibulocerebellar disorders. Patients may consider participating in research to characterize the natural history and genetic correlation of hereditary vestibulocerebellar syndromes. A concerted effort between patients and researchers will likely facilitate new gene discovery to improve the diagnosis and understanding of idiopathic disorders. Those with a firm genetic diagnosis may take part in clinical trials (http://clinicaltrials.gov), as researchers continue to develop new tools and approaches to measure treatment outcome and patient satisfaction.

References

1. Harding AE (1982). The clinical features and classification of the late onset autosomal dominant cerebellar ataxias. A study of 11 families, including descendants of the 'the Drew family of Walworth'. *Brain*, 105(Pt 1), 1–28.

2. Banfi S, Servadio A, Chung MY, et al. (1994). Identification and characterization of the gene causing type 1 spinocerebellar ataxia. *Nat Genet*, 7(4), 513–20.

3. Pulst SM, Nechiporuk A, Nechiporuk T, et al. (1996). Moderate expansion of a normally biallelic trinucleotide repeat in spinocerebellar ataxia type 2. *Nat Genet*, 14(3), 269–76.

4. Kawaguchi Y, Okamoto T, Taniwaki M, et al. (1994). CAG expansions in a novel gene for Machado–Joseph disease at chromosome 14q32.1. *Nat Genet*, 8(3), 221–8.

5. Ikeda Y, Dick KA, Weatherspoon MR, et al. (2006). Spectrin mutations cause spinocerebellar ataxia type 5. *Nat Genet*, 38(2), 184–90.

6. Zhuchenko O, Bailey J, Bonnen P, et al. (1997). Autosomal dominant cerebellar ataxia (SCA6) associated with small polyglutamine expansions in the alpha 1A–voltage-dependent calcium channel. *Nat Genet*, 15(1), 62–9.

7. Koob MD, Moseley ML, Schut LJ, et al. (1999). An untranslated CTG expansion causes a novel form of spinocerebellar ataxia (SCA8). *Nat Genet*, 21(4), 379–84.

8. Matsuura T, Yamagata T, Burgess DL, et al. (2000). Large expansion of the ATTCT pentanucleotide repeat in spinocerebellar ataxia type 10. *Nat Genet*, 26(2), 191–4.

9. Houlden H, Johnson J, Gardner-Thorpe C, et al. (2007). Mutations in TTBK2, encoding a kinase implicated in tau phosphorylation, segregate with spinocerebellar ataxia type 11. *Nat Genet*, 39(12), 1434–6.

10. Holmes SE, O'Hearn EE, McInnis MG, et al. (1999). Expansion of a novel CAG trinucleotide repeat in the 5' region of PPP2R2B is associated with SCA12. *Nat Genet*, 23(4), 391–2.

11. Waters MF, Minassian NA, Stevanin G, et al. (2006). Mutations in voltage-gated potassium channel KCNC3 cause degenerative and developmental central nervous system phenotypes. *Nat Genet*, 38(4), 447–51.

12. van de Leemput J, Chandran J, Knight MA, et al. (2007). Deletion at ITPR1 underlies ataxia in mice and spinocerebellar ataxia 15 in humans. *PLoS Genet*, 3(6), e108.

13. Miyoshi Y, Yamada T, Tanimura M, et al. (2001). A novel autosomal dominant spinocerebellar ataxia (SCA16) linked to chromosome 8q22.1–24.1. *Neurology*, 57(1), 96–100.

14. Koide R, Kobayashi S, Shimohata T, et al. (1999). A neurological disease caused by an expanded CAG trinucleotide repeat in the TATA-binding protein gene: a new polyglutamine disease? *Hum Mol Genet*, 8(11), 2047–53.

15. Anna Duarri, Justyna Jezierska, Michiel Fokkens, Michel Meijer, Helenius J Schelhaas, Wilfred F A den Dunnen, Freerk van Dijk, Corien Verschuuren-Bemelmans, Gerard Hageman, Pieter van de Vlies, Benno Küsters, Bart P van de Warrenburg, Berry Kremer, Cisca Wijmenga, Richard J Sinke, Morris A Swertz, Harm H Kampinga, Erik Boddeke and Dineke S Verbeek Mutations in potassium channel KCND3 cause spinocerebellar ataxia type 19 Accepted manuscript online: Annals of Neurology 23 JUL 2012 06:29AM EST | DOI: 10.1002/ana.23700.

16. Yi-chung Lee, Alexandra Durr, Karen Majczenko, Yen-hua Huang, Yu-chao Liu BS, Cheng-chang Lien, Pei-chien Tsai PhD, Yaeko Ichikawa, Jun Goto, Marie-Lorraine Monin, Jun Z Li, Ming-yi Chung, Emeline Mundwiller, Vikram Shakkottai, Tze-tze Liu, Christelle Tesson, Yi-chun Lu, Alexis Brice, Shoji Tsuji, Margit Burmeister, Giovanni Stevanin and Bing-wen Soong Mutations in KCND3 cause spinocerebellar ataxia type 22. Accepted manuscript online: 23 JUL 2012 06:29AM EST | DOI: 10.1002/ana.23701.

17. Bakalkin G, Watanabe H, Jezierska J, et al. (2010). Prodynorphin mutations cause the neurodegenerative disorder spinocerebellar ataxia type 23. *Am J Hum Genet*, 87(5), 593–603.

18. Stevanin G, Bouslam N, Thobois S, et al. (2004). Spinocerebellar ataxia with sensory neuropathy (SCA25) maps to chromosome 2p. *Ann Neurol*, 55(1), 97–104.

19. Yu GY, Howell MJ, Roller MJ, Xie TD, Gomez CM (2005). Spinocerebellar ataxia type 26 maps to chromosome 19p13.3 adjacent to SCA6. *Ann Neurol*, 57(3), 349–54.

20. Di Bella D, Lazzaro F, Brusco A, et al. (2010). Mutations in the mitochondrial protease gene AFG3L2 cause dominant hereditary ataxia SCA28. *Nat Genet*, 42(4), 313–21.

21. Coutinho P, Cruz VT, Tuna A, Silva SE, Guimarães J (2006). Cerebellar ataxia with spasmodic cough: a new form of dominant ataxia. *Arch Neurol*, 63(4), 553–5.

22. Storey E, Bahlo M, Fahey M, Sisson O, Lueck CJ, Gardner RJ (2009). A new dominantly inherited pure cerebellar ataxia, SCA 30. *J Neurol Neurosurg Psychiatry*, 80(4), 408–11.

23. Sato N, Amino T, Kobayashi K, et al. (2009). Spinocerebellar ataxia type 31 is associated with 'inserted' penta-nucleotide repeats containing (TGGAA)n. *Am J Hum Genet*, 85(5), 544–57.

24. Jiang H, Zhu, H-P, Gomez, CM (2010). SCA32: an autosomal dominant cerebellar ataxia with azoospermia maps to chromosome 7q32-q33. *Mov Disord*, 25(S2), S192.

25. Wang JL, Yang X, Xia K, et al. (2010). TGM6 identified as a novel causative gene of spinocerebellar ataxias using exome sequencing. *Brain*, 133(Pt 12), 3510–8.

26. Kobayashi H, Abe K, Matsuura T, et al. (2011). Expansion of intronic GGCCTG hexanucleotide repeat in NOP56 causes SCA36, a type of spinocerebellar ataxia accompanied by motor neuron involvement. *Am J Hum Genet*, 89(1), 121–30.

27. VanDyke DH, Griggs RC, Murphy MJ, Goldstein MN (1975). Hereditary myokymia and periodic ataxia. *J Neurol Sci*, 25(1), 109–18.

28. Brunt ER, van Weerden TW (1990). Familial paroxysmal kinesigenic ataxia and continuous myokymia. *Brain*, 113(Pt 5) 1361–82.

29. Hanson PA, Martinez LB, Cassidy R (1977). Contractures, continuous muscle discharges, and titubation. *Ann Neurol*, 1(2), 120–4.

30. Gancher ST, Nutt JG (1986). Autosomal dominant episodic ataxia: a heterogeneous syndrome. *Mov Disord*, 1(4), 239–53.

31. Kramer PL, Yue Q, Gancher ST, et al. (1995). A locus for the nystagmus-associated form of episodic ataxia maps to an 11-cM region on chromosome 19p. *Am J Hum Genet*, 57(1), 182–5.

32. Jen JC, Graves TD, Hess EJ, et al. (2007). Primary episodic ataxias: diagnosis, pathogenesis and treatment. *Brain*, 130(Pt 10), 2484–93.

33. Browne DL, Gancher ST, Nutt JG, et al. (1994). Episodic ataxia/myokymia syndrome is associated with point mutations in the human potassium channel gene, KCNA1. *Nat Genet*, 8(2), 136–40.

34. Zuberi SM, Eunson LH, Spauschus A, et al. (1999). A novel mutation in the human voltage-gated potassium channel gene (Kv1.1) associates with episodic ataxia type 1 and sometimes with partial epilepsy. *Brain*, 122(Pt 5) 817–25.

35. Lubbers WJ, Brunt ER, Scheffer H, et al. (1995). Hereditary myokymia and paroxysmal ataxia linked to chromosome 12 is responsive to acetazolamide. J Neurol Neurosurg Psychiatry, 59(4), 400–5.

36. Eunson LH, Rea R, Zuberi SM, et al. (2000). Clinical, genetic, and expression studies of mutations in the potassium channel gene KCNA1 reveal new phenotypic variability. Ann Neurol, 48(4), 647–56.

37. Ophoff RA, Terwindt GM, Vergouwe MN, et al. (1996). Familial hemiplegic migraine and episodic ataxia type-2 are caused by mutations in the Ca2+ channel gene CACNL1A4. Cell, 87(3), 543–52.

38. Engel KC, Anderson JH, Gomez CM, Soechting JF (2004). Deficits in ocular and manual tracking due to episodic ataxia type 2. Mov Disord, 19(7), 778–87.

39. Wiest G, Tian JR, Baloh RW, Crane BT, Demer JL (2001). Otolith function in cerebellar ataxia due to mutations in the calcium channel gene CACNA1A. Brain, 124(Pt 12), 2407–16.

40. Baloh RW, Yue Q, Furman JM, Nelson SF (1997). Familial episodic ataxia: clinical heterogeneity in four families linked to chromosome 19p. Ann Neurol, 41(1), 8–16.

41. Denier C, Ducros A, Vahedi K, et al. (1999). High prevalence of CACNA1A truncations and broader clinical spectrum in episodic ataxia type 2. Neurology, 52(9), 1816–21.

42. Griggs RC, Moxley RT, Lafrance RA, McQuillen J (1978). Hereditary paroxysmal ataxia: response to acetazolamide. Neurology, 28(12), 1259–64.

43. Strupp M, Kalla R, Dichgans M, Freilinger T, Glasauer S, Brandt T (2004). Treatment of episodic ataxia type 2 with the potassium channel blocker 4-aminopyridine. Neurology, 62(9), 1623–5.

44. Steckley JL, Ebers GC, Cader MZ, McLachlan RS (2001). An autosomal dominant disorder with episodic ataxia, vertigo, and tinnitus. Neurology, 57(8), 1499–502.

45. Cader MZ, Steckley JL, Dyment DA, McLachlan RS, Ebers GC (2005). A genome–wide screen and linkage mapping for a large pedigree with episodic ataxia. Neurology, 65(1), 156–8.

46. Farmer TW, Mustian VM (1963). Vestibulocerebellar ataxia. A newly defined hereditary syndrome with periodic manifestations. Arch Neurol, 8, 471–80.

47. Damji KF, Allingham RR, Pollock SC, et al. (1996). Periodic vestibulocerebellar ataxia, an autosomal dominant ataxia with defective smooth pursuit, is genetically distinct from other autosomal dominant ataxias. Arch Neurol, 53(4), 338–44.

48. Burgess DL, Jones JM, Meisler MH, Noebels JL (1997). Mutation of the Ca2+ channel beta subunit gene Cchb4 is associated with ataxia and seizures in the lethargic (lh) mouse. Cell, 88(3), 385–92.

49. Escayg A, De Waard M, Lee DD, et al. (2000). Coding and noncoding variation of the human calcium-channel beta4-subunit gene CACNB4 in patients with idiopathic generalized epilepsy and episodic ataxia. Am J Hum Genet, 66(5), 1531–9.

50. Jen JC, Wan J, Palos TP, Howard BD, Baloh RW (2005). Mutation in the glutamate transporter EAAT1 causes episodic ataxia, hemiplegia, and seizures. Neurology, 65(4), 529–34.

51. De Fusco M, Marconi R, Silvestri L, et al. (2003). Haploinsufficiency of ATP1A2 encoding the Na+/K+ pump alpha2 subunit associated with familial hemiplegic migraine type 2. Nat Genet, 33(2), 192–6.

52. Kerber KA, Jen JC, Lee H, Nelson SF, Baloh RW (2007). A new episodic ataxia syndrome with linkage to chromosome 19q13. Arch Neurol, 64(5), 749–52.

53. Cha YH, Lee H, Jen JC, Kattah JC, Nelson SF, Baloh RW (2007). Episodic vertical oscillopsia with progressive gait ataxia: clinical description of a new episodic syndrome and evidence of linkage to chromosome 13q. J Neurol Neurosurg Psychiatry, 78(11), 1273–5.

54. Campuzano V, Montermini L, Molto MD, et al. (1996). Friedreich's ataxia: autosomal recessive disease caused by an intronic GAA triplet repeat expansion. Science, 271(5254), 1423–7.

55. Savitsky K, Bar-Shira A, Gilad S, et al. (1995). A single ataxia telangiectasia gene with a product similar to PI-3 kinase. Science, 268(5218), 1749–53.

56. Engert JC, Bérubé P, Mercier J, et al. (2000). ARSACS, a spastic ataxia common in northeastern Québec, is caused by mutations in a new gene encoding an 11.5-kb ORF. Nat Genet, 24(2), 120–5.

57. Bomar JM, Benke PJ, Slattery EL, et al. (2003). Mutations in a novel gene encoding a CRAL-TRIO domain cause human Cayman ataxia and ataxia/dystonia in the jittery mouse. Nat Genet, 35(3), 264–9.

58. Moreira MC, Barbot C, Tachi N, et al. (2001). The gene mutated in ataxia-ocular apraxia 1 encodes the new HIT/Zn-finger protein aprataxin. Nature genetics, 29(2), 189–93.

59. Duquette A, Roddier K, McNabb-Baltar J, et al. (2005). Mutations in senataxin responsible for Quebec cluster of ataxia with neuropathy. Ann Neurol, 57(3), 408–14.

60. Swartz BE, Burmeister M, Somers JT, Rottach KG, Bespalova IN, Leigh RJ (2002). A form of inherited cerebellar ataxia with saccadic intrusions, increased saccadic speed, sensory neuropathy, and myoclonus. Ann N Y Acad Sci, 956, 441–4.

61. Gros-Louis F, Dupré N, Dion P, et al. (2007). Mutations in SYNE1 lead to a newly discovered form of autosomal recessive cerebellar ataxia. Nat Genet, 39(1), 80–5.

62. Régal L, Ebberink MS, Goemans N, et al. (2010). Mutations in PEX10 are a cause of autosomal recessive ataxia. Ann Neurol, 68(2), 259–63.

63. Vermeer S, Hoischen A, Meijer RP, et al. (2010). Targeted next-generation sequencing of a 12.5 Mb homozygous region reveals ANO10 mutations in patients with autosomal-recessive cerebellar ataxia. Am J Hum Genet, 87(6), 813–9.

64. Amor DJ, Delatycki MB, Gardner RJ, Storey E (2001). New variant of familial cerebellar ataxia with hypergonadotropic hypogonadism and sensorineural deafness. Am J Med Genet, 99(1), 29–33.

65. Myerowitz R, Costigan FC (1988). The major defect in Ashkenazi Jews with Tay-Sachs disease is an insertion in the gene for the alpha-chain of beta-hexosaminidase. J Biol Chem, 263(35), 18587–9.

66. Barnes D, Misra VP, Young EP, Thomas PK, Harding AE (1991). An adult onset hexosaminidase A deficiency syndrome with sensory neuropathy and internuclear ophthalmoplegia. J Neurol Neurosurg Psychiatry, 54(12), 1112–3.

67. Jacquemont S, Hagerman RJ, Leehey M, et al. (2003). Fragile X premutation tremor/ataxia syndrome: molecular, clinical, and neuroimaging correlates. Am J Hum Genet, 72(4), 869–78.

68. Bronstein AM, Mossman S, Luxon LM (1991). The neck-eye reflex in patients with reduced vestibular and optokinetic function. Brain, 114(Pt 1A), 1–11.

69. Wagner JN, Glaser M, Brandt T, Strupp M (2008). Downbeat nystagmus: aetiology and comorbidity in 117 patients. Journal Neuro Neurosurg Psychiatry, 79(6), 672–7.

70. Migliaccio AA, Halmagyi GM, McGarvie LA, Cremer PD (2004). Cerebellar ataxia with bilateral vestibulopathy: description of a syndrome and its characteristic clinical sign. Brain, 127(Pt 2), 280–93.

71. Szmulewicz DJ, Waterston JA, MacDougall HG, et al. (2011). Cerebellar ataxia, neuropathy, vestibular areflexia syndrome (CANVAS): a review of the clinical features and video-oculographic diagnosis. Ann N Y Acad Sci, 1233(1), 139–47.

72. Steinlin M (1998). Non-progressive congenital ataxias. Brain Dev, 20 (4), 199–208.

73. Nicolas E, Poitelon Y, Chouery E, et al. (2010). CAMOS, a nonprogressive, autosomal recessive, congenital cerebellar ataxia, is caused by a mutant zinc-finger protein, ZNF592. Eur J Hum Genet, 18(10), 1107–13.

74. Illarioshkin SN, Tanaka H, Markova ED, Nikolskaya NN, Ivanova-Smolenskaya IA, Tsuji S (1996). X-linked nonprogressive congenital cerebellar hypoplasia: clinical description and mapping to chromosome Xq. Ann Neurol, 40(1), 75–83.

75. Zanni G, Bertini E, Bellcross C, et al. (2008). X-linked congenital ataxia: a new locus maps to Xq25–q27.1. Am J Med Genet A, 146A(5), 593–600.

76. Dudding TE, Friend K, Schofield PW, Lee S, Wilkinson IA, Richards RI (2004). Autosomal dominant congenital non–progressive ataxia overlaps with the SCA15 locus. *Neurology*, 63(12), 2288–92.

77. Jen JC, Lee H, Cha YH, Nelson SF, Baloh RW (2006). Genetic heterogeneity of autosomal dominant nonprogressive congenital ataxia. *Neurology*, 67(9), 1704–6.

78. Strupp M, Schuler O, Krafczyk S, *et al.* (2003). Treatment of downbeat nystagmus with 3,4-diaminopyridine: a placebo-controlled study. *Neurology*, 61(2), 165–70.

79. Kalla R, Glasauer S, Schautzer F, *et al.* (2004). 4-aminopyridine improves downbeat nystagmus, smooth pursuit, and VOR gain. *Neurology*, 62(7), 1228–9.

CHAPTER 26

Bilateral Vestibular Failure: Causes and Courses

Thomas Brandt, Marianne Dieterich, and Michael Strupp

Clinical characteristics, pathophysiology, and aetiology

The key symptoms of bilateral vestibulopathy are:

- oscillopsia with blurred vision during head movements or locomotion
- unsteadiness of gait, particularly in the dark and on uneven ground
- impairment of spatial memory and navigation.

Bilateral vestibular failure (BVF) is by no means a rare vestibular disorder, particularly in the elderly. It accounts for more than 7% of 14,589 outpatients in our dizziness unit (1). BVF is characterized by the impaired or lost function of both peripheral vestibular labyrinths or of the VIIIth nerves. The most frequent complaint of patients with BVF is an unsteadiness of gait that worsens in darkness and on uneven ground due to deficient vestibulospinal function. About 40% of the patients complain of oscillopsia (i.e. apparent motion of the visual scene during head movements or when walking) (2). Oscillopsia is caused by involuntary retinal slip as a result of an insufficient vestibulo-ocular reflex (VOR). It has been shown that patients with BVF have impaired visual motion perception (3) and raised motion coherence thresholds across all velocities tested (4). This allows them to partially compensate for the oscillopsia. Patients with BVF show impaired performance in mental transformation tasks involving bodies or body parts in space (5).

BVF can also lead to impaired spatial memory and navigation associated with hippocampal atrophy (6; Figure 26.1). When tested with a virtual variant of the Morris water task these patients exhibit significant spatial memory and navigation deficits that closely match the pattern of hippocampal atrophy but are not associated with general memory deficits. This revives the idea that a major—and probably phylogenetically ancient—function of the archicortical hippocampal tissue is still evident in spatial aspects of memory processing for navigation, which critically depends on preserved vestibular function (6). The findings in humans were confirmed in a rat model of bilateral labyrinthectomy (7). No significant deficits

of spatial memory were found in patients with chronic unilateral vestibular deafferentation (8).

The diagnosis of BVF is based on the head impulse test (9–12) (Chapter 12), a simple bedside test for high-frequency VOR function, and bithermal caloric testing with oculographic recordings to detect a low-frequency VOR deficit. Saccular function, which is tested by vestibular-evoked myogenic potentials, is less affected than canal function in BVF (13).

The pathophysiology of BVF depends on various aetiologies (e.g. ototoxic drugs, in particular aminoglycosides (14), meningitis, Ménière's disease, neurofibromatosis type II, Cogan's syndrome, or rarely superficial cerebral haemosiderosis; Figures 26.2–26.4). The aetiology remains unclear in approximately half of the patients. To determine the causative factors and epidemiology of BV, the cases of 255 patients (mean age, 62 ± 16 years) diagnosed to have BVF in our dizziness unit between 1988 and 2005 were retrospectively reviewed (2) (Table 26.1). All patients had undergone a standardized neuro-ophthalmological and neuro-otological examination, electronystagmography with caloric irrigation, cranial magnetic resonance imaging, or computed tomography (n = 214), and laboratory tests. Sixty-two per cent of the study population was male. Previous vertigo attacks had occurred in 36%, indicating a sequential manifestation. The definite cause of BVF was determined in 24% and the probable cause in 25%. The most common causes were ototoxic aminoglycosides (13%), Ménière's disease (7%), and meningitis (5%). Strikingly, 25% exhibited cerebellar signs. Cerebellar dysfunction was associated with peripheral polyneuropathy in 32%, compared with 18% in BVF patients without cerebellar signs. Hypoacusis occurred bilaterally in 25% and unilaterally in 6% of all patients. It appeared most often in patients with BVF caused by Cogan's syndrome, meningitis, or Ménière's disease. Thus, the cause of BVF remains unclear in about half of all patients despite extensive examinations. A large subgroup of these patients have associated cerebellar dysfunction, downbeat nystagmus (15), and peripheral polyneuropathy. This suggests a new syndrome that may be caused by neurodegenerative or less likely autoimmune processes (2, 15). An association between bilateral vestibulopathy, cerebellar ataxia, and polyneuropathy has been described in several studies (16, 17), and evidence has been reported for a neurodegenerative disorder affecting multiple systems (18).

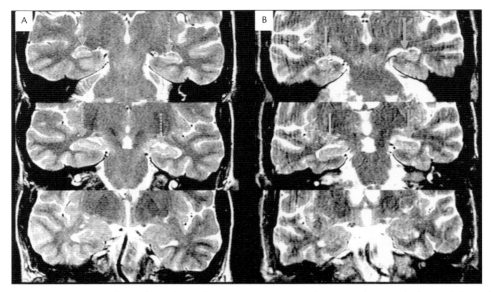

Fig. 26.1 A 16.9% volume loss in the hippocampus (arrows) was observed in BVF patients, compared to age- and sex-matched controls (normal hippocampus: dotted arrows).Volume loss was similar for the left and right hippocampus. Analysis of variance (ANOVA) with BVF status and sex confirmed a significant difference in hippocampal volume between BVF patients and controls. Examples of coronal 3-mm MRI T2-weighted images with a distance of 6 mm are shown. (A) A 39-year-old female volunteer. (B) A 40-year-old female BVF patient (6).

Other rare aetiologies for BVF are anticancer chemotherapy, loop diuretics, aspirin (19), non-Hodgkin's lymphoma, meningitis carcinomatosa, neurosarcoidosis, Behçet's disease, cerebral vasculitis, systemic lupus erythematosus, polychondritis, rheumatoid arthritis, polyarteritis nodosa, Wegener's granulomatosis, giant cell arteritis, primary antiphospholipid syndrome, B6 deficiency, hereditary sensory and autonomic neuropathy (HSAN IV), herpes simplex virus type I, congenital malformations, vertebrobasilar dolichoectasia, bilateral temporal bone fractures, or Paget's disease (11, 12, 20).

Differential diagnosis and clinical problems

Considerations for the differential diagnosis proceed along two lines (11, 12, 20). On the one hand, it is important to look for the causes (listed in Table 26.1) if clinical signs of a bilateral vestibulopathy are present. On the other, it is necessary to differentiate the illness from other vestibular and non-vestibular diseases, which are also characterized by oscillopsia and/or instability of posture and gait.

The following steps are important for the differential diagnosis:

- Differentiate the various causes and mechanisms of BVF.

- Differentiate from illnesses with similar key symptoms:
  - cerebellar or eye movement disorders without bilateral vestibulopathy (16–18)
  - phobic postural vertigo
  - intoxications

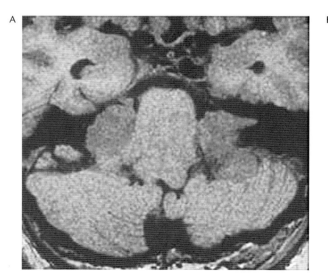
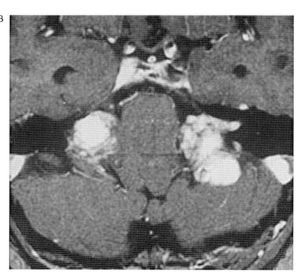

Fig. 26.2 Patient with neurofibromatosis type II and bilateral vestibular schwannomas. MRI axial projection before (A) and after (B) application of intravenous Gd-DTPA.

Table 26.1 Aetiology of bilateral vestibulopathy (n = 255): definite cause in 24%, probable cause in 25% (2)

Cause of Bilateral Vestibulopathy	Definite Cause		Probable Cause		Σ	
	n	%[a]	n	%[a]	n	%[a]
Antibiotics	27	11	5	2	32	13
Meniére's disease	4	2	13	5	17	7
Meningitis/encephalitis/cerebellitis	12	5	1	0	13	5
Two different causes	1	0	11	4	12	5
Spinocerebellar ataxia type 3 and 6/episodic ataxia type II/multiple system atrophy	0	0	9	4	9	4
Systemic autoimmune disease	2	1	6	3	8	3
Deficit of vitamin B12/folic acid	3	1	1	0	4	2
Creutzfeldt-Jakob disease	3	1	0	0	3	1
Cogan's syndrome	3	1	0	0	3	1
Positive family history for inner ear diseases	0	0	3	1	3	1
Miscellaneous	7	3	14	5	21	8

[a] Frequency of each cause is given as percentage of all included patients (N= 255); some of the percentages have been rounded up, others rounded down.

- vestibular paroxysmia
- perilymph fistulas
- orthostatic hypotension
- hyperventilation syndrome
- visual disorders
- unilateral vestibular deficit.

Prevention and treatment

Prevention is most important for the group of patients with ototoxic labyrinthine damage, above all damage due to aminoglycosides. Patients with renal insufficiency, advanced age, or familial susceptibility to aminoglycoside ototoxicity are at particular risk. The mitochondrial 12S rRNA is considered a hotspot for mutations associated with aminoglycoside-induced hearing loss; however, no mutations with a confirmed pathogenicity were found in patients with BVF and prior exposure to aminoglycosides (21). Careful monitoring of the hearing and vestibular function is necessary during treatment, as the ototoxic effects of gentamycin have a delayed onset, often appearing only after days or weeks. High doses of steroids are recommended for patients with Cogan's syndrome. If the response is inadequate or relapses occur, treatment with azathioprine or cyclophosphamide is recommended. The effectiveness of immunosuppressive treatment of patients with BVF and inner ear antibodies was moderate in four of 12 patients and proved only transient in two (22).

In addition, it is important to treat the causative underlying disease, for in individual cases this is also successful. Patients respond quite positively to physical therapy with gait and balance training.

This therapy accelerates adaptation to loss of function by promoting visual and somatosensory substitution (Chapter 17). The efficacy of vestibular exercises for peripheral vestibular disorders has been confirmed in a Cochrane analysis (23). It is important to inform the patients carefully about the type, mechanism, and course of their illness. It is our experience that the diagnosis of a bilateral vestibulopathy is still established much too late, despite many visits to the physician, a fact that only exacerbates the patients' complaints. Frequently, these subjective complaints are reduced by simply informing the patient about their illness.

Treatment of the various forms of BVF follows three lines of action (24):

- Prophylaxis of progressive vestibular loss,
- Recovery of vestibular function,
- Promotion of the compensation and substitution of missing vestibular input by physical therapy.

The development and clinical application of vestibular prostheses are promising and exciting, but currently still in their infancy (25–29).

Long-term course

The following is the most relevant question for these afflicted patients: does the long-term progression or recovery of vestibular function depend on the aetiology?

Little is known about the course of the disease, especially recovery (1). A few small case series have reported contradictory recovery rates (22, 30–32). In a report on 11 patients with idiopathic BVF (eight patients with simultaneous and three patients with sequential

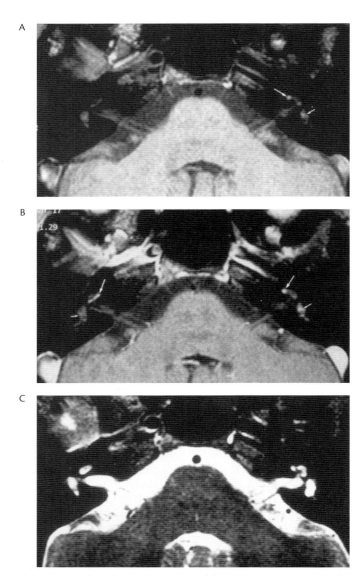

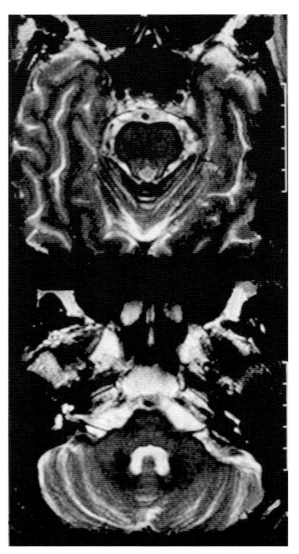

Fig. 26.3 Cogan's syndrome, subacute stage. (A) Axial projection, T1-weighted, two-dimensional fast low angle shot (2D-FLASH), no contrast medium. Signs of subacute haemorrhages are the signal increases in the vestibule (short arrow) and in the cochlea (long arrow); (B) axial projection, T1-weighted 2D-FLASH after administration of Gd-DTPA in the same patient. Clear enhancement by contrast medium in the area of the haemorrhage, namely in the cochlea (long arrow) and in the vestibule (short arrow); (C) axial projection, T2-weighted turbo-spin-echo imaging, no contrast medium, in a patient with Cogan's syndrome. The canals cannot be delimited; this is a sign of obliteration from scarring. (20)

Fig. 26.4 MRI of a patient with BVF due to cerebral haemosiderosis exhibiting the superficial siderosis as a hypointense rim of haemosiderin deposits around the brainstem and the VIIIth nerves.

onset of BVF), partial recovery was detected in four patients with simultaneous onset and in all three patients with sequential BVF after a follow-up of 1–7 years. Complete recovery did not occur in any of the patients (30). Improvement of vestibular function has also been described in single cases of different aetiologies, in particular when the cause of BVF was serous rather than suppurative destructive labyrinthitis (33–35). In contrast, a 5-year follow-up study (31) reported that seven patients with BVF did not show significant improvement in vestibular excitability. Also in our clinical experience, the prognosis of BVF is less favourable than hitherto reported. We examined 82 patients with BVF of various aetiologies and clinically re-evaluated them after a mean follow-up time

of 51 months (range 3 months to 13 years) (36). The initial diagnosis of BVF and clinical re-evaluation were made according to a standardized protocol, including a neuro-ophthalmological and neuro-otological workup. We not only determined the frequency and extent of recovery or worsening of vestibular function and their dependence on the aetiology of BVF, but also the impairment of the quality of life.

Statistical analysis of the mean peak slow-phase velocity (SPV) of caloric-induced nystagmus revealed a non-significant worsening over time (initial mean peak SPV $3.0 \pm 3.5°/s$ vs. $2.1 \pm 2.8°/s$). As regards the aetiological subgroups, only those patients with BVF due to meningitis exhibited an increasing, but non-significant SPV ($1.0 \pm 1.4°/s$ vs. $1.9 \pm 1.6°/s$). Vestibular outcome was independent of age, gender, time course of manifestation, and severity of BVF. Single analysis of all patients showed that a substantial improvement $\geq 5°/s$ occurred in two patients on both sides (idiopathic n = 1, Sjögren's syndrome n = 1) and in eight patients on one side (idiopathic n = 6, meningitis n = 1, Ménière's disease n = 1). In 84% of patients there was impairment of their health-related quality of life (42% slight, 24% moderate, 18% severe). Forty-three per cent of the patients rated the course of their disease as stable, 28% as worsened, and 29% as improved.

Conclusions

Bilateral vestibulopathy not only causes oscillopsia and unsteadiness of gait, but it also impairs spatial memory and navigation, the ability to perform mental transformation tasks of body position in space, as well as visual motion perception. The defects of spatial memory involve vestibulo-hippocampal connections, and the raised thresholds for motion detection involve vestibulo-visual connections. The latter connections are beneficial to the extent that they alleviate the distressing oscillopsia due to involuntary retinal slip during head movements. The challenge of treating BVF has led to the promising development of vestibular prostheses, prototypes of which are already available for first clinical studies.

References

1. Brandt T, Huppert D, Hüfner K, Zingler VC, Strupp M (2010). Long-term course and relapses of vestibular and balance disorders. *Restor Neurol Neurosci*, 28, 65–78.

2. Zingler VC, Cnyrim C, Jahn K, *et al.* (2007). Causative factors and epidemiology of bilateral vestibulopathy in 255 patients. *Ann Neurol*, 61, 524–32.

3. Grünbauer WM, Dieterich M, Brandt T (1998). Bilateral vestibular failure impairs visual motion perception even with the head still. *Neuroreport*, 9, 1807–10.

4. Kalla R, Muggleton N, Spiegel R, *et al.* (2011). Adaptive motion processing in bilateral vestibular failure. *J Neurol Neurosurg Psychiatry*, 82, 1212–16.

5. Grabherr L, Cuffel C, Guyot JP, Mast FW (2011). Mental transformation abilities in patients with unilateral and bilateral vestibular loss. *Exp Brain Res*, 209, 205–14.

6. Brandt T, Schautzer F, Hamilton DA, *et al.* (2005). Vestibular loss causes hippocampal atrophy and impaired spatial memory in humans. *Brain*, 128, 2732–41.

7. Besnard S, Machado ML, Vignaux G, *et al.* (2012). Influence of vestibular input on spatial and nonspatial memory and on hippocampal NMDA receptors. *Hippocampus*, 22, 814–26.

8. Hüfner K, Hamilton DA, Kalla R, *et al.* (2007). Spatial memory and hippocampal volume in humans with unilateral vestibular deafferentation. *Hippocampus*, 17, 471–85.

9. Halmagyi GM, Curthoys IS (1988). A clinical sign of canal paresis. *Arch Neurol*, 45, 737–9.

10. Jorns-Häderli M, Straumann D, Palla A (2007). Accuracy of the bedside head impulse test in detecting vestibular hypofunction. *J Neurol Neurosurg Psychiatry*, 78, 1113–18.

11. Jen JC (2009). Bilateral vestibulopathy: clinical, diagnostic, and genetic considerations. *Semin Neurol*, 29, 528–33.

12. Kim S, Oh YM, Koo JW, Kim JS (2011). Bilateral vestibulopathy: clinical characteristics and diagnostic criteria. *Otol Neurotol*, 32, 812–17.

13. Zingler VC, Weintz E, Jahn K, *et al.* (2008). Saccular function less affected than canal function in bilateral vestibulopathy. *J Neurol*, 255, 1332–6.

14. Ishiyama G, Ishiyama A, Kerber K, Baloh RW (2006). Gentamicin ototoxicity: clinical features and the effect on the human vestibulo-ocular reflex. *Acta Otolaryngol*, 126, 1057–61.

15. Wagner JN, Glaser M, Brandt T, Strupp M (2008). Downbeat nystagmus: aetiology and comorbidity in 117 patients. *J Neurol Neurosurg Psychiatry*, 79, 672–7.

16. Migliaccio AA, Halmagyi GM, McGarvie LA, Cremer PD (2004). Cerebellar ataxia with bilateral vestibulopathy: description of a syndrome and its characteristic clinical sign. *Brain*, 127, 280–93.

17. Kirchner H, Kremmyda O, Hüfner K, *et al.* (2011). Clinical, electrophysiological and MRI findings in patients with cerebellar ataxia and a bilaterally pathological head-impulse test. *Ann N Y Acad Sci*, 1233, 127–38.

18. Szmulewicz DJ, Waterston JA, Halmagyi GM, *et al.* (2011). Sensory neuropathy as part of the cerebellar ataxia neuropathy vestibular areflexia syndrome. *Neurology*, 76, 1903–10.

19. Strupp M, Jahn K, Brandt T (2003). Another adverse effect of aspirin: bilateral vestibulopathy. *J Neurol Neurosurg Psychiatry*, 74, 691.

20. Brandt T, Dieterich M, Strupp M (2013). *Vertigo and Dizziness—Common Complaints*. 2nd Edn. London: Springer.

21. Elstner M, Schmidt C, Zingler VC, *et al.* (2008). Mitochondrial 125 rRNA susceptibility mutations in aminoglycoside-associated and idiopathic bilateral vestibulopathy. *Biochem Biophys Res Commun*, 377, 379–83.

22. Deutschländer A, Glaser M, Strupp M, Dieterich M, Brandt T (2005). Immunosuppressive treatment in bilateral vestibulopathy with inner ear antibodies. *Acta Otolaryngol*, 125, 848–51.

23. Hillier SL, McDonnell M (2011). Vestibular rehabilitation for unilateral peripheral vestibular dysfunction. *Cochrane Database Syst Rev*, 2, CD005397.

24. Brandt T (1996). Bilateral vestibulopathy revisited. *Eur J Med Res*, 1, 361–8.

25. Della Santina CC, Migliaccio AA, Hayden R, *et al.* (2010). Current and future management of bilateral loss of vestibular sensation—an update on the Johns Hopkins Multichannel Vestibular Prosthesis Project. *Cochlear Implants Int*, 11(Suppl 2), 2–11.

26. Barros CG, Bittar RS, Danilov Y (2010). Effects of electrotactile vestibular substitution on rehabilitation of patients with bilateral vestibular loss. *Neurosci Lett*, 476, 123–6.

27. Dai C, Fridman GY, Chiang B, *et al.* (2011). Cross-axis adaptation improves 3D vestibulo-ocular reflex alignment during stimulation via a head-mounted multichannel vestibular prosthesis. *Exp Brain Res*, 210, 595–606.

28. Hayden R, Sawyer S, Frey E, Mori S, Migliaccio AA, Della Santina CC (2011). Virtual labyrinth model of vestibular afferent excitation via implanted electrodes: validation and application to design of a multichannel vestibular prosthesis. *Exp Brain Res*, 210, 623–40.

29. van de Berg R, Guinand N, Guyot J-P, Stokroos R, Kingma H (2011). The vestibular implant: Quo vadis? *Front Neurol*, 2, 47.

30. Vibert D, Liard P, Häusler R (1995). Bilateral idiopathic loss of peripheral vestibular function with normal hearing. *Acta Otolaryngol*, 115, 611–15.

31. Baloh RW, Enrietto J, Jacobson KM, Lin KM (2001). Age-related changes in vestibular function: a longitudinal study. *Ann N Y Acad Sci*, 942, 210–19.

32. Frese KA, Reker U, Maune S (2003). Der beidseitige Vestibularisausfall. *HNO*, 51, 221–5.

33. Rinne T, Bronstein AM, Rudge P, Gresty MA, Luxon LM (1998). Bilateral loss of vestibular function: clinical findings in 53 patients. *J Neurol*, 245, 314–21.

34. Fortnum HM (1982). Hearing impairment after bacterial meningitis. *Arch Dis Child*, 67, 1128–33.

35. Bronstein AM, Morland AB, Ruddock KH, Gresty MA (1995). Recovery from bilateral vestibular failure: implications for visual and cervico-ocular function. *Acta Otolaryngol Suppl*, 520, 405–7.

36. Zingler VC, Weintz E, Jahn K, *et al.* (2008). Follow-up of vestibular function in bilateral vestibulopathy. *J Neurol Neurosurg Psychiatry*, 79, 284–8.

CHAPTER 27

Vertigo and Dizziness in General Medicine

Kevin Barraclough and Barry Seemungal

Dizziness is a common presenting complaint to the hospital or community-based generalist, e.g. 2% of all primary care consultations relate to dizziness (1). Regarding the dizzy patient, perhaps the biggest frustration for the generalist is the failure to make a confident diagnosis underlying the patient's complaint. As with most other neurological complaints, an accurate history obtained from the dizzy patient can render the rest of the diagnostic process redundant. Unfortunately the ambiguity of language, compounded by the different lexicons of the dizzy patient and doctor, leads to a situation of general confusion (Chapter 16). Indeed such a situation is reflected in the lament of the neurologist, W. B. Matthews (2) that 'few (are the) physicians (who) do not experience a slight decline in spirits when they learn...their patient's complaint is giddiness...(and) frequently...after exhaustive inquiry it (is)...not clear what...the patient feels (or) why he feels it'.

In our search for diagnostic clarity, the first step should be lexical harmonization. Although it is important for doctors to be consistent amongst themselves in their definitions, more important is for the patient in front of the doctor to understand what the doctor means by 'dizzy' or 'vertigo' (see Chapter 11 for approaching a dizzy patient). Given that the word dizzy comes from old English meaning 'stupid' and vertigo derives from 'vertere' meaning 'to turn' in Latin, it can be argued that vertigo is the more precise. We suggest using 'vertigo' to mean the sensation of spinning of self or the environment. We base this not only on linguistic but also on neuroscientific grounds; Blanke (3) reported a patient who, during electrocortical stimulation, experienced sensations of self- and environmental motion (spinning) and whose *sensations* (of self- or environmental motion) were not modulated by eye closure nor accompanied by any nystagmus. This latter point is important, i.e. vertigo (a symptom) is quite separate from nystagmus (a sign) and its sequelae. Indeed when vertigo is accompanied by nystagmus then the patient sees the room spin.

Summary of approach to dizziness for the generalist

The generalist should begin by distinguishing vertigo from presyncope, 'lightheadedness' and disequilibrium of the elderly (4). Thus

the history should occupy 75% of the doctor's time with the patient. Since the generalist is the patient's first port of call, we advise that all dizzy patients have their postural blood pressure assessed and a 12-lead ECG. The generalist should then always perform a Hallpike manoeuvre and assess gait. In this way, the generalist will have screened for dizziness due to cardiovascular causes (blood pressure and ECG), BPPV (positive Hallpike) and central causes of 'dizziness' (gait ataxia and/or atypical Hallpike). This chapter deals with conditions encountered in general medicine that are frequently (or sometimes rarely) associated with the 'dizzy' patient. For the clinical approach to distinguishing between peripheral and central causes of dizziness the reader should refer to Chapters 11 and 29.

Drug-induced 'dizziness' and vestibular symptoms

A cursory examination of any pharmacopoeia (such as the *British National Formulary*) will demonstrate that legions of drugs have 'dizziness' as a side effect. Drugs are one of the commonest causes of 'dizziness' in generalist practice. 'Dizziness' is usually due to drug-induced orthostatic hypotension, sedation, or cerebellar intoxication. Most drug-induced dizziness occurs soon after the prescription was started or the dose changed (hence giving a clue to the diagnosis).

A careful drug history is a crucial component of the assessment of the dizzy patient, particularly the elderly dizzy patient who may be on multiple drug therapy. It is helpful to break down the drugs that cause 'dizziness' into four main groups (see Table 27.1) because the subjective nature of the 'dizziness' is different with each group:

The history of dizziness commencing on standing is obviously typical of orthostatic hypotension. However, particularly in the elderly, the symptomatic hypotension may come on at any time that the person is on their feet (5). The key in the history is that the 'dizziness' rarely happens when sitting and never happens when lying. The symptoms are also typically of a transient presyncopal type ('I feel I might faint'). Clinically significant postural drop of systolic blood pressure is 20 mmHg or more. It can, however, be very difficult to 'catch' and measure the postural drop. Another difficulty is that many elderly patients may have a significant postural drop

Table 27.1 Types of drugs causing 'dizziness'

	Type of drug	Notes
Drugs causing orthostatic hypotension	Therapeutic antihypertensive drugs	Alpha blockers are the most problematic but it occurs frequently with all six basic groups
	'Older' antipsychotic drugs	Particularly phenothiazines such as chlorpromazine
	'Atypical' antipsychotics	These also cause postural hypotension, particularly at initial dose titration and are increasingly used as an adjunct in refractory depression
	Tricyclic antidepressants	
	Antiparkinsonian dopaminergic drugs	
Drugs causing sedation	Benzodiazepines and 'Z drugs'	
	Antipsychotics	
	Vestibular sedatives such as antihistamines	
Cerebellar toxicity	Alcohol (acutely and chronically)	
	Antiepileptic drugs	(Especially carbamazepine—acutely and valproate—comes on subacutely) Antiepileptic drugs used for neuropathic pain or mood disorders in the elderly can be particularly problematic
	Lithium	
Ototoxic drugs	Aminoglycosides	Suspect if previous admission to ITU or renal dialysis unit. May have episodic, brief vertigo during loss of vestibular function. Symptoms manifest in mobilizing/rehabilitation with oscillopsia and gait problems
	Chemotherapy agents	Especially platinum drugs
	Non-steroidal anti-inflammatory drugs (acutely)	Overusage of aspirin
	Quinine or quinidine (acutely)	Remember overusage with nocturnal leg cramps
Extrapyramidal (gait) syndromes: antidopamine drugs	Includes vestibular sedatives such as stemetil (after chronic use in elderly)	

without symptoms, although such patients may present with collapse episodes. The 'gold standard' of diagnosis of orthostatic hypotension is to measure the drop in systolic blood pressure of more than 20 mmHg at a time of subjective 'dizziness'. In practice this is often difficult without prolonged monitoring with, for example, ambulatory blood pressure monitoring used in conjunction with a symptoms diary (6). Pragmatically, the general clinician often stops the drug to see if the symptoms resolve.

Any sedating drug can cause non-specific unsteadiness on the feet, particularly in the elderly. Typically some degree of drowsiness or cognitive slowness will usually be apparent to the patient and the observer. However, in the elderly alterations in levels of alertness can be less clear.

The elderly frail patient may exhibit 'disequilibrium of the elderly' (7). This is postural unsteadiness aggravated by muscle weakness, poor joint position sense, and delay of postural correcting reflexes. Small-vessel disease affecting the cerebral white matter also impairs balance. These patients typically display a 'subcortical gait' pattern characterized by small steps. Some patients with small-vessel disease may develop a parkinsonian-type gait with slow shuffling steps. These patients can be differentiated from Parkinson's disease by a relative sparing of the upper limbs and normal facial expression. Patients with small-vessel disease may also display gait ataxia (due to involvement of cerebellar white matter pathways) with broad-based gait, impaired tandem walking, and positional nystagmus (on Hallpike testing) of 'central' type. Irrespective of the aetiology, elderly patients with gait problems often deteriorate when sedating drugs are prescribed, often inappropriately for 'dizziness' (e.g. prochlorperazine). These drugs impair cognitive function and additionally impair extrapyramidal function. Such drugs may

increase falls by impairing frontal executive function with consequent impairment in decision-making and risk assessment (e.g. patients may climb a ladder to change a light bulb when in fact they are unsteady on a flat surface). Additionally, many such drugs have dopamine antagonistic properties and hence may unmask extrapyramidal gait dysfunction in patients with subcortical white matter small-vessel disease or in patients with early Parkinson's disease. Hence we do not advise chronic prescription of these drugs (except in a palliative care setting) as they usually worsen balance and increase falls.

Many drugs, including the antiepileptic drugs (AEDs), can cause an acute dose-dependent cerebellar toxicity. Less commonly, some AEDs (e.g. phenytoin) may induce an irreversible cerebellar syndrome (with cerebellar atrophy) with chronic usage. In the more common acute drug-intoxication, a simple clinical cerebellar screen would be to assess tandem walking and looking for gaze-evoked nystagmus (avoid extremes of gaze when assessing nystagmus). If the patient's epilepsy is well controlled but shows signs of cerebellar toxicity then a small AED dose reduction may be all that is required. Certainly abruptly stopping the patient's AED should be avoided lest status epilepticus be triggered. The generalist should think about obtaining neurological advice if in doubt about changing a patient's AED medication but certainly if there is poor epileptic control combined with cerebellar toxicity. Routine AED levels are not usually required so if the generalist thinks that checking AED levels would be a good idea then this usually indicates a non-routine situation requiring neurological advice.

Lithium toxicity, which is potentially fatal, is another cause of cerebellar toxicity. Missing a diagnosis of lithium toxicity is also a relatively common cause of litigation in the United Kingdom (8).

Acute alcohol intoxication is usually clear but the chronic alcohol may be very much less obvious clinically. In the emergency situation blood alcohol levels will help to clarify the matter.

Ototoxic drugs which cause vestibular failure may have their deleterious effect at any point in treatment, but usually the onset of symptoms is subacute. The commonest cause of in-hospital ototoxicity is gentamicin (9). An important point is that most cases of gentamicin-induced ototoxicity will have preserved hearing (10). This is because vestibular hair cells are much more sensitive to gentamicin than cochlear hair cells. This means that patients who show signs of hearing loss as a result of gentamicin will almost certainly have already suffered total and irreversible vestibular loss. Susceptible patients are often on intensive care or renal dialysis units. Patients may report brief episodes of vertigo (10), an unexplained phenomenon since systemic ototoxicity should ablate both peripheral vestibular organs symmetrically and it is the asymmetry of vestibular function which engenders dizziness and nystagmus. After this initial period, patients may be asymptomatic and their deficit only revealed on trying to mobilize or rehabilitate. In this case their 'dizziness' is predominantly oscillopsia precipitated by head motion (although sensations of self motion can be evoked from oscillopsia itself (11).

When the relationship of drug therapy to 'dizziness' is not clear, the clinician will need to balance the risks and benefits of maintaining the potentially offending drug with that of assessing the patient's response to drug withdrawal and subsequent reintroduction (12).

Cardiovascular causes of 'dizziness' and vestibular symptoms

In practice, once the clinician has considered the possibility of drug-induced 'dizziness' the next consideration is usually whether there is a cardiovascular cause.

Cardiovascular causes of dizziness are mediated by episodes of hypotension causing presyncopal symptoms. These can be orthostatic hypotension caused by drugs (see earlier), hypovolaemia, prolonged bed rest, or (more rarely) autonomic failure in a diabetic or parkinsonian patient. The other common cause of recurrent hypotensive episodes are cardiac arrhythmias. Rarer causes (but easily missed if not looked for) are critical aortic stenosis and critical bilateral carotid disease.

Orthostatic hypotension

As discussed earlier, the key to the diagnosis is that the episodes of dizziness rarely, if ever, occur when the patient is not standing (see Figure 9.2, Chapter 9). The episodes may occur within seconds of standing but can be delayed. In the elderly they can occur at any time when the patient is standing (5). The symptoms are typically presyncopal rather than vertiginous or unsteadiness of gait. However, the symptom may be described merely as 'lightheadedness'.

The commonest cause of recurrent orthostatic hypotension is drug therapy, particularly antihypertensive drugs. Often, if drug therapy is not the culprit there may be a fairly clear cause such as hypovolaemia (from dehydration or drugs) or prolonged bed rest (sometimes exacerbated by heat or prolonged standing).

If drugs or hypovolaemia are excluded as causes of orthostatic hypotension (and the postural drop is demonstrated) it is necessary to consider rarer causes such as an autonomic neuropathy,

hypoadrenalism (see later). Orthostatic hypotension in the patient with parkinsonism is typically due to the dopaminergic drugs, although, idiopathic Parkinson's disease patients may develop autonomic failure as part of the neurodegenerative process and exacerbated by the deconditioning consequent upon immobility. Less commonly parkinsonism and autonomic failure signifies multisystem atrophy, a neurodegenerative disorder. An autonomic neuropathy causing orthostatic hypotension should also be considered in patients with longstanding type 1 diabetes.

Other symptoms of an autonomic neuropathy may be erectile or ejaculatory impotence in a man, gustatory sweating (particularly in diabetics), constipation, and upper abdominal 'bloating' (due to gastric stasis). The main physical sign is orthostatic hypotension but other features may be a fixed resting heart rate greater than 90 beats/min (bpm) without normal variability (for example, sinus arrhythmia disappears from the rhythm strip on a 12-lead ECG, though this usually absent in any case in the older patient), and hyperhidrosis of the palms. In the parkinsonian patient there will be extrapyramidal signs of rigidity, bradykinesia, and tremor. In the diabetic patient there will be peripheral sensory loss and loss of tendon reflexes.

There is some evidence that hypoadrenalism in the elderly may be a commoner cause of orthostatic hypotension than is realized. This may sometimes be secondary to slow growing pituitary adenomas (a relatively common incidental finding at postmortem in the elderly) rather than primary adrenal failure. Hypoadrenalism should be suspected with persistently low systolic blood pressures (typically <110 mmHg) and particularly if an elderly patient has been very hypotensive postoperatively. The only manifestations of chronic hypoadrenalism may be postural dizziness, a lowish systolic blood pressure, and hyponatraemia (13).

Cardiac arrhythmias

Both tachyarrhythmias and bradyarrhythmias can cause 'dizziness' or more clearly defined episodes of presyncope or syncope. Clues to the cardiac nature of the episodes of dizziness may be the awareness of palpitations, the concurrence of chest pain or breathlessness, the sudden onset and offset of paroxysmal arrhythmias, or the presence of an already known cardiac history.

Unfortunately both palpitations (with a prevalence as high as 16% in medical outpatients (14)) and dizziness are common in the general population and their concurrence as symptoms often does not indicate causation (15).

Cardiac arrhythmias can be classified into the types shown in Table 27.2.

In the young patient with an atrial tachyarrhythmia without other heart muscle or valvular disease the patient is unlikely to be symptomatically hypotensive because of the large functional reserve of the young heart. Thus, a young man with fast atrial fibrillation secondary to an episode of 'binge' alcohol consumption will usually be aware of palpitations and may be aware of being breathless on exertion, but he is unlikely to have symptomatic hypotension. The main exception would be re-entrant supraventricular tachycardia with pre-excitation and extremely fast ventricular rates of 200 bpm or more.

On the other hand, the elderly patient without significant cardiac reserve may become symptomatically hypotensive with the onset of episodes of paroxysmal atrial fibrillation or otherwise asymptomatic ventricular tachycardia. The clue to the episodes of sinoatrial

Table 27.2 Types of cardiac arrhythmias

	Bradyarrhythmias	Tachyarrhythmias
Supraventricular	Sinoatrial arrest	Re entrant SVT
	Atrioventricular block	Atrial fibrillation/flutter
	Sick sinus syndrome	Pre-excitation syndromes
	Slow atrial fibrillation or atrial fibrillation with AV nodal block	
Ventricular		Ventricular tachycardia

or atrioventicular nodal heart block is the paroxysmal nature of the symptoms and the lack of warning ('Stokes–Adams attacks').

Cardiac examination may demonstrate a tachycardia or bradycardia but is mainly to detect valvular disease, particularly a critical stenosis. A well-known caution in clinical examination is that critical aortic stenosis may have a soft systolic murmur due to low volume flow. The same phenomenon (lack of a bruit) occurs with critical carotid stenosis.

Away from the event a 12-lead ECG may be normal. Modern ambulatory monitors allow for routine monitoring of up to 7 days (rather than the old 24-h Holter tapes that had a relatively poor sensitivity for detecting significant arrhythmias). Implantable loop recorders may be necessary to capture the events that occur very infrequently.

Dysfunctional breathing

Dysfunctional breathing (previously called 'hyperventilation' is very common in the general population (16). Symptoms often include 'dizziness' or non-specific 'lightheadedness'. When associated with non-specific, non-cardiac type chest discomfort it is known as Da Costa's syndrome (17). A high score on the Nijmegen questionnaire is suggestive of the diagnosis (18).

Traumatic brain injury

Traumatic brain injury (TBI) is the commonest cause of death and disability in young people (19). TBI occurs following blunt trauma to the cranium (i.e. closed head injury) and may cause two types of injury: 1) brain contusions arising from the percussive effect of the blunt trauma or 2) shearing injuries where rotational acceleration leads to shearing of white matter tracts within the brain. Traditional brain imaging sequences are sensitive at discerning contusions (and associated parenchymal haemorrhage) but shearing injury of white matter tracts is usually radiologically invisible except for some sensitive sequences (e.g. diffusion tensor imaging; 20). Traumatic brain injury may also be accompanied by neck injury thus the effects of head injury are often confounded with neck injury and vice versa.

Following recovery from the acute phase of TBI (e.g. recovery from coma and/or other life-threatening organ injuries) the commonest chronic symptoms following TBI is headache and dizziness. In our experience, the two commonest causes of vertigo in TBI are migrainous vertigo and BPPV and the two diagnoses often coexist. TBI appears to trigger migraine *de novo*, i.e. in individuals with no past migraine history perhaps suggesting that at least in some cases, TBI provokes the pathological cascade that may result in migraine as well as that for BPPV.

In mild TBI (i.e. no brain contusions or temporal bone injury) there are usually no measurable vestibular deficits. Although there is evidence in mild TBI for deficits in smooth pursuit gain, the

degree reported is too small to be clinically apparent (21). Patients with significant cerebral cortical injury however, often display abnormalities of smooth pursuit ipsilateral to the cortical lesion although for more subtle

Positional vertigo is usually related to BPPV and clinical assessment of any dizzy patient should in any case *always* include the Hallpike manoeuvre even when there is no obvious history of BPPV. Occasionally patients have both BPPV and migrainous vertigo. Since migrainous vertigo can provoke positional vertigo, and acute vertigo per se (including that from BPPV) may trigger migraine, establishing an exact causal relationship for positional vertigo may be difficult.

Always ask about visual vertigo symptoms (Chapter 13) which are common if the dizziness has become chronic. Visual vertigo is amenable to vestibular 'OKN' therapy (see Chapter 13); however, we advise treating any active migraine prior to considering visuo-vestibular therapy. In general, we have a low threshold for treating any concurrent migraine. We encourage patients in who there is suspected or confirmed BPPV, to incorporate a 5-min session of Brandt–Daroff exercises into their bedtime routine.

Whiplash

There is no convincing evidence that neck injury per se is casual in dizziness. It goes without saying that any significant whiplash injury involves significant accelerations of the head. In patients with an acute head/neck injury presenting with vertigo one should always consider a vertebral artery dissection (see Chapter 23). However 'chronic whiplash syndrome' is recognized as one of the 'functional somatic syndromes' (22) and, particularly within the context of litigation, quite severe symptoms may remain unexplained (23).

Endocrine and metabolic disease

Hypoglycaemia

Since the brain is an obligate glucose consumer, glucose metabolism, excretion, and delivery is highly regulated with a tight regulation of plasma glucose levels. Even during periods of fasting, blood glucose levels are maintained by gluconeogenesis; i.e. the process of metabolizing lipids (and protein in periods of starvation) to glucose. Significant hypoglycaemia can thus only occur if there is at least one of the following: 1) excessive exogenous insulin administration; 2) pathological insulin secretion; 3) impaired gluconeogenesis (e.g. hepatic failure).

Hypoglycaemia may cause any neurological symptom or sign including dizziness, vertigo, or spontaneous nystagmus. The diagnosis should be suspected in patients with recurrent dizziness who are on insulin therapy and those with hepatic insufficiency. Rarely recurrent hypoglycaemia may be due to an insulinoma. In such cases symptoms typically occur with fasting hence the propensity for symptoms to occur in early morning (i.e. with overnight fasting). Hypoglycaemia can be readily confirmed with finger prick testing. Rare cases of inulsinoma require additional blood tests of blood insulin and C-peptide taken concurrently with confirmed episodes of hypoglycaemia.

The treatment is acute intravenous glucose. If there is any risk of thiamine deficiency (see section 'Acute Wernicke's encephalopathy') then thiamine should be administered ideally before glucose administration or at the very least, thiamine and glucose therapy should be commenced in parallel.

Acute Wernicke's encephalopathy

This is due to thiamine deficiency. Patients classically present with a triad of ophthalmoplegia (almost any eye movement abnormality can occur), ataxia, and encephalopathy. Patients with spontaneous nystagmus may complain of oscillopsia with dizziness and imbalance due to gait ataxia. Patients with significant encephalopathy may however have 'no complaints'.

Patients at risk include alcoholics with a poor diet, patients on artificial nutrition (clinicians should have independent verification of adequate thiamine intake in such cases), and patients with eating disorders or with refractory vomiting (e.g. hyperemesis gravidarum).

Treatment is with a course of intravenous thiamine (followed by adequate dietary thiamine intake). Acute thiamine replacement may not be sufficient, however, to avert permanent neurological sequelae including ocular motility, gait, and cognitive deficits.

Thyroid disease

The commonest cause of thyroid dysfunction is organ-specific auto-immune disease. Chronic hypothyroidism causes a potentially reversible cerebellar syndrome including gait ataxia. Thyrotoxicosis (e.g. Graves disease) does not typically result in problems of dizziness and gait ataxia. Occasionally supraventricular tachycardias (due to thyrotoxicosis) may result in episodic dizziness.

Adrenal insufficiency

The commonest cause of adrenal insufficiency is inadequate replacement of exogenous corticosteroids in patients on long-term steroid therapy (either due to increased steroid requirement during periods of physiological stress or too rapid a reduction of steroid dosage). Less common causes are auto-immunity and rarely (at least in the developed world) infection such as tuberculosis or cytomegalovirus adrenalitis (the latter is particularly seen in AIDS cases). In some patients with a depleted adrenal reserve (e.g. exogenous steroids, infective or auto-immune adrenalitis) administration of enzyme inducing drugs (e.g. rifampicin) may precipitate an Addisonian crisis. As mentioned earlier, in the elderly, functional hypoadrenalism due to benign pituitary adenomas should be considered.

Addisonian crises may present with postural dizziness (e.g. due to cardiovascular insufficiency). Patients with chronic hypo-adrenalism do not typically complain of postural dizziness unless there are additional aggravating factors (since cardiovascular effects of hypoadrenalism are only seen in acute crises).

In critically ill patients, treatment and diagnosis should occur concurrently; a random blood cortisol should be obtained (albeit this is only informative if taken in the morning and levels should be interpreted in the context of physiological need—i.e. higher cortisol levels are required in critical illness) followed by intravenous corticosteroid replacement. In subacute cases a 30-min Synacthen test can be followed by steroid administration.

Guillain–Barré syndrome—Miller Fisher variant

The Miller Fisher (MFS) variant of Guillain–Barré syndrome (GBS) presents with the classical triad of ophthalmoplegia, ataxia, and areflexia. Occasionally there may be diagnostic confusion with an acute Wernicke's encephalopathy but in the MFS there should be no mental obtundation (note however, some GBS patients with ophthalmoplegia may be an encephalopathic—'Bickerstaff'encephalitis; 24). Typical MFS patients complain of head movement-induced oscillopsia and dizziness due to ophthalmoplegia.

A full description of the diagnosis and management of MFS is beyond the scope of this article, however, important investigations include lumbar puncture (typically one finds an acellular CSF with elevated protein), brain MRI, an appropriately timed nerve conduction study, and antiganglioside antibodies (anti-GM1 antibodies are associated with MFS). Treatment for GBS/MFS includes supportive therapy (e.g. ventilator support for respiratory insufficiency) and specific therapy, e.g. intravenous immunoglobulin.

Chronic follow-up of patients with MFS has demonstrated that symptoms of dizziness and oscillopsia parallel changes in vestibular perception rather than persisting deficits in ocular motility (11). This suggests that cases of MFS with persisting symptoms may benefit from appropriate Cawthorne–Cooksey exercises since these exercises promote central adaptation (see Chapter 6).

Renal disease

Patients with renal insufficiency are more at risk of drug-related dizziness (see section 'Drug-induced dizziness') due to problems of renal clearance. Such patients are particularly susceptible to gentamicin-induced vestibular failure. Occasionally patients with gentamicin-related vestibular failure develop episodic spontaneous vertigo in the initial process of vestibular failure (9) but often this phase is asymptomatic. Following vestibular ablation however, patients complain of head-movement related oscillopsia and dizziness.

Patients on renal dialysis experience significant fluid shifts that may lead to postural hypotension (see earlier section on postural hypotension). There is no evidence that renal dysfunction leads to increased BPPV through an effect on the endolymphatic milieu.

Epilepsy

Vestibular epilepsy is rare but does occur with a handful of cases reported in the literature. That focal brain stimulation can induce sensations of dizziness (from rocking to spinning) was demonstrated initially by Penfield (25). Kahane et al. (26) have provided a large database of cerebral loci producing vestibular symptoms with the main areas producing such features in the superior inferior temporal gyrus and contiguous temporo-parietal cortex. Vestibular features, however, do not provide a reliable indication of the ictal focus since the clinical manifestations may represent spread of cortical electrical activity rather than signifying the origin of the ictal focus.

Summary

In practice, the clinician faced with the dizzy patient usually has to initially assess whether the patient has a primary vestibular disorder or whether the dizziness is presyncopal in nature, due to cardiovascular disorders, or whether it could be related to existing drug therapy. The latter is a particularly common cause of dizziness that can be overlooked.

References
1. Bird JC, Beynon GJ, Prevost AT, Baguley DM (1998). An analysis of referral patterns for dizziness in the primary care setting. *Br J Gen Pract*, 48(437), 1828–32.

2. Matthews WB (1963). *Practical Neurology*. Oxford: Blackwell.

3. Blanke O, Perrig S, Thut G, Landis T, Seeck M (2000). Simple and complex vestibular responses induced by electrical cortical stimulation of the parietal cortex in humans. *J Neurol Neurosurg Psychiatry*, 69(4), 553–6.

4. Drachman DA, Hart CW (1972). An approach to the dizzy patient. *Neurology*, 22(4), 323–34.

5. Baloh RW, Ying SH, Jacobson KM (2003). A longitudinal study of gait and balance dysfunction in normal older people. *Arch Neurol* 60(6), 835–39.

6. Bath AP, Walsh RM, Ranalli P, *et al.* (2000). Experience from a multidisciplinary 'dizzy' clinic. *Am J Otol*, 21(1), 92–7.

7. Belal, A Jr, Glorig A (1986). Dysequilibrium of ageing. *J Laryngol Otol*, 100, 1037–41.

8. National Patient Safety Agency. *Patient Safety Alert – Safer lithium therapy (NPSA/2009/PSA005)*. London: NPSA.

9. Seemungal BM, Bronstein AM (2007). Aminoglycoside ototoxicity: Vestibular function is also vulnerable. *BMJ*, 335, 952.

10. Ishiyama G, Ishiyama A, Kerber K, Baloh RW (2006). Gentamicin ototoxicity: clinical features and the effect on the human vestibulo-ocular reflex. *Acta Otolaryngol*, 126(10), 1057–61.

11. Seemungal BM, Masaoutis P, Green DA, Plant GT, Bronstein AM (2011). Symptomatic recovery in Miller Fisher syndrome parallels vestibular-perceptual and not vestibular-ocular reflex function. *Front Neurol*, 2, 2.

12. Madlon-Kay D (1985). Evaluation and outcome of the dizzy patient. *J Fam Pract*, 21(2), 109–13.

13. Bornstein SR (2009). Predisposing factors for adrenal insufficiency. *N Engl J Med*, 360, 2328–39.

14. Barsky AJ, Ahern DK, Bailey ED, Delamater BA (1996). Predictors of persistent palpitations and continued utilisation. *J Fam Pract*, 42(5), 465–72.

15. Thavendiranathan P, Bagai A, Khoo C, Dorian P, Choudhry NK (2009). Does this patient with palpitations have a cardiac arrhythmia? *JAMA*, 302(16), 2135–43.

16. Thomas M, Price D, McKeever T, Lewis S, Hubbard R (2003). Dysfunctional breathing in adults with and without asthma – a prevalence survey. *Am J Respir Crit Care Med*, 167(7), 1578–9.

17. Paul O (1987). Da Costa's syndrome or neurocirculatory asthenia. *Br Heart J*, 58(4), 306–15.

18. van Dixhoorn J, Duivenvoorden HJ (1985). Efficacy of Nijmegen questionnaire in recognition of the hyperventilation syndrome. *J Psycosom Res*, 29, 199–206.

19. Ghajar, J (2000). Traumatic brain injury. *Lancet*, 356, 923–9.

20. Niogi SN, Mukherjee P (2010). Diffusion tensor imaging of mild traumatic brain injury. *J Head Trauma Rehabil*, 25(4), 241–55.

21. Heitger MH, Jones RD, Macleod AD, Snell DL, Frampton CM, Anderson TJ (2009). Impaired eye movements in post-concussion syndrome indicate suboptimal brain function beyond the influence of depression, malingering or intellectual ability. *Brain*, 132(10), 2850–70.

22. Hennigsen P, Zipfel S, Herzog W (2007). Management of functional somatic syndromes. *Lancet*, 369, 946–55.

23. Lankester BJA, Garneti N, Gargan MF, Bannister GC (2006). Factors predicting outcome after whiplash injury in subjects pursuing litigation. *Eur Spine J*, 15(6), 902–7.

24. Odaka, M, Yuki N, Yamada M, *et al.* (2003). Bickerstaff's brainstem encephalitis: clinical features of 62 cases and a subgroup associated with Guillain-Barré syndrome. *Brain*, 126(10), 2279–90.

25. Penfield W, Jasper H (1954). *Epilepsy and the functional anatomy of the human brain* (2nd ed). Boston, MA: Little, Brown and Co.

26. Kahane P, Hoffmann D, Minotti L, Berthoz A (2003). Reappraisal of the human vestibular cortex by cortical electrical stimulation study. *Ann Neurol*, 54(5), 615–24.

CHAPTER 28

Motion Sickness and Disorientation in Vehicles

John F. Golding and Michael A. Gresty

General introduction

Much of the content of this book concerns the characteristics of the person who has become ill as a consequence of vestibular or related disease. By contrast, we discuss the response of the normal person in environments beyond everyday pedestrian experience. This dichotomy could be thought of 'The sick person in the healthy environment *versus* the healthy person in a sick environment'. We first deal with motion sickness, a universal experience which may become a problem in the susceptible individual or in extreme environments. Secondly we address the problem of disorientation. Spatial disorientation is familiar in the specialized occupations of pilots, astronauts, and divers. However, recently we have observed similar problems in users of road vehicles which have been severe enough to have attracted clinical attention.

Motion sickness

Introduction

'Sailing on the sea proves that motion disorders the body ...' observed the Greek physician Hippocrates over 2000 years ago. 'Nausea' derives from the Greek root word 'naus', hence 'nautical' meaning a ship. Nowadays there is a potential to cause motion sickness in a wide range of situations—in cars, tilting trains, funfair rides, aircraft, weightlessness in outer-space, virtual reality, and simulators (Table 28.1). The general term 'motion sickness' embraces car-sickness, air-sickness, space-sickness, sea-sickness, etc. The following short review is arranged as the what, how, why of motion sickness, followed by predictors and preventions.

Signs and symptoms

The aversive nature of motion sickness was exploited in historical times both as an unusual form of punishment (1) and also as a strange type of therapy (2). The primary signs and symptoms of motion sickness are nausea and vomiting, together with a host of other related symptoms including stomach awareness, sweating, and facial pallor (sometimes called 'cold sweating'), increased salivation, sensations of bodily warmth, dizziness, drowsiness (also denoted as the 'sopite syndrome'), sometimes headache, and,

unsurprisingly, loss of appetite and increased sensitivity to odours. A typical motion sickness questionnaire shown in Table 28.2 lists the more frequent symptoms excluding vomiting and facial pallor. This is an adaptation of the simulator sickness questionnaire (3). The occurrence of oculomotor symptoms is relatively higher in situations where visual mismatches may be the provoking stimulus such as in simulators and virtual reality systems, as opposed to motion sickness due to whole body accelerative stimuli such as during ship motion. For a more rapid assessment the following global sickness rating scale has proved reliable and useful: 1 = no symptoms; 2 = initial symptoms of motion sickness but no nausea; 3 = mild nausea; 4 = moderate nausea; 5 = severe nausea and/or retching; 6 = vomiting (4). Physiological responses associated with motion sickness may vary between individuals. These often include autonomic changes such as sweating and vasoconstriction of the skin causing pallor (less commonly skin vasodilation and flushing in some individuals) with the simultaneous opposite effect of vasodilation and increased blood flow of deeper blood vessels, changes in heart rate which are often an initial increase followed by a rebound decrease, and inconsistent changes in blood pressure (5). For the stomach gastric stasis occurs and increased frequency and reduced amplitude of the normal electogastric rhythm (6). A whole host of hormones are released mimicking a generalized stress response amongst which vasopressin is thought to be most closely associated with the time course of motion sickness (7). The observation of cold sweating suggests that motion sickness may disrupt aspects of temperature regulation (8), a notion also consistent with the observation that motion sickness reduces deep core body temperature during cold water immersion, accelerating onset of hypothermia (9).

Although motion sickness is unpleasant in its own right, under some circumstances it may have adverse consequences for performance and even survival. Motion sickness preferentially causes decrements on performance of tasks which are complex, require sustained performance, and offer the opportunity to the person to control the pace of their effort (10). For pilots and aircrew it can slow training in the air and in simulators and even cause a minority to fail training (5). Approximately 70% of novice astronauts will suffer space sickness in the first 24 hours of flight. Although

Table 28.1 Provocative stimuli

Context	Examples of provocative stimuli
Land	Cars, coaches, tilting trains, ski, camels, elephants, funfair rides
Sea	Boats, ferries, survival rafts, divers' lines undersea
Air	Transport planes, small aircraft, hovercraft, helicopters, parabolic flight
Space	Shuttle, spacelab
Optokinetic	Wide-screen cinemas, microfiche-readers, 'haunted swing', simulators, virtual reality (HMD), rotating visual drums or spheres, pseudo-coriolis, reversing prism spectacles
Laboratory	Cross-coupled (Coriolis), low-frequency translational oscillation (vertical or horizontal), off vertical axis rotation (OVAR), counter-rotation, *g*-excess in human centrifuges
Associated stimuli	Emetic toxins, chemotherapy, PONV, extreme arousal (fear increases/fight decreases)

Notes: (1) 'Laboratory' stimuli evoking motion sickness are simply refined elements of those provocative stimuli found in the outside world; (2) 'Optokinetic' stimuli are classed separately since they do not need additional physical transportation of the person under all definitions, although some might be also classed under 'Laboratory'; (3) 'Associated' stimuli are included to indicate the basic evolutionary functions served by nausea and vomiting.

vomiting in space is doubtless unpleasant, the possibility of vomiting while in a spacesuit in microgravity is potentially life threatening, consequently precluding extravehicular activity for at least the first 24 hours of spaceflight (11). For survival-at-sea, such as in lifecrafts, seasickness can reduce survival chances by a variety of mechanisms, including reduced morale and the 'will to live', failure to consistently perform routine survival tasks, dehydration due to loss of fluids through vomiting (5), and possibly due to the increased risk of hypothermia (9).

Table 28.2 Motion Sickness Symptom Questionnaire (excludes vomiting and facial pallor). Do you have any of the following symptoms right now? (tick boxes)

	0	1	2	3
	None	**Slight**	**Moderate**	**Severe**
General discomfort				
Fatigue				
Headache				
Eye strain				
Difficulty focusing				
Increased salivation				
Sweating				
Nausea				
Difficulty concentrating				
Fullness of head				
Blurred vision				
Dizziness (eyes open)[a]				
Dizziness (eyes closed)[a]				
Vertigo				
Stomach awareness				
Burping				

[a] Illusory feelings of motion.

Causes

The wide range of stimuli that can provoke motion sickness can be seen in Table 28.1. The key observation in understanding the most probable mechanism for the cause of motion sickness is that the physical intensity of the stimulus is not necessarily related to the degree of nauseogenicity. For example, with optokinetic stimuli the motion is implied but not real. When a person sitting at the front in a wide-screen cinema experiences self-vection and 'cinerama sickness', there is no physical motion of the body in the real world. In this example, the vestibular and somatosensory systems are signalling that the person is sitting still, but the visual system is signalling illusory movement or self-vection. Consequently the generally accepted explanation of the 'how' of motion sickness is based on some form of sensory conflict or sensory mismatch. The sensory conflict or sensory mismatch is between actual versus expected invariant patterns of vestibular, visual, and kinaesthetic inputs (1). These also include intravestibular conflicts between rotational accelerations sensed by the semicircular canals and linear-translational accelerations (including gravitational) sensed by the otoliths. A variety of detailed models have been developed to explain the nature of sensory conflict or sensory mismatch (12, 13). Benson (5) categorized neural mismatch into two main types: 1) conflict between visual and vestibular inputs or 2) mismatch between the canals and the otoliths. An even more simplified model was proposed by Bos and Bles (14). This is that there is only one conflict: between the subjective expected vertical and the sensed vertical. However, despite this apparent simplification the underlying model is necessarily complex and finds difficulty in accounting for the observation that motion sickness can be induced by types of optokinetic stimuli which pose no conflict concerning the earth vertical (15).

The 'rule of thumb' model originally advanced by Stott (16) may not be the most elegant in theoretical terms but arguably is still the most practical. This model proposes a set of simple rules, which if broken, will lead to motion sickness:

Rule 1. Visual-vestibular: motion of the head in one direction must result in motion of the external visual scene in the opposite direction.

Rule 2. Canal-otolith: rotation of the head, other than in the horizontal plane, must be accompanied by appropriate angular change in the direction of the gravity vector.

Rule 3. Utricle-saccule: any sustained linear acceleration is due to gravity, has an intensity of 1 *g* and defines 'downwards'.

In other words, the visual world should remain space stable, and gravity should always point down and average over a few seconds to 1 *g*.

In some environments there may be only one provocative stimulus. For example, at sea it is the low-frequency 'heave' motion of the vessel that provokes seasickness. However, in many environments multiple stimuli and conflicts may be involved. For example, airsickness in a pilot produced by the flight of an agile military aircraft may be due to up to five sources. Flying through air turbulence produces low-frequency translational oscillation of the aircraft, which may cause airsickness. In addition, during aircraft turns there may be provocation from the four following sources: visual-vestibular mismatches as the pilot senses 'down' to remain through the axis of the body but the external visual world to be tilted; sustained changes in the scalar magnitude of gravitoinertial force (GIF) due to centripetal acceleration; cross-coupling (Coriolis) due to head movements during rotation of the aircraft if the turn is tight enough; and also the g-excess illusion if the pilot tilts the head during increased GIF.

In virtual reality systems and simulators, self-vection, retinal slip, and poor eye collimation may be an important provocative stimulus, but phase lag between real motion and the corresponding update of the visual display may be equally or more important. Compensatory vestibule-ocular reflexes (VORs) to head movements are as fast as 10 ms or so, consequently visual update lag disparities not much longer than this may be easily detectable by subjects. If visual display update lags are much longer than this then they may provoke sickness, since it has been shown that virtual reality sickness has been induced with update lags as short as 48 ms.

Low-frequency translational motion is a major source of motion sickness in land vehicles, ships, and aircraft and has been sufficiently well described to provide engineering design parameters (exposure time, acceleration, frequency) for standards regulated by the International Organization for Standardization (17). The frequency weighting function is of theoretical as well as applied interest. Laboratory experiments (18, 19) and ship motion surveys (20) have shown that nauseogenicity increases as a function of exposure time and acceleration intensity as might be expected, but more unusually that nauseogenicity peaks at the low frequency motion of around 0.2 Hz. Such low-frequency motions are present in transportation in ships, coaches, aircraft flying through air turbulence, and on camels and elephants, all of which can provoke motion sickness. This frequency relationship also explains why some forms of transport are not provocative, for example people do not experience 'horse-sickness'. During horse riding, walking, running, riding off-road trail bikes, the frequencies are higher than 1 Hz. Consequently, although these motions can be quite severe (capable of bruising the person), they are not nauseogenic. Hypotheses for the frequency dependence of nauseogenicity of translational oscillation are a phase-error in signalling motion between canal-otolith and somatosensory systems (13, 21), or a frequency-dependent phase-error between the sensed vertical and the subjective or expected vertical (14). It has also been proposed that a zone of perceptuo-motor ambiguity around 0.2 Hz triggers sickness, since at higher frequencies imposed accelerations are usually interpreted as translation of self through space, whereas at lower frequencies imposed accelerations are usually interpreted as a shift in the main force vector, i.e. tilt of self with respect to the assumed gravity vertical (4, 22). The region of 0.2 Hz would be a cross-over between these two interpretations and, thus, a frequency region of maximal uncertainty concerning the correct frame of reference for spatial orientation. More recently Gresty et al (23) proposed a somewhat related 'ecological' explanation, that this frequency tuning of motion sickness is related to mechanical limitations on human body motion. This proposes that a cause of MS may be difficulty in selecting appropriate tactics to maintain body stability at vehicle motion circa 0.2 Hz, between whole-body GIF alignment seen at lower frequencies versus lateropulsion seen at higher frequencies.

The previous paragraphs describe what might be termed the 'how' of motion sickness in terms of mechanisms. By contrast it is necessary to look elsewhere for an understanding of the 'why' of motion sickness. The primary functions of the vestibular system are spatial orientation, maintenance of balance, and stabilizing of vision through VORs. An additional vestibular function has been proposed, which is that it acts as a toxin detector. Thus, the evolutionary purpose of what we call 'motion sickness' is postulated to be the same as for any emetic response, which is to protect the organism from the toxic effects of potentially harmful substances that it may have ingested (24). The 'toxin detector' hypothesis proposes that the brain has evolved to recognize any derangement of expected patterns of vestibular, visual, and kinaesthetic information as evidence of central nervous system malfunction and to initiate vomiting as a defence against a possible ingested neurotoxin, i.e. it provides a 'backup' to the main toxin detector system of chemoreceptors of the afferent vagal nerves and the chemoreceptor trigger zone of the brainstem. According to this hypothesis, motion sickness in pedestrian man or other animals is simply the inadvertent activation of this ancient defence reflex by the sensory conflicts induced by the novel altered visual and force environments of sea, air, land transport, virtual reality, etc. This evolutionary-based hypothesis is consistent with the observation that motion sickness is evolutionarily well preserved from man down to the level of the fish (ironically, fish can become seasick during aquarium transport) (1). It is also consistent with the observation that people who are more susceptible to motion sickness are also more susceptible to toxins, chemotherapy, and postoperative nausea and vomiting (PONV) (25). Finally, this theory has been experimentally tested with evidence of reduced emetic response to challenge from toxins after bilateral vestibular ablation (26).

A number of alternative hypotheses have been proposed. One alternative hypothesis is based on the observation that tilt stimulation of the otoliths in the cat, which transduce linear accelerations, provoke a pressor response (increased blood pressure and cardiac output) mediated via vestibular-cardiovascular projections. It has been proposed that motion sickness is caused by the inappropriate activation of such vestibular-cardiovascular reflexes. This proposes that the vestibular and visual systems influence autonomic control for the purpose of maintaining homeostasis during movement and changes in posture. Thus motion sickness arises from an aberrant activation of neural pathways that serve to maintain a stable internal environment (27). A somewhat similar, non-functional explanation has been proposed by Balaban (28) that motion sickness might be regarded as referred visceral discomfort after activation of vestibular autonomic reflexes due to the convergence of vestibular and autonomic afferent information in the brainstem and cerebellum. The vestibular-cardiovascular reflex hypothesis has a good historical pedigree in the 19th-century concept of 'cerebral anaemia' as the cause of motion sickness (29). Although some support is provided by the observation that cerebral hypoperfusion preceded nausea during GIF variation induced by centrifugation (30), the situation is unclear since there is considerable overlap between sick and non-sick individuals' pressor responses to motion sickness induced by the GIF variation of parabolic flight (31). The importance of the vestibular-cardiovascular reflexes in maintaining blood pressure seems limited since bilateral labyrinthectomized patients' pressor responses to rapid tilts are only minimally slower than normals (<500 ms) (32) and also by the observation that these patients do not appear to be fainting frequently as they adjust their posture during everyday activity as they walk around, lay down, and stand up. Moreover, although not a formal disproof, this hypothesis does not predict the relative nauseogenicity of the various gravity and body referenced directions of nauseogenic provocative motion, which would be expected to alter blood pressure (4, 33). Another hypothesis, which has received less attention, postulates that motion sickness is a punishment system which has evolved to discourage development of perceptual-motor programmes that are inefficient or cause spatial disorientation (34). All of these hypotheses remain in contention to provide explanations for the 'why' of motion sickness, but at present, the balance of evidence would seem to favour the toxin detector hypothesis.

Predictors of motion sickness susceptibility

Although individuals vary widely in their susceptibility, nearly all people can be made motion sick given a sufficiently provocative stimulus. Almost the only individuals who are immune to motion sickness are those who have complete bilateral loss of labyrinthine (vestibular apparatus) function. Even this may not be absolutely true under all circumstances since there is evidence that bilateral labyrinthine defective individuals are still susceptible to motion sickness provoked by visual stimuli designed to induce self-vection during pseudo-coriolis stimulation, i.e. pitching head movements in a rotating visual field (35). Blind or blindfolded normally sighted individuals can be made motion sick using real motion, although obviously optokinetic stimuli (Table 28.1) are ineffective. With regard to the contribution of aspects of other individual differences in vestibular function to motion sickness susceptibility, the evidence is limited. Otolith asymmetry between left and right labyrinths, as measured during parabolic flight, has been proposed as an indicator of susceptibility for space sickness (36). Mal-de-debarquement is the sensation of unsteadiness and tilting of the ground when a sailor returns to land. A similar effect is observed in astronauts returning to 1 g on Earth after extended time in weightlessness in space. In severe cases this can lead to motion sickness but symptoms usually resolve within a few hours as individuals readapt to the normal land environment. Individuals susceptible to mal-de-debarquement may have reduced reliance on vestibular and visual inputs and increased dependence on the somatosensory system for the maintenance of balance (37). However, in a more general sense, individual variation in sensory thresholds to angular or translational accelerations does not seem to relate to susceptibility in any obvious fashion. The evidence that individual differences in postural stability or perceptual style (38) are major predictors of motion sickness susceptibility seems limited (22). Similarly, individual variation in the VOR does not seem to be a reliable predictor of susceptibility. Some authors assert that shorter time constants of the central vestibular velocity store predict reduced motion sickness susceptibility (39), but others have found no evidence of such a relationship (40). It has been suggested that it is not duration of the time constant per se, but the ability to modify readily the time constant that may be a candidate marker for success in motion sickness habituation (22).

Certain groups with medical conditions may be at elevated risk. Many patients with vestibular pathology and disease and vertigo can be especially sensitive to any type of motion. The well known association among migraine, motion sickness sensitivity, and Ménière's disease dates back to the initial description of the syndrome by Prosper Ménière in 1861. It has been proposed that there may be a genetic link caused by defective calcium ion channels shared by the brain and inner ear leading to reversible hair cell depolarization, producing vestibular symptoms and that the headache might just

be a secondary phenomenon (41). An alternative explanation has been proposed based upon different functioning of the serotonergic system in the brains of migraineurs (42, 43).

There is a large genetic contribution to the individual differences in susceptibility. This is to be expected since motion sickness has been evolutionary well preserved and is postulated to be of survival advantage as a poison detector (see above). Mono- and dizygotic twin studies indicate that the heritability of motion sickness is high, at around 70% in childhood, and declines through puberty and the early adult years to around 55% (44). This decline of heritability with age may be due to varying exposure between individuals to provocative environments and habituation. Multiple genes are probably involved, however the nature of the genes involved is as yet undefined. One example is the observation that a single-nucleotide polymorphism of the alpha2-adrenergic receptor increases autonomic responses to stress and contributes to individual differences in autonomic responsiveness to provocative motion (45). However, it is unclear whether this is a marker for motion sickness susceptibility, per se, or a general marker for autonomic sensitivity. There is some evidence for Chinese hypersusceptibility to motion sickness, and this may provide some indirect evidence for a genetic contribution to such differences (46, 47).

Sex and age are two main predictors in the general population of individual susceptibility. Surveys of transportation by sea, land, and air, indicate that women are more susceptible to motion sickness than men; women show higher incidences of vomiting and reporting a higher incidence of symptoms such as nausea (48). This increased susceptibility is likely to be objective and not subjective because women vomit more than men. For example, large-scale surveys of passengers at sea indicate a 5:3 female to male risk ratio for vomiting (20). It does not seem related to extra habituation to greater ranges of motion environments experienced by risk-taking males (49), nor to gender biased differential self-selection between males and females when volunteering for laboratory motion sickness experiments (50). Moreover, this sex difference is not exclusive to humans because in animals, such as *Suncus murinus* (house musk shrew), females show significantly more emetic episodes and shorter latencies to emesis in experimental exposures to motion (51). The cause of greater motion sickness susceptibility in women has been suggested to involve the female hormonal cycle. However, although susceptibility varies over the menstrual cycle, peaking around menstruation, it is unlikely that this can fully account for the greater susceptibility in females because the magnitude of fluctuation in susceptibility across the cycle is only around one-third of the overall difference between male and female susceptibility (52). The elevated susceptibility of females to motion sickness or indeed to PONV or chemotherapy-induced nausea and vomiting (25, 53), may serve an evolutionary function. Thus, more sensitive sickness thresholds in females may serve to prevent exposure of the fetus to harmful toxins during pregnancy, or subsequently through milk. This elevated susceptibility in females may be 'hard-wired' but capable of upregulation albeit variably by hormonal influences during the menstrual cycle and even further during pregnancy.

Infants and very young children are immune to motion sickness. However, they have no difficulty vomiting. Motion sickness susceptibility begins from perhaps around 6–7 years of age (1) and peaking around 9–10 years (54). The reasons for this are uncertain. Puberty begins later (around 10–12 years) than the age 6–7 years for onset of motion sickness susceptibility. This implies that sex hormonal changes per se are not a direct explanation for the onset of motion sickness susceptibility. Another possibility is that the perceptuo-motor map is still highly plastic and not fully formed until around 7 years of age. Most models of motion sickness propose that this perceptuo-motor map provides the 'expected' invariant patterns for detecting possible sensory mismatches in the relationships between vestibular, visual and kinaesthetic inputs. Following the peak susceptibility, there is a subsequent decline of susceptibility during the teenage years towards adulthood around 20 years. This doubtless reflects habituation. Although it is often stated that this decline in susceptibility continues in a more gradual fashion throughout life towards old age, the evidence is weak given that older people may avoid motion environments if they know that they are susceptible. Indeed, longitudinal evidence from individuals who have been studied objectively in the laboratory suggests that towards older age, susceptibility may increase in some individuals.

A multiplicity of other possible predictors of susceptibility have been examined over the years, with relatively few being found to be of significance. Cross-sectional surveys show that individuals with high levels of aerobic fitness appear to be more susceptible to motion sickness, and experiments show aerobic fitness training increases motion sickness susceptibility (55). The reasons are unclear, with one suggestion being that a more reactive autonomic nervous system (including hypothalamic–pituitary–adrenal axis) in aerobically fit individuals may sensitize them. Psychological variables such as mood may modify susceptibility in contradictory directions: 'state' variables such as extreme fear or anxiety conditioned to motion, may contribute indirectly to motion sickness susceptibility, although by contrast, extreme arousal 'fight-flight' such as observed in warfare may suppress motion sickness (1). Personality 'trait' variables such as extraversion or neuroticsm do not strongly predict motion sickness susceptibility, with only minor correlations being observed between extraversion or similar personality traits with reduced susceptibility (1, 56).

Motion sickness Susceptibility Questionnaires MSSQ (sometimes called Motion History Questionnaires) enable an estimate to be made of an individual's susceptibility. A typical questionnaire is shown in Table 28.3, which has been validated for exposure to motion stimuli in the laboratory and in transport environments (57). An overall indicator of susceptibility, may be calculated as the MSSQ score = (total sickness score) × (18)/(18 − number of types not experienced), this formula corrects for differing extent of exposure to different motion stimuli in individuals. For the normal population, the median MSSQ score is 11.3, where higher scores indicate greater susceptibility and vice versa, more details are given in the original reference (57).

Table 28.3 Motion Sickness Susceptibility Questionnaire Short-form (MSSQ-Short) (adapted from Golding (57))
This questionnaire is designed to find out how susceptible to motion sickness you are, and what sorts of motion are most effective in causing that sickness. Sickness here means feeling queasy or nauseated or actually vomiting.
Your childhood experience only (before 12 years of age), for each of the following types of transport or entertainment please indicate:
1. As a child (before age 12), how often you felt sick or nauseated (tick boxes):

	Not applicable— never travelled	Never felt sick	Rarely felt sick	Sometimes felt sick	Frequently felt sick
Cars					
Buses or coaches					
Trains					
Aircraft					
Small boats					
Ships, e.g. channel ferries					
Swings in playgrounds					
Roundabouts in playgrounds					
Big dippers, funfair rides					
	t	0	1	2	3

Your experience over the last 10 years (approximately), for each of the following types of transport or entertainment please indicate:
2. Over the last 10 years, how often you felt sick or nauseated (tick boxes):

	Not applicable— never travelled	Never felt sick	Rarely felt sick	Sometimes felt sick	Frequently felt sick
Cars					
Buses or coaches					
Trains					
Aircraft					
Small boats					
Ships, e.g. channel ferries					
Swings in playgrounds					
Roundabouts in playgrounds					
Big dippers, funfair rides					
	t	0	1	2	3

Behavioural countermeasures

Behavioural countermeasures to motion sickness may be broadly classified into habituation versus more immediate short-term behavioural modifications such as changes in body posture, visual attention, etc. Habituation offers the surest counter measure to motion sickness but by definition is a long-term approach. Habituation is superior to antimotion sickness drugs, and it is free of side effects (58). The most extensive habituation programmes, often denoted 'motion sickness desensitization', are run by the military, where antimotion sickness medication is contraindicated for pilots because of side effects including drowsiness and blurred vision. These programmes have success rates exceeding 85% (13) but can be extremely time consuming, lasting many weeks. Critical features include: 1) the massing of stimuli (exposures at intervals greater than a week almost prevents habituation), 2) use of graded stimuli to enable faster recoveries and more sessions to be scheduled, which may help avoid the opposite process of sensitization, and 3) maintenance of a positive psychological attitude to therapy (59).

Antimotion sickness drugs are of little use in this context, since both laboratory (60) and sea studies (61) show that although such medication may speed habituation compared to placebo in the short term, in the longer term it is disadvantageous. This is because when the antimotion sickness medication is discontinued, the medicated group relapses and is worse off than those who were habituated under placebo. Habituation, itself, is often stimulus specific, producing the problem of lack of generalization and transfer of habituation from one type of motion to another. Thus, to foster transfer, it is useful to use as wide a variety of provocative motions as possible (see Table 28.1 'Laboratory' stimuli). The studies by Kaufman (62) underline the specificity of habituation to different types of motion, with different anatomical patterns of neuronal functional changes (presumably reflecting learning) in the vestibule–olivo–cerebellar network to different classes of provocative stimuli. Neural structures such as the amygdala as well as such areas as the nucleus tractus solitarius are thought to be important in processes of induction of and habituation to motion sickness (63, 64). The scope of applications extends to habituation training to reduce motion sickness produced by short arm rotors intended to provide artificial gravity in future space flight (65). Research continues to optimize habituation approaches (39, 66, 67).

Immediate short-term behavioural counter measures include reducing head movements, aligning the head and body with GIF (4) or laying supine (33). However, such protective postures may be incompatible with task performance. It is usually better to be in control, i.e. to be the driver or pilot rather than a passenger (68). Obtaining a stable external horizon reference is helpful (69). With regard to the latter, a direct view out of a car window reduced sickness but a real-time video display of the view ahead failed to reduce sickness in rear-seat car passengers (70). Controlled regular breathing has been shown to increase significantly motion tolerance to provocative motion, being approximately half as effective as standard antimotion sickness drugs yet rapid to implement and free of side effects. The mechanism by which controlled breathing has its effect is uncertain but may involve activation of the known inhibitory reflex between respiration and vomiting (71, 72). Supplemental oxygen may be effective for reducing motion sickness in patients during ambulance transport. By contrast, it does not alleviate motion sickness in individuals who are otherwise healthy. This

apparent paradox is perhaps explained by the suggestion that supplemental oxygen may work by ameliorating a variety of internal states that sensitize for motion sickness (73). Some report acupuncture and acupressure to be effective against motion sickness (74). However, well-controlled trials find no evidence for their value (75). Anecdotally, modification of diet has been said to alter susceptibility to motion sickness. Unfortunately, the evidence is contradictory; for example, a recent study suggesting that protein-rich meals may inhibit motion sickness (76) may be contrasted with a study which drew the opposite conclusion that any meal of high protein or dairy foods 3–6 h prior to flight should be avoided to reduce airsickness susceptibility (77). It has been suggested that ginger (main active agent gingerol) acts to calm gastrointestinal feedback (78), but studies of its effects on motion sickness have been equivocal making it an unlikely potent antimotion sickness agent. For habitual smokers the temporary abstinence and consequent withdrawal from nicotine provides significant protection against motion sickness (79). Indeed this finding may explain why smokers are at reduced risk for PONV whereas non-smokers have elevated risk, the other main PONV risk factors being female sex, greater motion sickness susceptibility, and previous episodes of PONV. Temporary nicotine withdrawal perioperatively and consequent increased tolerance to sickness may explain why smokers have reduced risk for PONV (79).

Pharmacological countermeasures

Most of the drugs currently used against motion sickness were identified and proven over 40 years ago (80). They may be divided into the categories: antimuscarinics (e.g. scopolamine), H_1 antihistamines (e.g. dimenhydrate), and sympathomimetics (e.g. amphetamine). Commonly used antimotion sickness drugs are shown in Table 28.4. However, these drugs, alone or in combination (e.g. scopolamine + dexamphetamine) are only partially effective. The more recently developed potent antiemetics are not effective against motion sickness, including D_2 dopamine receptor antagonists and $5HT_3$ antagonists used for side effects of chemotherapy (81). This is probably because their sites of action may be at vagal afferent receptors or the brainstem chemoreceptor trigger zone (CTZ), whereas antimotion sickness drugs act elsewhere.

All antimotion sickness drugs can produce unwanted side effects, drowsiness being the most common. Promethazine is a classic example (58). Scopolamine may cause blurred vision in a minority of individuals, especially with repeated dosing. The antimotion sickness combination drug amphetamine + scopolamine (so-called 'scopdex') is probably the most effective with the fewest side-effects, at least for short-term use. This is because both scopolamine and amphetamine are proven antimotion sickness drugs, doubtless acting through different pathways so they have additive efficacy, and their side effects of sedation and stimulation cancel each other out. Unfortunately for legal reasons (drug abuse potential) the scopdex combination is no longer available apart from specialized military use. Although it is generally accepted that some drugs such as transdermal scopolamine or the calcium channel antagonist cinnarizine, are significantly less sedating than others (82), the consequent performance decrements may still not be acceptable in challenging occupations such as piloting aircraft.

Oral administration must anticipate motion since motion sickness induces gastric stasis consequently preventing drug absorption

Table 28.4 Common antimotion sickness drugs

Drug	Route	Adult dose	Time of onset	Duration of action (h)
Scopolamine	Oral	0.3–0.6 mg	30 min	4
Scopolamine	Injection	0.1–0.2 mg	15 min	4
Scopolamine	Transdermal patch	one	6–8 h	72
Promethazine	Oral	25–50 mg	2 h	15
Promethazine	Injection	25 mg	15 min	15
Promethazine	Suppository	25 mg	1 h	15
Dimenhydrinate	Oral	50–100 mg	2 h	8
Dimenhydrinate	Injection	50 mg	15 min	8
Cyclizne	Oral	50 mg	2 h	6
Cyclizne	Injection	50 mg	15 min	6
Meclizine	Oral	25–50 mg	2 h	8
Buclizne	Oral	50 mg	1 h	6
Cinnarizine	Oral	15–30 mg	4 h	8

Adapted from Benson (5).

by this route (83). Injection overcomes the various problems of slow absorption kinetics and gastric stasis or vomiting. Other routes such as transdermal also offer advantages providing protection for up to 72 h with low constant concentration levels in blood, thus reducing side effects. However, transdermal scopolamine has a very slow onset time (6–8 h), which can be offset by simultaneous administration of oral scopolamine enabling protection from 30 min onwards (84). There may be variability in absorption via the transdermal route which alters effectiveness between individuals (85). Buccal absorption is effective with scopolamine but an even faster route is via nasal scopolamine spray. Although not yet available for routine use, with higher (alkaline) pH buffered formulations to promote absorption, peak blood levels may be achieved in 9 min (86), and this route has been shown to be effective against motion sickness (87). 'Chewing gum' formulations offer the prospect of adequate motion sickness prophylaxis with reduced side effects compared to tablets, due to a more sustained release (88).

Investigations of new antimotion sickness drugs include re-examination of old drugs such as phenytoin, as well as the development of new agents such as neurokinin 1 antagonists. The range of drugs is wide and the list is long. Such drugs include phenytoin, betahistine, chlorpheniramine, cetirizine, fexofenadine, benzodiazepines and barbiturates, the antipsychotic droperidol, corticosteroids such as dexamethasone, tamoxifen, opioids such as the u-opiate receptor agonist loperamide, neurokinin NK_1 receptor antagonists, vasopressin V_{1a} receptor antagonists, N-methyl-D-aspartate (NMDA) antagonists, 3-hydroxypyridine derivatives, $5HT_{1a}$ receptor agonists such as the antimigraine triptan rizatriptan, selective muscarinic M_3/m5 receptor antagonists such as zamifenacin and darifenacin. So far none of these drugs have proven to be of any major advantage over those currently available for motion sickness (89). The reasons are various and include relative lack of efficacy, complex and variable pharmacokinetics, or in those that are effective, unacceptable side effects. Future development of drugs with highly selective affinities to receptor subtypes relevant to motion sickness may produce an antimotion sickness drug of high efficacy with few side-effects. A good candidate would be a selective antagonist for the M5 muscarinic receptor (90).

Motorists' (vestibular) disorientation

Introduction

A state of 'spatial disorientation' is created when sensory signals relating orientation and motion in space are inadequate or interpreted inappropriately with the potential consequence of dysfunctional behaviour. Although more familiar in the aerospace theatre (91), disorientation occurs also in road vehicles (92). Here, we describe individuals who suffer persistent and disabling disorientation when driving which usually manifests as a perceived threat of veering or rolling over (93). Few have identifiable diseases which could account for their symptoms although anxiety frequently appears to be a potential triggering factor in the development of disorientation. The symptoms of disorientation accord with an inappropriate interpretation of the complex sensory signals that arise from the complex, dynamic environment of modern highway motoring as a consequence of ambiguous force and motion signals (94). The misperceptions of orientation can be considered as a primitive naïve way of interpreting sensory signals whereas driving is a highly cognitive learned skill (95). As with disorientation in aviators, desensitization and retraining in a framework of cognitive therapy, relearning driving skills, is the treatment of choice.

Disorientation and road traffic incidents

The majority of motoring accidents are caused by loss of control attributable to attentional shifts, perhaps due to distraction, and inappropriate speed (96, 97). Spatial disorientation, arguably the most frequent cause of accidents involving aircraft (98, 99), is rarely considered by investigators as a possible causal factor in road traffic incidents (RTIs). This is undoubtedly a serious omission because maintenance of spatial orientation is a prime imperative and disorientation is a threat to survival. A moment's reflection on common and shared experience of the road illustrates how state of orientation determines attentional state. Consider driving at high speed in an orderly column of vehicles on a motorway. Since the relative speeds between vehicles are low with little demands on driving tactics and in a modern car, vibration and sound are minimized the awareness of speed is downregulated; the experience can even be relaxing. Now project oneself to be standing at the side of the motorway, viewing the traffic rushing past at 70 miles an hour a few metres distant: an alarming experience revealing the true speeds and dangers inherent in motorway driving. Such a degree of apprehension on the part of a driver would substantially modify driving behaviour. In this example, awareness of spatial orientation whilst driving is down regulated with the possible consequence that vigilance is lowered. Positive misperceptions of orientation in road vehicles may also influence driving manoeuvres leading to mishap.

Characteristics of spatial disorientation in road vehicles

Disorientation in vehicles, specifically cars, is a commonplace but a neglected phenomenon. It may affect driving by changing driving tactics or through effects on attention (97).

The steep hill

Many readers will have experienced the perception of extreme inclination ascending steep hills in a car; in extreme cases wondering if the climb is achievable. The steepness is an illusion: roads do not have extreme inclines; the steepest metalled roads in Europe involve only 18–20° of tilt above horizontal. The appearance of gradient derives from visual foreshortening, engine load, misperception of subjective tilt due to seated posture, and redistribution of blood volume from the legs to the trunk.

The tilted horizon

The sea horizon, the only true horizontal, may appear to be tilted when driving coastal roads involving steep hills and bends. Similarly, plains can appear tilted when viewed from mountain roads and rivers may appear to be flowing uphill. For example, the sea horizon tilt illusion is produced reliably in observers at 1° 51° 0.6^1 45.20^{11} N, 1° 12.10^1 16^{11} E on the A20 on the south coast of England which affords a view of the English Channel (visible on 'Google Earth' together with a photograph showing the sea to be apparently tilted). The apparent tilt of the horizon could be caused by both a visual 'frame effect' of the road and vehicle structure giving false cues to orientation and also by ocular counter-rolling of the eyes provoked by the lateral acceleration rounding a bend. Ocular counter-rolling, say to the left, induces an apparent rightwards tilt of the visual world; which the reader can verify by pressing gently inwards and upwards on the outer soft tissue of the orbit and observing the resulting the apparent tilt of the visual scene. Illusions of horizon tilt could induce the perception of rolling over in vehicles (100, 101) and may be part of the mechanism, evoked later in the chapter, explaining serious, persistent disorientation.

Apparent drift when stationary

A version of the railway train illusion of self-motion in a stationary carriage provoked by the sight of an adjacent moving train, illusory drift in a vehicle is often provoked when traffic is coming to a halt at a red light. Cars moving slowly on either side of one's own stationary vehicle can induce a perception of inappropriate self-motion, which is often countered by a reflex thrust on the brake. This is a manifestation of visually induced 'vection' (102).

Veering and rolling over

Inappropriate perceptions of threatened veering and rolling over are the dominant features of the 'motorist's vestibular disorientation syndrome' as first described by Page and Gresty (93). These symptoms are the main clinical topic of this article for they cause particular distress when they become a frequent experience, prompting the sufferer to seek medical opinion. In all the patients who have presented to our clinics over the years with complaints of disorientation during driving, perceptions of threatened veering and rolling are universal complaints with remarkably uniform characteristics. The inappropriate perceptions are so systematic and realistic that a number of patients reported changing cars before realizing that the problem was not one of individual vehicles' driving characteristics. The patients' experiences of veer and rolling described next are from the author's own history taking.

Feeling that the car is threatening to veer occurs typically on open fast roads such as motorways. Veering is usually to the side of the road (for both right- and left-hand side driving). It may also occur when traffic such as large trucks are passing by, in which case the threatened veer is into the traffic. Veering is rare on smaller roads, presumably because of the proximity of multiple surrounding cues to appropriate interpretation of orientation. Most often there is a threat of veering and the driver may believe that he has to hold the steering wheel to avoid a veer. In one instance of a female

taxi driver, a perceived threat of veering provoked an inappropriate steering correction leaving the driver facing the wrong way on the opposite side of the road. Threat of veering eventually (the actual time course of development is unclear) becomes a reliable occurrence on all open highways, thereby confining the driver to lesser town and suburban roads.

Perceptions of threatened rolling over occur on bends in the road; typically on fast open highways and apparently made worse if the bend is embedded in a hill descent. The perception is so alarming that the driver is compelled to slow down. In two patients interviewed the perceptions of threatened rolling on bends increased in frequency and generalized to all roads, eventually making driving impossible.

Prevalence

Precise documentation of prevalence of systematic disorientation during driving has not been reported. In 10 years' experience in a neuro-otological clinic in a London tertiary referral centre, the consultants had seen 4–5 patients per year with specific complaints of driving, amongst an average of 450–500 new patients referred with complaints of *dizziness of possible vestibular origin*. The caveat to be borne in mind for future surveys of prevalence is that spatial disorientation may be overlooked as a possible diagnosis.

Diagnosis

The characteristics of motorists ('vestibular') disorientation are so stereotypical that once reported, diagnosis is almost certain, with the obvious caveat that the *cause for the emergence of the symptoms* is not! Spatial disorientation in motorists may be missed or fail to be considered as a diagnosis in people with driving problems. For example, one female patient's complaints of veering had been dismissed by an otologist as a failure to realize that roads have a camber.

Patient characteristics

Disoriented drivers are typically young and middle-aged adults who drive frequently. The onset of disorientation is frequently marked by a single alarming episode; for example, in one patient a perception of extreme instability and veering when driving on a high motorway bridge which crosses the river Thames. Thereafter the subject becomes increasingly aware of disorientation until it becomes a reliable occurrence. The experience of disorientation is usually confined to driving but occasional sufferers also report disorientation when travelling as passengers. State anxiety can be identified in many but the level may not be exceptionally high. No relationship to motion sickness has been identified.

Illustrative case histories

A 36-year-old male 'on the road' rescue automobile engineer who spent all his working day on the road developed perceptions of threatened veering to the side of the road and rolling over when on bends when driving on motorways. He was well (a long history was available from his GP), neither drank alcohol nor smoked and denied any significant anxiety. He was slightly overweight, unfit, and admitted to a bad driving posture.

A 45-year-old male developed veering and threat of rolling over on highways he used to travel between work and home. Although physically well, he admitted to high anxiety due to failing in business and was retraining for a professional career.

A 30-year-old male, 'special forces' helicopter pilot when flying in mist developed a sensation of extreme instability. Thereafter he felt that the craft was about to 'tip out of the sky' with the slightest turbulence and he could not function as a pilot. The perception of instability extended to driving his car. He was extremely fit but had anxiety related to family relationships. A member of his wing had been recently beheaded by a rotor blade but he did not think this was particularly stressing: 'part of what you have trained for'. There were no findings on neurological and otological examination and testing.

A 30-year-old female developed disorientation when driving on major roads between work, home, and schools which rendered her unable to function. She had recently been deserted by her husband leaving her in sole responsibility for the family including having to drive the children to school and herself to work. The symptoms were not of general anxiety about driving. They were classified as motorist's disorientation because of stereotyped incidents of disorientation.

Comment: these cases illustrate the wide range of medical and social contexts within which patients have presented with motorist's disorientation. Driving rehabilitation would clearly have to be targeted within the context of therapy for anxiety, phobia, and lifestyle change according to individual patient needs.

Mechanisms

The symptoms described are not vague, reflective of general anxiety about driving. As with disorientation scenarios in flight, their characteristics and reproducibility point to specific mechanisms.

Page and Gresty (93) originally proposed that asymmetries of canal and otolithic function, unmasked by the general instability of the highway environment, were responsible for sensations of rolling over and veering. A demonstration of this possibility is that

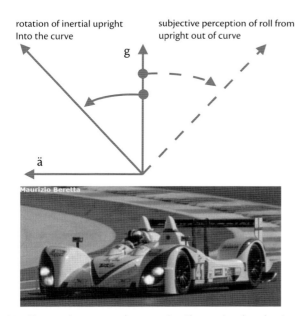

Fig. 28.1 Forces acting on a car when cornering. The centripetal acceleration causes a tilt of the inertial vertical into the bend. In terms of the inertial forces acting the driver is tilted away from inertial upright out of the bend. This possible resulting perception of tilt is suppressed by the cognitive framework of the car being held on the road by weight and its suspension (g = acceleration of gravity, ä centripetal acceleration). With kind permission of Maurizio Beretta and Martin Krejci.

patients with unilateral vestibular loss 'fly' flight simulators in an attitude tilted over to the side of lesion when exposed to simulated turbulence (103). However, although vestibular asymmetry may be a factor in some dizzy drivers, it is unlikely to be the predominate mechanism; otherwise many vestibular patients would experience similar symptoms, which is simply not the case. Similarly, tendencies to veer in one patient had been ascribed by an otologist to her scoliosis creating a potential source of misleading sensory input.

A perceived threat of rolling over is a well identified aspect of perceptions associated with lateral linear acceleration and tilt with respect to gravity (or an inertial force field) (104) and with rolling of the visual scene (100, 101). The lateral, 'centripetal', acceleration experienced when rounding a bend causes a tilt of the gravitoinertial vertical from earth upright to inclination in the direction of the centre of rotation. This earth tilted direction of the GIFs acting on the car is 'physical uprightness': witness the cyclist who leans into the bend to balance his bike; an attempt to remain earth upright would throw the bike and rider out of the bend. However, the weight and suspension of a four-wheeled vehicle keeps it oriented approximately earth upright. A driver normally learns to interpret the centripetal acceleration of cornering as a lateral force on his flank but an alternative perception and one which is feasible in physics, is that the driver is tilted out of the bend away from the gravitoinertial upright. The possibility of perceiving threatened rolling has some wisdom, for cornering at too high a speed will indeed result in the car rolling as road adhesion fails. It seems that some individuals come to interpret the sensory signals engendered by cornering in a vehicle as threatened rolling. This perception is perhaps facilitated by the lack of structure on open highways to reinforce the cognitive framework being in a vehicle which is maintained road and earth upright by weight and suspension (Figure 28.1). It is probably also facilitated by banking of the road, typical of motorway curves, which acts to protect against actual rolling at speed (105). Curiously, a perception of rolling in tilt from upright in a car on a bend is the more primitive, 'physiological' interpretation of sensations. Car drivers must *learn* to interpret sensory signals in terms of the framework of a car held to earth horizontal by a suspension and road adhesion (95).

A perception of threatened veering when the vehicle is at uniform speed on an open road is also likely to be provoked by visual stimulation, particularly since somatosensory cues to orientation may be masked by vibration, downregulated because of monotony and adapted because of immobility of the seated driver. Visual flow can induce body reorientations of which the protagonist is unaware, the visually induced perception of self-motion as experienced in the railway train illusion (102). Visual flow induces a sense of self-motion in the opposite direction to the flow which is some combination of rotation and linear translation. Vection is enhanced when the field of view contains a reference which is fixed to the subject, such as a finger held out in front of the eyes; in the case of a car this could be the frame of the windows and screen.

When proceeding at speed on an open straight highway the dominant rapid optic flow derives from the driver's view of the proximal road and roadside. Optic flow in the driver's view out of the opposite side of the car is of lower angular velocity and not so compelling. A possible perception induced in the driver is of a rotation away from the origin of the visual flow which is interpreted as veering. This effect is enhanced because the apparent size of objects is distorted by velocity and distance with more rapidly approaching objects seeming to be smaller (Helmholtz in James (102)). Alternatively, the driver may unconsciously correct the car's direction creating an actual veer, responding to subliminal cues to orientation (106). Passing traffic may enhance vection (Figure 28.2), in particular, overtaking traffic on the nearside provides an overall unidirectional motion of the visual field resulting in veering into the passing vehicles; a symptom often reported by sufferers. Traffic moving at the same speed may remove the vection potential of the view out of the nearside of the vehicle thus enhancing the vection induced by the view to the driver's side. Finally, any tendency to veer or perceive the threat of veering would be enhanced by road camber and perception that other vehicles, barriers, or road edges are perilously close.

Why do such symptoms emerge?

The patient histories described above demonstrate a wide spectrum of psychological and sociological comorbidities. Significant state anxiety is a frequent but not universal occurrence in patients complaining of disorientation during driving. Similarly, phobia is also implicated in some but by no means all patients (107, 108). In any case such psychological states would not alone explain the specificity of the symptoms.

The authors favour the hypothesis that perceptions of rolling and veering are alternative interpretations of the inherently ambiguous sensory information derived from the highway and vehicle environment. This interpretation is consistent with current concepts of interpretation of sensory input in terms of statistical likelihood (109) of correctness. Misperception of orientation within the context of vehicle and highway can be understood as reversion to primitive interpretations of the patterns of sensory input eschewing the cognitive framework that has been constructed when learning and practising driving and this may be the key to appropriate rehabilitation! All who experience vehicle motion are undoubtedly capable of perceiving motion in similar ways to these patients for such susceptibility is exploited in fairground rides. For some reason dizzy drivers are particularly susceptible to deconstruction of the cognitive framework of highway driving. It is not known how dizzy

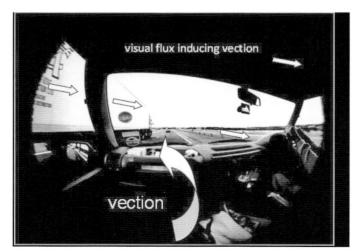

Fig. 28.2 A view taken with a fish-eye lens from within the cockpit of a car driving on a UK motorway and being overtaken by a truck. The dominant visual flow is to the driver's right inducing a perception of self-motion, 'vection' of the driver to the left with the result that he perceives that he may be turning into the truck.

drivers respond to other perceptual ambiguities, such as the Necker cube or visual frame effects.

Treatment

The model for driving rehabilitation is adopted from experience with rehabilitating pilots from disorientation during flight.

- Exclusion of organic disease.
- Treatment of general state anxiety/phobia.
- Explanation of how disorientation may occur. (Although our current understanding of how disorientation symptoms arise may be partially wrong, explanation of physiological principles has been found to be a useful anchor for treatment which the patients are willing to accept, at least as a way of illustrating how the senses can mislead.)
- Progressive desensitization following a planned, preferably written, schedule of driving commencing with short duration exposures driving on small local roads at quiet times and eventually progressing to long trips on the highway. This is done 'piece by piece', always stopping for 'time out' if driving becomes significantly stressful.
- Within each desensitization exposure the protagonist gives himself an explicit verbal briefing of the planned journey and talks himself through driving.
- During the session the protagonist gives himself a continual verbal appraisal of the actual road conditions and strengthens cognitive context. For example, if he feels his lane and be too narrow a check that the vehicle ahead negotiates the lane with ease assures the driver that he can follow; if he feels veering he checks the steering wheel and sides of the vehicle against lane markings.
- Anxiety is managed by stopping 'taking time out' by the roadside during which the driver seeks fresh air and performs anxiolytic controlled breathing and postural relaxation and undertakes exercises such as stretching.
- The driver should always adopt a 'command' posture, at the same time maintaining a relaxed muscle tone.
- A log should be kept of the progress of rehabilitation so that the sufferer can better objectify his experiences.

A note of caution: desensitization by 'immersion', the driver forcing himself to continue driving in one long session challenge, as advocated by some psychotherapists, is not to be recommended. Should disorientation fail to be resolved, anxiety, panic, and more severe disorientation may result with negative consequences for rehabilitation and safety. A female driver who persisted with long driving sessions on the recommendation of her therapist incurred a serious RTI which she attributed to overwhelming disorientation.

Implications for road safety

The authors recall only one serious accident resulting directly from a motorist's disorientation together with one report of veering across the centre of the road creating a potential for collision. It is likely that few significant incidents are reported because the experience of disorientation is so alarming that the driver slows or stops, thereafter proceeding with extreme caution. Currently there are no guidelines on fitness for dizzy drivers to drive.

References

1. Reason JT, Brand JJ (1975). *Motion sickness*. London: Academic Press.

2. Harsch V (2006). Centrifuge 'therapy' for psychiatric patients in Germany in the early 1800s. *Aviat Space Environ Med*, 77, 157–60.

3. Kennedy RS, Fowlkes JE (1992). Simulator sickness is polygenic and poly-symptomatic: Implications for research. *Int J Aviat Psychol*, 2, 23–38.

4. Golding JF, Bles W, Bos JE, Haynes T, Gresty MA (2003). Motion sickness and tilts of the inertial force environment: active suspension systems versus active passengers. *Aviat Space Environ Med*, 74, 220–7.

5. Benson AJ (2002). Motion sickness. In Pandolf K, Burr R (Eds) *Medical Aspects of Harsh Environments vol. 2*, pp. 1048–83. Washington, DC: Walter Reed Army Medical Center.

6. Stern RM, Koch KL, Leibowitz HW, Linblad IM, Shupert CL, Stewart WR (1985). Tachygastria and motion sickness. *Aviat Space Environ Med*, 56, 1074–7.

7. Eversmann T, Gottsmann M, Uhlich E, Ulbrecht G, von Werder K, Scriba PC (1978). Increased secretion of growth hormone, prolactin, antidiuretic hormone and cortisol induced by the stress of motion sickness. *Aviat Space Environ Med*, 49, 55.

8. Golding JF (1992). Phasic skin conductance activity and motion sickness. *Aviat Space Environ Med*, 63, 165–71.

9. Cheung B, Nakashima AM, Hofer KD (2011). Various anti-motion sickness drugs and core body temperature changes. *Aviat Space Environ Med*, 82, 409–15.

10. Hettinger LJ, Kennedy RS, McCauley ME (1990). Motion and human performance. In Crampton GH (Ed) *Motion and Space Sickness*, pp. 412–41. Boca Raton, FL: CRC Press.

11. Heer M, Paloski WH (2006). Space motion sickness: incidence, etiology, and countermeasures. *Auton Neurosci*, 129, 77–9.

12. Oman CM (1990). Motion sickness: a synthesis and evaluation of the sensory conflict theory. *Comp J Physiol Pharmacol*, 68, 294–303.

13. Benson AJ (1999). Motion sickness. In Ernsting J, Nicholson AN, Rainford DS (Eds) *Aviation Medicine*, pp. 455–71. Oxford: Butterworth Ltd.

14. Bos JE, Bles W (1998). Modelling motion sickness and subjective vertical mismatch detailed for vertical motions. *Brain Res Bull*, 47, 537–42.

15. Bubka A, Bonato F, Urmey S, Mycewicz D (2006). Rotation velocity change and motion sickness in an optokinetic drum. *Aviat Space Environ Med*, 77, 811–15.

16. Stott JRR (1986). Mechanisms and treatment of motion illness. In Davis CJ, Lake-Bakaar GV, Grahame-Smith DG (Eds) *Nausea and vomiting: mechanisms and treatment*, pp. 110–29. Berlin: Springer-Verlag.

17. ISO 2631 (1997). *International Standard ISO 2631–1:1997(E). Mechanical vibration and shock. Evaluation of human exposure to whole-body vibration. Part 1: General Requirements. 2nd ed. Corrected and reprinted.* Geneva: International Organization for Standardization.

18. O'Hanlon JF, McCauley ME (1974). Motion sickness incidence as a function of the frequency and acceleration of vertical sinusoidal motion. *Aviat Space Environ Med*, 45, 366–9.

19. Golding JF, Mueller AG, Gresty MA (2001). A motion sickness maximum around 0.2 Hz frequency range of horizontal translational oscillation. *Aviat Space Environ Med*, 72, 188–92.

20. Lawther A, Griffin MJ (1988). A survey of the occurrence of motion sickness amongst passengers at sea. *Aviat Space Environ Med*, 59, 399–406.

21. Von Gierke HE, Parker DE (1994). Differences in otolith and abdominal viscera graviceptor dynamics: implications for motion sickness and perceived body position. *Aviat Space Environ Med*, 65, 747–51.

22. Golding JF, Gresty MA (2005). Motion sickness. *Curr Opin Neurol*, 18, 29–34.

23. Gresty MA, Golding JF, Darwood A, Powar JS, Gresty J (2011). Do biomechanical constraints on human movement determine the frequency tuning of vehicular motions that provoke motion sickness ? *Aviat Space Environ Med*, 82, 242.

24. Triesman M (1977). Motion sickness: an evolutionary hypothesis. *Science*, 197, 493–95.

25. Morrow GR (1985). The effect of a susceptibility to motion sickness on the side effects of cancer chemotherapy. *Cancer*, 55, 2766–70.

26. Money KE, Cheung BS (1983). Another function of the inner ear: facilitation of the emetic response to poisons. *Aviat Space Environ Med*, 54, 208–11.

27. Yates BJ, Miller AD, Lucot JB (1998). Physiological basis and pharmacology of motion sickness: an update. *Brain Res Bull*, 47, 395–406.

28. Balaban CD (1999). Vestibular autonomic regulation (including motion sickness and the mechanism of vomiting). *Curr Opin Neurol*, 12, 29–33.

29. Nunn PWG (1881). Seasickness, its causes and treatment. *Lancet* ii, 1151–52.

30. Serrador JM, Schlegel TT, Black FO, Wood SJ (2005). Cerebral hypoperfusion precedes nausea during centrifugation. *Aviat Space Environ Med*, 76, 91–6.

31. Schelgel TT, Brown TE, Wood SJ, Benavides EW, Bondar RL, Stein F, Moradshahi P, Harm DL, Fritsch-Yelle JM, Low PA (2001). Orthostatic intolerance and motion sickness after parabolic flight. *J Appl Physiol*, 90, 67–82.

32. Radtke A, Popov K, Bronstein AM, Gresty MA (2003). Vestibular-autonomic control in man: short- and long- latency effects on cardiovascular function. *J Vestib Res*, 13, 25–37.

33. Golding JF, Markey HM, Stott JRR (1995). The effects of motion direction, body axis, and posture, on motion sickness induced by low frequency linear oscillation. *Aviat Space Environ Med*, 66, 1046–51.

34. Guedry FE, Rupert AR, Reschke MF (1998). Motion sickness and development of synergy within the spatial orientation system. A hypothetical unifying concept. *Brain Res Bull*, 47, 475–80.

35. Johnson WH, Sunahara FA, Landolt JP (1999). Importance of the vestibular system in visually induced nausea and self-vection. *J Vestib Res*, 9, 83–87.

36. Diamond SG, Markham CH (1991). Prediction of space motion sickness susceptibility by disconjugate eye torsion in parabolic flight. *Aviat Space Environ Med*, 62, 201–5.

37. Nachum Z, Shupak A, Letichevsky V, *et al.* (2004). Mal de debarquement and posture: reduced reliance on vestibular and visual cues. *Laryngoscope*, 114, 581–6.

38. Riccio GE, Stoffregen TA (1991). An ecological theory of motion sickness and postural instability. *Ecol Psych*, 3, 195–240.

39. Dai M, Raphan T, Cohen B (2011). Prolonged reduction of motion sickness sensitivity by visual-vestibular interaction. *Exp Brain Res*, 210, 503–13.

40. Furman JM, Marcus DA, Balaban CD (2011). Rizatriptan reduces vestibular-induced motion sickness in migraineurs. *J Headache Pain*, 12, 81–8.

41. Baloh RW (1998). Advances in neuro-otology. *Curr Opin Neurol*, 11, 1–3.

42. Drummond PD (2005). Effect of tryptophan depletion on symptoms of motion sickness in migraineurs. *Neurology*, 65, 620–2.

43. Brey RL (2005). Both migraine and motion sickness may be due to low brain levels of serotonin. *Neurology*, 65, E9–10.

44. Reavley CM, Golding JF, Cherkas LF, Spector TD, MacGregor AJ (2006). Genetic influences on motion sickness susceptibility in adult females: a classical twin study *Aviat Space Environ Med*, 77, 1148–52.

45. Finley JC Jr, O'Leary M, Wester D, *et al.* (2004). A genetic polymorphism of the alpha2-adrenergic receptor increases autonomic responses to stress. *J Appl Physiol*, 96, 2231–9.

46. Stern RM, Hu S, LeBlanc R, Koch KL (1993). Chinese hyper-susceptibility to vection-induced motion sickness. *Aviat Space Environ Med*, 64, 827–30.

47. Klosterhalfen S, Kellermann S, Pan F, Stockhorst U, Hall G, Enck P (2005). Effects of ethnicity and gender on motion sickness susceptibility. *Aviat Space Environ Med*, 76, 1051–7.

48. Kennedy RS, Lanham DS, Massey CJ, Drexler JM (1995). Gender differences in simulator sickness incidence: implications for military virtual reality systems. *SAFE J*, 25, 69–76.

49. Dobie T, McBride D, Dobie T Jr, May J (2001). The effects of age and sex on susceptibility to motion sickness. *Aviat Space Environ Med*, 72, 13–20.

50. Flanagan MB, May JG, Dobie TG (2005). Sex differences in tolerance to visually-induced motion sickness. *Aviat Space Environ Med*, 76, 642–6.

51. Javid FA, Naylor RJ (1999). Variables of movement amplitude and frequency in the development of motion sickness in Suncus murinus. *Pharmacol Biochem Behav*, 64, 115–22.

52. Golding JF, Kadzere PN, Gresty MA (2005). Motion sickness susceptibility fluctuates through the menstrual cycle. *Aviat Space Environ Med*, 76, 970–3.

53. Golding JF (1998). Motion sickness susceptibility questionnaire revised and its relationship to other forms of sickness. *Brain Res Bull*, 47, 507–16.

54. Turner M, Griffin MJ (1999). Motion sickness in public road transport: passenger behaviour and susceptibility. *Ergonomics*, 42, 444–61.

55. Cheung BSK, Money KE, Jacobs I (1990). Motion sickness susceptibility and aerobic fitness: a longitudinal study. *Aviat Space Environ Med*, 61, 201–4.

56. Gordon CR, Ben-Aryeh H, Spitzer O, Doweck A, Melamed Y, Shupak A (1994). Seasickness susceptibility, personality factors, and salivation. *Aviat Space Environ Med*, 65, 610–14.

57. Golding JF (2006). Predicting Individual Differences in Motion Sickness Susceptibility by Questionnaire. *Pers Indiv Dif*, 41, 237–48.

58. Cowings PS, Toscano WB (2000). Autogenic-feedback training exercise is superior to promethazine for control of motion sickness symptoms. *J Clin Pharmacol*, 40, 1154–65.

59. Yen Pik Sang F, Billar J, Gresty MA, Golding JF (2005). Effect of a novel motion desensitization training regime and controlled breathing on habituation to motion sickness. *Percept Mot Skills*, 101, 244–56.

60. Wood CD, Manno JE, Manno BR, Odenheimer RC, Bairnsfather LE (1986). The effect of antimotion sickness drugs on habituation to motion. *Aviat Space Environ Med*, 57, 539–42.

61. van Marion WF, Bongaerts MC, Christiaanse JC, Hofkamp HG, van Ouwerkerk W (1985). Influence of transdermal scopolamine on motion sickness during 7 days' exposure to heavy seas. *Clin Pharmacol Ther*, 38, 301–5.

62. Kaufman GD (2005). Fos expression in the vestibular brainstem: what one marker can tell us about the network. *Brain Res Rev*, 50, 200–211.

63. Nakagawa A, Uno A, Horii A, et al. (2003). Fos induction in the amygdala by vestibular information during hypergravity stimulation. *Brain Res*, 986, 114–23.

64. Pompeiano O, d'Ascanio P, Balaban E, Centini C, Pompeiano M (2004). Gene expression in autonomic areas of the medulla and the central nucleus of the amygdala in rats during and after space flight. *Neuroscience*, 124, 53–69.

65. Young LR, Sienko KH, Lyne LE, Hecht H, Natapoff A (2003). Adaptation of the vestibulo-ocular reflex, subjective tilt, and motion sickness to head movements during short-radius centrifugation. *J Vestib Res*, 13, 65–77.

66. Cheung B, Hofer K (2005). Desensitization to strong vestibular stimuli improves tolerance to simulated aircraft motion. *Aviat Space Environ Med*, 76, 1099–104.

67. Stroud KJ, Harm DL, Klaus DM (2005). Preflight virtual reality training as a countermeasure for space motion sickness and disorientation. *Aviat Space Environ Med*, 76, 352–6.

68. Rolnick A, Lubow RE (1991). Why is the driver rarely sick? The role of controllability in motion sickness. *Ergonomics*, 34, 867–79.

69. Bos JE, MacKinnon SN, Patterson A (2005). Motion sickness symptoms in a ship motion simulator: effects of inside, outside, and no view. *Aviat Space Environ Med*, 76, 1111–18.

70. Griffin MJ, Newman MM (2004). Visual field effects on motion sickness in cars. *Aviat Space Environ Med*, 75, 739–48.

71. Yen-Pik-Sang F, Billar JP, Golding JF, Gresty MA (2003). Behavioral methods of alleviating motion sickness: effectiveness of controlled breathing and music audiotape. *J Travel Med*, 10, 108–12.

72. Yen-Pik-Sang F, Golding JF, Gresty MA (2003). Suppression of sickness by controlled breathing during mild nauseogenic motion. *Aviat Space Environ Med*, 74, 998–1002.

73. Ziavra NV, Yen Pik Sang FD, Golding JF, Bronstein AM, Gresty MA (2003). Effect of breathing supplemental oxygen on motion sickness in healthy adults. *Mayo Clinic Proc*, 78, 574–8.

74. Bertalanffy P, Hoerauf K, Fleischhackl R, et al. (2004). Korean hand acupressure for motion sickness in prehospital trauma care: a prospective, randomized, double-blinded trial in a geriatric population. *Anesth Analg*, 98, 220–3.

75. Miller KE, Muth ER (2004). Efficacy of acupressure and acustimulation bands for the prevention of motion sickness. *Aviat Space Environ Med*, 75, 227–34.

76. Levine ME, Muth ER, Williamson MJ, Stern RM (2004). Protein-predominant meals inhibit the development of gastric tachyarrhythmia, nausea and the symptoms of motion sickness. *Aliment Pharmacol Ther*, 19, 583–90.

77. Lindseth G, Lindseth PD (1995). The relationship of diet to airsickness. *Aviat Space Environ Med*, 66, 537–41.

78. Lien HC, Sun WM, Chen YH, Kim H, Hasler W, Owyang C (2003). Effects of ginger on motion sickness and gastric slow-wave dysrhythmias induced by circular vection. *Am J Physiol Gastrointest Liver Physiol*, 284, G481–9.

79. Golding JF, Prosyanikova O, Flynn M, Gresty MA (2011). The effect of smoking nicotine tobacco versus smoking deprivation on motion sickness. *Autonomic Neurosci*, 160, 53–8.

80. Wood CD, Graybiel A (1969). Evaluation of 16 antimotion sickness drugs under controlled laboratory conditions. *Aerospace Med*, 39, 1341–4.

81. Levine ME, Chillas JC, Stern RM, Knox GW (2000). The effects of serotonin (5-HT3) receptor antagonists on gastric tachyarrhythmia and the symptoms of motion sickness. *Aviat Space Environ Med*, 71, 1111–4.

82. Gordon CR, Gonen A, Nachum Z, Doweck I, Spitzer O, Shupak A (2001). The effects of dimenhydrinate, cinnarizine and transdermal scopolamine on performance. *J Psychopharmacol*, 15, 167–72.

83. Stewart JJ, Wood MJ, Parish RC, Wood CD (2000). Prokinetic effects of erythromycin after antimotion sickness drugs. *J Clin Pharmacol*, 40, 347–53.

84. Nachum Z, Shahal B, Shupak A, et al. (2001). Scopolamine bioavailability in combined oral and transdermal delivery. *J Pharmacol Exp Ther*, 296, 121–3.

85. Gil A, Nachum Z, Dachir S, et al. (2005). Scopolamine patch to prevent seasickness: clinical response vs. plasma concentration in sailors. *Aviat Space Environ Med*, 76, 766–70.

86. Ahmed S, Sileno AP, deMeireles JC, et al. (2000). Effects of pH and dose on nasal absorption of scopolamine hydrobromide in human subjects. *Pharm Res*, 17, 974–7.

87. Simmons RG, Phillips JB, Lojewski RA, Wang Z, Boyd JL, Putcha L (2010). The efficacy of low-dose intranasal scopolamine for motion sickness. *Aviat Space Environ Med*, 81, 405–12.

88. Seibel K, Schaffler K, Reitmeir P (2002). A randomised, placebo-controlled study comparing two formulations of dimenhydrinate with respect to efficacy in motion sickness and sedation. *Arzneimittelforschung*, 52, 529–36.

89. Golding JF (2006). Motion sickness susceptibility. *Autonomic Neurosci*, 30, 67–76.

90. Golding JF, Stott JRR (1997). Comparison of the effects of a selective muscarinic receptor antagonist and hyoscine (scopolamine) on motion sickness, skin conductance and heart rate. *Br J Clin Pharmacol*, 43, 633–7.

91. Benson AJ, Stott JRR (2006). Spatial disorientation in flight. In Rainford DR, Gradwell DP (Eds) *Ernsting's Aviation Medicine*, pp 433–58. London: Hodder Education.

92. NATO RT-MPO-086 HFM (2002). Spatial Disorientation in Military Vehicles: Causes, Consequences and Cures RTO-MP-086 AC/323(HFM-085)TP/42. RTO Human Factors and Medicine Panel (HFM). Symposium held in La Coruña, Spain, 15–17 April 2002.

93. Page NGR Gresty MA (1985). Motorist's vestibular disorientation syndrome. *J Neurol Neurosurg Psychiat*, 48, 729–35.

94. Probst T, Straube A, Bles W (1985). Differential effects of ambivalent visual-vestibular-somatosensory stimulation on the perception of self-motion. *Behav Brain Res*, 16, 71–9.

95. Wertheim AH, Mesland BS, Bles W (2001). Cognitive suppression of tilt sensations during linear horizontal self-motion in the dark. *Perception*, 30, 733–41.

96. The 100-Car Naturalistic Driving Study (2005). Virginia Tech Transportation Institute (VTTI) and sponsored by the National Highway Traffic Safety Administration (NHTSA). Report available from Virginia Tech, Virginia Department of Transportation (VDOT), and Virginia Transportation Research Council (VTRC).

97. Liang Y, Lee JD (2010). Combining cognitive and visual distraction: Less than the sum of its parts. *Acid Anal Prev*, 42, 881–90.

98. Li G, Baker SP, Grabowski JG, Rebok GW (2001). Factors associated with pilot error in aviation crashes. *Aviat Space Environ Med*, 72, 52–8.

99. Matthews RJS, Previc F, Bunting A. USAF Spatial Disorientation Survey. NATO RT-MPO-086 HFM (2002). *Spatial Disorientation in Military Vehicles: Causes, Consequences and Cures*, Chapter 7, pp. 1–13. NATO.

100. Dichgans J, Held R, Young LR, Brandt T (1972). Moving visual scenes influence the apparent direction of gravity. *Science*, 178, 1217–9.

101. Previc FH, Kenyon, RV, Boer, ER, Johnson, BH (1993). The effects of background visual roll stimulation on postural and manual control and self-motion perception. *Perception Psychophys*, 54, 93–107.

102. James W (1892). *Psychology. The Briefer Course*. Chapter 11, Perception, pp. 187–8. New York: Henry Holt. Reproduced by Dover, Toronto, 2001.

103. Aoki M, Ito Y, Burchill P, Brookes GB, Gresty MA (1999). Tilted perception of the subjective 'upright' in unilateral loss of vestibular function. *Am J Otol*, 20, 741–7.

104. Lichtenberg BK, Young LR, Arrott AP (1982). Human ocular counter-rolling induced by varying linear accelerations. *Exp Brain Res*, 48, 127–36.

105. Previc FH, Varner DC, Gillingham KK (1992). Visual scene effects on the somatogravic illusion. *Aviat Space Environ Med*, 63, 1060–64.

106. K. Mogg, B.Bradley (1998). A cognitive-motivational analysis of anxiety. *Behav Res Ther*, 36, 809–48.

107. Brandt T, Huppert D, Dieterich M (1994). Phobic postural vertigo: a first follow-up. *J Neurol*, 241, 191–5.

108. Brandt T (1996). Phobic postural vertigo. *Neurology*, 46, 1515–19.

109. MacNeilage PR, Banks MS, Berger DR, Bülthoff HH (2007). A Bayesian model of the disambiguation of gravito-inertial force by visual cues. *Exp Brain Res*, 179, 263–90.

CHAPTER 29

Fits, Faints, Funny Turns, and Falls in the Differential Diagnosis of the Dizzy Patient

Alexander A. Tarnutzer and
David E. Newman-Toker

Introduction

Clinicians who evaluate patients with vestibular disorders or vertigo are often faced with patients who have atypical 'spells,' loss of consciousness, or unexplained falls. In such cases, there is often uncertainty about the underlying cause. Vestibular or balance disorders are almost always part of the differential diagnosis, but these are accompanied by cardiovascular, neurological, and psychiatric disorders that can produce similar symptoms. Some of these problems are benign (e.g. vasovagal syncope), although others are more dangerous and urgent (e.g. transient ischaemic attack (TIA)). The challenge for the vestibular clinician is to identify which patients are likely to have non-vestibular causes and to determine the most appropriate referral and degree of urgency. Sometimes this is easy, but sometimes the distinction is less obvious. For instance, patients with underlying cardiac causes may present with true spinning vertigo more often than previously imagined (1, 2), or those with benign paroxysmal positional vertigo (BPPV) may present with postural lightheadedness, near faint, and imbalance that could be mistaken for orthostatic hypotension (3, 4). The difficulty in diagnosis has led some groups to create multidisciplinary diagnostic clinics for the assessment of falls and syncope (3).

This chapter presents a framework for approaching the adult patient with 'fits, faints, funny turns, or falls.' We begin with definitions, symptom prevalence, and general diagnostic considerations before offering an overall approach to diagnosis for three major categories of patients: 1) those with transient loss of consciousness (TLOC) with or without dizziness or vertigo, 2) those with transient dizziness, vertigo, or presyncope without clear loss of consciousness, and 3) those with unexplained falls. We consider the differential diagnosis within each category. Where possible, we identify specific history and examination features that predict the underlying aetiology; particularly those that help differentiate benign from dangerous causes. We close with some general recommendations about diagnostic testing, referrals, and instructions for patients (e.g. regarding driving or other activities).

Definitions

Most clinicians are familiar with terms such as 'syncope', 'seizure', and 'drop attacks', but consistent use of such terminology is the exception rather than the rule. Recently, attempts have been made by various international expert working-groups to develop consensus definitions for many of these terms. Box 29.1 offers definitions used in this chapter, relying on consensus definitions whenever possible. In particular, we emphasize use of definitions proposed by the International Classification of Vestibular Disorders (ICVD), currently being developed by the Classification Committee of the Bárány Society (5). For example, the terms dizziness and vertigo are usually defined separately in Europe, while American use of these terms identifies dizziness as an umbrella term that includes vertigo as a subset (5). We have followed ICVD practice here and define them separately. Different authors have used the term *drop attack* variably, sometimes in a broad way that includes falls with TLOC and sometimes in a very narrow way referring only to a specific clinical presentation of falls without TLOC in middle-aged women (6). Unlike cardiologists, neurologists, and generalist physicians, neuro-otologists often restrict 'drop attacks' to falls resulting from vestibular disorders. Because of this ambiguity, and in accordance with ICVD terminology, drop attacks of apparent vestibular origin are categorized as either balance-related falls or balance-related near falls, but the term 'drop attack' is generally avoided (5).

Box 29.1 Glossary of key terms related to 'fits, faints, funny turns, and falls'*

Cataplexy
Sudden loss of muscle tone resulting from strong emotions. It is common in narcolepsy, otherwise called narcolepsy–cataplexy. The emotional trigger is usually laughter such that cataplexy occurs either when hearing a joke or telling one. The loss of tone has a cephalo-caudal progression, beginning in (and sometimes only present in) the muscles of the face and neck (7, 8).

Concussion
A complex pathophysiological process affecting the brain, induced by traumatic biomechanical forces. Several common features that incorporate clinical, pathological, and biomechanical injury constructs that may be utilized in defining the nature of a concussive head injury include: 1) concussion may be caused either by a direct blow to the head, face, neck, or elsewhere on the body with an 'impulsive' force transmitted to the head; 2) concussion typically results in the rapid onset of short-lived impairment of neurological function that resolves spontaneously; 3) concussion may result in neuropathological changes but the acute clinical symptoms largely reflect a functional disturbance rather than a structural injury; 4) concussion results in a graded set of clinical symptoms that may or may not involve loss of consciousness. Resolution of the clinical and cognitive symptoms typically follows a sequential course, however, it is important to note that in a small percentage of cases post-concussive symptoms may be prolonged; 5) no abnormality on standard structural neuroimaging studies is seen in concussion (9).

Directional pulsion
Feeling of being unstable with a tendency to veer or fall in a particular direction while seated, standing, or walking. The direction should be specified as latero-, retro, or anteropulsion. If lateropulsion, the direction (right or left) should be specified (5). If there is no specific directional bias to the sensation, it is referred to as *unsteadiness* (see later definition). Directional pulsion may predispose to falls.

Dizziness
Sensation of disturbed or impaired spatial orientation without a false or distorted sense of motion (5). This term includes sensations sometimes referred to as *giddiness, lightheadedness*, or *non-specific dizziness*, but does not include *vertigo* (5).

Drop attack
A sudden fall without loss of consciousness (10, 11). The term 'drop attack' is variably used for Ménière's disease, atonic epileptic seizures, and unexplained falls (11). Some authors have adopted a very narrow usage to describe rare subpopulations (6), while others include any fall associated with loss of consciousness (12). Ambiguous and inconsistent application in the literature has led to its non-use in consensus definitions for vestibular symptoms (5). In this review, we generally avoid using the term 'drop attacks' and primarily substitute the terms 'sudden' or 'unexplained' falls, as appropriate (see definition of 'fall').

Fall
Loss of postural stability from an upright, antigravity position or posture (e.g. standing or sitting), generally resulting in an uncontrolled, gravity-driven postural shift. *Completed falls* are usually terminated by uncontrolled impact with immovable objects such as the floor, and often result in physical injury. *Near falls* are 'caught' (i.e. self-corrected before undesired impact, as by a reflexive postural correction or deliberate outstretched arm) (5). A *balance-related fall* is one related to strong unsteadiness, directional pulsion, or other vestibular symptom (e.g. vertigo) (5). We here define a *sudden* fall as one with absent or brief (seconds) prodrome or warning. We further define an *unexplained* fall as one without obvious environmental (e.g. collision, slip, trip) or symptomatic (e.g. TLOC, severe vertigo) cause.

Otolithic crisis (also 'Tumarkin's otolithic crisis' or 'Tumarkin's crisis')
Sudden fall without loss of consciousness ('drop attack') of vestibular origin (13). These events are presumed secondary to aberrant signalling in the otolithic graviceptive afferents from the vestibular system. Patients sometimes experience strong directional pulsion as if being pushed over or drawn to the floor (5), resulting in what we here refer to as a 'symptomatic balance-related fall'. In other cases, the fall is associated with an unheralded lapse of postural tone and the link to a vestibular/otolithic pathogenesis is merely inferred. In keeping with consensus recommendations (5), we generally avoid using the term 'otolithic crisis' and refer to this latter group instead as 'sudden, balance-related falls' if the link to a vestibular or otolithic pathogenesis has been established with confidence.

Presyncope (also 'near syncope' or 'faintness')
Sensation of impending loss of consciousness (5). This sensation may or may not be accompanied by a completed syncope. When followed by syncope, the presyncope is one of several possible prodromal symptoms. Although the definition for completed syncope incorporates a mechanistic understanding, presyncope is defined here without regard to underlying cause or mechanism.

Seizure (also 'fit')
Transient and short-lived attack linked to an abnormal excessive or synchronous neuronal activity in the brain (14). Seizures resulting in loss of consciousness are generalized or complex partial events, since simple partial seizures, by definition, involve no alteration of consciousness (15). *Psychogenic non-epileptic seizures*, also known as *pseudo-seizures*, are non-epileptic paroxysmal events without an organic or somatic cause. They consist of paroxysmal behavioural, motor, or sensory episodes associated with a variety of other phenomena (e.g. vocalizations, crying, other expressions of emotion) that do not result from abnormal electrical activity of the brain (16). These non-epileptic events may cause apparent unconsciousness.

Startle reaction
Motor response to a surprising stimulus. The normal reaction to a surprising stimulus is a sudden increase in muscle tone, and a *pathological startle reaction* (as in the clinical syndrome of hyperekplexia) involves a gross increase in muscle activity. Some authors have also included sudden *loss* of tone in their definition of pathological startle reactions (7, 17). This approach, however, muddles the distinction with cataplexy, so we restrict the definition here to cases with reflexively *increased* postural tone. These alterations of muscular tone due to startle may result in loss of postural stability and falls.

(Continued)

Syncope (also 'Faint')

TLOC due to transient global cerebral hypoperfusion characterized by rapid onset, short duration, and spontaneous complete recovery (11). Syncope usually leads to loss of postural control and falling. This definition clearly distinguishes between syncope and other causes of TLOC such as seizure and brain concussion as well as falls that occur without TLOC (e.g. slip/trip). *Convulsive syncope* presents with brief involuntary, non-rhythmic and multifocal jerking movements of the limbs (myoclonus) after the TLOC and may be mistaken for a generalized seizure (18). *Pseudo-syncope* represents an apparent loss of consciousness without transient global cerebral hypoperfusion that is caused by psychiatric disease or other psychogenic factors (19).

Transient ischaemic attack (TIA)

A transient episode of neurological dysfunction caused by focal brain, spinal cord, or retinal ischaemia, without acute infarction and with return to normal neurological function (20). This definition does not identify or restrict the duration of the episode, abandoning the previous definition's 24-h limitation (20). It generally requires neuroimaging and excludes any patient with clinical, radiographic, or pathological evidence of completed infarction who is then said to have 'stroke' rather than TIA. When symptoms are transient or mild and imaging reveals a stroke, the preferred term is now *minor stroke*, and when diagnostic uncertainty exists as to the presence of infarction (but not the cerebrovascular aetiology), the term *acute neurovascular syndrome* is now recommended (20).

Transient loss of consciousness (TLOC)

A transient, self-limited loss of consciousness, usually leading to falling (21). Unconsciousness that is transient but post-traumatic (e.g. concussion) is excluded, as are states of unconsciousness that are not self-limited (e.g. coma). A distinction is made between 'true' (e.g. syncope, generalized seizure, basilar TIA, hypoglycaemia) and 'apparent' (e.g. otological drop attacks/falls, spinal cord TIA, cataplexy, psychogenic

pseudo-syncope) loss of consciousness, although it is acknowledged that this distinction cannot always be made confidently in clinical practice due to lack of medical history or confusing clinical features (11).

Transient neurological deficit (TND) (also 'transient neurological episode' (20) or 'attack' (22))

A transient episode of neurological dysfunction, generally lasting less than 24 h. The neurological dysfunction may be 'focal' (e.g. hemiparesis, aphasia) or 'non-focal' (e.g. dizziness, confusion). The definition for TND used here is neutral with respect to the underlying aetiology, and spells may be linked to various pathomechanisms, including those associated with hypoperfusion (e.g. syncope, TIA), primary electrical disturbance (e.g. seizure, migraine), and abnormal mechanical states (e.g. concussion, canalolithiasis).

Unsteadiness

Feeling of being unstable while seated, standing, or walking without a particular directional preference (5). If there is specific directional bias to the sensation, it is referred to as *directional pulsion* (see earlier definition). Unsteadiness may predispose to falls.

Vertigo

The sensation of self-motion when no self-motion is occurring or to the sensation of distorted self-motion during an otherwise normal head movement. This includes both false spinning sensations (spinning vertigo) and other false sensations of motion such as swaying, tilting, bobbing, bouncing, or sliding (non-spinning vertigo) (5). When spatial orientation is disturbed without a false sense of motion, the term *dizziness* is instead applied.

* Authors fond of alliterative titles have combined patients with related symptoms under headings such as 'fits, faints, and funny turns' (18, 23, 24). *Fits* and *faints* refer to seizures and syncope, respectively. *Funny turns* are typically the least well defined (23), but may include spells of dizziness, vertigo, or related balance complaints.

Readers should note that some of these terms are defined as pure symptoms (e.g. dizziness, vertigo, TND), while others combine clinical phenomenology with mechanistic understanding (e.g. concussion, seizure, syncope, TIA). In the latter case, an initial diagnostic assessment must be completed before the patient can appropriately be categorized, and the classification is subject to subsequent revision based on additional diagnostic testing (e.g. an event initially referred to as a 'seizure' might later be reclassified as a 'syncope,' or vice versa).

Some nuances of these clinical categories are worth noting. First, there is not an obligate, one-to-one directional relationship between TLOC and falls. A *fall* occurs only while upright and unsupported (whether associated with TLOC or not), but TLOC may occur even lying down (e.g. in the case of blood donors (25)). Thus, TLOC only results in symptomatic loss of postural stability when adequate postural/motor tone is required to stabilize the patient's physical position. Conversely, many falls are not caused by TLOC (18), but are linked instead to a disturbance of posture related to other internal (e.g. vertigo, directional pulsion,

cataplexy) or external (e.g. accidental collisions, slips/trips) factors (19, 26). Second, 'true' and 'apparent' TLOC may be difficult to distinguish based on available historical information, since patients may be uncertain and witnesses may be unavailable or only offer uninformative descriptions of the event. In some cases, even direct expert clinical observation during an episode may be inadequate to discern true from apparent unconsciousness (e.g. in some cases of non-epileptic seizures (27)). Complicating matters further, the temporal sequence of events and the causal relationship between TLOC and fall, even when both are known to have occurred, may also be difficult to discern. TLOC may precede a fall (i.e. TLOC causes fall) and similar transient unconsciousness may follow a fall (i.e. fall causes transient unconsciousness, generally due to head trauma with concussion). Amnesia resulting either from the TLOC itself or concussion may obscure the order of events and make it difficult to determine the direction of causality. Figure 29.1 demonstrates a conceptual model for the relationships among terms linked to real or apparent loss of consciousness and falls.

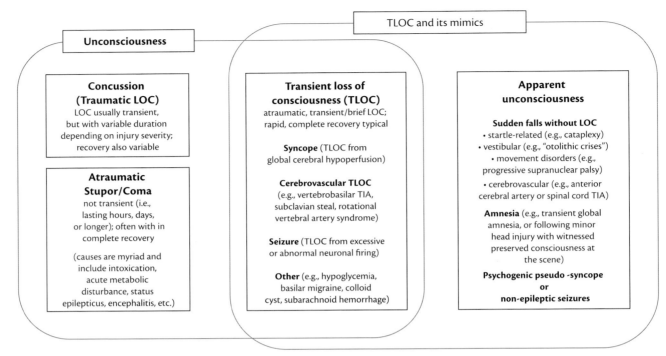

Fig. 29.1 Relationships among different categories of impaired consciousness and mimics with respect to duration (transient vs. prolonged unconsciousness) and mechanism (e.g. traumatic vs. atraumatic). Adapted from Thijs et al. (21). For detailed definitions of individual terms, see Box 29.1. LOC, loss of consciousness; TIA, transient ischaemic attack; TLOC, transient loss of consciousness.

General diagnostic considerations

Epidemiology and diagnostic approach

'Fits, faints, funny turns, and falls' are frequent complaints in daily practice across settings, but particularly in frontline healthcare settings such as the emergency department (ED). Seizures account for an estimated 0.6% of ED visits (28) with about half of these visits (0.3%) linked to a first ever seizure (14). Syncope accounts for another 0.9–1.7% of ED referrals (11, 29). Roughly 3–6% of US ED visits (and a similar fraction of primary care visits) are attributed to dizziness or vertigo (30, 31). In a nationally representative sample, the annual rate for fall-related ED-visits (including syncope- or seizure-related falls) was 3.1 per 100 persons, corresponding to 9% of all ED visits (32). Thus, more than one of every ten ED patients is affected by one or more of these clinical presentations.

The differential diagnoses for seizures ('fits'), syncope ('faints'), dizziness/vertigo ('funny turns'), and unexplained falls are broad and partially overlapping. Regardless of the category, benign, self-limited conditions that do not require an extensive work-up must be distinguished from acute, life-threatening causes where immediate, correct management affects outcome (Table 29.1). Because dangerous underlying causes are not rare in patients with these symptoms, early and accurate risk stratification should be a major focus of initial diagnostic evaluation (29, 33, 34). In addition to determining acute management, proper diagnosis is essential to reduce fall recurrence and resulting injuries, and to prevent subsequent morbidity or mortality from the underlying disease causing the initial clinical presentation (19, 35). Because of the high prevalence of these symptoms in clinical practice, the approach to bedside diagnostic assessment and laboratory testing must generally also be efficient and parsimonious.

The general approach to the patient with 'fits, faints, funny turns, or falls' requires first determining whether the patient suffered TLOC (Figure 29.1). Those with clear TLOC usually have seizure or syncope, which must be distinguished from one another. Guidelines for the specific diagnostic approach to a patient with seizure (14) or syncope (11) have been developed by expert panels and are discussed in greater detail in the sections that follow. Some consideration must also be given to cerebrovascular and other uncommon causes, particularly when dizziness or vertigo is present as a prodromal symptom and especially when residual neurological deficits are present after consciousness is regained.

For those without clear TLOC but who suffer brief, atypical 'spells' or 'funny turns,' most have underlying benign vestibular or benign cardiovascular causes, but dangerous diseases (especially TIA and cardiac arrhythmia) must be considered, as in those with TLOC. As yet, no fully developed diagnostic guidelines are available for unselected patients with 'funny turns,' although recent evidence syntheses for the diagnosis and management of BPPV (36, 37) mark an important milestone towards more general diagnostic guidance. In this chapter we offer some basic principles of diagnosis for this latter group but refer readers to other chapters for a more detailed treatment of the approach to specific vestibular disorders.

Those presenting with falls may be thought of as having environmental, symptomatic, or unexplained falls (Figure 29.2), discussed in greater detail in the sections that follow. We are not aware of any consensus standards for the diagnostic approach to unexplained falls. Key disorders likely to present clinically with unexplained falls are described in greater detail below, along with more specific suggestions for diagnostic evaluation of these patients. Patients with unexplained TLOC or falls after bedside clinical assessment may undergo a variety of diagnostic tests to help identify the underlying

Table 29.1 Causes of 'fits, faints, funny turns, and falls' by degree of medical urgency

	Benign or less urgent	Dangerous or more urgent
TLOC with or without vertigo or dizziness	**Seizures** ('idiopathic') • Idiopathic generalized seizures (e.g. atonic, myoclonic–astatic)[a] • Idiopathic focal seizures with secondary generalization **Syncope** • Reflex syncope • Vasovagal syncope • Situational syncope • Carotid sinus syncope • Orthostatic syncope • Medication-related • Chronic autonomic failure (e.g. multiple systems atrophy, diabetes mellitus) **Other true or apparent TLOC** • Cerebrovascular • Subclavian steal syndrome • Rotational vertebral artery syndrome • Other structural/functional • Chiari malformation, type I • Basilar migraine • Hyperventilation syndrome • Psychogenic pseudo-syncope or non-epileptic seizures[a]	**Seizures** ('symptomatic') • Encephalitis (e.g. herpetic) • Hypoglycaemia, hyperglycaemia • Stroke, intracranial haemorrhage • Intracranial neoplasm **Syncope** • Cardiopulmonary • Cardiac arrhythmia • Myocardial ischaemia • Structural heart disease • Pulmonary embolism • Aortic dissection • Orthostatic syncope • Hypovolaemia (haemorrhage, diuretics, severe diarrhoea) **Other true or apparent TLOC** • Cerebrovascular • Vertebrobasilar TIA[b] • Carotid artery occlusion[c] • Subarachnoid haemorrhage • Other structural/functional • Obstructive hydrocephalus (e.g. colloid cyst) • Metabolic (e.g. hypoxia, hypoglycaemia) • Neuroendocrine neoplasm
Transient vertigo or dizziness without TLOC	As with TLOC[d] plus… • Simple partial seizures (e.g. focal sensory seizure) • Vestibular conditions (e.g. vestibular migraine, Ménière's disease, benign paroxysmal positional vertigo) • Autonomic conditions (e.g. initial orthostatic hypotension, postural orthostatic tachycardia syndrome, postprandial hypotension) • Other (panic attack, drug intoxication)	As with TLOC[d] plus… • Urgent vestibular conditions (e.g. bacterial labyrinthitis, autoimmune inner ear disease, perilymphatic fistula)
Unexplained falls without TLOC	'Other' category from TLOC[d] plus… • Simple partial seizures (e.g. focal motor seizure) • Vestibular conditions (e.g. Ménière's disease, vestibular migraine, superior canal dehiscence syndrome) • Motor tone disorders (cataplexy, hyperekplexia, focal dystonia) • Neurodegenerative postural disorders (e.g. Parkinson's disease, progressive supranuclear palsy) • Psychogenic gait disorder/falls • Cryptogenic falls	'Other' category from TLOC[d] plus… • Acute dystonic reactions (e.g. neuroleptic-induced)

TIA, transient ischaemic attack; TLOC, transient loss of consciousness

[a] Likely to present with TLOC or unexplained falls but unlikely to complain of vertigo or dizziness.

[b] The prevalence of TIA-related syncope is uncertain, since many studies deliberately exclude patients with focal neurological symptoms. Series of patients presenting with acute syncope where neurological symptoms were not uniformly excluded a priori have found rates of TIA-related syncope as low as 0.4% and as high as 8% (141, 142).

[c] In carotid occlusion there may be true or apparent TLOC. True TLOC may result from carotid sinus distension with resulting reflex syncope or from global cerebral hypoperfusion in the context of marginal cerebrovascular reserve (e.g. with combined bilateral carotid and basilar stenoses). Apparent TLOC may result from sudden falls due to leg weakness or amnesia related to transient aphasia.

[d] Almost all of the disorders listed in the 'TLOC' row (TLOC with or without vertigo or dizziness) may also present with vertigo, dizziness, or presyncope, but without frank TLOC. Some of these disorders (listed as 'Other' than Seizure or Syncope) may also present with unexplained falls without TLOC.

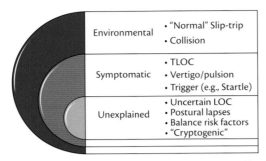

Fig. 29.2 The spectrum of falls. Many falls are purely environmental (without disease), many are symptomatic (with disease), and relatively few lack an obvious cause.

cause such as tilt table testing, prolonged ambulatory electrocardiography (ECG) or event monitoring, and video-electroencephalography (video-EEG).

Principles of bedside history and examination

In the following sections we address the causes and diagnostic evaluation of TLOC ('fits and faints'), atypical spells of dizziness or vertigo ('funny turns'), and unexplained falls, focusing wherever possible on symptoms and signs that allow a distinction between the most frequent and the most dangerous underlying causes. While not all diagnoses may be made confidently at the bedside, a detailed history about the event and a clinical examination is often the cornerstone for achieving a final diagnosis. Key elements of the history and exam must determine the choice and urgency of any advanced diagnostic testing that follows. Some general principles of bedside inquiry are described in the paragraph that follows.

The patient should be asked if she can recall all the details of the event or if there is a gap in memory for events (i.e. amnesia). The patient should be asked about the timeline (e.g. prior episodes and their frequency; rapidity of onset and episode duration) and context of the event (e.g. activity and posture at the onset; presence of prodromal symptoms; and any apparent triggers). Particularly when amnesia for the event is present, directly asking the patient about the presence of TLOC may be less informative than asking witnesses, since the patient may not remember or even take notice of having been unconscious (38, 39). Whenever possible, eyewitnesses should be interviewed about the event to help determine if the patient lost responsiveness or consciousness. Specific inquiry should be made about whether the patient uttered any vocalizations, made any gestures, or tried to steady themselves at the onset of the event; had abnormal eye, eyelid, face, mouth, jaw, or limb movements; or manifested changes in overall appearance, skin colour/temperature, postural tone (e.g. stiff, flaccid, or both). When available, acute measurements of pulse, blood pressure, or cardiac rhythm should be sought. If the patient believes an episode can be replicated at the bedside, this should be attempted under controlled conditions with the necessary safety precautions in place (e.g. to prevent a fall; or monitor and reverse a life-threatening cardiac arrhythmia, should it occur). The remainder of the examination should be targeted to the suspected cause or mechanism, although, generally, this should include bedside tests across organ systems (i.e. cardiovascular, neurological, and oto-vestibular signs) rather than being restricted to one.

Transient loss of consciousness with or without dizziness/vertigo

In this section we discuss the epidemiology, pathogenesis, clinical presentation, differential diagnosis, and bedside approach to the patient with a clear history of loss of consciousness, whether or not the patient experienced a prodrome comprising dizziness, vertigo, or other neurological symptoms, and whether or not the event led to a fall. We avoid discussion of those with clear head trauma as the inciting event, since concussion, seizure, and even syncope (e.g. due to pain) may result from acute head injury, and these mechanisms may be comorbid or difficult to distinguish. Here we restrict ourselves to those with 'spontaneous' presentations (i.e. where the symptoms do not clearly follow and result from head trauma). In this section, we emphasize the two most common types of TLOC (i.e. syncope and seizure), highlighting their specific relationship to vestibular symptoms and focusing on clinical features that help distinguish between them ('fit versus faint').

Case series describing patients presenting to the ED with TLOC report vasovagal syncope, psychogenic pseudo-syncope, and seizure to be the most frequent causes, accounting for up to 70% of cases (40). The chief diagnostic concerns are dangerous causes of syncope (e.g. cardiac arrhythmia, myocardial ischaemia) or seizure (e.g. meningitis or encephalitis) along with TIA or minor stroke. Acute, life-threatening metabolic disturbances such as hypoxia, hypoglycaemia, hyperglycaemia, hyponatraemia, and drug intoxication usually result in stupor or coma, rather than TLOC, but occasional exceptions occur, especially for transient hypoglycaemia. Transient, sudden increases in intracranial pressure, as with temporary cerebrospinal fluid flow obstruction (e.g. colloid cyst) or aneurysmal subarachnoid haemorrhage may also lead to LOC or collapse that mimics benign forms of syncope or seizure (41). Readers should note that the relative prevalence of benign and dangerous causes likely varies across consulting practices depending on referral patterns.

TLOC of any cause is often preceded by vestibular sensations such as dizziness or vertigo lasting seconds to minutes. Less commonly it is preceded by headache or other, more specific neurological symptoms (e.g. weakness, numbness, diplopia) that narrow the differential diagnosis more effectively. TLOC almost invariably leads to loss of muscle tone and results in a fall if the event occurs while the patient is in an upright and unsupported position. Typically, the fall is followed by a period of variable length of lack of response to external stimuli and amnesia. Irrespective of the underlying disease, falls from TLOC may cause major soft-tissue injuries as well as bony fractures. For example, recurrent syncopal falls (even of benign aetiology) are associated with fractures in 5% (42). In conditions where prodromal symptoms are typically absent or the patient population is disproportionately older (e.g. falls related to carotid sinus hypersensitivity), fractures are even more common, affecting up to one in four patients (43, 44). If TLOC results in a fall with secondary head trauma, complications of traumatic brain injury may obscure or confound identification of the initial cause of TLOC.

Syncope ('faints')

Lifetime prevalence for a single syncope in the general population almost reaches 50% (11). Updated guidelines for the diagnosis and management of syncope have been published by The Task Force for the Diagnosis and Management of Syncope of the European Society of Cardiology (11). Syncope can be divided into several major categories based on pathophysiology: *reflex syncope, orthostatic syncope (hypovolaemia, medications, autonomic failure)*, and *cardiac syncope* (21). Each is dealt with in greater detail in the following sections. The relative frequency of different underlying causes for syncope varies by patient age. Reflex syncope accounts for 73% of cases in those under age 40 but only 45% among those over age 60 (45). Vasovagal syncope, a form of reflex syncope, is, by far, the most common cause among younger patients. By contrast, carotid sinus syncope, another form of reflex syncope, and cardiac syncope account for a larger fraction in patients over the age of 40–50 years (46). The prevalence of different causes also varies somewhat by the clinical setting from which they are recruited.

Clinical symptoms of syncope vary from patient to patient and may vary from event to event in a single individual. Preceding a syncope the patient will usually notice prodromal neurological (e.g. dizziness, blurred vision, lightheadedness, loss of colour vision, narrowing of the visual field, hearing loss) or autonomic (e.g. nausea, palpitations, warmth, cold) symptoms (47), some of which may be quite difficult to distinguish from the symptoms of seizure, migraine, or TIA (22). Contrary to popular belief (48), even in those with underlying cardiac or cardiovascular causes, vertigo is just as likely a symptom as dizziness (1). Prodromal symptoms classically start shortly before the actual loss of consciousness and last just 30–60 s (49) but presyncope sometimes lasts several minutes (50). Readers should note that presyncope is notoriously variable in its duration, with many patients experiencing symptoms that last many minutes or even hours (51); extended, 'stable' presyncopal symptoms, however, are often not followed by TLOC (i.e. completed syncope). The patient or bystanders may notice autonomic signs such as pallor, cyanosis, flushing, sweating, or pupillary dilatation (47). The duration of unconsciousness is typically 10–20 s as observed in laboratory-induced reflex syncope and in prospective studies with blood-donors (25, 52, 53), but the event may last up to several minutes, depending on the underlying mechanism and whether the patient achieves a supine position promptly (which speeds restoration of cerebral blood flow). Note that patient or witness-estimated durations for syncope are generally longer, with fewer than half of cases said to resolve in less than a minute (45). Overall recovery from syncope is usually spontaneous, prompt and often complete within about 30 s, although post-event fatigue or confusion lasting longer than a minute are both extremely common (45, 50). The duration of postictal confusion is closely correlated with the duration of TLOC and the duration of the underlying circulatory arrest responsible for TLOC (49). A small subset of patients takes more than an hour to recover fully (50, 54). Despite otherwise complete neurological recovery, permanent retrograde amnesia for a brief period prior to uncomplicated syncope is not unusual (11), especially in elderly patients. Retrograde amnesia for up to 20 s prior to the faint has been documented under controlled conditions (52), and amnesia for the TLOC is believed to account for many patients who present with unexplained falls, rather than syncope, per se (38, 39).

Both flaccid (mostly forwards) and stiff (mostly backwards) falls are noted in syncope with about equal frequency (55). The presence of myoclonic jerks, although often considered by witnesses and physicians alike to be a sign of seizure, does not exclude the possibility of syncope. In fact, short-lasting, synchronous bilateral, non-rhythmic, multifocal myoclonic jerks of small amplitude are frequently observed in syncope (18) (often called 'convulsive syncope'). Myoclonic jerks after the fall lasting more than 15 s, however, are rare (55). Based on the underlying pathophysiological mechanism, myoclonic jerks always *follow* loss of consciousness in syncope (unlike seizures where they may either precede or follow unconsciousness, or even occur without unconsciousness). These syncopal myoclonic jerks are believed to represent hypoxic spinal myoclonus, a so-called 'release' phenomenon resulting from cortical disinhibition secondary to global cerebral hypoperfusion. Convulsive syncope is observed in 12% of blood donors presenting with syncope (53) and in 90% of cases when inducing syncope in healthy volunteers by a sequence of hyperventilation, orthostasis, and Valsalva manoeuvre (55). Other seizure-like features that may occur with syncope such as tongue biting (particularly the tip of the tongue) and incontinence (particularly for urine) are described further later in the chapter.

Bedside evaluation of the patient with suspected syncope should initially focus on confirming a typical history for syncope (as opposed to seizure or other mimic), followed by a search for triggers or other clinical features that might differentiate between benign (especially reflex syncope) and potentially dangerous (especially cardiac syncope) causes (Table 29.2). When taking the patient's history, specific triggers (e.g. pain, fear) should be sought along with predisposing factors such as volume depletion (e.g. due to dehydration, diarrhoea) or medication use (e.g. antihypertensive therapy) that might have contributed to baseline systemic hypotension. Any treatment should be directed at the underlying cause.

Reflex syncope

The most common cause of TLOC, reflex syncope (also referred to as neurocardiogenic syncope or neurally-mediated syncope), affects up to 40% of the population (56–58). In reflex syncope, an inappropriate lack of sympathetic vasoconstriction ('vasodepressor' mechanism) and an excess of vagally-mediated bradycardia ('cardioinhibitory' mechanism) can both contribute to systemic hypotension (11). One or both mechanisms occur as part of an abnormal reflex response to a normal physiological stimulus in the presence of an otherwise normal autonomic system. Classic clinical subtypes include vasovagal syncope, situational syncope (e.g. micturition, defecation, cough), and carotid sinus syncope. The presence of particular triggers helps identify the 'reflex' mechanism and defines the clinical subtype. Vasovagal syncope is noted in contexts where pain or fear predominates, particularly in the context of heat, dehydration, or prolonged standing. Situational syncope is diagnosed when episodes are tightly linked to urination, defecation, cough, or swallowing. Carotid sinus syncope results from head/neck turning or direct carotid pressure. The modern understanding of these disorders, however, suggests that the underlying reflex pathophysiology (vasodepressor, cardioinhibitory, or mixed) is largely independent of the specific trigger (11). Thus, identifying syncope triggers is usually more relevant to confirming a reflex cause than defining the precise mechanism or choosing therapy. Readers should note that some triggers such as exertion/exercise or Valsalva do not necessarily point to a benign, reflex syncope and may result from dangerous disorders such as anaemia, myocardial ischaemia, or severe aortic stenosis.

Subtypes of reflex syncope are clinically similar, although vasovagal forms predominate in younger populations and carotid sinus

Table 29.2 Clinical predictors of benign (reflex) vs. dangerous (cardiac) causes in syncope

Clinical finding	Predictor	Strength	Notes
Presence of 'benign' triggers	Reflex syncope	Strong	'Benign' triggers (pain, fear, medical procedure, fasting, prolonged standing, warm room) or situational occurrences are moderately predictive of vasovagal syncope (81), although these triggers are absent in up to 50% of reflex syncope patients (226). Note that triggers do not uniformly suggest a benign disorder. Cardiogenic syncope may be triggered by exercise or Valsalva due to obstructive cardiac outflow disease or myocardial ischaemia. Startle (e.g. loud noise, fright, extreme emotional stress) may also occur in cardiac disease, particularly in paediatric patients at risk for rare disorders such as the long QT syndrome (3)
Spontaneous episodes without trigger or situational occurrence	Cardiogenic syncope	Moderate	Lack of triggers or situational occurrence favours cardiogenic syncope, though obvious triggers may be absent in up to 50% of patients with benign, reflex causes (226). Thus, those with spontaneous episodes identify a higher risk population that may warrant additional testing to exclude cardiac causes
Gradual onset	Reflex syncope	Weak	Prodromal symptoms classically start 30–60 s before the actual vasovagal loss of consciousness, but are notoriously variable in their duration (49, 51). While gradual onset with a more protracted prodrome is rare in complete heart block (mean prodrome 1.4 ± 1.8 s), it is fairly typical for cardiac syncope associated with ventricular tachycardia (mean prodrome 34 ± 79 s) (226). Thus, gradual onset is a relatively weak differentiator between reflex syncope and ventricular tachycardia
Abrupt onset without prodrome or sudden offset	Cardiogenic syncope	Moderate	Warning periods of few seconds or less favour cardiogenic syncope, particularly due to heart block (226). Likewise, absent fatigue during recovery also favours cardiogenic syncope, particularly due to heart block (226)
First episode at age <35–40 years	Reflex syncope	Moderate	The prevalence of dangerous causes for syncope is low in young adults. Greater care should be taken in paediatric or early teen patients, especially if symptoms are triggered by startle or exertion; these patients may have congenital cardiac syndromes such as pre-excitation or long QT syndrome (3)
First episode at age >40–50 years	Cardiogenic syncope	Moderate	Age >54 years is a strong predictor for cardiac syncope (226). First episodes of reflex syncope are rarely observed beyond the age of 35 years and should raise suspicion for a cardiogenic cause (45, 81). The age association is muted somewhat if the duration since the first episode is greater than 4 years
Syncope while supine or sleeping	Cardiogenic syncope	Strong	Reflex syncope and orthostatic syncope are extremely rare while supine or sleeping (3). Almost all syncope while supine is cardiac in origin (54). Occasional rare cases are due to unusual dangerous disorders such as systemic mastocytosis or other endocrine release syndrome
Cardiorespiratory symptoms (chest pain, dyspnoea, palpitations)	Cardiogenic syncope	Weak	Prodromal symptoms of chest pain or dyspnoea may suggest a cardiac or other dangerous aetiology (e.g. aortic dissection, pulmonary embolus) (79). Similar symptoms may also occur in reflex syncope (45, 50). Palpitations are more frequent in reflex syncope overall (226), but may favour cardiogenic syncope when there is suspected structural heart disease or abnormal electrocardiogram (18, 54)
Facial cyanosis during syncope or syncope >2 min in duration	Cardiogenic syncope	Moderate	Facial cyanosis may favour seizure; however, if syncope is already the more likely cause, facial cyanosis supports a cardiac origin of syncope over a reflex cause (81). A prolonged loss of consciousness again favours seizure, but, if known to be syncopal, supports a cardiac origin over a reflex cause

TIA, transient ischaemic attack; TLOC, transient loss of consciousness.

forms predominate in older populations. In reflex syncope, dizziness is a frequent prodromal symptom, present in 73% in one study (45). In a study reporting vasovagal syncope in blood donors, dizziness was noted in 67% of patients (25). Autonomic symptoms (nausea, palpitations, pallor, diaphoresis or pupillary dilatation ((47)) are typically prominent and frequent findings in reflex syncope, and characteristic prodromal symptoms (including dizziness or vertigo) are often recalled by the patient after the event. By contrast, some cardiac causes (especially complete heart block) tend to produce syncope without memorable prodrome (47, 50). Mild or severe fatigue lasting more than a minute after termination of syncope is a very prominent symptom following reflex syncope, being reported by greater than 90% of patients with reflex syncope (50). This contrasts with patients with cardiac syncope (particularly that due to brief atrioventricular block) in which residual symptoms, including fatigue, are very uncommon (50, 59). Thus, fatigue or tiredness that outlasts the first minute after regaining consciousness favours reflex over cardiogenic syncope (60).

Carotid sinus syncope (also known as carotid sinus hypersensitivity or carotid sinus syndrome) deserves special consideration from a neuro-otological perspective since symptoms may appear to be induced by head movements, initially suggesting the possibility of vestibular disease. Triggers are typically lateral neck rotations or direct neck compressions (e.g. due to a tight neck collar or tie) and sometimes swallowing, all believed to mechanically stimulate hypersensitive baroreceptors of the carotid sinus, leading to the reflex syncope. A recent report of bradycardia and brief asystole following vestibular stimulation as applied during the head-impulse test (61) likely occurred via a similar mechanism, since more direct vestibular-vagal reflex pathways do not appear to have major cardiac effects (62).

Provocation by direct carotid sinus pressure or massage is used for diagnostic purposes, although care should be taken in older patients with atherosclerotic risk factors or known vascular disease, since stroke is a potential complication of this bedside procedure (11). Autonomic testing during carotid sinus massage may help confirm a reflexive pattern of cardiovascular responses. Peripheral vestibular disorders that might be confused for carotid sinus syncope or vice versa include horizontal canal BPPV and partially-compensated unilateral vestibular failure (e.g. postvestibular neuritis or in chronic Ménière's disease). Patients with these disorders typically experience dizziness or vertigo with lateral head movements, similar to those with carotid sinus syncope, but the trigger is the head movement rather than the neck movement, per se. Thus, if symptoms can be reproduced at the bedside using an en bloc head/neck movement (i.e. without rotating the head relative to shoulders), then carotid sinus syncope is effectively excluded. A more challenging differential diagnosis is between carotid sinus syncope and rotational vertebral artery syndrome. In this rare disorder of mechanical occlusion of a lone or dominant vertebral artery, symptoms such as syncope, near syncope, transient vertigo, or nystagmus result from intermittent cerebellar or brainstem ischaemia, linked to the same trigger as carotid sinus syncope (i.e. far lateral neck rotation) (63). Since vertigo (1) and even nystagmus (64) have been reported in cardiovascular syncope, their presence alone does not exclude a reflex syncopal cause. If the patient lacks other triggers such as tight neck collars or swallowing, reproduction of symptoms by carotid sinus massage may be the only differentiating feature.

Treatment options for reflex syncope are usually non-pharmacological and emphasize trigger avoidance and mechanical or behavioural strategies to decrease any underlying orthostasis. Patients should be advised to avoid provocative situations and rapid postural shifts in vasovagal syncope and instructed on limiting use of tight neckties or shirt collars in carotid sinus syndrome. Anti-orthostatic manoeuvres such as squatting or standing with the legs crossed may help reduce venous pooling, thereby decreasing symptomatic syncope (65, 66).

Orthostatic syncope (hypovolaemia, medications, and autonomic failure)

Orthostatic hypotension (an abnormal drop of blood pressure in response to a gravitational postural challenge) accounts for 24% of all acute syncopal presentations (67) and is the most frequent presentation of autonomic failure (68). Orthostatic hypotension is defined as a sustained decline in blood pressure of at least 20 mmHg systolic or 10 mmHg diastolic within 3 min of standing (69). The most commonly identified causes of orthostatic hypotension are medications and hypovolaemia (67), while other conditions leading to autonomic failure such as diabetes, neurodegenerative disorders, or idiopathic pure autonomic failure are less frequent. Initial orthostatic hypotension and postural orthostatic tachycardia syndrome (POTS) usually cause presyncopal symptoms of dizziness or vertigo rather than frank syncope, so will be discussed in the section describing transient dizziness without TLOC.

Premonitory symptoms are usually less prominent in orthostatic hypotension than reflex syncope, though patients can report pain in the neck and shoulders while standing due to local ischaemia of these muscles at the onset of complaints ('coat hanger pain') (68), as well as light-headedness, greying out, and hearing loss. Again, vertigo is a common symptom (1).

The cardinal difference between autonomic failure and reflex syncope is that in autonomic failure, the autonomic nervous system attempts correctly to control blood pressure but is unable to do so, while in reflex syncope the autonomic nervous system is capable, but acts incorrectly (18). When standing up an increase in the heart rate and in blood pressure allow appropriate response to the higher demands placed on the vascular system by gravity. Sympathetic vasoconstriction is a key component of this response. When standing up, blood pressure drops in orthostatic hypotension, often in association with an appropriate tachycardic response

as an (insufficient) attempt to compensate for the hypotension. This is distinct from reflex syncope where bradycardia develops inappropriately, despite the presence of hypotension. Care should be taken, however, to avoid inferring too much about the underlying diagnosis from the patient's heart rate. Classically, volume depletion results in tachycardia. However, absence of tachycardia or even relative bradycardia do not exclude catastrophic underlying conditions such as ruptured ectopic pregnancy (70). Overt clues to dangerous conditions presenting with severe orthostatic hypotension may be lacking in some cases of myocardial infarction, occult sepsis, or diabetic ketoacidosis (71).

Symptomatic autonomic failure and syncope is usually delayed after a postural challenge ('classic orthostatic hypotension') and presents typically only after prolonged standing. The time to develop symptoms of orthostatic hypotension after standing up can be used as a parameter to quantify the severity of autonomic failure (19). Sometimes the drop in pressure is delayed until after exertion or effort, such as with walking up a flight of stairs ('post exercise' hypotension). Although syncope may also occur during (as opposed to after) exercise, this co-incident timing makes a cardiac origin (19) or anaemia (72) more likely.

Postprandial hypotension constitutes a context-specific form of syncope with a related, yet distinct, pathomechanism. It results from blood pooling in the splanchnic system that is not compensated for adequately to support the cerebrovascular circulation. Whereas symptoms are mild in the majority of patients, they may be severe enough to cause syncope in high-risk groups such as those with autonomic failure (19). It is readily recognized because of the close temporal relationship between eating and resulting presyncope-syncope.

Autonomic failure may be caused by neurodegenerative disease (e.g. 'pure' autonomic failure, multiple systems atrophy (73)), systemic disease (e.g. diabetes mellitus, systemic amyloidosis), or be pharmacologically-induced (e.g. antihypertensives, antihistamines, dopaminergic drugs, tricyclic antidepressants, diuretics) (68, 74). In patients with idiopathic Parkinson's disease autonomic failure is rare. Nevertheless, these patients may faint due to medication-related orthostatic hypotension, and they may present with apparent TLOC due to falls linked to postural imbalance and unsteadiness (75).

Treatments should be focused on the underlying pathomechanism, whenever possible. Volume depletion is only directly responsible for syncope in cases with substantial volume loss (e.g. gastrointestinal bleeding), but lesser degrees of volume depletion are frequently a contributing factor in patients with reflex or orthostatic syncope. Volume replacement should always be considered if the patient has signs of hypovolaemia (e.g. reduced jugular venous pressure or decreased skin turgor). If medication-related orthostatic hypotension is suspected (74), potentially offending drugs should be reduced in dosage or withdrawn if underlying medical conditions permit. In cases where non-pharmacological autonomic failure predominates or when other interventions fail, midodrine or fludrocortisone combined with increased salt intake may provide helpful drug treatments of orthostatic hypotension.

Cardiac syncope

Although syncope usually has a good prognosis, patients with underlying cardiac disease have a substantially worse prognosis compared to those with other forms of syncope (11, 76, 77), reaching a mortality of up to 30% at 1 year (78). Therefore, assessing for a cardiac origin of syncope substantially influences both prognosis and treatment. Cardiac syncope may result from outflow obstruction linked to structural heart disease (e.g. hypertrophic cardiomyopathy, aortic stenosis) or arrhythmia. Both bradyarrhythmias and tachyarrhythmias due to various causes (e.g. myocardial infarction, cardiac conduction system disease, pro-arrhythmic medication) may trigger syncope and should be sought as possible causes, especially in elderly patients with known prior cardiac disease.

Higher age (>45 years), known cardiac disease, and male sex increase the likelihood of potentially dangerous underlying cardiogenic syncope (50). By contrast, young age (<35 years), absence of suspected or known heart disease, and female sex together dramatically reduce the risk (54). Since dangerous causes often lead to major adverse events within a matter of a few years, those with duration of less than 1 year are at greatest risk (60). Patients with a longstanding history over many years with numerous (3 or more) recurrent episodes of syncope are more likely to have a benign cause (54). Although older age and short illness duration are clear risk factors for more dangerous causes, a cardiogenic origin should not be excluded a priori in the young or in those whose initial symptoms began at a young age. Congenital structural heart disease (e.g. congenital valvular stenosis) or conduction system disease (e.g. accessory bypass tract (Wolff–Parkinson–White syndrome) or long-QT syndrome) may be occult prior to presentation with syncope in childhood or early adulthood.

Certain clinical features suggest cardiac syncope. For example, syncope while supine is uncommon but strongly favours a cardiac cause (54). Triggers in cardiogenic syncope are usually absent, and this may be the most consistent differentiating feature between benign (reflex or benign orthostatic) and dangerous cardiac causes. Syncope occurring during exercise (e.g. myocardial ischaemia), Valsalva (e.g. aortic stenosis), or startle (long QT-syndrome) may be exceptions. Although classically cardiac causes are said to occur abruptly and without prodromal symptoms, this prototypic presentation of cardiac syncope is generally seen with complete heart block (sometimes called 'Stokes–Adams attacks' (59)), but not necessarily with ventricular tachycardia (50). Thus, the *absence* of prodrome is a 'red flag' for cardiac syncope (47) but the *presence* of prodrome should not prevent consideration of cardiac causes, particularly in a patient without a benign trigger for syncope. Prodromal symptoms of chest pain or dyspnoea may suggest a cardiac or other dangerous aetiology (e.g. aortic dissection, pulmonary embolus) (79). Some studies suggest palpitations favour cardiogenic syncope in those with known or suspected structural heart disease (18, 54), but other studies differ (50). Palpitations frequently occur in benign types of syncope, including about one in four patients with reflex syncope (45, 50) and virtually all patients with POTS. Therefore, care should be taken to avoid drawing strong inferences from the presence or absence of palpitations in syncope. Facial flushing at regaining consciousness has been described in cardiac syncope. This symptom, however, is not definitive, as it may also be observed in abrupt reflex syncope (80). Facial cyanosis may favour seizure; however, if syncope is already the more likely mechanism, facial cyanosis appears to support a cardiac origin (81). Similarly, if not due to seizure, loss of consciousness greater than 2 min in duration (82) may also predict a cardiac cause. Recovery after cardiac syncope is variable, but generally prompt and asymptomatic (i.e. without fatigue), particularly in complete heart block (50).

All patients should be investigated for the possibility of structural heart disease, at a minimum by electrocardiography, searching for a frankly abnormal cardiac rhythm or evidence of conduction system disease (e.g. bundle branch block, pre-excitation, or prolonged QT interval). Patients with a normal electrocardiogram who have suffered three or more syncopal spells over a period longer than 4 years, whose symptoms began prior to age 35, have clear reflex or orthostatic triggers, include a prodrome longer than 10 s with dizziness and autonomic symptoms but no chest pain or dyspnoea, never occur while supine, recover in less than 2 min without facial cyanosis or flushing, but leave them with substantial post-syncopal fatigue, almost certainly have a non-threatening cause. Head-up tilt table testing can help confirm cases where features are suggestive but not confirmatory of a reflex mechanism. Those with recent-onset symptoms, who appear acutely ill, or have known cardiac risk factors or 'red flag' features should be urgently evaluated and generally hospitalized. Those at higher risk but with less acute symptoms should be referred expeditiously to a cardiologist for consideration of further testing such as echocardiography, prolonged ambulatory electrocardiography, or cardiac loop recorder placement.

Seizures ('fits')

Epileptic seizures (or 'epileptic attacks') have variable manifestations, depending on the location and type of seizure. Those with TLOC (with or without loss of motor tone) are discussed here and include primary and secondary generalized seizures (e.g. tonic–clonic or absence seizures), as well as complex partial seizures (e.g. temporal lobe seizures). Seizures are pathophysiologically linked to an abnormal excessive or synchronous neuronal activity in the brain. The most recent definitions are provided by the International League Against Epilepsy (ILAE) (83) and can be found in Box 29.1. Roughly 4–5% of the general population will suffer from one or more non-febrile seizures during their lifetime (84, 85).

A typical generalized, tonic–clonic generalized seizure usually does not present a diagnostic challenge with regards to the fall. It is the less obvious seizures that may be mistaken for syncope or falls due to other causes. These include atonic and myoclonic-astatic generalized seizures and partial seizures with secondary generalization. Atonic seizures by definition do not present with convulsions, but control over postural muscles is temporarily lost. These episodes are usually long enough so that the patient falls limply to the ground, so such episodes might be mistaken for syncope or present as unexplained falls. Determining the state of consciousness in these patients may prove difficult. Fortunately, in the general population, atonic seizures are rare; such seizures are typically part of specific childhood epilepsy syndromes such as Lennox–Gastaut syndrome and juvenile myoclonic epilepsy (86). Both idiopathic and symptomatic seizures need to be considered and further evaluated based on clinical findings. Metabolic changes including both hyper- and hypoglycaemia (e.g. due to insulin overdose) may trigger seizures. Hypnagogic myoclonus, narcolepsy, psychogenic seizures, hyperventilation syndrome and some medication reactions may imitate generalized seizures, so must also be considered in the differential diagnosis of an apparent TLOC with what appear to be 'epileptic' clinical features. Limb-shaking TIA due to stenosis or occlusion of one or both internal carotid arteries (87) may present with myoclonic limb movements, apparent TLOC, and falls (88), a clinical picture that might also be confused for a seizure.

The bedside approach to the patient with suspected seizure should focus on identifying signs and symptoms associated with seizure that reliably differ from those seen in syncope, as discussed further later in detail (see section 'Fit or faint'). Clinically, the presentation of a seizure depends on the functional properties of the cortical areas affected. Premonitory symptoms in epileptic seizures are known as epileptic aura phenomena. Typical epileptic auras that might precede TLOC include rising epigastric sensations, an unpleasant taste or smell, déjà-vu, and macropsia (89, 90). Various prodromal symptoms may emerge in the hours before a seizure occurs. In a study of 100 randomly-selected adult epileptic patients, behavioural changes, cognitive, sleep or speech disturbances, anxiety and fatigue within hours before the seizure were reported by 39% of patients (91). Such non-specific 'irritability' symptoms are rarely helpful diagnostically, since similar symptoms are common in the general population and in other disease populations (e.g. migraine). The vast majority of seizures are not related to specific environmental triggers. In reflex epilepsy, however, visual, acoustic (music or startling sounds), or kinaesthetic stimuli trigger seizures (19).

Dizziness or vertigo as a premonitory symptom is frequent in syncope, but can also occur prior to TLOC due to seizure. Historically vertigo was closely linked with epilepsy and was considered a harbinger of chronic epilepsy (92). While such historical thinking has generally given way to modern concepts of primary vestibular pathology unrelated to epilepsy, data from patients with documented epilepsy still suggests a real association. Case series data suggest that dizziness or vertigo is a frequent symptom among randomly-selected patients visiting an epilepsy clinic (71% (34/48)) (93), a figure which certainly exceeds the general population prevalence of the symptom. Rotatory vertigo appears to be a specific symptom in 6–19% of patients with various forms of epilepsy, including those with temporal lobe, parietal lobe, occipital lobe, and generalized epilepsy (94–98). While some such patients likely have anticonvulsant medication side effects or comorbid vestibular pathology to explain their vestibular symptoms, well-documented cases of dizziness or vertigo during an evolving epileptic aura indicate that vertigo can be a direct manifestation of seizure (99). As described later in this chapter, some such patients may initially present with brief, isolated dizziness or vertigo lasting seconds that occurs for weeks or months prior to the onset of obvious generalized seizures (99). A careful inquiry regarding any possible cognitive, motor, or somatosensory manifestations is therefore warranted in such patients.

Fit or faint?

Differentiation between syncope and seizure generally relies on a careful history of the event, including obtaining information from eyewitnesses (11, 50, 56, 100). Table 29.3 lists clinical features that may help distinguish seizures from syncope in patients with TLOC. The presence or absence of triggers often helps in the differential diagnosis. The presence of a specific trigger for the event strongly suggests syncope (particularly reflex syncope) as the underlying cause for TLOC (11). The exception may be startling auditory stimuli, which may induce seizures (reflex epilepsy), sudden falls

Table 29.3 Clinical predictors of syncope vs. seizure in patients with 'fits, faints, funny turns, falls'

Symptom / sign	Seizure	Syncope
Triggers	Uncommon (emotional stress, sleeplessness, menses; rarely auditory stimuli in reflex epilepsy)	Common (prolonged sitting/standing, fear, pain, urination, defecation, cough, swallowing, exertion, etc.; rarely auditory stimuli in long QT or related syndromes)
Prodromal symptoms	Rising epigastric sensation, unpleasant taste or smell, prodromal déjà vu, macropsia, mood changes, visual or auditory hallucinations,[a] dizziness, vertigo, lightheadedness (89, 90, 104)	Presyncope, lightheadedness, dizziness, vertigo, diaphoresis, pallor, chest pain, dyspnoea, palpitations, nausea (89, 104, 227)
Duration of prodrome	Seconds ('a few') (99)	Seconds to minutes (226)
Duration of loss of consciousness	Minutes (usually >1–2) (104)	Seconds (usually <30 s) (18, 55); if longer, usually cardiac in origin
Facial cyanosis (witnessed)	Fairly common in generalized seizures (89, 104)	Rare with reflex syncope (104); sometimes present in cardiac syncope; pallor typical for reflex syncope
Frothing at the mouth (witnessed)	Fairly common in generalized seizures (104)	Uncommon in syncope (104)
Myoclonic jerking movements (witnessed)	Seconds–minutes; synchronous and rhythmic, may precede TLOC (89)	Seconds (usually <15 s), asynchronous, arrhythmic, always follow TLOC (55, 89)
Mental status after the event (witnessed or self-reported)	Moderate disorientation and confusion very common (89, 104), sometimes lasting >5 min	Brief confusion fairly common (89, 104), rarely lasts more than 2 min in the absence of head trauma
Tongue biting	Common, lateral side (105)	Rare (4), tip of tongue (105, 228)
Urinary incontinence	Common, may include bedwetting (89)	Common, rarely includes bedwetting (89)
Recovery	Postictal confusion (but may be clearheaded immediately) and headaches (89, 104)	Oriented immediately on regaining consciousness (18, 49), but fatigue, sweating, confusion may occur (60, 226)
Electroencephalography	Generalized or focal epileptic discharges	Sequence of generalized wave slowing high amplitudes and eventual flattening (55, 106, 212)
Electrocardiography	Rarely ictal bradycardia (111, 229) or asystole (230)	Sinus tachycardia, sinus bradycardia or cardiac arrhythmia are frequent

TLOC, transient loss of consciousness

[a] If hallucinations occur in syncope, it is usually during recovery as the individual regains consciousness (109).

without TLOC (hyperekplexia), dizziness or vertigo (superior canal dehiscence syndrome), or true syncope (long QT-syndrome). Even under the best of circumstances, however, the two syndromes may be confused clinically, and some cases may require prolonged physiological monitoring for accurate differentiation (101).

Syncope appears to be misdiagnosed as seizure in an estimated 20–30% of patients with convulsive episodes (101). Zaidi and colleagues studied 74 patients previously diagnosed with epilepsy and found an alternative diagnosis in 31 patients (42%) pointing either to reflex or cardiac syncope or psychogenic origin (102). Many misdiagnoses of epilepsy may be due to partially overlapping clinical features and the high prevalence of reflex syncope (102). Other misdiagnoses may relate to inaccurate reporting of patients or eyewitnesses. Some degree of retrograde amnesia prior to the TLOC event is typical in patients with complex partial or generalized seizures, but it is frequent in syncope as well (38, 39); this amnesia may limit the ability of patients to accurately report prodromal symptoms that might otherwise be helpful or diagnostic. To assess eyewitness accounts, Thijs and colleagues showed a video of either a generalized tonic–clonic seizure or a reflex syncope to psychology students then interviewed them about clinical features; students could reliably report the muscle tone (stiff in seizure vs. flaccid in syncope), but many other features of TLOC were overlooked or inaccurately reported (103).

Readers should note that several clinical findings and tests promoted in textbooks as distinctive for either seizure or syncope, are, in fact, non-discriminative or only discriminate well when additional symptom details are considered. For example, the presence *myoclonic jerks* is not specific for seizure, as jerking is seen frequently in syncope; however, jerking lasting more than 15 s is highly suggestive of seizure. *Urinary incontinence* alone is not a helpful distinguishing feature, as this occurs in 17% of generalized seizures and in 26% of syncopal events (45, 89, 104, 105), but *bedwetting* is highly predictive of seizures (89), presumably because syncope rarely occurs while in bed. The presence of tongue biting, often sought as a predictor of seizure, is only a strong predictor after one considers the location of the tongue bite. A *lateral tongue bite* has a very high specificity (99%) for a seizure, whereas a tongue bite at the tip of the tongue favours syncope, despite its relative rarity (105). *Lateral head turning*, classically linked only to seizure, may be observed in syncope as well (89, 106, 107), although it is probably still a strong predictor of seizure along with any unusual posturing of the limbs or body (89). *Postictal confusion* is another classical symptom of seizure (104), but is probably only confirmatory when it is prolonged, since brief confusion is non-specific, occurring in 10–30% of patients with syncope (89, 108). So-called 'aura' symptoms are said to suggest seizure, but prodromal neurological symptoms of presyncope may seem superficially (e.g. micropsia in seizure versus tunnel vision or the sense of 'things moving away' in syncope) or profoundly (e.g. depersonalization or epigastric 'rising' sensations in either syndrome) similar (47). Even frank *hallucinations*, often thought of as exclusive to seizures, are sometimes reported by patients suffering syncope. Typically, however, unlike epileptic hallucinations, these *syncopal hallucinations* do not precede or occur during the attack, but instead occur when the attack has ended and the patient is regaining consciousness (109, 110).

The rare association of cardiac arrhythmia caused by seizure may occasionally complicate differentiation between syncope and seizure, since both may be present even during a single TLOC event.

Symptomatic bradycardia and cardiac asystole provoked by epileptic seizures (preferentially with temporal lobe location) are rare but important complications in epilepsy and appear to be relevant in the pathogenesis of sudden unexplained death in epilepsy (SUDEP) (111–116). In a recent review of the literature ictal asystole was found in 0.27% of patients who underwent video-EEG (117).

Mimics of TLOC: pseudo-syncope and pseudo-seizure

Syncope-like or seizure-like episodes may be due to (presumptive) functional or psychogenic causes. Such cases are most clearly defined by the presence of symptomatic episodes without corresponding physiological changes required for a syncope or seizure diagnosis (e.g. by EEG video telemetry (118)). These events have been labelled with various terms, including pseudo-syncope, pseudo-non-epileptic seizures, psychogenic non-epileptic attack (PNEA), psychogenic pseudo-TLOC, among others (119). A psychogenic non-epileptic attack disorder often coexists with epilepsy, and can be encountered in as many as 20% of patients with epilepsy (120–122). Estimates among patients with syncope range as high as 24% (123), although other series have suggested much lower rates (0.3–2.2%) (124, 125).

It is presumed in such cases that the TLOC is apparent, rather than actual (Figure 29.1), but this may not be evident clinically. Some clinical features may help distinguish these cases. Previous unexplained medical symptoms, a psychiatric history, and a history of childhood traumatic experiences are conditions that favour a diagnosis of dissociative seizure or a psychogenic cause of blackouts (120). The likelihood of psychogenic non-epileptic seizures varies with the time of occurrence—they are rarely observed between midnight and 6:00 am and do not arise during sleep (126). Long duration of unconsciousness, very frequent episodes, and severe psychosocial stressors favour a diagnosis of psychogenic seizure (19). Suggestibility of attacks is said to be highly predictive of a functional cause (127). Pseudo-seizures typically present with asynchronous, waxing-and-waning, convulsion-like movements, sometimes with pelvic thrusting (27, 118). Whereas during syncope and seizure the eyes are usually open and tonically deviated upwards, patients with pseudo-seizure typically have the eyes closed (55, 64, 128, 129). When examining pupil reflexes in these patients, the examiner may observe forceful eye closure and avoidance of gaze (although care should be taken with this sign, since reflex blepharospasm can occur in neurological disease (130)). On examination, a limb stopping mid-flight when lifted and released by the examiner above the subject's head has sometimes been proposed to be a distinguishing feature (18), but in patients with psychogenic origin, responses to avoid pain may be suppressed, limiting the value of this observation in differential diagnosis (18). At the end of the attack these patients may be immediately alert and oriented (131), but may become very emotional. It is a misconception, however, that serious injuries are rare features in psychogenic non-epileptic seizures (18, 132).

Increased blood levels of prolactin measured early (10–20 min) after presumed seizure support the diagnosis of a true epileptic pathogenesis (133, 134), although some studies suggest lower accuracy than one might hope (135, 136). Prolactin measurements do not adequately distinguish syncope from seizure (134) as marked elevations of serum prolactin levels may occur within 30 min of syncope induced by head up-tilt (137, 138). Lack of elevation does not accurately identify non-epileptic or psychogenic TLOC, since only about half of epileptic seizures are associated with a clear pro-lactin elevation (134).

In patients with known psychiatric diagnosis and TLOC the search for an underlying somatic origin must be pursued with the same elaborateness as in all other patients. This holds especially true for psychiatric patients under medication, as drugs such as antidepressants and neuroleptics may increase the likelihood of somatic causes such as cardiac arrhythmia or autonomic dysfunc-tion. For a firm diagnosis of psychogenic syncope or seizure, ictal monitoring with video-EGG (including heart rate and preferably blood pressure recording) is mandatory (118). The documenta-tion of unresponsiveness with lack of abnormal slow activity and a normal alpha rhythm is diagnostic of a psychogenic episode (139). Although occasionally questioned on ethical grounds, some clini-cians and researchers have proposed induction and suggestion as a means to provoke psychogenic pseudo-TLOC in order to increase the likelihood of typical events during video-EEG monitoring (27).

Other causes of TLOC

While seizure and reflex syncope are by far the most frequent causes of TLOC, a broad variety of other, less frequent, but potentially dangerous conditions are associated with TLOC. These disorders are not related to low systemic blood pressure and include cases of TLOC due to cerebrovascular disease (vertebrobasilar TIA, vascu-lar steal syndromes, carotid artery occlusion, subarachnoid haem-orrhage), basilar migraine, structural nervous system disorders, and metabolic problems (especially hypoglycaemia and hypoxia). Vertebral artery compression as observed in rotational vertebral artery syndrome generally leads to presyncope rather than actual TLOC and is discussed in the section 'transient dizziness without TLOC'.

While syncope is associated with a global state of cerebral hypop-erfusion due to failure of systemic blood pressure, transient ischae-mic attacks (TIA) and steal syndromes are associated with regional cerebral hypoperfusion. About 10% of patients with vertebrobasilar insufficiency and vertigo or dizziness as a dominant symptom also have syncope (140). Series of patients presenting with acute syn-cope have found 0.4–8% of patients with TIA as a cause (141, 142). In vertebrobasilar TIA, TLOC is said not to occur in the absence of focal neurological symptoms or signs (143). This observation may, in part, be circular—most definitions of TIA-related syncope require associated focal vertebrobasilar symptoms to confirm the diagnosis. In support of the contention, however, are longitudinal data suggesting that patients with truly isolated syncope (including no history of prior or concurrent neurological, coronary, or other cardiovascular disease stigmata) are at no increased risk of stroke over time (144). These findings are countered by longitudinal stud-ies in patients with a history of vascular risk factors or (non-focal) vertebrobasilar symptoms such as vertigo or dizziness who may, in fact, be at meaningful risk for TIA as a cause (141).

Syncope in the subclavian steal syndrome is also classically associated with focal neurological symptoms or signs (145, 146). Whether and how often subclavian steal syndrome results in TLOC without focal neurological signs remains unclear (18). The most frequent symptoms are vertigo (61%), syncope (44%), and arm claudication (33%). Blood pressure differences between the two arms and appearance of symptoms after upper extremity exercise may be clues (147). The risk of completed stroke is uncertain and

debated, but probably quite low (148); thus, diagnosis of mild or atypical cases may not be terribly important.

Other central disorders are occasionally associated with TLOC. Contrary to conventional wisdom, anterior circulation cerebrovas-cular disease may also be associated with syncope, with or without vertigo or dizziness (149). Some such cases presumably represent sudden falls without true TLOC due to leg weakness (88), but other cases may result, instead, from true TLOC due to a carotid sinus syncope-type mechanism (150) or perhaps 'steal vertebrobasilar insufficiency' (151). In patients presenting with acute headache, the presence of TLOC is a strong predictor of subarachnoid haemor-rhage as a cause (152). In basilar-type migraine (roughly 10% of migraine with aura), TLOC is among the presenting symptoms in 16% (6/38) (153). Neurological TLOC has also been reported in structural nervous system disorders such as type I Chiari malfor-mation (154, 155); some structural disorders causing intermittent obstructive hydrocephalus (e.g. due to colloid or pineal cyst) have been associated with both true TLOC and sudden, unexplained falls without TLOC.

Transient dizziness or vertigo without loss of consciousness

In this section we briefly discuss patients with transient dizziness, vertigo, or presyncope without clear loss of consciousness. We again restrict ourselves to those with 'spontaneous' presentations (i.e. where the symptoms do not clearly follow and result from head trauma or clear drug or alcohol exposure). We mention the most common vestibular causes of transient dizziness or vertigo with-out TLOC, referring readers to the prior section or other chapters for additional details where appropriate. We emphasize benign, non-vestibular and important, dangerous causes not described in the earlier section.

Transient dizziness or vertigo without loss of consciousness has a broad differential diagnosis that cuts across organ systems, includ-ing transient vestibular, cardiovascular, cerebrovascular, haemato-logical, and metabolic disorders. In acute care settings such as the ED, benign oto-vestibular causes account for 33% of dizziness or vertigo presentations, but half are due to medical disorders, includ-ing about 20% cardiovascular (30). More importantly, at least 15% are due to dangerous conditions including fluid and electrolyte dis-turbances, cerebrovascular disease, cardiac arrhythmia, acute coro-nary syndrome, anaemia, and hypoglycaemia (30). Although the risk of dangerous disorders is presumed to be lower in outpatient or primary care clinics, current best evidence does not seem to sup-port this view (156).

Most experts recommend a bedside approach that combines careful history taking, a focused clinical examination, and selected follow-up testing in cases where a benign disorder cannot be con-firmed. Since the quality or 'type' of vestibular symptom (vertigo, dizziness, unsteadiness, other) is not reliably reported by patients (157), other symptom attributes and historical features such as duration (seconds vs. minutes vs. hours vs. days), onset (abrupt vs. gradual), triggers (e.g. head position or posture), prior episodes (first episode vs. single prodrome vs. recurrent episodic dizziness) and associated symptoms (e.g. headache, auditory symptoms) are crucial. Thus, 'timing and triggers' (rather than 'type') can be used to classify transient dizziness or vertigo into (a) brief, positional vs. (b) transient, episodic spontaneous.

Patients classified as having brief, positional or postural dizziness or vertigo without TLOC usually have either BPPV or orthostatic hypotension. BPPV may be confused for orthostatic hypotension if patients complain of dizziness on arising (3). Nevertheless, the two can be differentiated by inquiring about symptoms that occur on reclining or when rolling in bed, which should only be present in those with BPPV. Different forms of BPPV, their diagnosis, and treatment are described elsewhere in this book. Dangerous mimics include serious causes of orthostatic hypotension that may not be obvious (e.g. internal bleeding) (71) and central paroxysmal positional vertigo (158) due to posterior fossa lesions (neoplasm, demyelination, infarction, haemorrhage, Chiari malformation (159)). Peripheral positional nystagmus and central positional nystagmus may be differentiated based on specific nystagmus features (158). Positional TIAs due to vertebrobasilar insufficiency (160) remain a controversial syndrome, although it is likely that haemodynamic TIAs after postural shifts can cause orthostatic dizziness even without systemic orthostatic hypotension (161). A similar phenomenon may occur with intracranial hypotension (162).

Patients with transient, episodic dizziness or vertigo without TLOC often have traditional neuro-otological disorders such as vestibular migraine or Ménière's disease, discussed in other chapters. Other patients, however, have reflex syncope, panic attacks, or occasionally seizures. Dangerous mimics include cerebrovascular (vertebrobasilar TIA), cardiorespiratory (cardiac arrhythmia, unstable angina pectoris, pulmonary embolus), endocrine (hypoglycaemia, neuro-humoral neoplasms), or toxic (intermittent carbon monoxide exposure) causes.

Vascular causes of transient dizziness or vertigo without TLOC

In some patients, an exaggeration of normal orthostatic reflex responses results in a benign syndrome of very brief dizziness on arising known as *initial orthostatic hypotension*. This syndrome is typically noted in teens of slight build or during growth spurts, and, though accompanied by presyncopal symptoms similar to those described above, only infrequently results in syncope (163). Unlike the more typical forms of orthostatic hypotension described above, the drop in blood pressure is usually not sustained long enough to result in syncope, and the pressure drop itself can only be measured with specialized equipment that allows continuous heart rate and blood pressure monitoring (163). Initial orthostatic hypotension is accompanied by an appropriate, mild tachycardia, rather than the inappropriate delayed bradycardia of reflex syncope (163). Unlike those with the more dangerous *immediate* orthostatic hypotension, whose symptoms occur on arising, persist, and may be due to life-threatening illnesses (71), symptoms of benign *initial* orthostatic hypotension generally abate within 30–60 s (163). Patients should be counselled to arise slowly in order to minimize symptoms.

In other patients, orthostatic dysregulation does not result in hypotension but does result in *orthostatic tachycardia* with an increase in heart rate of more than 30 beats per minute on arising, despite a preserved blood pressure. If accompanied by symptoms of cerebral hypoperfusion, this syndrome is known as *postural orthostatic tachycardia syndrome* (POTS). While presyncope, lightheadedness, and dizziness are common in patients with POTS, only a minority will actually lose consciousness (164). Palpitations are the second most frequent symptom (165). Other symptoms include visual blurring, tunnel vision, tremulousness, and weakness of the legs; less common symptoms include hyperventilation, anxiety, chest wall pain, acral coldness, or pain and headaches (166). POTS usually develops between the ages of 15–50 and is more common in women (165). Some have comorbid migraine, sleep disorders, or fibromyalgia, and about half appear to have a limited form of autonomic neuropathy (165).

Vertebrobasilar TIAs can present with isolated episodes of dizziness lasting weeks to months, even years, prior to completed stroke (140, 167). Dizziness is the most common symptom in basilar artery occlusion (occurring without other neurological symptoms in 20% of cases) and vertebral artery dissection (168). Because 5% of TIA patients suffer a stroke within 48 h, prompt diagnosis is critical (169). Clinical findings that may prove useful in the distinction between benign (e.g. vestibular migraine, Ménière's disease) and dangerous (vertebrobasilar TIA) causes of dizziness or vertigo without TLOC are discussed in Table 29.4.

The rare and controversial (170) *rotational vertebral artery syndrome* (RVAS) can present with dizziness or vertigo triggered by far lateral neck rotation causing posterior circulation TIA due to mechanical occlusion of a sole or dominant vertebral artery contralateral to the head turn (63, 171). In the extreme, this syndrome is said to lead to completed infarction due to repetitive vertebral artery injury, sometimes called *bow hunter's stroke* (172, 173). Some recent evidence suggests vertebral artery hypoplasia or stenosis might interact with other vascular risk factors to produce dizziness during such head rotations (160). Possible cases of RVAS must first be assessed for carotid sinus syndrome or horizontal canal BPPV (described earlier), as all three conditions may be triggered by head rotation (174).

Systemic hypertension is frequently diagnosed as a cause of dizziness, but evidence of a causal relationship in uncomplicated chronic hypertension (i.e. without hypertensive encephalopathy or intracerebral haemorrhage) is generally lacking. Acute hypertension, as that seen with phaeochromocytoma, can cause dizziness or vertigo, though generally in association with other symptoms such as acute headache or autonomic hyperactivity (175). Other cardiovascular causes such as cardiac arrhythmia, unstable angina pectoris, and pulmonary embolus often result in syncope and are described in greater detail earlier in the chapter.

Non-vascular causes of transient dizziness or vertigo without TLOC

Dizziness or vertigo as a premonitory symptom of generalized seizure is well described. Although rare, there have been reports of truly *isolated epileptic vertigo*, sometimes called 'tornado epilepsy,' mimicking vestibular disorders (176). It is presumed that such seizures involve activation of vestibular-associated cortical regions in the superior temporal and anteroinferior parietal lobes or posterior insula (177, 178). It is likely that patients with isolated epileptic dizziness represent less than 1% of all new cases of epilepsy (99). In one case series, 30 patients presented with a chief complaint of dizziness (53%) or vertigo (47%) found to be epileptic in origin (99). Symptoms were very brief, lasting only seconds. Most had other clinical features of epilepsy, including brief absences (50%), generalized convulsions (23%), or depersonalization (23%); additional features included headaches, déjà vu, anxiety/panic, automatisms, auditory hallucinations, and gustatory hallucinations (99). Nevertheless, many of these patients experienced dizziness at times

Table 29.4 Clinical predictors of benign (vestibular migraine/Ménière's) vs. dangerous (vertebrobasilar TIA) causes in transient dizziness

Clinical finding	Predictor	Strength	Notes
Age >50 years	TIA	Weak	Age is a known risk factor for TIA, although vestibular migraine may shift from headache earlier in life to isolated dizziness or vertigo later in life (231)
Age <50 years	Migraine > Ménière's	Moderate	Migraine and Ménière's disease are the more common aetiologies in younger patients, but vertebral artery dissection is the most common identifiable cause of TIA and stroke in patients age 18–45 years (168)
Stroke risk factors	TIA	Moderate	Patients with at least one stroke risk factor (smoking, hypertension, diabetes, hyperlipidaemia, atrial fibrillation, eclampsia, hypercoagulable state, prior stroke or myocardial infarction) appear to have an increased risk of TIA and stroke (34)
Recent history of prior episodes of dizziness or vertigo	Non-predictive	–	Vestibular migraine, Ménière's disease, and TIA all may present with a first episode OR recurrent, episodic vertigo/dizziness over weeks to months; TIA presentations rarely have a history of episodes >2 years (34)
History of migraine headaches	Migraine > Ménière's	Weak	Typical presentation of migraine may shift from headache to isolated dizziness (231); migraine affects 15–20% of the general population but headaches are believed to be present in the vast majority of vestibular migraine sufferers, so its absence is a stronger predictor against migraine than its presence is for migraine
Sudden, severe, or sustained headache or neck pain	TIA	Moderate	Headaches at the time of vestibular migraine tend to be relatively mild; sudden, severe, or sustained pain may be a sign of vertebral artery dissection, especially located in posterior neck or trapezius (34)
Prodromal visual symptoms	Migraine	Weak	Classical migraine aura symptoms (slowly-expanding, arc-shaped, geometric, scintillating scotoma) are infrequent as a prodrome of vestibular migraine, but only rarely occur in TIA; other visual symptoms (hemianopsia, homonymous scotoma, etc.) are non-specific and do not discriminate
Aural fullness or tinnitus before or during the episode	Ménière's > migraine	Weak	Aural fullness and ringing are typical in Ménière's and also occur in basilar migraine (232); these symptoms can occur in TIA, generally in the AICA territory due to cochlear or cochlear nucleus ischaemia (233)
Hearing loss during the episode	Non-predictive	–	Hearing loss occurs in Ménière's and in basilar migraine (232), but it is also typical in AICA TIA (233); if the hearing loss is sudden, severe, or bilateral at onset, TIA is probably more likely
Absence of aural or auditory symptoms or signs	Non-predictive	–	Absent aural/auditory symptoms reduces the likelihood of Ménière's (though there may be isolated vestibular spells, particularly early in the illness course); it does not alter the likelihood of migraine or TIA
Presence of 'focal' neurological symptoms or signs	TIA	Moderate	Neurological symptoms (e.g. diplopia, incoordination, weakness), signs (e.g. ocular misalignment) are present in the majority of vertebrobasilar TIAs (140); similar symptoms are often seen in basilar migraine (232, 234), but not in the more common, isolated vestibular migraine or in Ménière's disease
Absence of 'focal' neurological symptoms or signs	Ménière's > migraine	Weak	Many vertebrobasilar TIAs present initially with isolated dizziness or vertigo that can go on for up to 2 years leading up to a completed infarction (140)

AICA, anterior inferior cerebellar artery; PICA, posterior inferior cerebellar artery; TIA, transient ischaemic attack

independent of their other epileptic symptoms, and some experienced isolated dizziness at the onset of their illness (99). In the recovery phase after these seizures, nausea was frequently reported (99), thus increasing the chances of confusion with a primary vestibular disorder. Since nystagmus has been demonstrated in epilepsy, generally with the fast phase directed away from the side of the lesion (179), a history of nystagmus during the episode cannot confidently exclude epilepsy as a cause. Since these epileptic dizziness or vertigo spells last only seconds and are spontaneous rather than positional or otherwise triggered, the differential diagnosis predominantly includes vestibular migraine (180) and vestibular paroxysmia (181). Inquiring about symptoms specific for epilepsy is an appropriate first step, although video-EEG telemetry may occasionally be necessary to exclude seizures as a cause for recurrent, unexplained, brief, spontaneous dizziness or vertigo.

Transient dizziness without TLOC is a common side effect of a variety of medications, many linked to orthostatic hypotension via cardiovascular mechanisms (182). Direct central nervous system effects may also cause transient symptoms (e.g. dose-dependent side effects in the hours after dosing the medication). Dangerous general medical disorders such as hypoglycaemia and intermittent carbon monoxide poisoning are also associated with transient dizziness or vertigo (30). Care should be taken to inquire for a history of relevant exposures and comorbid symptoms such as mental confusion or headaches.

Unexplained falls

In this section we briefly discuss the epidemiology, pathogenesis, differential diagnosis, clinical presentation, and bedside approach to the patient with unexplained falls. By definition (Box 29.1), we restrict ourselves to those without clear loss of consciousness and without obvious environmental (e.g. collision, slip, trip) or symptomatic (e.g. TLOC, severe vertigo) causes for the fall or falls. We emphasize the most common classes of unexplained falls, including those related to transient disruptions of postural control through vestibular or vascular mechanisms (e.g. 'otolithic crises,' carotid hypersensitivity, TIA), baseline problems of gait and stance (e.g. movement disorders, ataxia syndromes), and psychogenic falls. We also discuss rare forms (e.g. narcolepsy-cataplexy, hyperekplexia, and cryptogenic falls) that may present with isolated falls that initially may not be of obvious cause.

With increasing age, falls (with or without TLOC) become more frequent (183, 184). Most of the falling elderly have one or more pathological predisposing conditions, and the chance of falling increases markedly with the number of identified risk factors (185). Falls in older subjects are associated with high levels of morbidity and healthcare resource utilization (e.g. due to hip fracture). Recurrent falls may result in employment restrictions and lifestyle changes, causing an impairment of quality of life. Most falls are linked to environmental or symptomatic causes, including TLOC, but some are sudden and initially unexplained. Using a structured clinical approach, Parry and colleagues were able to determine a diagnosis in 90% of patients with recurrent, sudden falls without TLOC (186). Cardiovascular diagnoses (53%) were most commonly implicated, with neurological (29%), gait and balance abnormalities (18%), and drug-related causes (12%) being the other most frequent diagnoses; 22% had more than one diagnosis believed to be contributing to the sudden falls.

All falls result from an interaction between environmental conditions and the individual's balance, coordination, and postural control mechanisms that maintain a stable upright posture. Some falls, however, are reasonably attributed entirely to an environmental cause without need to invoke consideration of a disease state or faulty balance mechanisms (e.g. pedestrian hit by a car; 'normal' fall while ice skating for the first time). Symptomatic falls are linked to TLOC, destabilizing acute vestibular symptoms (e.g. severe vertigo, otolithic crises), or specific diseases known to cause

falls through reflex mechanisms (e.g. startle/hyperekplexia, laughter/cataplexy). It is important to remember that multiple falls in a single patient are sometimes attributable to more than one cause or mechanism (e.g. orthostatic syncope from autonomic failure and non-orthostatic balance-related falls without TLOC, both in a patient with multiple systems atrophy) (19). Especially in elderly people, multiple contributing factors can be identified when searching for an underlying cause of a fall or a TLOC (187). For the elderly, drug-related falls need to be evaluated carefully since antipsychotics, tricyclic antidepressants, and benzodiazepines may lead to sudden falls without TLOC (188). For those who fall without frank explanation, less common or less obvious disorders must be considered, including carotid sinus hypersensitivity, cardiac arrhythmias, atonic seizures, psychiatric mimics of seizure or syncope, and various chronic vestibular and neurological conditions characterized by impaired balance, postural, and motor mechanisms.

Those who present with a fall or falling as the primary symptom should first be assessed for the presence of an obvious environmental or symptomatic cause (Figure 29.2). Vertigo as a cause for falls will usually be reported, as will severe directional pulsion (e.g. a feeling of being pushed to one side or thrown to the ground). TLOC may be more difficult to determine. In unheralded syncope due to carotid sinus hypersensitivity, complete heart block, or atonic epileptic seizures, the presence of TLOC may be uncertain or unwitnessed. Therefore, these conditions should be considered even if falls reportedly occur without TLOC. Traditionally, sudden falls without TLOC have been called 'drop attacks,' although recommended terminology suggests that they instead be referred to simply as *sudden falls* with or without TLOC (Box 29.1). Triggers and clinical contexts that discriminate among various causes for sudden falls are found in Table 29.5.

Table 29.5 Triggers and clinical context for various causes of unexplained falls (11, 17–19, 56, 200–203, 235–241)

Triggers, clinical context	Vasovagal & situational syncope	Carotid sinus syncope	Autonomic & orthostatic syncope	Cardiac syncope	Epilepsy	Cataplexy	Hyperekplexia	Psychogenic falls	Sudden balance-related falls	Obstructive intracranial masses	TIA
Emotional stress, fear, pain as triggers	++			+	+	+++	+	++			
Valsalva (urination, cough, straining)	++		+	+						+	
Arising quickly	++		+++	+					++	+	+
Prolonged standing	+++		++	+							+
Head turning, neck compression		+++							+	+	+
Startling auditory stimuli				+	+		+++				
During exercise	+		+	+++	+						+
After exercise	++		++	+	+						
Hypovolaemia	++	+	+++	+							+
Menstruation	+		+		+						
Sleep deprivation	+				+						

Scale (+, ++, +++) denotes degree of association between a particular context and specific aetiology; grey boxes indicate no well-described association

Vascular causes of apparently unexplained falls

Cardiovascular causes of sudden falls include cardiac arrhythmias (particularly complete heart block) and carotid sinus syncope, both of which are described in greater detail above. Whether these disorders can lead to sudden falls without TLOC less uncertain, but, since the TLOC is not always obvious, these disorders may present clinically as unexplained falls.

Cerebrovascular causes of sudden falls include carotid occlusion and vertebrobasilar TIA. Although either may lead to TLOC, both tend to cause sudden falls with preserved consciousness. Consciousness is clearly preserved in those with cerebrovascular causes for leg weakness and falling. Anterior cerebral artery ischaemia in the parasagittal premotor and motor regions controlling the lower extremities can cause falls without TLOC (189). Patients with a common origin for the blood supply of both anterior cerebral arteries from the same internal carotid artery are predisposed to this condition. Likewise, spinal cord ischaemia can cause sudden leg weakness and falls; this has been reported in aortic dissection (190). In general, sudden falls of cerebrovascular cause are usually accompanied by other neurological symptoms or signs, some of which may persist after the fall (e.g. leg weakness (190)). Subarachnoid haemorrhage can cause sudden falls, but most often with TLOC (41).

Common non-vascular causes of apparently unexplained falls

Neuro-otologists are familiar with vestibular causes of unexplained or sudden falls. Falling in the context of severe vertigo hardly presents a diagnostic challenge, but other patients with inner ear vestibular disorders can present with falls as the dominant or sole manifestation (10). Classically, sudden falls are seen in the advanced stages of Ménière's disease, but may present as the initial symptom and can also be seen in other vestibular disorders. Other vestibular disorders associated with sudden unexplained and unprovoked falls without TLOC include vestibular migraine (191), BPPV (4, 192), and superior canal dehiscence (193) syndrome. The last of these presents with sound- and pressure-induced vertigo due to the absence of normal bone coverage at the apex of the superior semicircular canal (194).

Sudden falls occur in an estimated 6% of patients with Ménière's disease (13, 195), although others have reported much higher rates (196). These attacks have been eponymously referred to as *otolithic crises of Tumarkin* (197). The reference to an otolithic mechanism derives from the inappropriate reflex postural adjustments that lead to the fall, as well as the linear and tilt-related (presumed otolithic) illusions of motion that frequently accompany the fall. For example, these may include a feeling of being pushed or thrown to the ground, or that the environment is tilting or even flipped upside down. In Ménière's disease, surgical ablation or intratympanic gentamicin are potential treatments for these sudden falls (198).

Falls without TLOC are common in patients with movement disorders and ataxic syndromes. Parkinson's disease, progressive supranuclear palsy, multiple systems atrophy, and normal pressure hydrocephalus may present with freezing of gait, narrowing of the base support, and sudden postural failures due to uncompensated shifts in the centre of mass (18, 199). Falls in Parkinson's disease tend to be forward because of the forward-stooped posture and festination of gait. By contrast, falls in progressive supranuclear palsy are more often backwards due to the hyperextended body and neck posture. Chronic ataxia syndromes tend to produce falls without a directional preference. Even if patients present initially with falling as the dominant disease manifestation, other neurological symptoms or signs are almost invariably present.

Case reports indicate sudden, initially unexplained falls can also be observed in normal pressure hydrocephalus, obstructive hydrocephalus, third ventricle colloid cysts, and tumours of the posterior cranial fossa. Abrupt neck flexion can precipitate drop attacks in patients with posterior fossa tumours (26). Neuroimaging is generally sufficient to identify these structural causes, which presumably relate to intracranial pressure dynamics.

Psychogenic falls include a broad spectrum of clinical presentations including complete falls and even physical injury. Expert opinion suggests that young age (200, 201), very frequent episodes (201), and falls occurring only in the presence of bystanders (19) favour a psychogenic origin. A history of psychiatric disease, signs of ongoing psychiatric disorders such as depression or anxiety, or a history of physical or sexual abuse provide further support for a psychogenic cause (18, 19, 202). Falls may occur more slowly and can be associated with postural or gait signs on examination that appear non-physiologic.

Rare non-vascular causes of apparently unexplained falls

Sudden bilateral loss of muscle tone due to strong emotions (laughter, anger, surprise, startle) (203) is known as *cataplexy*. While these falls are triggered and therefore 'symptomatic' rather than 'unexplained', the association with strong emotions may not be apparent very early in the illness course. Partial attacks with loss of muscle tone in certain muscle groups only (e.g. dropping of the jaw or head nodding) are more common than generalized loss of muscle tone (i.e. resulting in a flaccid fall to the ground). Episodes usually last less than a minute (26) and rarely exceed several minutes. Depending on the temporal evolution during an episode, cataplectic attacks may either resemble TLOC (rapid fall) or psychogenic falling (with slow onset, patients may stop falling mid-flight). Cataplexy is one of the mandatory findings in patients with narcolepsy (together with excessive daytime sleepiness, sleep paralysis, and hypnagogic hallucinations). Cataplexy may occur independently from narcolepsy only in association with structural brain disease (e.g. Niemann–Pick disease, brainstem or hypothalamic lesions). Sudden vestibular falls and atonic seizures are in the differential diagnosis of cataplexy. Atonic seizures usually occur in a different clinical context (i.e. symptomatic generalized epilepsies of the Lennox–Gastaut type (27)). However, sudden falls have also been described in association with longstanding temporal lobe seizures; these falls appear to be atonic seizures, rather than secondary generalization into a tonic–clonic form (204). In these cases, the presence or absence of TLOC may be unclear.

Both inherited (autosomal dominant) and symptomatic forms of *hyperekplexia* (also termed 'startle disease') have been described. They are characterized by exaggerated startle reactions to unexpected auditory, some aesthetic and visual stimuli (205) and may lead to sudden unexplained falls without loss of consciousness. These falls typically start with momentary stiffening followed by 'falling like a log' and may be confused with startle-induced cataplexy. Hyperekplexia (stiff falls) and cataplexy (flaccid falls) can be differentiated on the basis of muscle tone at the time of the fall. Symptomatic hyperekplexia has been observed in patients with traumatic brain injury, post-anoxic encephalopathy, viral encephalitis, and paraneoplastic syndromes (19). In the differential diagnosis of stiff falls are generalized tonic seizures, although TLOC is typically present. Pain, fear, and anxiety, which may trigger reflex epilepsy, are rarely related to initiation of cataplectic attacks or hyperekplexia (19).

Cryptogenic drop attacks in middle aged women have been described as a specific clinical syndrome (6). The authors identified a distinct clinical profile in women over age 40 who suffered sudden falls to the knees without TLOC while walking termed 'maladie des genoux bleus.' These patients lack prodromal or postictal symptoms such as dizziness or imbalance, and report no triggers. Whether this syndrome represents a discrete disorder or merely reflects inadequate diagnostic testing in search of an alternate aetiology remains unclear.

Laboratory-based diagnostic testing and referrals

While most vestibular specialists will refer patients with presumed non-vestibular causes to other providers for further evaluation and testing, it is generally helpful for the referring physician to have a sense for which tests might be performed and are likely to offer the greatest diagnostic benefit. This knowledge allows for an anticipatory explanation to the patient as well as a fact check for the referring physician with regard to the appropriateness of any work-up subsequently obtained by the patient's primary care provider or other specialist.

As described earlier, the diagnostic evaluation for the patient with a 'fit, faint, fall, or funny turn' should include a detailed history and a careful otological, neurological, and cardiovascular exam. Unfortunately, the cause for an estimated 20–30% of these episodes will remain unclear after the initial bedside evaluation. In pursuing further testing or referral, the physician should bear in mind that ordering ancillary studies to search for low-prevalence conditions in patients with unexplained 'spells' carries the risk of a high rate of false-negative and false-positive test results. Thus, indiscriminate use of multiple tests is likely an inefficient (and perhaps ineffective) strategy for arriving at a final diagnosis and management strategy.

Vestibular evaluation

Vestibular testing is described extensively elsewhere in this volume. In addition to bedside tests for those with unexplained TLOC, vertigo, dizziness, or falls, a battery of physiological assessments may be performed if vestibular disease is suspected or must be 'ruled out.' Quantitative tests might include electro-oculography or video-oculography in the setting of various vestibular testing paradigms (e.g. positional tests, caloric or impulsive tests, rotational tests, vestibular-evoked myogenic potentials). Other related tests might include audiometry and dynamic posturography.

Cardiac evaluation

Cardiac work-up should be obtained in patients with unexplained TLOC, vertigo, dizziness, or falls if symptoms are triggered by exertion, are associated with cardiorespiratory symptoms (e.g. chestpain, dyspnoea, palpitations), or occur in the context of known cardiac or pulmonary disease. Cardiac diagnostics should probably

also be performed in those who lack clear evidence of a specific vestibular or other neurological or medical cause, particularly if TLOC is present, and especially if it occurs without prodrome or while supine or sleeping (11).

Electrocardiography is a typical first step. If abnormalities are found suggesting a cardiogenic origin (e.g. arrhythmias, signs of ventricular hypertrophy or atrial enlargement, long QT-interval), *echocardiography* is required. In a prospective observational study of patients with syncope, systolic dysfunction was found in 27% of patients with a positive cardiac history or abnormal electrocardiography but in 0% of patients with a negative cardiac history and a normal ECG. This finding is highly predictive of an underlying arrhythmia (67). Patients with abnormal ECGs or echocardiograms are at much higher risk of dangerous arrhythmias and should be evaluated promptly, sometimes as inpatients.

If no structural heart disease sufficient to explain the symptoms is evident by a single electrocardiogram and cardiac ultrasound, a search for a potential cardiac arrhythmia by prolonged monitoring is often warranted. This typically includes prolonged ambulatory monitoring by *holter-ECG* or loop recorder. There is still debate about the overall diagnostic yield or cost-effectiveness of such monitoring. In unselected syncope or drop attack patients, diagnostic yield on relevant arrhythmias ranges from about 2–15% (206–208). Extending the ambulatory monitoring period to 72 h increases the yield by a factor of nearly two, but, as one might expect, with diminishing marginal yield over time (day 1: 15%; day 2: 10%; day 3: 4%) (208). Loop recorders retain a continuous recent electrocardiographic trace and store a 'snapshot' of the recent trace when the patient notes that a spell has occurred and 'activates' the device. Loop recorders may be worn externally for a month or implanted under the skin for up to 2 years or more. It appears that the yield of continuous electrocardiography continues to rise for up to 1 year and that the 12-month monitoring period has an estimated sensitivity for detecting arrhythmias of greater than 90% in unexplained syncope (209). Recent recommendations suggest that earlier use of implantable recorders than is typical in current practice may be warranted (210). Ambulatory blood pressure monitoring can also sometimes be a diagnostic aid if diurnal or situational (e.g. postprandial) blood pressure fluctuations are suspected (11).

Tilt-table testing has been extensively studied in the setting of TLOC and may prove helpful in identifying patients with reflex syncope as underlying cause. It aims to provoke syncopal episodes under controlled conditions and is helpful in the diagnostic approach to syncope of presumed vasovagal origin. The focus is on identifying a cardioinhibitory (bradycardia) or a vasodepressor (hypotension) response to tilt and various testing protocols have been proposed and are reviewed elsewhere (19). Some protocols involve use of provoking manoeuvres (e.g. carotid sinus massage, eyeball compression) or pharmacological challenge. Because some of these protocols aggressively seek to provoke syncope which might not correlate with spontaneous syncopal episodes, the specificity of tilt table findings has sometimes been called into question (211). Thus, exclusion of more dangerous causes (e.g. arrhythmia) is generally warranted as a first step if there are any concerning or atypical features, and care should be taken before relying too heavily on tilt table results for a final diagnosis. In addition to diagnosis of reflex syncope, tilt testing may help in identifying psychogenic spells—patients who suffer apparent TLOC or make convulsive movements during head-upright tilt without any associated change in physiological parameters are more likely to have a psychogenic origin (201). It should also be remembered that tilt testing could provoke BPPV symptoms, and might not be recognized as a cause in a typical cardiology laboratory.

Neurological evaluation: stroke

A stroke work-up should be obtained in patients with unexplained TLOC, vertigo, dizziness, or falls if symptoms are associated with stroke-like neurological manifestations (particularly hemiparesis or hemisensory loss), or occur in the context of prior strokes or vascular disease. Stroke diagnostics should probably also be performed in those who lack clear evidence of a specific vestibular or other neurological or medical cause.

Non-enhanced computed tomography (CT) scans of the brain are generally unhelpful because of the low sensitivity for CT in assessing the posterior cranial fossa, where much of the relevant pathology is located in those with vestibular-type symptoms. CT with or without CT angiography may be appropriate if an urgent stroke treatment decision is required (e.g. decision for acute thrombolysis) or when magnetic resonance imaging (MRI) is unavailable and immediate risk of repeat stroke must be assessed. Under more typical circumstances, if neuroimaging is required, MRI with diffusion-weighted-imaging for acute ischaemia and magnetic resonance angiography for vascular stenoses in the head, neck, or chest is generally the preferred study. Magnetic susceptibility sequences searching for small, old haemorrhages may be relevant in cases where old traumatic brain injury or cerebral amyloid angiopathy is a diagnostic consideration. Contrast-enhanced images or special sequences focused on cranial nerve imaging (e.g. constructive interference in steady state (CISS)) may be appropriate if structural lesions of the VIIIth cranial nerve are suspected, but are generally unnecessary if stroke or TIA is the diagnosis under investigation.

Vascular ultrasound of the carotid (anterior) and vertebrobasilar (posterior) circulation could be performed if the more sensitive and specific forms of vascular imaging described above are unavailable. Additional tests to assess the likelihood of a TIA or measure risk of stroke recurrence should also include a search for atrial fibrillation, routes for paradoxical embolism (e.g. patent foramen ovale), hypercoagulable state, and chronic risks for atherosclerosis.

Neurological evaluation: seizure

A seizure work-up should be obtained in patients with unexplained TLOC, vertigo, dizziness, or falls if symptoms involve loss of awareness or are associated with seizure-like neurological manifestations (particularly hallucinations or jerking movements), or occur in the context of a known seizure disorder. Seizure diagnostics should probably also be performed in those who lack clear evidence of a specific vestibular or other neurological or medical cause.

The diagnostic approach to presumed seizure almost invariably includes *electroencephalography* (EEG). During an episode, seizure and syncope have distinct patterns of EEG physiology. In seizure, epileptiform activity is observed. In syncope, EEG recordings show a typical sequence of slowing of background rhythms, high amplitude delta activity, followed by flattening of the EEG if the syncope persists long enough (212, 213).

Routine EEGs are performed while awake and for a limited period. Performing an EEG-recording during sleep increases the diagnostic sensitivity, and sleep deprivation (for all or most of the night) increases it even further (214–216). EEGs may also be repeated. The most sensitive, non-invasive strategies involve prolonged ambulatory EEG monitoring or inpatient video-EEG monitoring. Timing matters with respect to the event. An EEG is ideally obtained within the first 24 h after the event (217). The diagnostic yield of an awake EEG in the first 24 h after a presumed generalized convulsion is about 50% for epileptiform activity, but drops down to 21–34% in the next 24 h (100). False negative interictal results may occur in as many as 50% of routine recordings, and false positive results are occasionally found as well, since epileptoform EEG findings occur in roughly 2–6% of non-epileptic individuals in the general population (218–220). Repeating the EEG recording reduces the false negative rate to 30% and sleep deprived recordings reduces them to 20% (221). In circumstances where it is difficult to distinguish between convulsive syncope and epilepsy, electroencephalogram during tilt-table provocation can be diagnostic (102, 222). However, this testing paradigm can probably be reserved for those patients with an atypical history (11). Video EEG monitoring is expensive but provides the most definitive diagnoses when typical episodes can be recorded any analyzed both phenomenologically and physiologically.

Neurological evaluation: movement or degenerative disorders

In cases where symptoms or signs may seem to suggest an underlying movement or neurodegenerative disorder, patients should be referred to an appropriate consultant for evaluation and treatment. Occasionally autonomic function studies (beyond those described as part of the tilt table evaluation above) may prove informative in diagnosing an early case of multiple systems atrophy, Shy–Drager variant. Rare disorders such as MELAS (mitochondrial encephalomyopathy, lactic acidosis, and stroke-like episodes) may require specialized genetic or other tests (e.g. muscle biopsy). In general, however, these diagnoses are made clinically.

Special issues

Demographic and referral pattern variations

Age is an important diagnostic variable. Very young patients may have causes, both benign and dangerous, unfamiliar to adult caregivers (e.g. long-QT syndrome or breath-holding spells (11)). Young adult patients are less likely than older individuals to have TIA or stroke, but more likely to be misdiagnosed when they do. Great care should be taken to avoid missing craniocervical vascular dissection in these patients, especially given its similarity to migraine-like symptoms. Elderly patients are at much higher risk of dangerous disorders such as cardiac arrhythmia and are more likely to have atypical clinical presentations (11). They are also more likely to have 'red herring' associated clinical findings that may have no causal relationship to the underlying cause for their symptoms (e.g. mild orthostatic hypotension in an elderly patient on anti-hypertensives who complains of lightheadedness on arising too quickly…but turns out to have BPPV).

Sex, race, and ethnicity may also influence clinical presentations. Syncope, dizziness, and vertigo are slightly more common in women than men, and dangerous causes are slightly more common in men than women. Care should be taken, however, since women are more likely to present with atypical symptoms (e.g. of myocardial ischaemia). Although relatively little is known about racial and ethnic differences in these clinical situations, it is clear that the use of descriptive terms around dizziness varies by native language as well as racial, geographic, or cultural background. Greater care is warranted when evaluating someone from an unfamiliar racial, ethnic, or cultural background.

Referral patterns are important sources of clinical variation, particularly regarding the relative prevalence of different disorders. Dangerous diseases are far more common in emergency care settings than in tertiary care referral clinics, even with identical-sounding symptoms. Referral biases may also affect the apparent sensitivity or specificity of certain clinical features. For example, vestibular disorders are more likely to present with vestibular-sounding symptoms when referred to a vestibular clinic than when seen in falls and syncope unit or general care setting (e.g. ED) (3). It is wise to adjust baseline prevalence estimates based on the setting in which the patient is being seen. It is also probably a good idea to maintain a healthy scepticism regarding the applicability of personal experience when practicing outside one's typical clinical care setting.

Driving with fits, faints, falls, and funny turns

When taking care of a patient's underlying cause of 'fits, faints, falls, or funny turns' it is the physician's responsibility to address issues related to fitness to operate a motor vehicle. Although laws vary across jurisdictions, most countries or provinces place certain restrictions on driving with a seizure disorder. While neurologists are generally familiar with the regulations for patients with seizures, they are left with less certain guidance for driving restrictions in patients with syncope, episodic vertigo, or sudden falls. From a purely risk-mitigation standpoint, it is probably ill-advised for patients at significant risk of sudden loss of motor tone or consciousness to operate a motorized vehicle. This holds especially true for public servants such as pilots and bus or cab drivers. But when balancing the public good with the severe impact on personal freedom imposed by such a restriction, decisions are less clear.

Syncope occurred while driving a vehicle in 3–10% of patients (223, 224), leading to accidents in one-third of these cases in one study (223). Nevertheless, the cumulative probability of recurrence of syncope while driving was only 7% in 8 years (224) and the risk for syncope-mediated driving accidents (0.8% per year) was less than in high-risk accident groups *without* known medical conditions (11). In the current European Society of Cardiology guidelines for private drivers with syncope, no restrictions are recommended for patients with reflex syncope, unexplained syncope, and cardiac arrhythmia, once successful treatment is established (11). For professional drivers, permanent restrictions may apply for severe and recurrent reflex syncope. Ultimately, most of these decisions are guided by medical judgement of risk and careful discussion with the patient, rather than legal mandates.

Fall precautions

In patients at risk for falls and fall-related injuries, a structured risk assessment is recommended (225). Fall prevention in individual patients may include medical approaches such as cataract surgery, cardiac pacing, and medication reduction in order to minimize potentially treatable risk factors. Generally these medical interventions should be accompanied by referral to a physical therapist (or physiatrist) for formal gait evaluation, balance training exercises, and needs assessment for ambulatory assistive devices (e.g. single-leg canes, four-leg canes, walkers).

References

1. Newman-Toker DE, Dy FJ, Stanton VA, Zee DS, Calkins H, Robinson KA (2008). How often is dizziness from primary cardiovascular disease true vertigo? A systematic review. *J Gen Intern Med*, 23(12), 2087–94.
2. Newman-Toker DE, Camargo CA, Jr. (2006). 'Cardiogenic vertigo' – true vertigo as the presenting manifestation of primary cardiac disease. *Nat Clin Pract Neurol*, 2(3), 167–72; quiz 73.
3. Lawson J, Johnson I, Bamiou DE, Newton JL (2005). Benign paroxysmal positional vertigo: clinical characteristics of dizzy patients referred to a Falls and Syncope Unit. *QJM*, 98(5), 357–64.
4. Lawson J, Bamiou DE, Cohen HS, Newton J (2008). Positional vertigo in a Falls Service. *Age Ageing*, 37(5), 585–9.
5. Bisdorff A, Von Brevern M, Lempert T, Newman-Toker DE (2009). Classification of vestibular symptoms: towards an international classification of vestibular disorders. *J Vestib Res*, 19(1–2), 1–13.
6. Stevens DL, Matthews WB (1973). Cryptogenic drop attacks: an affliction of women. *Br Med J*, 1(5851), 439–42.
7. Stephenson JB, Hoffman MC, Russell AJ, et al. (2005). The movement disorders of Coffin-Lowry syndrome. *Brain Dev*, 27(2), 108–13.
8. Billiard M, Bassetti C, Dauvilliers Y, et al. (2006). EFNS guidelines on management of narcolepsy. *Eur J Neurol*, 13(10), 1035–48.
9. McCrory P, Meeuwisse W, Johnston K, et al. (2009). Consensus statement on Concussion in Sport – the 3rd International Conference on Concussion in Sport held in Zurich, November 2008. *J Sci Med Sport*, 12(3), 340–51.
10. Ishiyama G, Ishiyama A, Jacobson K, Baloh RW (2001). Drop attacks in older patients secondary to an otologic cause. *Neurology*, 57(6), 1103–6.
11. Moya A, Sutton R, Ammirati F, et al. (2009). Guidelines for the diagnosis and management of syncope (version 2009). *Eur Heart J*, 30(21), 2631–71.
12. Lee H, Yi HA, Lee SR, Ahn BH, Park BR (2005). Drop attacks in elderly patients secondary to otologic causes with Meniere's syndrome or non-Meniere peripheral vestibulopathy. *J Neurol Sci*, 232(1–2), 71–6.
13. Black FO, Effron MZ, Burns DS (1982). Diagnosis and management of drop attacks of vestibular origin: Tumarkin's otolithic crisis. *Otolaryngol Head Neck Surg*, 90(2), 256–62.
14. Krumholz A, Wiebe S, Gronseth G, et al. (2007). Practice Parameter: evaluating an apparent unprovoked first seizure in adults (an evidence-based review), report of the Quality Standards Subcommittee of the American Academy of Neurology and the American Epilepsy Society. *Neurology*, 69(21), 1996–2007.
15. Commission on Classification and Terminology of the International League Against Epilepsy (1981). Proposal for revised clinical and electroencephalographic classification of epileptic seizures. *Epilepsia*, 22(4), 489–501.
16. Carreno M (2008). Recognition of nonepileptic events. *Semin Neurol*, 28(3), 297–304.
17. Bakker MJ, van Dijk JG, van den Maagdenberg AM, Tijssen MA (2006). Startle syndromes. *Lancet Neurol*, 5(6), 513–24.
18. Thijs RD, Bloem BR, van Dijk JG (2009). Falls, faints, fits and funny turns. *J Neurol*, 256(2), 155–67.
19. Bloem BR, Overeem S, Van Dijk JG (2004). Syncopal falls, drop attacks and their mimics. In Bronstein AM, Brandt T, Woollacott MH (Eds) *Clinical disorders of balance, posture and gait*, pp. 286–316. London: Arnold Publ.
20. Easton JD, Saver JL, Albers GW, et al. (2009). Definition and evaluation of transient ischemic attack: a scientific statement for healthcare professionals from the American Heart Association/American Stroke Association Stroke Council; Council on Cardiovascular Surgery and Anesthesia; Council on Cardiovascular Radiology and Intervention; Council on Cardiovascular Nursing; and the Interdisciplinary Council on Peripheral Vascular Disease. The American Academy of Neurology affirms the value of this statement as an educational tool for neurologists. *Stroke*, 40(6), 2276–93.
21. Thijs RD, Wieling W, Kaufmann H, van Dijk G (2004). Defining and classifying syncope. *Clin Auton Res*, 14(Suppl 1), 4–8.

22. Fonseca AC, Canhao P (2011). Diagnostic difficulties in the classification of transient neurological attacks. *Eur J Neurol*, 18(4), 644–8.

23. Mackay M (2005). Fits, faints and funny turns in children. *Aust Fam Physician*, 34(12), 1003–8.

24. Murtagh J (2003). Fits, faints and funny turns. A general diagnostic approach. *Aust Fam Physician*, 32(4), 203–6.

25. Newman BH, Graves S (2001). A study of 178 consecutive vasovagal syncopal reactions from the perspective of safety. *Transfusion*, 41(12), 1475–9.

26. Remler BF, Daroff RB (2007). Falls and drop attacks. In Bradley WG, Daroff RB, Fenichel GM, Jankovic J (Eds) *Neurology in Clinical Practice* (5th ed), pp. 23–7. Oxford: Butterworth-Heinemann.

27. Benbadis S (2009). The differential diagnosis of epilepsy: a critical review. *Epilepsy Behav*, 15(1), 15–21.

28. Martikainen K, Seppa K, Viita P, Rajala S, Laippala P, Keranen T (2003). Transient loss of consciousness as reason for admission to primary health care emergency room. *Scand J Prim Health Care*, 21(1), 61–4.

29. Kessler C, Tristano JM, De Lorenzo R (2010). The emergency department approach to syncope: evidence-based guidelines and prediction rules. *Emerg Med Clin North Am*, 28(3), 487–500.

30. Newman-Toker DE, Hsieh YH, Camargo CA, Jr., Pelletier AJ, Butchy GT, Edlow JA (2008). Spectrum of dizziness visits to US emergency departments: cross-sectional analysis from a nationally representative sample. *Mayo Clin Proc*, 83(7), 765–75.

31. Kroenke K, Mangelsdorff AD (1989). Common symptoms in ambulatory care: incidence, evaluation, therapy, and outcome. *Am J Med*, 86(3), 262–6.

32. Mathers LJ, Weiss HB (1998). Incidence and characteristics of fall-related emergency department visits. *Acad Emerg Med*, 5(11), 1064–70.

33. Cheung CS, Mak PS, Manley KV, et al. (2010). Predictors of important neurological causes of dizziness among patients presenting to the emergency department. *Emerg Med J*, 27(7), 517–21.

34. Tarnutzer AA, Berkowitz AL, Robinson KA, Hsieh YH, Newman-Toker DE (2011). Does my dizzy patient have a stroke? A systematic review of bedside diagnosis in acute vestibular syndrome. *CMAJ*, 183(9), E571–92.

35. Edlow JA, Newman-Toker DE, Savitz SI (2008). Diagnosis and initial management of cerebellar infarction. *Lancet Neurol*, 7(10), 951–64.

36. Bhattacharyya N, Baugh RF, Orvidas L, et al. (2008). Clinical practice guideline: benign paroxysmal positional vertigo. *Otolaryngol Head Neck Surg*, 139(5 Suppl 4), S47–81.

37. Fife TD, Iverson DJ, Lempert T, et al. (2008). Practice parameter: therapies for benign paroxysmal positional vertigo (an evidence-based review), report of the Quality Standards Subcommittee of the American Academy of Neurology. *Neurology*, 70(22), 2067–74.

38. Parry SW, Steen IN, Baptist M, Kenny RA (2005). Amnesia for loss of consciousness in carotid sinus syndrome: implications for presentation with falls. *J Am Coll Cardiol*, 45(11), 1840–3.

39. O'Dwyer C, Bennett K, Langan Y, Fan CW, Kenny RA (2011). Amnesia for loss of consciousness is common in vasovagal syncope. *Europace*, 13(7), 1040–5.

40. Day SC, Cook EF, Funkenstein H, Goldman L (1982). Evaluation and outcome of emergency room patients with transient loss of consciousness. *Am J Med*, 73(1), 15–23.

41. Seet CM (1999). Clinical presentation of patients with subarachnoid haemorrhage at a local emergency department. *Singapore Med J*, 40(6), 383–5.

42. Kapoor WN, Peterson J, Wieand HS, Karpf M (1987). Diagnostic and prognostic implications of recurrences in patients with syncope. *Am J Med*, 83(4), 700–8.

43. Kenny RA, Richardson DA (2001). Carotid sinus syndrome and falls in older adults. *Am J Geriatr Cardiol*, 10(2), 97–9.

44. McIntosh SJ, Lawson J, Kenny RA (1993). Clinical characteristics of vasodepressor, cardioinhibitory, and mixed carotid sinus syndrome in the elderly. *Am J Med*, 95(2), 203–8.

45. Romme JJ, van Dijk N, Boer KR, et al. (2008). Influence of age and gender on the occurrence and presentation of reflex syncope. *Clin Auton Res*, 18(3), 127–33.

46. Davies AJ, Steen N, Kenny RA. Carotid sinus hypersensitivity is common in older patients presenting to an accident and emergency department with unexplained falls. *Age Ageing*, 30(4), 289–93.

47. Benke T, Hochleitner M, Bauer G (1997). Aura phenomena during syncope. *Eur Neurol*, 37(1), 28–32.

48. Stanton VA, Hsieh YH, Camargo CA, Jr., et al. (2007). Overreliance on symptom quality in diagnosing dizziness: results of a multicenter survey of emergency physicians. *Mayo Clinic Proc*, 82(11), 1319–28.

49. Wieling W, Thijs RD, van Dijk N, Wilde AA, Benditt DG, van Dijk JG (2009). Symptoms and signs of syncope: a review of the link between physiology and clinical clues. *Brain*, 132(Pt 10), 2630–42.

50. Calkins H, Shyr Y, Frumin H, Schork A, Morady F (1995). The value of the clinical history in the differentiation of syncope due to ventricular tachycardia, atrioventricular block, and neurocardiogenic syncope. *Am J Med*, 98(4), 365–73.

51. Sheldon RS, Amuah JE, Connolly SJ, et al. (2009). Design and use of a quantitative scale for measuring presyncope. *J Cardiovasc Electrophysiol*, 20(8), 888–93.

52. Karp HR, Weissler AM, Heyman A (1961). Vasodepressor syncope: EEG and circulatory changes. *Arch Neurol*, 5, 94–101.

53. Lin JT, Ziegler DK, Lai CW, Bayer W (1982). Convulsive syncope in blood donors. *Ann Neurol*, 11(5), 525–8.

54. Alboni P, Brignole M, Menozzi C, et al. (2001). Diagnostic value of history in patients with syncope with or without heart disease. *J Am Coll Cardiol*, 37(7), 1921–8.

55. Lempert T, Bauer M, Schmidt D (1994). Syncope: a videometric analysis of 56 episodes of transient cerebral hypoxia. *Ann Neurol*, 36(2), 233–7.

56. Colman N, Nahm K, van Dijk JG, Reitsma JB, Wieling W, Kaufmann H (2004). Diagnostic value of history taking in reflex syncope. *Clin Auton Res*, 14(Suppl 1), 37–44.

57. Ganzeboom KS, Colman N, Reitsma JB, Shen WK, Wieling W (2003). Prevalence and triggers of syncope in medical students. *Am J Cardiol*, 91(8), 1006–8, A8.

58. Ganzeboom KS, Mairuhu G, Reitsma JB, Linzer M, Wieling W, van Dijk N (2006). Lifetime cumulative incidence of syncope in the general population: a study of 549 Dutch subjects aged 35–60 years. *J Cardiovasc Electrophysiol*, 17(11), 1172–6.

59. Scherf D, Bornemann C (1970). The Stokes-Adams syndrome. *Cardiovasc Clin*, 2(2), 101–16.

60. Sheldon R, Hersi A, Ritchie D, Koshman ML, Rose S (2010). Syncope and structural heart disease: historical criteria for vasovagal syncope and ventricular tachycardia. *J Cardiovasc Electrophysiol*, 21(12), 1358–64.

61. Ullman E, Edlow JA (2010). Complete heart block complicating the head impulse test. *Arch Neurol*, 67(10), 1272–4.

62. Kasbekar AV, Baguley DM, Knight R, et al. (2010). Heart rate and blood pressure effects during caloric vestibular testing. *J Laryngol Otol*, 124(6), 616–22.

63. Vilela MD, Goodkin R, Lundin DA, Newell DW (2005). Rotational vertebrobasilar ischemia: hemodynamic assessment and surgical treatment. *Neurosurgery*, 56(1), 36–43; discussion -5.

64. Lempert T, von Brevern M (1996). The eye movements of syncope. *Neurology*, 46(4), 1086–8.

65. Krediet CT, van Dijk N, Linzer M, van Lieshout JJ, Wieling W (2002). Management of vasovagal syncope: controlling or aborting faints by leg crossing and muscle tensing. *Circulation*, 106(13), 1684–9.

66. van Lieshout JJ, ten Harkel AD, Wieling W (1992). Physical manoeuvres for combating orthostatic dizziness in autonomic failure. *Lancet*, 339(8798), 897–8.

67. Sarasin FP, Junod AF, Carballo D, Slama S, Unger PF, Louis-Simonet M (2002). Role of echocardiography in the evaluation of syncope: a prospective study. *Heart*, 88(4), 363–7.

68. Mathias CJ (2003). Autonomic diseases: clinical features and laboratory evaluation. *J Neurol Neurosurg Psychiatry*, 74(Suppl 3), iii31–41.

69. Freeman R, Wieling W, Axelrod FB, et al. (2011). Consensus statement on the definition of orthostatic hypotension, neurally mediated syncope and the postural tachycardia syndrome. *Clin Auton Res*, 21(2), 69–72.

70. Birkhahn RH, Gaeta TJ, Van Deusen SK, Tloczkowski J (2003). The ability of traditional vital signs and shock index to identify ruptured ectopic pregnancy. *Am J Obstet Gynecol*, 189(5), 1293–6.

71. Gilbert VE (1993). Immediate orthostatic hypotension: diagnostic value in acutely ill patients. *South Med J*, 86(9), 1028–32.

72. Lasch KF, Evans CJ, Schatell D (2009). A qualitative analysis of patient-reported symptoms of anemia. *Nephrol Nurs J*, 36(6), 621–4, 31–2; quiz 33.

73. Wenning GK, Ben Shlomo Y, Magalhaes M, Daniel SE, Quinn NP (1994). Clinical features and natural history of multiple system atrophy. An analysis of 100 cases. *Brain*, 117(Pt 4), 835–45.

74. Gupta V, Lipsitz LA (2007). Orthostatic hypotension in the elderly: diagnosis and treatment. *Am J Med*, 120(10), 841–7.

75. Bloem BR, Grimbergen YA, Cramer M, Willemsen M, Zwinderman AH (2001). Prospective assessment of falls in Parkinson's disease. *J Neurol*, 248(11), 950–8.

76. Middlekauff HR, Stevenson WG, Saxon LA (1993). Prognosis after syncope: impact of left ventricular function. *Am Heart J*, 125(1), 121–7.

77. Soteriades ES, Evans JC, Larson MG, et al. (2002). Incidence and prognosis of syncope. *N Engl J Med*, 347(12), 878–85.

78. Kapoor WN, Karpf M, Wieand S, Peterson JR, Levey GS (1983). A prospective evaluation and follow-up of patients with syncope. *N Engl J Med*, 309(4), 197–204.

79. Quinn JV, Stiell IG, McDermott DA, Sellers KL, Kohn MA, Wells GA (2004). Derivation of the San Francisco Syncope Rule to predict patients with short-term serious outcomes. *Ann Emerg Med*, 43(2), 224–32.

80. Wieling W, Krediet CT, Wilde AA (2006). Flush after syncope: not always an arrhythmia. *J Cardiovasc Electrophysiol*, 17(7), 804–5.

81. Sheldon RS, Sheldon AG, Connolly SJ, et al. (2006). Age of first faint in patients with vasovagal syncope. *J Cardiovasc Electrophysiol*, 17(1), 49–54.

82. Oh JH, Hanusa BH, Kapoor WN (1999). Do symptoms predict cardiac arrhythmias and mortality in patients with syncope? *Arch Intern Med*, 159(4), 375–80.

83. Fisher RS, van Emde Boas W, et al. (2005). Epileptic seizures and epilepsy: definitions proposed by the International League Against Epilepsy (ILAE) and the International Bureau for Epilepsy (IBE). *Epilepsia*, 46(4), 470–2.

84. Hauser WA, Annegers JF, Kurland LT (1993). Incidence of epilepsy and unprovoked seizures in Rochester, Minnesota: 1935–1984. *Epilepsia*, 34(3), 453–68.

85. Forsgren L, Bucht G, Eriksson S, Bergmark L (1996). Incidence and clinical characterization of unprovoked seizures in adults: a prospective population-based study. *Epilepsia*, 37(3), 224–9.

86. Grunewald RA, Panayiotopoulos CP (1993). Juvenile myoclonic epilepsy. A review. *Arch Neurol*, 50(6), 594–8.

87. Baquis GD, Pessin MS, Scott RM (1985). Limb shaking – a carotid TIA. *Stroke*, 16(3), 444–8.

88. Gerstner E, Liberato B, Wright CB (2005). Bi-hemispheric anterior cerebral artery with drop attacks and limb shaking TIAs. *Neurology*, 65(1), 174.

89. Sheldon R, Rose S, Ritchie D, et al. (2002). Historical criteria that distinguish syncope from seizures. *J Am Coll Cardiol*, 40(1), 142–8.

90. Theodore WH, Porter RJ, Penry JK (1983). Complex partial seizures: clinical characteristics and differential diagnosis. *Neurology*, 33(9), 1115–21.

91. Scaramelli A, Braga P, Avellanal A, et al. (2009). Prodromal symptoms in epileptic patients: clinical characterization of the pre-ictal phase. *Seizure*, 18(4), 246–50.

92. Bladin PF (1998). History of 'epileptic vertigo': its medical, social, and forensic problems. *Epilepsia*, 39(4), 442–7.

93. Hughes JR, Drachman DA (1977). Dizziness, epilepsy and the EEG. *Dis Nerv Syst*, 38(6), 431–5.

94. Gowers WR (1885). *Epilepsy and other chronic convulsive diseases*. New York: William Wood & Co.

95. Currie S, Heathfield KW, Henson RA, Scott DF (1971). Clinical course and prognosis of temporal lobe epilepsy. A survey of 666 patients. *Brain*, 94(1), 173–90.

96. Salanova V, Andermann F, Rasmussen T, Olivier A, Quesney LF (1995). Parietal lobe epilepsy. Clinical manifestations and outcome in 82 patients treated surgically between 1929 and 1988. *Brain*, 118 (Pt 3), 607–27.

97. Williamson PD, Thadani VM, Darcey TM, Spencer DD, Spencer SS, Mattson RH (1992). Occipital lobe epilepsy: clinical characteristics, seizure spread patterns, and results of surgery. *Ann Neurol*, 31(1), 3–13.

98. Taylor DC, Lochery M (1987). Temporal lobe epilepsy: origin and significance of simple and complex auras. *J Neurol Neurosurg Psychiatry*, 50(6), 673–81.

99. Kogeorgos J, Scott DF, Swash M (1981). Epileptic dizziness. *Br Med J (Clin Res Ed)*, 282(6265), 687–9.

100. McKeon A, Vaughan C, Delanty N (2006). Seizure versus syncope. *Lancet Neurol*, 5(2), 171–80.

101. Kanjwal K, Karabin B, Kanjwal Y, Grubb BP (2009). Differentiation of convulsive syncope from epilepsy with an implantable loop recorder. *Int J Med Sci*, 6(6), 296–300.

102. Zaidi A, Clough P, Cooper P, Scheepers B, Fitzpatrick AP (2000). Misdiagnosis of epilepsy: many seizure-like attacks have a cardiovascular cause. *J Am Coll Cardiol*, 36(1), 181–4.

103. Thijs RD, Wagenaar WA, Middelkoop HA, Wieling W, van Dijk JG (2008). Transient loss of consciousness through the eyes of a witness. *Neurology*, 71(21), 1713–8.

104. Hoefnagels WA, Padberg GW, Overweg J, van der Velde EA, Roos RA (1991). Transient loss of consciousness: the value of the history for distinguishing seizure from syncope. *J Neurol*, 238(1), 39–43.

105. Benbadis SR, Wolgamuth BR, Goren H, Brener S, Fouad-Tarazi F (1995). Value of tongue biting in the diagnosis of seizures. *Arch Intern Med*, 155(21), 2346–9.

106. Gastaut H, Fischer-Williams M (1957). Electro-encephalographic study of syncope; its differentiation from epilepsy. *Lancet*, 273(7004), 1018–25.

107. Robillard A, Saint-Hilaire JM, Mercier M, Bouvier G (1983). The lateralizing and localizing value of adversion in epileptic seizures. *Neurology*, 33(9), 1241–2.

108. Calkins H, Shyr Y, Frumin H, Schork A, Morady F (1995). The value of the clinical history in the differentiation of syncope due to ventricular tachycardia, atrioventricular block, and neurocardiogenic syncope. *Am J Med*, 98(4), 365–73.

109. Lempert T, Bauer M, Schmidt D (1994). Syncope and near-death experience. *Lancet*, 344(8925), 829–30.

110. Stephenson JBP (2002). Fainting and syncope. In Maria BL (Ed) *Current management in pediatric neurology*, pp. 345–51. Hamilton: BC Decker.

111. Rocamora R, Kurthen M, Lickfett L, Von Oertzen J, Elger CE (2003). Cardiac asystole in epilepsy: clinical and neurophysiologic features. *Epilepsia*, 44(2), 179–85.

112. Phizackerley PJ, Poole EW, Whitty CW (1954). Sino-auricular heart block as an epileptic manifestation; a case report. *Epilepsia*, 3, 89–91.

113. Kiok MC, Terrence CF, Fromm GH, Lavine S (1986). Sinus arrest in epilepsy. *Neurology*, 36(1), 115–6.

114. Blumhardt LD, Smith PE, Owen L (1986). Electrocardiographic accompaniments of temporal lobe epileptic seizures. *Lancet*, 1(8489), 1051–6.

115. Wilder-Smith E (1992). Complete atrio-ventricular conduction block during complex partial seizure. *J Neurol Neurosurg Psychiatry*, 55(8), 734–6.

116. van Rijckevorsel K, Saussu F, de Barsy T (1995). Bradycardia, an epileptic ictal manifestation. *Seizure*, 4(3), 237–9.

117. Schuele SU, Bermeo AC, Alexopoulos AV, *et al.* (2007). Video-electrographic and clinical features in patients with ictal asystole. *Neurology*, 69(5), 434–41.

118. Cuthill FM, Espie CA (2005). Sensitivity and specificity of procedures for the differential diagnosis of epileptic and non-epileptic seizures: a systematic review. *Seizure*, 14(5), 293–303.

119. Bodde NM, Brooks JL, Baker GA, *et al.* (2009). Psychogenic non-epileptic seizures – definition, etiology, treatment and prognostic issues: a critical review. *Seizure*, 18(8), 543–53.

120. Mellers JD (2005). The approach to patients with 'non-epileptic seizures'. *Postgrad Med J*, 81(958), 498–504.

121. Smith PE (2001). If it's not epilepsy. *J Neurol Neurosurg Psychiatry*, 70 Suppl 2:II9–14.

122. Hadjikoutis S, Smith PE (2005). Approach to the patient with epilepsy in the outpatient department. *Postgrad Med J*, 81(957), 442–7.

123. Linzer M, Felder A, Hackel A, *et al.* (1990). Psychiatric syncope: a new look at an old disease. *Psychosomatics*, 31(2), 181–8.

124. Luzza F, Pugliatti P, di Rosa S, Calabro D, Carerj S, Oreto G (2003). Tilt-induced pseudosyncope. *Int J Clin Pract*, 57(5), 373–5.

125. Petersen ME, Williams TR, Sutton R (1995). Psychogenic syncope diagnosed by prolonged head-up tilt testing. *QJM*, 88(3), 209–13.

126. Bazil CW, Walczak TS (1997). Effects of sleep and sleep stage on epileptic and nonepileptic seizures. *Epilepsia*, 38(1), 56–62.

127. Lancman ME, Asconape JJ, Craven WJ, Howard G, Penry JK (1994). Predictive value of induction of psychogenic seizures by suggestion. *Ann Neurol*, 35(3), 359–61.

128. Stephenson JBP. Anoxic seizures or syncopes. In Stephenson JBP (Ed) *Fits and faints*, pp. 41–58. Oxford: Mac Keith Press.

129. Chung SS, Gerber P, Kirlin KA (2006). Ictal eye closure is a reliable indicator for psychogenic nonepileptic seizures. *Neurology*, 66(11), 1730–1.

130. Jankovic J, Havins WE, Wilkins RB (1982). Blinking and blepharospasm. Mechanism, diagnosis, and management. *JAMA*, 248(23), 3160–4.

131. Ettinger AB, Weisbrot DM, Nolan E, Devinsky O (1999). Postictal symptoms help distinguish patients with epileptic seizures from those with non-epileptic seizures. *Seizure*, 8(3), 149–51.

132. Voermans NC, Zwarts MJ, van Laar T, Tijssen MA, Bloem BR (2005). Fallacious falls. *J Neurol*, 252(10), 1271–3.

133. Bauer J (1996). Epilepsy and prolactin in adults: a clinical review. *Epilepsy Res*, 24(1), 1–7.

134. Chen DK, So YT, Fisher RS (2005). Use of serum prolactin in diagnosing epileptic seizures: report of the Therapeutics and Technology Assessment Subcommittee of the American Academy of Neurology. *Neurology*, 65(5), 668–75.

135. Willert C, Spitzer C, Kusserow S, Runge U (2004). Serum neuron-specific enolase, prolactin, and creatine kinase after epileptic and psychogenic non-epileptic seizures. *Acta Neurol Scand*, 109(5), 318–23.

136. Alving J (1998). Serum prolactin levels are elevated also after pseudo-epileptic seizures. *Seizure*, 7(2), 85–9.

137. Oribe E, Amini R, Nissenbaum E, Boal B (1996). Serum prolactin concentrations are elevated after syncope. *Neurology*, 47(1), 60–2.

138. Pohlmann-Eden B, Stefanou A, Wellhausser H (1997). Serum prolactate in syncope. *Neurology*, 48(5), 1477–8.

139. Benbadis SR, Chichkova R (2006). Psychogenic pseudosyncope: an underestimated and provable diagnosis. *Epilepsy Behav*, 9(1), 106–10.

140. Grad A, Baloh RW (1989). Vertigo of vascular origin. Clinical and electronystagmographic features in 84 cases. *Arch Neurol*, 46(3), 281–4.

141. Davidson E, Rotenbeg Z, Fuchs J, Weinberger I, Agmon J (1991). Transient ischemic attack-related syncope. *Clin Cardiol*, 14(2), 141–4.

142. Quinn J, McDermott D, Stiell I, Kohn M, Wells G (2006). Prospective validation of the San Francisco Syncope Rule to predict patients with serious outcomes. *Ann Emerg Med*, 47(5), 448–54.

143. Savitz SI, Caplan LR (2005). Vertebrobasilar disease. *N Engl J Med*, 352(25), 2618–26.

144. Savage DD, Corwin L, McGee DL, Kannel WB, Wolf PA (1985). Epidemiologic features of isolated syncope: the Framingham Study. *Stroke*, 16(4), 626–9.

145. Hennerici M, Klemm C, Rautenberg W (1988). The subclavian steal phenomenon: a common vascular disorder with rare neurologic deficits. *Neurology*, 38(5), 669–73.

146. Taylor CL, Selman WR, Ratcheson RA (2002). Steal affecting the central nervous system. *Neurosurgery*, 50(4), 679–88; discussion 88–9.

147. Smith JM, Koury HI, Hafner CD, Welling RE (1994). Subclavian steal syndrome. A review of 59 consecutive cases. *J Cardiovasc Surg (Torino)*, 35(1), 11–14.

148. Bornstein NM, Norris JW (1986). Subclavian steal: a harmless haemodynamic phenomenon? *Lancet*, 2(8502), 303–5.

149. Zhou Y, Lee SH, Therani AS, Robinson KA, Newman-Toker D (2011). Anterior Circulation Stroke Causing Dizziness or Vertigo: A Systematic Review. 136th Annual Meeting of the American Neurological Association, 25–27 September, 2011, San Diego, CA.

150. Dulay D, Gould PA, Leung A, Krahn AD (2008). Images in cardiovascular medicine. A sensitive dissection: profound bradycardia complicating carotid dissection. *Circulation*, 118(11), e152–3.

151. Bogousslavsky J, Regli F (1985). Vertebrobasilar transient ischemic attacks in internal carotid artery occlusion or tight stenosis. *Arch Neurol*, 42(1), 64–8.

152. Perry JJ, Stiell IG, *et al.* (2010). High risk clinical characteristics for subarachnoid haemorrhage in patients with acute headache: prospective cohort study. *BMJ*, 341:c5204.

153. Kirchmann M, Thomsen LL, Olesen J (2006). Basilar-type migraine: clinical, epidemiologic, and genetic features. *Neurology*, 66(6), 880–6.

154. Weig SG, Buckthal PE, Choi SK, Zellem RT (1991). Recurrent syncope as the presenting symptom of Arnold-Chiari malformation. *Neurology*, 41(10), 1673–4.

155. Prilipko O, Dehdashti AR, Zaim S, Seeck M (2005). Orthostatic intolerance and syncope associated with Chiari type I malformation. *J Neurol Neurosurg Psychiatry*, 76(7), 1034–6.

156. Kruschinski C, Hummers-Pradier E, Newman-Toker D, Camargo CA, Jr., Edlow JA (2008). Diagnosing dizziness in the emergency and primary care settings. *Mayo Clin Proc*, 83(11), 1297–8; author reply 8–9.

157. Newman-Toker DE, Cannon LM, Stofferahn ME, Rothman RE, Hsieh YH, Zee DS (2007). Imprecision in patient reports of dizziness symptom quality: a cross-sectional study conducted in an acute care setting. *Mayo Clin Proc*, 82(11), 1329–40.

158. Buttner U, Helmchen C, Brandt T (1999). Diagnostic criteria for central versus peripheral positioning nystagmus and vertigo: a review. *Acta Otolaryngol*, 119(1), 1–5.

159. Leigh RJ, Zee DS (2006). *The Neurology of Eye Movements* (4th ed). New York: Oxford University Press.

160. Moubayed SP, Saliba I (2009). Vertebrobasilar insufficiency presenting as isolated positional vertigo or dizziness: a double-blind retrospective cohort study. *Laryngoscope*, 119(10), 2071–6.

161. Stark RJ, Wodak J. Primary orthostatic cerebral ischaemia. *J Neurol Neurosurg Psychiatry*, 46(10), 883–91.

162. Blank SC, Shakir RA, Bindoff LA, Bradey N (1997). Spontaneous intracranial hypotension: clinical and magnetic resonance imaging characteristics. *Clin Neurol Neurosurg*, 99(3), 199–204.

163. Stewart JM, Clarke D (2011). 'He's dizzy when he stands up': an introduction to initial orthostatic hypotension. *J Pediatr*, 158(3), 499–504.

164. Raj SR (2006). The Postural Tachycardia Syndrome (POTS), pathophysiology, diagnosis & management. *Indian Pacing Electrophysiol J*, 6(2), 84–99.

165. Low PA, Sandroni P, Joyner M, Shen WK (2009). Postural tachycardia syndrome (POTS). *J Cardiovasc Electrophysiol*, 20(3), 352–8.

166. Low PA, Opfer-Gehrking TL, Textor SC, *et al.* (1995). Postural tachycardia syndrome (POTS). *Neurology*, 45(4 Suppl 5), S19–25.

167. Gomez CR, Cruz-Flores S, Malkoff MD, Sauer CM, Burch CM (1996). Isolated vertigo as a manifestation of vertebrobasilar ischemia. *Neurology*, 47(1), 94–7.

168. Gottesman RF, Sharma P, Robinson KA, *et al.* (2012). Clinical characteristics of symptomatic vertebral artery dissection. A systematic review. *Neurologist* (in press)

169. Shah KH, Kleckner K, Edlow JA (2008). Short-term prognosis of stroke among patients diagnosed in the emergency department with a transient ischemic attack. *Ann Emerg Med*, 51(3), 316–23.

170. Brandt T, Baloh RW (2005). Rotational vertebral artery occlusion: a clinical entity or various syndromes? *Neurology*, 65(8), 1156–7.

171. Kuether TA, Nesbit GM, Clark WM, Barnwell SL (1997). Rotational vertebral artery occlusion: a mechanism of vertebrobasilar insufficiency. *Neurosurgery*, 41(2), 427–32; discussion 32–3.

172. Shimizu T, Waga S, Kojima T, Niwa S (1988). Decompression of the vertebral artery for bow-hunter's stroke. Case report. *J Neurosurg*, 69(1), 127–31.

173. Sorensen BF (1978). Bow hunter's stroke. *Neurosurgery*, 2(3), 259–61.

174. Heidenreich KD, Carender WJ, Heidenreich MJ, Telian SA (2010). Strategies to distinguish benign paroxysmal positional vertigo from rotational vertebrobasilar ischemia. *Ann Vasc Surg*, 24(4), 553 e1–5.

175. Mannelli M, Ianni L, Cilotti A, Conti A (1999). Pheochromocytoma in Italy: a multicentric retrospective study. *Eur J Endocrinol*, 141(6), 619–24.

176. Nielsen JM (1959). Tornado epilepsy simulating Meniere's syndrome: report of 4 cases. *Neurology*, 9, 794–6.

177. Penfield W, Erickson TC (1941). *Epilepsy and Cerebral Localization*. London: Bailliere.

178. Brandt T, Dieterich M (1999). The vestibular cortex. Its locations, functions, and disorders. *Ann N Y Acad Sci*, 871, 293–312.

179. Kaplan PW, Tusa RJ (1993). Neurophysiologic and clinical correlations of epileptic nystagmus. *Neurology*, 43(12), 2508–14.

180. Neuhauser H, Leopold M, von Brevern M, Arnold G, Lempert T (2001). The interrelations of migraine, vertigo, and migrainous vertigo. *Neurology*, 56(4), 436–41.

181. Hufner K, Barresi D, Glaser M, *et al.* (2008). Vestibular paroxysmia: diagnostic features and medical treatment. *Neurology*, 71(13), 1006–14.

182. Shoair OA, Nyandege AN, Slattum PW (2011). Medication-related dizziness in the older adult. *Otolaryngol Clin North Am*, 44(2), 455–71.

183. Black SE, Maki BE, Fernie GR (1993). Aging, imbalance and falls. In Sharpe A, Barber HO (Eds) *The Vestibulo-Ocular Reflex and Vertigo*, pp. 317–35. New York: Raven.

184. Wolfson L (1992). Falls and gait. In Katzman R, Rowe IW (Eds) Principles of Geriatric *Neurology*, Philadelphia: FA Davis.

185. Tinetti ME, Baker DI, McAvay G, *et al.* (1994). A multifactorial intervention to reduce the risk of falling among elderly people living in the community. *N Engl J Med*, 331(13), 821–7.

186. Parry SW, Kenny RA (2005). Drop attacks in older adults: systematic assessment has a high diagnostic yield. *J Am Geriatr Soc*, 53(1), 74–8.

187. O'Mahony D, Foote C (1998). Prospective evaluation of unexplained syncope, dizziness, and falls among community-dwelling elderly adults. *J Gerontol A Biol Sci Med Sci*, 53(6), M435–40.

188. Lee MS, Marsden CD (1995). Drop attacks. *Adv Neurol*, 67, 41–52.

189. Meissner I, Wiebers DO, Swanson JW, O'Fallon WM (1986). The natural history of drop attacks. *Neurology*, 36(8), 1029–34.

190. Lin BF, Chen YS, Weng HF, Chia WT (2009). Acute aortic dissection presenting as case of accidental falling with flaccidity of left lower extremity. *Am J Emerg Med*, 27(1), 127 e1–2.

191. Ishiyama G, Ishiyama A, Baloh RW (2003). Drop attacks and vertigo secondary to a non-meniere otologic cause. *Arch Neurol*, 60(1), 71–5.

192. Lawson J, Johnson I, Bamiou DE, Newton JL (2005). Benign paroxysmal positional vertigo: clinical characteristics of dizzy patients referred to a Falls and Syncope Unit. *QJM*, 98(5), 357–64.

193. Brantberg K, Ishiyama A, Baloh RW (2005). Drop attacks secondary to superior canal dehiscence syndrome. *Neurology*, 64(12), 2126–8.

194. Minor LB, Solomon D, Zinreich JS, Zee DS (1998). Sound- and/or pressure-induced vertigo due to bone dehiscence of the superior semicircular canal. *Arch Otolaryngol Head Neck Surg*, 124(3), 249–58.

195. Baloh RW, Jacobson K, Winder T (1990). Drop attacks with Meniere's syndrome. *Ann Neurol*, 28(3), 384–7.

196. Kentala E, Havia M, Pyykko I (2001). Short-lasting drop attacks in Meniere's disease. *Otolaryngol Head Neck Surg*, 124(5), 526–30.

197. Tumarkin A (1936). The otolithic catastrophe: a new syndrome. *BMJ*, 1, 175–7.

198. Odkvist LM, Bergenius J (1988). Drop attacks in Meniere's disease. *Acta Otolaryngol Suppl*, 455, 82–5.

199. Boonstra TA, van der Kooij H, Munneke M, Bloem BR (2008). Gait disorders and balance disturbances in Parkinson's disease: clinical update and pathophysiology. *Curr Opin Neurol*, 21(4), 461–71.

200. van Dijk JG, Thijs RD, Benditt DG, Wieling W (2009). A guide to disorders causing transient loss of consciousness: focus on syncope. *Nat Rev Neurol*, 5(8), 438–48.

201. Grubb BP, Gerard G, Wolfe DA, *et al.* (1992). Syncope and seizures of psychogenic origin: identification with head-upright tilt table testing. *Clin Cardiol*, 15(11), 839–42.

202. Reuber M, Howlett S, Khan A, Grunewald RA (2007). Non-epileptic seizures and other functional neurological symptoms: predisposing, precipitating, and perpetuating factors. *Psychosomatics*, 48(3), 230–8.

203. Overeem S, Mignot E, van Dijk JG, Lammers GJ (2001). Narcolepsy: clinical features, new pathophysiologic insights, and future perspectives. *J Clin Neurophysiol*, 18(2), 78–105.

204. Gambardella A, Reutens DC, Andermann F, *et al.* (1994). Late-onset drop attacks in temporal lobe epilepsy: a reevaluation of the concept of temporal lobe syncope. *Neurology*, 44(6), 1074–8.

205. Gaitatzis A, Kartsounis LD, Gacinovic S, *et al.* (2004). Frontal lobe dysfunction in sporadic hyperekplexia – case study and literature review. *J Neurol*, 251(1), 91–8.

206. Gibson TC, Heitzman MR (1984). Diagnostic efficacy of 24-hour electrocardiographic monitoring for syncope. *Am J Cardiol*, 53(8), 1013–7.

207. Luxon LM, Crowther A, Harrison MJ, Coltart DJ (1980). Controlled study of 24-hour ambulatory electrocardiographic monitoring in patients with transient neurological symptoms. *J Neurol Neurosurg Psychiatry*, 43(1), 37–41.

208. Bass EB, Curtiss EI, Arena VC, *et al.* (1990). The duration of Holter monitoring in patients with syncope. Is 24 hours enough? *Arch Intern Med*, 150(5), 1073–8.

209. Assar MD, Krahn AD, Klein GJ, Yee R, Skanes AC (2003). Optimal duration of monitoring in patients with unexplained syncope. *Am J Cardiol*, 92(10), 1231–3.

210. Brignole M, Vitale E (2010). Implantable loop recorders in clinical practice. [Online article] http://www.escardio.org/communities/councils/ccp/e-journal/volume9/Pages/Implantable-Loop-Recorders-clinical-practice.aspx

211. Brignole M, Menozzi C (1997). Methods other than tilt testing for diagnosing neurocardiogenic (neurally mediated) syncope. *Pacing Clin Electrophysiol*, 20(3 Pt 2), 795–800.

212. Aminoff MJ, Scheinman MM, Griffin JC, Herre JM (1988). Electrocerebral accompaniments of syncope associated with malignant ventricular arrhythmias. *Ann Intern Med*, 108(6), 791–6.

213. Brenner RP (1997). Electroencephalography in syncope. *J Clin Neurophysiol*, 14(3), 197–209.

214. Ellingson RJ, Wilken K, Bennett DR (1984). Efficacy of sleep deprivation as an activation procedure in epilepsy patients. *J Clin Neurophysiol*, 1(1), 83–101.

215. Mendez M, Radtke RA (2001). Interactions between sleep and epilepsy. *J Clin Neurophysiol*, 18(2), 106–27.

216. Roupakiotis SC, Gatzonis SD, *et al.* (2000). The usefulness of sleep and sleep deprivation as activating methods in electroencephalographic recording: contribution to a long-standing discussion. *Seizure*, 9(8), 580–4.

217. King MA, Newton MR, Jackson GD, *et al.* (1998). Epileptology of the first-seizure presentation: a clinical, electroencephalographic, and magnetic resonance imaging study of 300 consecutive patients. *Lancet*, 352(9133), 1007–11.

218. Leniger T, Isbruch K, von den Driesch S, Diener HC, Hufnagel A (2001). Seizure-associated headache in epilepsy. *Epilepsia*, 42(9), 1176–9.

219. Zivin L, Marsan CA (1968). Incidence and prognostic significance of 'epileptiform' activity in the eeg of non-epileptic subjects. *Brain*, 91(4), 751–78.

220. Gregory RP, Oates T, Merry RT (1993). Electroencephalogram epileptiform abnormalities in candidates for aircrew training. *Electroencephalogr Clin Neurophysiol*, 86(1), 75–7.

221. Hopkins A, Garman A, Clarke C (1988). The first seizure in adult life. Value of clinical features, electroencephalography, and computerised tomographic scanning in prediction of seizure recurrence. *Lancet*, 1(8588), 721–6.

222. Grubb BP, Gerard G, Roush K, *et al.* (1991). Differentiation of convulsive syncope and epilepsy with head-up tilt testing. *Ann Intern Med*, 115(11), 871–6.

223. Maas R, Ventura R, Kretzschmar C, Aydin A, Schuchert A (2003). Syncope, driving recommendations, and clinical reality: survey of patients. *BMJ*, 326(7379), 21.

224. Sorajja D, Nesbitt GC, Hodge DO, *et al.* (2009). Syncope while driving: clinical characteristics, causes, and prognosis. *Circulation*, 120(11), 928–34.

225. Panel on Prevention of Falls in Older Persons, American Geriatrics Society and British Geriatrics Society (2011). Summary of the Updated American Geriatrics Society/British Geriatrics Society clinical practice guideline for prevention of falls in older persons. *J Am Geriatr Soc*, 59(1), 148–57.

226. Calkins H, Shyr Y, Frumin H, Schork A, Morady F (1995). The value of the clinical history in the differentiation of syncope due to ventricular tachycardia, atrioventricular block, and neurocardiogenic syncope. *Am J Med*, 98(4), 365–73.

227. Graham LA, Kenny RA (2001). Clinical characteristics of patients with vasovagal reactions presenting as unexplained syncope. *Europace*, 3(2), 141–6.

228. van der Sluijs BM, Bloem BR (2006). Neurological picture. Diagnosis at the tip of the tongue. *J Neurol Neurosurg Psychiatry*, 77(6), 718.

229. Reeves AL, Nollet KE, Klass DW, Sharbrough FW, So EL (1996). The ictal bradycardia syndrome. *Epilepsia*, 37(10), 983–7.

230. Devinsky O, Pacia S, Tatambhotla G (1997). Bradycardia and asystole induced by partial seizures: a case report and literature review. *Neurology*, 48(6), 1712–4.

231. Lempert T, Neuhauser H, Daroff RB (2009). Vertigo as a symptom of migraine. *Ann N Y Acad Sci*, 1164, 242–51.

232. Sturzenegger MH, Meienberg O (1985). Basilar artery migraine: a follow-up study of 82 cases. *Headache*, 25(8), 408–15.

233. Lee H, Baloh RW (2005). Sudden deafness in vertebrobasilar ischemia: clinical features, vascular topographical patterns and long-term outcome. *J Neurol Sci*, 228(1), 99–104.

234. Baloh RW (1997). Neurotology of migraine. *Headache*, 37(10), 615–21.

235. Lee MS, Choi YC, Heo JH, Choi IS (1994). 'Drop attacks' with stiffening of the right leg associated with posterior fossa arachnoid cyst. *Mov Disord*, 9(3), 377–8.

236. Kapoor WN (1989). Syncope with abrupt termination of exercise. *Am J Med*, 87(5), 597–9.

237. Mathias CJ, Holly E, Armstrong E, Shareef M, Bannister R (1991). The influence of food on postural hypotension in three groups with chronic autonomic failure – clinical and therapeutic implications. *J Neurol Neurosurg Psychiatry*, 54(8), 726–30.

238. Somerville ER (1994). Orthostatic transient ischemic attacks: a symptom of large vessel occlusion. *Stroke*, 15(6), 1066–7.

239. Vates GE, Wang KC, Bonovich D, Dowd CF, Lawton MT (2002). Bow hunter stroke caused by cervical disc herniation. Case report. *J Neurosurg*, 96(1 Suppl), 90–3.

240. Sturm JW, Fedi M, Berkovic SF, Reutens DC (2002). Exercise-induced temporal lobe epilepsy. *Neurology*, 59(8), 1246–8.

241. Simpson RK, Jr., Grossman RG. Seizures after jogging (1989). *N Engl J Med*, 321(12), 835.

CHAPTER 30

Behavioural Neuro-Otology

Jeffrey P. Staab

Introduction—what is behavioural neuro-otology?

One goal of this chapter is to eliminate the legacy of dichotomous thinking that characterized medical-psychiatric discourse throughout the 20th century and replace it with a pragmatic, integrated approach that is applicable to neuro-otological clinical care, teaching, and research in the 21st century. Dichotomous thinking is a line of reasoning in which physical symptoms are first considered from medical and surgical perspectives, and then if no explanation is forthcoming, are assumed to be caused by psychological factors, even if the relationship of physical symptoms to psychological factors is supported by nothing more than anecdote and theory (1). One shortcoming of dichotomous thinking is that no entity, clinical or otherwise, has ever been adequately understood by defining it by what it is not. Behavioural factors in neuro-otology are no exception. They must be defined by empirical research, not presumed by the absence of pathophysiological mechanisms from medicine or surgery, which are themselves incompletely understood. Another shortcoming of dichotomous thinking specific to neuro-otology is that behavioural factors are integral to locomotion. They are not separate phenomena, but are pivotal components of neural systems that control gait, posture, and oculomotor activity in health and disease. This chapter attempts to synthesize decades of clinical observations and research about behaviour factors in neuro-otology and vestibular physiology. Its title reflects that effort.

Consider Figure 30.1, a stylized depiction of two individuals in a large warehouse. One is on the floor, the other on a raised catwalk. Research involving normal subjects in similar settings has shown that the person on the catwalk instinctively walks slower and takes shorter strides than the person on the floor. This effect is more noticeable in older adults than younger ones (2). The person on the catwalk slows down even more if asked to perform a cognitive task while walking (i.e. walking and talking). His or her response latency during the task is a fraction of a second longer than the person on the floor (3). If asked to stand on tiptoes, the person on the catwalk rises up more slowly than the person on the floor, although both use the same motor paradigms. The individual on the catwalk rises to tiptoes even more slowly if performing the task on the edge of the walkway (4). The physics of walking and talking or standing on tiptoes are no different on the catwalk than on the floor, but the

consequences of failure are greater. In the normal subjects of these studies, adjustments to gait and posture coincided with increased anxiety about falling, reduced confidence in balance, and greater subjective sensations of unsteadiness (3). State, not trait, anxiety appears to correlate with balance confidence in such circumstances (5). Thus, the instantaneous and automatic perception of threat alters locomotor function. Normal individuals instinctively change motor control strategies based on situational risk. Cognitive resources such as attention and concentration are diverted to locomotion and away from tasks of lesser importance in high-demand environments. These adjustments are so instantaneous and natural that most individuals are not aware of them, except in extreme circumstances or when they fail. The influence of threat on postural control does not require conscious mental effort. People do not fall out of bed at night because they retain spatial awareness about the location of the edge of the bed and their position relative to it, even while asleep.

A group of French investigators has developed an animal model to study the effects of threat/anxiety systems on locomotion (6–8). Animals from a strain of mice that demonstrate highly anxious behaviours had more difficulty traversing a raised, rotating beam

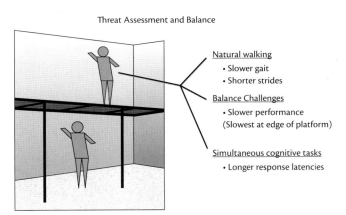

Fig. 30.1 Stylized depiction of two individuals in a large warehouse, one walking on the floor, the other on a raised catwalk. Please see text for a discussion of research findings on differences between the two in gait, balance challenges, and simultaneous cognitive tasks.

than mice from a non-anxious strain. Anxious mice slipped and paused on the beam more often than non-anxious mice. Treatment with anxiolytic antidepressants from the selective serotonin reuptake inhibitor (SSRI) class (fluoxetine or paroxetine) or a benzodiazepine (diazepam) improved the performance of anxious mice to the level of non-anxious mice. Administration of an anxiogenic agent to normal mice caused their balance function to deteriorate (8). These results demonstrate that threat systems have potent effects on locomotion across highly mobile species.

An integrated concept of locomotion— peripheral, central, and behavioural systems

The research reviewed in the previous section cannot be understood by focusing on peripheral and central vestibular systems alone. Subjects on the catwalk had no histories of vestibular, visual, proprioceptive, or somatosensory deficits or problems with central processing of stimuli from these peripheral systems. From a neurophysiological perspective, peripheral and central vestibular pathways do not contain a threat detector. Rather, they are connected to the brain's threat systems at several important junctures from the cortex to brainstem (see (9) for a review). As a result, circuits through the central nucleus of the amygdala that instinctively assess threat, those of closely-linked limbic association areas that direct attention to novel or unexpected stimuli, and pathways through the orbitofrontal cortex, which modify instinctive fear responses based on individual temperament, are well positioned to adjust locomotor control. These adjustments may be reflexive, conditioned by experience, or thoughtfully directed by conscious contemplation. Figure 30.2 is a three-part schematic of brain systems that participate in control of locomotion. They include peripheral vestibular, visual, and somatosensory systems and central vestibular pathways that are well known to neuro-otologists and vestibular physiologists. On top of this is a layer that encompasses neural pathways responsible for threat evaluation and conscious control of movement. Within this third layer, the behavioural layer, is neural circuitry that affects posture, gait, locomotion, and oculomotor control as fundamentally as the more familiar peripheral and central vestibular systems.

Applications of the integrated principles of behavioural neuro-otology

The observation that behavioural factors play an integral role in normal locomotion raises the possibility that they may cause or contribute to balance disorders when they go awry. Behavioural factors also would be expected to interact with peripheral and central vestibular diseases, altering the clinical manifestations of those conditions. These effects occur commonly in clinical practice, though they often are unrecognized. Figure 30.3 shows the difference in consultation outcomes between a typical tertiary neuro-otological practice with a focus on detecting central and peripheral vestibular diseases and one that systematically integrated methods for identifying behavioural factors into the evaluation process. These data were obtained from Mayo Clinic in Rochester, Minnesota, which shifted from a traditional tertiary model of neurology and otology examinations accompanied by vestibular laboratory testing to an integrated neuro-otology consultation process in 2008. Prior to the change, 25% of patients referred for evaluation were discharged with consultation reports stating that their examination and test findings were unrevealing and no cause for their vestibular symptoms could be determined. After the change, in which simple, but systematic screening processes were instituted to identify behavioural factors, fewer than 2% of patients were discharged without a diagnosis. Chronic subjective dizziness (CSD) and vestibular migraine (VM) became the second and third most common problems identified in patients referred for evaluation of vestibular symptoms. Comorbid behavioural factors were recognized more consistently in patients with primary vestibular disorders, resulting in more comprehensive treatment recommendations. This change vastly improved quality of care for the 500 patients annually whose problems were undetected by the previous practice. The former process was not deficient from a medical-surgical standpoint. It simply had not been informed by behavioural neuro-otological research conducted over the last decade. The Mayo Clinic experience is not unique. Its former approach is still considered the standard of care in many neuro-otology practices. Fortunately, the benefits of integrated care are being realized in a growing number of institutions worldwide. Successful integrated care does not require extensive time, resources, retraining,

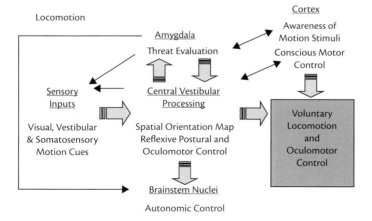

Fig. 30.2 An integrated model of control systems for voluntary locomotion and oculomotor control. The model has three layers: 1) peripheral sensory inputs, 2) central vestibular processing, and 3) behavioural systems that include threat evaluation and conscious control of movement.

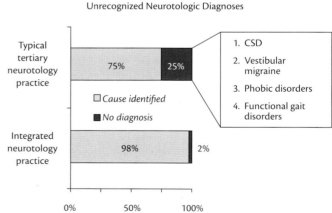

Fig. 30.3 A comparison of consultation outcomes between traditional models of tertiary neurotology evaluations and integrated neurotology care. Data are from the Mayo Clinic experience before and after developing an integrated process of care in 2008. Diagnoses in the box were previously underrecognized.

or the services of a dedicated psychiatrist or psychologist. It does require a broadened concept of vestibular and balance disorders to include peripheral, central, and behavioural factors (Figure 30.2) and a willingness to employ an expanded list of therapeutic strategies to include medical, surgical, and behavioural interventions. The remainder of this chapter provides data to support this broader concept and the interventions that accompany it. Behavioural factors cause or contribute to the most common and easily remedied aberrations of balance function. For the foreseeable future, the data of Figure 30.3 suggest that no practice improvement is as likely to help as many patients with vestibular symptoms as the full integration of behavioural concepts into neuro-otology. An integrated approach to research may yield insights into mechanisms of balance function that might otherwise be overlooked.

Anxiety disorders, vestibular symptoms, and balance function

The evidence cited in the discussion of Figure 30.1 demonstrates the positive effects that behavioural factors exert on locomotor control, introducing caution in potentially dangerous situations and diverting cognitive resources to challenging balance tasks as needed. However, the threat system may have deleterious effects as well. Anxiety disorders, in particular, may cause vestibular symptoms, adversely affect postural control, and confound the presentation and treatment of vestibular diseases.

Figure 30.4 was constructed from the results of a detailed investigation of anxiety disorders, tolerance for space and motion stimuli, and vestibular symptoms. Jacob and colleagues (10) recruited 25 subjects with panic disorder, 50 subjects with other anxiety disorders (mostly generalized anxiety disorder and social phobia), and 30 subjects without pathological anxiety. All subjects were free of neuro-otological problems. Subjects completed standardized questionnaires about height phobia, discomfort with complex space and motion stimuli (e.g. travelling across bridges, shopping in busy malls, riding in vehicles), and the presence of dizziness. The majority of subjects with anxiety disorders reported uneasiness with heights, including 80% of subjects with panic disorder and 60% of subjects with other anxiety disorders (Figure 30.4, darker bars in the panic and anxiety groups). These rates did not differ statistically between the anxiety groups. Subjects with height phobia were excluded from the control group. Subjects with anxiety disorders also had higher scores on a questionnaire about space and motion

discomfort than control subjects (Figure 30.4, SMD scores). A possible interaction between height phobia and space and motion discomfort was observed. Subjects with height phobia had greater space and motion discomfort than subjects without height phobia. There were no significant differences in this finding across anxiety disorders. Finally, most subjects with an anxiety disorder, including 80% in the panic group and 50% in the other anxiety disorders group experienced constant or fluctuating dizziness (striped bars). Again, there was an intriguing potential interaction. Complaints of dizziness were far more likely to occur in subjects with an anxiety disorder who also had height phobia or high scores for space and motion discomfort. These results indicate that patients with anxiety disorders frequently experience uneasiness with a wide variety of space, motion, and height stimuli. This effect is not specific to any particular anxiety disorder, though it may be more pronounced in patients with panic and generalized anxiety. For the most part, however, it appears to be a fundamental trait of individuals with an anxiety diathesis.

Starting in the early 1990s, several investigators published studies of vestibular function tests in patients with anxiety disorders, particularly panic disorder with or without agoraphobia (11–16). Most reported that patients with anxiety disorders were more likely than normal control subjects to have one or more test parameters outside the normal range on caloric, optokinetic, or autorotation tests (i.e. tests of basic vestibular reflexes). These investigators concluded that patients with anxiety disorders, particularly panic disorder, might have subtle vestibular deficits that made them more aware of motion stimuli and more anxious about their balance. However, a careful examination of the results showed that reported abnormalities varied from subject to subject, both within and between studies. No consistent pattern emerged and results were not indicative of any central or peripheral vestibular disorder (1). Furthermore, Jacob and colleagues (10) found no differences between patients with anxiety disorders and normal controls in otolith-ocular reflexes or canal-otolith interactions generated by off-vertical axis rotations. The two most detailed investigations of this topic (12, 16) suggested a possible link between past vestibular events and current physical and behavioural symptoms. Jacob et al. (12) found an association between past (compensated) peripheral vestibular deficits, present hypersensitivity to motion stimuli, and phobic avoidance of situations that patients related to their symptoms. Tecer et al. (16) found a link between non-specific balance test abnormalities and persistent dizziness, but not phobic avoidance. In sum, patients with anxiety disorders may demonstrate non-specific, non-diagnostic abnormalities on tests of basic vestibular reflexes (e.g. caloric, rotary chair, or autorotation). The source of these abnormalities is uncertain, but they are not consistent with known peripheral or central vestibular disorders.

In contrast to these essentially negative results on tests of basic vestibular reflexes, investigations employing measures of higher order, integrated balance function, such as static and dynamic posturography and the Sensory Organization Test (SOT), revealed a more consistent pattern of dysfunction due to anxiety disorders. On static (17) and dynamic (18) posturography, patients with panic disorder swayed more than normal control subjects. The degree of postural instability correlated with severity of phobic avoidance and anticipatory anxiety about situations associated with dizziness. Perna et al. (19) were able to normalize instability on static posturography in 15 subjects with panic disorder by treating them

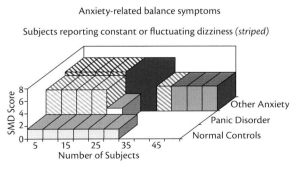

Anxiety-related balance symptoms

Subjects reporting constant or fluctuating dizziness (striped)

Fig. 30.4 Anxiety-related vestibular symptoms in patients with panic disorder, other anxiety disorders, and normal subjects. See text for details. SMD, space and motion discomfort. Data are from Jacob et al. (10).

with paroxetine, a result that paralleled the French investigations with anxious mice (8). Patients with anxiety disorders demonstrate visual or somatosensory preference patterns on the SOT. Cevette and colleagues (20) found that patients with anxiety or somatoform disorders had lower scores on Conditions III–VI than normal subjects and lower scores on Conditions III and IV than patients with peripheral or central vestibular deficits. Jacob and colleagues (10, 13) also found that patients with anxiety disorders fared poorer on Conditions III and IV than normal individuals. Redfern et al. (21) took these findings a step further. They showed that subjects with anxiety disorders were more susceptible than normal individuals to the destabilizing effects of optic flow while standing on a stable platform, even when adequate vestibular and somatosensory data were available. This effect was mediated by subjects' space and motion discomfort. Thus, patients with anxiety disorders, especially those who report high levels of uneasiness with space and motion stimuli, do not seem to integrate visual, vestibular, and somatosensory information in a normal manner. Instead, they develop an over-reliance on visual and, to a lesser extent, somatosensory cues. This leaves them vulnerable to the potentially destabilizing effects of highly active or complex visual motion stimuli.

The adverse effects of anxiety disorders on locomotion may be observed in childhood. Erez et al. (22) queried grade school children about experiences with challenging balance situations at home and school and measured their performance on laboratory balance tasks. Although all children had normal neuro-otological examinations, those with anxiety disorders were more sensitive than those without anxiety disorders to challenging balance situations in the natural environment. Children with anxiety disorders performed more slowly and made more mistakes on laboratory balance tasks. Child development researchers have observed manifestations of anxiety disorders as early as toddlerhood, especially in those with anxious temperaments and strong family histories of anxiety (23), so it is not surprising that the adverse effects of anxiety disorders on locomotor skills may be apparent at a young age, too.

The Behavioral Subcommittee for the International Classification of Vestibular Disorders (ICVD) reviewed these findings and similar data from other studies and concluded that panic attacks and generalized anxiety may cause dizziness, unsteadiness, and mild vertigo (24). The prevalence of panic and generalized anxiety is quite remarkable in neuro-otology settings. They were identified as the primary diagnosis in 8–10% of all patients and 35% of patients with chronic, non-vertiginous dizziness referred to tertiary neuro-otology centres in Germany and the United States (25–28). These rates far exceed the prevalence of panic (2.7%) and generalized anxiety (3.1%) in the general populace (29). Another large group of neuro-otology patients has anxiety disorders that coexist with peripheral and central vestibular diseases, as described in more detail in a later section. The Behavioral Subcommittee for the ICVD is in the process of writing diagnostic criteria that will help neuro-otologists identify pathological anxiety that affects patients with dizziness and unsteadiness (Chapter 16).

Functional neurological conditions

The most common behavioural causes of vertigo and ataxia are functional neurological conditions, particularly functional gait disorders. These conditions are more common in neurology than otology practices, with prevalence estimates as high as 12% in neurology (26) and as low as 0.6% in otology (28). Patients with

these conditions may complain of vertigo, gait abnormalities, or inability to walk. However, the unusual spinning sensations that they describe (e.g. constant whirling of the environment) and peculiar gait abnormalities that they manifest (e.g. atasia abasia) reveal the behavioural origins of their problems (30). These conditions are classified as conversion disorders in the current edition of the Diagnostic and Statistical Manual of Mental Disorders (DSM-IV-TR) (31), but the term 'functional' will be added in the next edition (DSM-5) (32), scheduled for publication in 2013. The pitfalls of dichotomous thinking should be kept in mind when consulting with patients who present with functional neurological or vestibular problems. It is quite common for functional disorders to coexist with, be triggered by, or even cause physical illnesses. Therefore, patients with obvious functional presentations deserve adequate evaluations for comorbid vestibular diseases. Fortunately, functional neurological disorders may be treated quite successfully when properly identified. Physical therapy, particularly when managed by a physical therapist experienced in treating functional conditions, is the mainstay of treatment in conjunction with cognitive behavioural psychotherapy (33).

Anxiety and depression in patients with vestibular diseases and disorders

Patients with vestibular diseases have far higher rates of anxiety and depressive disorders (30–50%) than patients in general medical practices (9–15%) and behavioural morbidity strongly affects their clinical outcomes (25–26, 34–38). In two separate studies (39, 40), 50% of patients contacted 3–5 years after an acute vestibular loss reported clinically significant anxiety or depression. Excluding individuals with pre-existing psychiatric illnesses, Godemann and colleagues (41) found that one of every eight patients (12.9%) who had an episode of vestibular neuritis developed new onset anxiety or somatoform disorders within 2 years after onset of their vestibular symptoms. In Ménière's disease, rates of anxiety and depression vary with the state of illness (42–44). In general, behavioural morbidity increases with illness duration and number of episodes, but it is not strictly associated with objective measures of auditory or vestibular dysfunction (43, 45). Some patients with Ménière's disease are quite resilient while others fare poorly. Patients with anxious temperaments report more psychological distress, rate their physical symptoms more severely, and are more preoccupied with being ill (45). They also may be more likely to have progression of low frequency hearing loss (44, 46). Vestibular migraine is receiving increased attention as a cause of episodic vestibular symptoms (21). Early data suggest that behavioural morbidity is quite common in vestibular migraine (35–50%) (47) and that anxiety predating the onset of vestibular migraine predisposes patients to chronic dizziness (48).

Behavioural factors may adversely affect the outcomes of medical or surgical treatment for vestibular diseases. For example, Boleas-Aguirre and colleagues (49) followed 103 patients with Ménière's disease prospectively for a mean of 5.3 years after treatment with transtympanic gentamicin. They achieved excellent vertigo control with 81% of patients free of vertigo spells during the last 6 months of the study. However, pretreatment anxiety and scores on the 1995 American Academy of Otolaryngology—Head and Neck Surgery Functional Level Scale (FLS) for Ménière's disease (50) significantly influenced overall outcomes. A close examination of data from that study (49), redrawn in Figure 30.5, showed that patients with pre-treatment FLS scores of 3, 4, or 5 had mean

Vertigo Symptom Scale (VSS) autonomic/anxiety scores ranging from 15–20 (51). Patients with pretreatment FLS scores of 6 had a mean VSS autonomic/anxiety score that was twice as high at 35. In contrast, VSS physical symptom scores were not different across four FLS categories (Figure 30.5, left panel). Patients with pretreatment FLS scores of 6 had the poorest outcomes overall. Sixteen patients (15.5%) developed chronic unsteadiness after gentamicin treatment, most of whom had pretreatment FLS scores of 6. These subjects reported no reduction in scores on Dizziness Handicap Inventory physical or functional subscales (52) or VSS autonomic/anxiety following treatment. In other words, patients with Ménière's disease who had high pretreatment anxiety were more functionally impaired than those with low pretreatment anxiety despite having similar levels of physical symptoms. They also achieved poorer results from transtympanic gentamicin, with a strong tendency to develop persistent unsteadiness despite good vertigo control. Post-treatment FLS scores improved across the board, but were still determined more by levels of autonomic/anxiety than physical symptoms on the VSS (Figure 30.5, right panel). Boleas-Aguirre et al. (49) concluded that patients with FLS scores of 6 require 'special care.' What their data show is that those patients require treatment of their anxiety, possibly before surgical intervention. The Mayo Clinic integrated neuro-otology team has adopted that approach, screening patients for anxiety and offering aggressive interventions for anxiety as part of a multidisciplinary treatment plan. Data on outcomes are not yet available, but anecdotal evidence suggests that adequate control of anxiety may obviate the need for surgical treatment for some patients.

Given the high prevalence of behavioural morbidity in patients with vestibular diseases and disorders, it is reasonable to inquire about the temporal relationship between behavioural and neuro-otological factors. Does behavioural morbidity always follow the onset of vestibular deficits or might there be behavioural factors that predispose patients to develop vestibular conditions? Retrospective (27) and prospective (48) studies have investigated this question. Figure 30.6 shows data from a retrospective study (27) in which investigators were asked to make a forced choice as to whether a vestibular deficit or psychiatric disorder

occurred first in patients with chronic dizziness. Consensus was achieved on a three-path, rather than two-path model. Approximately one-third of patients had anxiety disorders as the only cause of their vestibular symptoms. This was dubbed true psychogenic dizziness. A second third of patients had anxiety or depressive disorders develop only after the occurrence of a vestibular or other medical crisis that triggered acute vestibular symptoms. They had otogenic anxiety. The final third had longstanding anxiety disorders or a strong anxiety diathesis (e.g. anxious temperament or family history of anxiety disorders), but did not developed vestibular symptoms until they had an acute vestibular or medical event. Then, they experienced an increase in anxiety along with persistent vestibular symptoms. An interaction of behavioural and physical factors produced their symptoms. The three paths were associated with different patterns of anxiety disorders. Panic disorder predominated among patients in the psychogenic path. Lower levels of panic or minor anxiety symptoms revolving only around dizziness were most common among patients in the otogenic path. Generalized anxiety was the primary psychiatric diagnosis in the interactive path. Response to treatment for dizziness and anxiety was less robust for patients in the interactive path, possibly reflecting their lifelong anxiety diathesis (53). A prospective study (48) confirmed the existence of these three paths and the importance of pre-existing behavioural factors as predictors of a more chronic course of illness after a vestibular event. That study found preliminary evidence that some vestibular conditions (e.g. vestibular migraine) may be more likely than others (e.g. benign paroxysmal positional vertigo (BPPV) to precipitate behavioural morbidity. All of these studies of behavioural factors in patients with vestibular diseases and disorders emphasize the importance setting aside dichotomous thinking and replacing it with strategies to identify clinically significant anxiety and depression in patients with dizziness in order to improve diagnostic rates and accuracy and improve treatment outcomes, including responses to medical and surgical interventions (25, 30, 39).

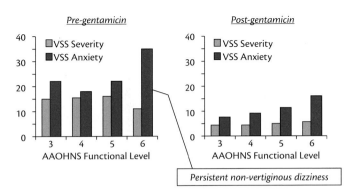

Fig. 30.5 Effects of anxiety on functional status in patients with Ménière's disease before and after treatment with transtympanic gentamicin. Severity of anxiety on the Vertigo Symptom Scale (VSS) was the primary determinant of functional level pre- and post-treatment. The highest levels of pre-treatment anxiety were linked to the poorest functional status and greatest likelihood of developing chronic dizziness after treatment. Redrawn from Boleas-Aguirre et al. (49).

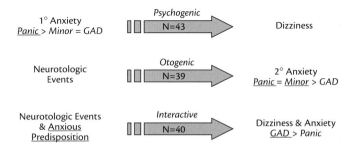

Fig. 30.6 Depiction of three longitudinal relationships between anxiety, vestibular diseases, and resultant vestibular symptoms. Anxiety disorders could be the primary causes of symptoms, secondary consequences of vestibular diseases, or pre-date vestibular diseases, but be exacerbated by them. Data are from Staab and Ruckenstein (27, 53).

Phobic postural vertigo and chronic subjective dizziness

In 1986, while detailed studies into the relationships among vestibular and psychiatric disorders were underway around the world, Brandt and Dieterich (54) described a clinical condition that they called Phobischer Attacken Schwank-schwindel or phobic postural vertigo (PPV). As reviewed by Brandt (55), PPV is defined by symptoms of postural dizziness and fluctuating unsteadiness that are provoked by environmental (bridge, staircase, busy street) or social (crowds, store, restaurant) stimuli. PPV may be triggered initially by vestibular disorders, medical illnesses, or psychological stress. Brandt and Dieterich included two behavioural criteria in the definition of PPV: 1) presence of an obsessive-compulsive personality, labile affect, and mild depression, and 2) anxiety and vegetative disturbance. They and their colleagues found PPV to be the second most common cause of dizziness in their university-based practice, behind BPPV (55). Longitudinal follow-up found PPV to be a stable, clinically recognizable construct. Huppert, et al. (56) contacted 105 patients who were diagnosed with PPV an average of 8.5 years earlier (range 5–16 years) and reaffirmed the diagnosis of PPV in all patients. None had been misdiagnosed or subsequently developed other neurological or vestibular conditions. The natural history of PPV was marked by chronic dizziness and unsteadiness that waxed and waned and trended gradually downward in severity, but did not resolve (56, 57). The behavioural outcome was less favourable.

Two-thirds of patients developed clinically problematic anxiety or depression (58).

Diagnostic studies were able to differentiate PPV from panic and other psychiatric disorders (55). As such, the concept of PPV was a step forward in understanding a segment of the patient population that had been previously included under the vaguely and dichotomously defined umbrella of psychogenic dizziness (i.e. dizziness without a clearly identifiable medical cause). However, the definition of PPV was never formally validated. Its amalgam of physical, behavioural, and personality features did not lend itself to easy pathophysiological inquiry or clinical application. As a result, PPV has been considered infrequently outside of a few European medical centres in the 25 years since it was first described. In the early-2000s, Staab and Ruckenstein began a series of studies to identify core clinical features (28, 30), streamline and validate diagnostic criteria (58), understand the relationship to other conditions (30, 32, 47, 53), and conduct treatment trials (59–61). Their work produced the clinical syndrome of chronic subjective dizziness (CSD) (28). The Behavioral Subcommittee of the ICVD was charged with reconciling PPV and CSD into one internationally acceptable definition based on empirical data for both conditions (24).

Consolidated features of PPV/CSD

Table 30.1 organizes PPV/CSD into five categories: 1) primary physical symptoms, 2) their relationship to posture, 3) provocative factors, 4) findings on physical examination and vestibular

Table 30.1 Consolidated clinical features of phobic postural vertigo–chronic subjective dizziness (PPV/CSD)

Feature	Description	Comments
Primary physical symptoms	Persistent unsteadiness, dizziness, or both are present for at least part of the day, on most days, for 3 months or more. Unsteadiness and dizziness may wax and wane	Vertigo is not part of PPV/CSD, but patients who have PPV/CSD plus another vestibular disorder may have episodic vertigo plus chronic unsteadiness and dizziness
Relationship to posture	Primary symptoms are related to body posture, being most severe when walking or standing, less severe when sitting, and absent (or minimally present) when recumbent	Postural and orthostatic symptoms differ. Postural symptoms are present while in an upright posture. Orthostatic symptoms occur on arising to an upright posture
Provocative factors	Symptoms are present without specific provocation, but are exacerbated by one or more of the following: • Active or passive motion of self without regard to direction or position (i.e. head-motion dizziness) • Exposure to large-field moving visual stimuli or complex visual patterns (i.e. visually-induced dizziness) • Performance of small-field, precision visual activities (e.g. using a computer, reading, needlework)	Provocative factors include motion of self, exposure to environments with challenging motion stimuli or complex visual cues and performance of precision visual tasks, such using a computer or reading. Symptoms of PPV/CSD may be present without provocation, but usually reflect the cumulative burden of provoking factors over preceding hours or days
Precipitating (triggering) factors	Precipitating factors include: • Acute or recurrent vestibular diseases or disorders • Acute or recurrent medical problems that produce unsteadiness or dizziness • Acute or recurrent psychiatric disorders that produce unsteadiness or dizziness	The most common triggers for PPV/CSD in order of prevalence are: previous acute vestibular disorders (compensated or not), panic attacks, vestibular migraine, mild traumatic brain injury or whiplash, generalized anxiety, dysautonomias, dysrhythmias, recurrent vestibular disorders, adverse drug reactions, and other medical events
Physical examination and laboratory findings	Physical examination and laboratory assessment are often normal, but may reveal evidence of a vestibular or other medical condition that may be active, treated, or resolved	PPV/CSD may be present alone or coexist with other neurotological or medical conditions. Positive exam findings do not exclude PPV/CSD, but rather identify comorbid conditions. Emerging data suggest that there may be a unique pattern of sway on posturography in PPV/CSD
Behavioural symptoms	Behavioural assessment may be normal or reveal evidence of clinically significant psychological distress or changes in activities of daily living	Research studies have shown that PPV/CSD is a unique clinical entity, not a forme fruste of a psychiatric illness. Patients with PPV/CSD may or may not have comorbid behavioural, mostly anxiety, disorders.

laboratory testing, and 5) behavioural factors. The primary physical symptoms contained in the original reports of PPV (54, 55) and CSD (28) are essentially the same. Initial findings from the Mayo Clinic validation study of CSD support the description given in Table 30.1 (58). Patients experience persistent sensations of rocking or swaying unsteadiness, non-vertiginous dizziness, or both. In most cases, unsteadiness and dizziness are present throughout the day, though they may wax and wane in severity, with quiescent periods, particularly in the morning or after an extended period of rest. PPV/CSD is generally quite chronic, often lasting for months or years. The average duration of illness in two large studies of CSD was 4.5 years (28, 58). Spontaneous remission does occur, but resolution is gradual (55). Unsteadiness in PPV/CSD is not visible on physical examination. Family members or friends may report that they have seen their loved one swaying or rocking when standing or veering from side to side when walking. If prominent, this observation raises the possibility of comorbid neurological or behavioural disorders (e.g. peripheral neuropathy, phobia of falling, functional gait disorder). Brandt (55) added that there may be fluctuations in unsteadiness or momentary illusions of body perturbations lasting seconds to minutes, but these symptoms also have been reported in vestibular migraine (21), making them non-specific. Vertigo is not part of PPV/CSD. However, patients with past vestibular crises may give histories of previous episodes of vertigo and individuals with coexisting vestibular diseases may report episodic vertigo superimposed on chronic unsteadiness and dizziness.

The definition of PPV contains a postural element. Symptoms are present when patients are standing or walking. A postural criterion is not part of the definition of CSD (28), but postural symptoms are recognized by CSD investigators who are reticent to make the diagnosis clinically in patients who do not give an indication that their symptoms are worst when upright and weak or absent when recumbent. The ICVD (64) draws a clear distinction between postural, orthostatic, and positional symptoms. Postural symptoms occur when patients are sitting, standing or walking upright, but not when recumbent. Orthostatic symptoms occur during or immediately after patients assume an upright posture after being recumbent. Positional symptoms occur when the head or moves into or through a specific orientation in space. Postural symptoms are an integral part of PPV/CSD. Orthostatic and positional symptoms are not.

Provoking factors have been a source of debate. The descriptions of PPV include examples of provocative situations (e.g. bridges, crowds) (54, 55), whereas the definitions of CSD include categories of provocative stimuli (head movement, complex visual stimuli) (28). The debate is not about these differences in definitions, because the PPV examples fit quite nicely into the CSD categories. Rather the controversy has been over how sensitive and specific these provocative factors are for PPV/CSD. Patients with other vestibular diseases (e.g. Ménière's disease, vestibular migraine, central vestibular disorders) find head movements and strong environmental motion to be quite provocative during flare-ups of illness. Patients with panic disorder, agoraphobia, and specific phobia of dizziness may feel worse in these same situations. Differences with PPV/CSD are as follows. Patients with other vestibular diseases are likely to experience vertigo with motion of self or surround. Vertigo is not a symptom of PPV/CSD. Patients with other vestibular diseases can reduce symptoms quite dramatically within seconds to

minutes of holding still or removing themselves from strong environmental motion, whereas patients with PPV/CSD are likely to experience exacerbations of symptoms lasting for hours or days even after modest exposure to provocative factors. Patients with PPV/CSD usually have chronic symptoms that reflect an accumulation of exposures to over hours or days, making them vulnerable to additional provocations at almost any time. Patients with other vestibular diseases are affected by provoking factors during acute episodes of illness, but are rather less susceptible otherwise. PPV/CSD differs from panic and other anxiety disorders because fear is not a prominent part of the response to provocative stimuli in PPV/CSD. Patients with PPV/CSD may avoid provocative situations because they do not want to exacerbate their physical symptoms. Patients with panic and other anxiety disorders avoid provocative situations because of fears about catastrophic consequences (e.g. becoming incapacitated or embarrassing themselves in public). Early results from the Mayo Clinic validation study of CSD (58) suggest that the prevalence of head motion-induced vestibular symptoms does not differ significantly among patients with PPV/CSD, Ménière's disease, vestibular migraine, and BPPV. The type and duration of provoked symptoms might be more discriminative. In contrast, the presence of visually induced symptoms appears to be more sensitive and specific for PPV/CSD. Further investigations of this topic may be needed.

Brandt and Dieterich identified previous vestibular disorders, other serious medical conditions, and periods of psychological stress as triggers for PPV (54, 55). Staab and colleagues provided more details in studies of CSD (28, 58). The most common triggering events included previous acute peripheral or central vestibular disorders such as BPPV or vestibular neuritis (25%), panic attacks, especially in young adults (15–20%), vestibular migraine (15–20%), generalized anxiety (15%), mild traumatic brain injury (concussion or whiplash), especially in young men (10–15%), and dysautonomias (7%). Dysrhythmias, recurrent vestibular disorders, adverse drug reactions, and other medical events complete the list at 1–2% each.

The possibility that PPV and CSD might coexist with other vestibular or medical disorders was not addressed in the original conceptualizations of either condition (28, 54). PPV and CSD were considered to be consequences of vestibular, medical, or psychiatric triggers. As a result, the definition of PPV states that the physical examination is normal (54, 55). The definition of CSD is a bit more lenient, allowing for non-specific abnormalities on physical examination or vestibular laboratory testing (28), but still excluding patients with clinically significant physical findings. Clinical experience suggests that this is an error. The current consensus among CSD investigators is that the syndrome coexists with a wide variety of other disorders, including the triggering illnesses listed above that are chronic or recurrent conditions themselves (e.g. panic and generalized anxiety, migraine, traumatic brain injury, dysautonomias, and dysrhythmias). Initial data from the Mayo Clinic validation study of CSD (58) supports this newer conceptualization of comorbidity in PPV/CSD and extends it to episodic vestibular disorders such as Ménière's disease. Therefore, positive findings on physical examination or vestibular laboratory testing do not exclude the diagnosis of CSD. Rather, they identify coexisting conditions.

The characteristic features of PPV include a diverse collection of behavioural factors such as obsessive compulsive personality traits, labile affect, anxiety, avoidance behaviours, mild depression, classical and operant conditioning, and stress (55). This is the most problematic aspect of PPV. No other clinical entity contains such an amalgam of physical and psychiatric symptoms, personality traits, and presumptive psychological mechanisms. Some are internally inconsistent. For example, the obsessive compulsive personality is usually associated with a restricted, not labile, affect. More importantly, these features give the impression that PPV is a psychiatric condition, despite Brandt's reasonable insistence to the contrary (55), doing little to interest neurologists or otologists in adopting it out of the dichotomously defined world of psychogenic dizziness (personal communications between the author and numerous leading otologists in the United States). In putting together the definition of CSD, Staab and Ruckenstein quickly realized that these behavioural factors were not core manifestations of the condition (28, 30). The diagnosis could be made quite readily on clinical grounds by identifying the characteristic pattern of primary physical symptoms, provoking factors, and precipitants listed in Table 30.1. Therefore, Staab and colleagues focused the definition of CSD on its key physical features (28) and began a series of systematic investigations into the links with behavioural factors and their role in the pathophysiological mechanisms of the condition (see (30) for review). The results of these studies coincide with the work of other recent investigators (48) to draw a coherent, albeit still tentative, picture of the behavioural factors that predispose individuals to PPV/CSD, play a crucial role in its onset, and add considerable morbidity for many patients.

Individuals with CSD are more likely to possess anxious and introverted, but not compulsive, personality traits than the general population as measured on the NEO Personality Inventory—Revised (NEO-PI-R) (65). A composite anxious, introverted temperament was identified significantly more often in patients with CSD than in subjects who had other vestibular diseases coexisting with anxiety disorders (e.g. comorbid vestibular migraine and generalized anxiety) (66). Psychiatric researchers have linked NEO-PI-R anxious and introverted traits to variations in monoamine neurotransmitter genes and vulnerability to develop anxious, depressive, and possibly somatic symptom disorders after exposure to adverse life events (67). These findings coincide with earlier observations about PPV/CSD being more likely to develop and have a more chronic course in individuals with a strong anxious diathesis (53). Perhaps the NEO-PI-R anxious, introverted temperament is the most specific marker to date of this predisposition, a step closer to the genetics of PPV/CSD.

Anxious and depressive symptoms are common in PPV/CSD, but far from universal. Data from Germany (55) and the United States (58) found clinically significant anxiety in about 60% of patients with PPV/CSD and clinically significant depressive symptoms in about 45%. Importantly, one-quarter of patients with PPV/CSD had neither anxiety, nor depression. The prevalence of psychiatric symptoms in PPV/CSD is significant greater than the rates of 35% and 20%, respectively for anxiety and depression, observed in patients with Ménière's disease, vestibular migraine, and BPPV. However, this numerical difference is not specific enough (39–46%) to distinguish PPV/CSD from the other diseases (58). These findings indicate that anxiety and depression are common in patients with PPV/CSD, as they are to a somewhat lesser extent in patients with other vestibular disorders. However, the results also demonstrate

that anxiety and mood symptoms are not an integral part of PPV/CSD, but rather a common co-occurrence.

A new pathophysiological model of PPV/CSD—magnified response, readaptation failure

Classical and operant conditioning have been hypothesized to be the primary mechanisms responsible for perpetuating PPV (55) and CSD (30). In general, this theory holds that because new onset vestibular symptoms are particularly anxiogenic (68), they are potent unconditioned stimuli for triggering classically conditioned, reflexive hypersensitivity to subsequent internal or external motion stimuli and operantly conditioned behavioural changes in motion-rich environments. This is thought to produce a self-sustaining vicious circle in which hypersensitive reflexes distort postural and oculomotor responses to motion, triggering increased awareness of postural control challenges, thereby reinforcing the heightened sensitivity of postural control reflexes and behavioural alterations in motion-rich environments. Cognitive distortions also are thought to perpetuate PPV/CSD via catastrophic thoughts (e.g. crashing the car) and dysphoric ruminations (e.g. becoming chronically handicapped) about vestibular symptoms (30).

This formulation of classical and operant conditioning as the pathophysiological mechanisms of PPV/CSD is grounded in well-established principles of behavioural and cognitive theories. However, there are no specific data to support it. Rather, several lines of evidence suggest an alternative mechanism. Patients afflicted by new onset vestibular symptoms must adapt quickly to their deficits to improve their capacity for safe mobility. During the early phases of an acute vestibular crisis, it would be necessary to suppress sensory input from damaged systems, shift preferences to intact sensory systems, employ high-demand postural control strategies (moving cautiously, using supports), and adopt a higher level of vigilance about the environment. These changes would be adaptive in the short run, but would be expected to revert to normal as the crisis remits and compensation occurs. The hypothesis offered here is that PPV/CSD arises from maladjustment during the early period of illness followed by failure to readapt as the acute injury resolves. Acute vestibular events are the most anxiety provoking of medical crises (68). They provide ample incentive for the threat system to alter postural control strategies. There are several lines of evidence to suggest that these alterations may be exaggerated and persist in patients who have highly anxious responses to acute vestibular symptoms. First of all, anxiety appears to reduce individuals' tolerance for postural disturbances. In one study of this effect (69), anxious individuals on a posture platform responded more quickly to rotational perturbations and made more postural corrections than less anxious subjects. In essence, they employed a stiffer and more reactive postural control strategy that resulted in narrower postural displacements, but required more corrective actions than their more relaxed counterparts. Another set of studies (70, 71) showed that vision interacts with state anxiety to alter the relative weighting of visual, vestibular, and proprioceptive inputs. Healthy college students with higher levels of anxiety swayed more than their less anxious classmates while standing on a posture platform with eyes open, but not eyes closed (70). The frequency content of postural sway suggested a stronger shift toward visual-vestibular inputs and away from somatosensory inputs in anxious than non-anxious individuals in the eyes open condition (71). Individuals with high trait anxiety (i.e. strong anxious temperaments) showed greater adaptation than individuals with low trait anxiety to visual feedback gains that were altered to one-half or two times normal in a virtual reality environment. They demonstrated a strong shift to the novel, but erroneous, visual change even when accurate vestibular and somatosensory data were available (72). These findings in normal individuals suggest that anxiety not only exerts protective effects on locomotion as discussed with Figure 30.1, but also may reduce the flexibility of postural control systems and diminish their adaptability.

Two prospective studies captured patients within the first few days of onset of vestibular neuronitis or BPPV and showed that 30% of subjects had persistent complaints of dizziness or unsteadiness at 3 (73) and 12 months after their illnesses began (74). Symptoms persisted despite the fact that vestibular laboratory testing demonstrated excellent recovery or compensation from peripheral deficits in 90% of subjects with ongoing complaints. High levels of anxiety at the onset of vertigo, vigilance about vestibular symptoms, and catastrophic thinking about possible outcomes were the primary predictors of a transition from acute vertigo to chronic unsteadiness and dizziness. Anxiety-related symptoms became stronger predictors of long-term outcome at each successive follow-up period during the yearlong study. These data show that patients destined to develop chronic unsteadiness and dizziness enter a highly anxious state early in the course of their acute vestibular crises and that high anxiety is associated with poor recovery. However, this observation does not identify a pathophysiological process to explain persistent symptoms. Data from two small investigations of anxiety, physical symptoms, and postural sway during recovery from acute vestibular neuronitis raise possible mechanisms (75, 76). Patients recovering from vestibular neuronitis who had coexisting generalized anxiety showed greater postural sway when standing with eyes closed or when exposed to optokinetic stimuli moving toward the side of their lesion (75). In a study of postural sway patterns, Alessandrini et al. (76) found that full recovery was marked by the emergence of a postural sway component that was outside of the vestibular frequency range, where sway was intensified by the vestibular deficit. The appearance of this recovery component, which was in the low end of the somatosensory range, coincided with the start of symptom resolution and reduction in the intensity of vestibular sway. Patients whose symptoms persisted through the 9-month study period showed no shift away from high intensity vestibular sway. These findings indicate that anxiety appears to magnify postural instability and responses to motion stimuli during acute vestibular crises and may inhibit the emergence of postural control strategies that are associated with recovery.

Patients with PPV/CSD may have a unique postural sway pattern. Krafczyk et al. (77) found increased sway at a frequency 3.53–8 Hz in patients with PPV, which they related to co-contraction of antigravity muscles. This is a postural control strategy that normal individuals employ when consciously aware of challenging balance situations. The existence of the 3.53–8-Hz sway pattern in PPV was confirmed in a second study (78). Patients with PPV were compared to individuals with cerebellar atrophy, acute vestibular neuronitis, primary orthostatic tremor, and normal controls. All groups of comparative subjects had different postural sway patterns. Patients with PPV were found to use unnecessarily high-demand postural control strategies during low-demand balance tasks (e.g. normal stance on foam with eyes open), a tactic that paradoxically produced more postural instability than normal individuals had in those situations.

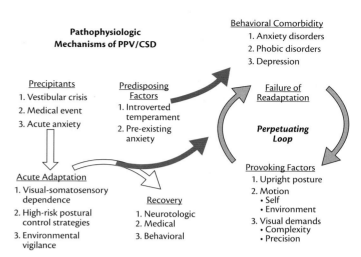

Fig. 30.7 A new conceptualization of pathophysiological processes underlying phobic postural vertigo–chronic subjective dizziness (PPV/CSD) and its medical and behavioural morbidity. Precipitating, predisposing, perpetuating, and provoking factors are identified. Please see text for additional discussion.

In contrast, the postural stability of patients with PPV was closer to that of normal individuals during more challenging balance tasks (e.g. tandem stance on foam with eyes closed), where high demand strategies were needed (79). It is not known how or when patients with PPV/CSD develop this potentially unique sway pattern. However, it suggests that a possible pathophysiological process that sustains PPV/CSD is the continued use of high-demand postural control strategies in everyday situations where they are no longer needed. Failure of postural and oculomotor control systems to readapt to the routine demands of locomotion could explain the two main features of PPV/CSD, postural unsteadiness and dizziness on the output side and hypersensitivity to motion stimuli on the input side.

Figure 30.7 is a schematic of this model. Precipitating events trigger the necessary elements of acute adaptation. For most patients, natural neuro-otological, medical, and behavioural recovery takes place over a time course determined by the nature of the triggering event. However, patients who posses predisposing factors such as an anxious, introverted temperament or strong anxiety diathesis have magnified acute responses and limited readaptation that drives them into a perpetual loop in which heightened reactivity to motion stimuli and continued use of high-demand postural control strategies turn previously benign circumstances into highly provocative situations. Those same predisposing factors simultaneously put patients at risk for behavioural comorbidity. This integrated model of PPV/CSD places it at the interface of neuro-otology and psychiatry. Behavioural factors are key components of its pathophysiology, but it is not a psychiatric or psychogenic disorder, even when panic attacks are the precipitating event. In the absence of known interactions between neural circuitry serving balance function and threat responses, it would not exist.

Detecting behavioural factors in patients with vestibular symptoms

As stated in the chapter introduction, dichotomous thinking is an outmoded approach to the patient with vestibular symptoms in the 21st century. Behavioural factors are simply too common, affect clinical course and medical-surgical therapies too much, and are too easily treated in their own right to relegate them to an after-thought or ignore them completely. It is easy to detect behavioural factors and patients are surprising open to considering them as part of an integrated management plan. This openness stands in marked contrast to patients' rejection of behavioural factors when presented in dichotomous terms. Patients have long resisted either/or think-ing about physical and psychological symptoms and research data have borne out their objections—behavioural factors are a major component of vertigo, unsteadiness, and dizziness, not separate phenomena. Neurologists and otologists may wonder why they should incorporate processes for identifying behavioural morbid-ity into their busy non-psychiatric practices. The answer is simple. That is where the patients are!

Figure 30.2 provide the conceptual model for well-integrated management plans, including diagnostic evaluations, treatment, and patient education. The site of the lesion may be peripheral, cen-tral, behavioural, or more than one. The treatment plan may include medical, surgical, and behavioural interventions (including physi-cal therapy). The key to detecting behavioural factors is the patient's clinical history (54). They key to interpreting physical and behav-ioural morbidity correctly is the answer to three questions (1):

1) Does the patient have an *active* peripheral or central vestibular deficit?

2) Does the vestibular deficit, if present, explain *all* of the patient's symptoms?

3) Has the patient described emotional distress or behavioural changes?

The first question focuses the diagnostic impression on attributing current symptoms to current illness (i.e. to what the patient *has* now, not what he or she *had* previously). A man with a 4-year history of vestibular symptoms that started with 2 weeks of acute vertigo and ataxia, but evolved into daily dizziness and motion sensitivity that are worst when upright had vestibular neuritis, but now has PPV/CSD. The second question abolishes dichotomous thinking and replaces it with an integrated thought process that seeks a full accounting of the patient's illness. A woman with positional vertigo and a positive Dix–Hallpike test who has been afraid to leave her house for 3 months has BPPV and a phobic disorder (agoraphobia). The final question tunes the clinician into behavioural factors that a patient may reveal, sometimes off-handedly, in his or her history. A woman being seen for routine follow-up of Ménière's disease who sadly says that she has never held her new grandson because she might get dizzy and drop him is not describing the state of her hydrops, but rather a phobic disorder (fear of vertigo).

Physical examinations and vestibular laboratory tests are more likely to reveal active vestibular deficits in patients with acute onset or recent recurrences of vestibular symptoms, than in individuals with chronic complaints (55). Exams and lab tests also are more likely to be positive in patients with complaints of vertigo, ataxia, diplopia, or oscillopsia than in those with symptoms of unsteadi-ness, dizziness, or non-specific visual changes. Positive physical exam or test findings identify vestibular deficits, but do not exclude behavioural morbidity unless the answer to the earlier question #2 is yes and the answer to question #3 is no. Patients with functional neurological disorders may show dramatic findings incompat-ible with medical illnesses. It is important to resist dichotomous thinking in these circumstances because functional disorders may coexist with medical conditions. True malingering is quite rare in patients with vestibular symptoms (1, 27).

Table 30.2 contains a description of six validated, self-report ques-tionnaires that can be used to detect behavioural factors in patients with vestibular symptoms. All of them are short, easy to score, and have been used in research conducted in neuro-otological settings

Table 30.2 Questionnaires for detecting behavioural morbidity in patients with vestibular symptoms

Tool	Description	Advantages and disadvantages
Dizziness Handicap Inventory (DHI)	• 25-item self-report of physical, functional, and emotional symptoms of dizziness • Functional and emotional scales capture behavioural symptoms • Versions in several languages	• Widely employed in dizziness research • Quantitative, can be used to track progress • Total score is more useful than subscales • Limited correlation with balance function tests
Vertigo Symptom Scale (VSS)	• 36-item self-report with 2 subscales, a Vertigo scale for vestibular symptoms and an Autonomic/Anxiety scale for anxiety • Versions in several European languages	• Not used as widely as the DHI, but has better psychometric properties • Subscales correlate with objective measures of vestibular symptoms and standard ratings of psychological symptoms
Activities-specific Balance Confidence Scale (ABC)	• Self-rated confidence in doing 16 activities of daily living involving movement	• Developed and validated for use in the elderly • Correlates reasonably well with the DHI and Dynamic Gait Index
Patient Health Questionnaire (PHQ-9)	• 9-item self-report of depressive symptoms • Validated in many languages	• Identifies significant depressive symptoms • Quantitative, can be used to track progress • Download free of charge at: http://www.phqscreeners.com
Generalized Anxiety Disorder Questionnaire (GAD-7)	• 7-item self-report of various anxiety symptoms, not just generalized anxiety • Validated in many languages	• Identifies significant anxiety symptoms • Quantitative, can be used to track progress • Download free of charge at: http://www.phqscreeners.com
Hospital Anxiety & Depression Scale (HADS)	• 14-item self-report of anxiety and depressive symptoms • Validated in many languages	• Identifies clinically significant symptoms • Quantitative, can be used to track progress • Request permission for use at: permissions@gl-assessment.co.uk

(35, 36, 47, 80). The simplest process is to incorporate one or more of these questionnaires into the medical history forms that most clinicians ask patients to complete at home or in the office prior to neuro-otological consultation. The questionnaires are not used to make psychiatric diagnoses, but high scores on the DHI functional or emotional subscales, VSS autonomic/anxiety subscale, Hospital Anxiety and Depression Scale (HADS) (81), Patient Health Questionnaire (PHQ-9) (82), or Generalized Anxiety Disorder Questionnaire (GAD-7) (83) provide quantitative data about the presence of behavioural morbidity. It is perfectly reasonable to choose the DHI or VSS and HADS or PHQ-9/GAD-7. The Activities-specific Balance Confidence Scale (ABC) (84) is used primarily by physical therapists. Vestibular deficits, behavioural factors, or both may cause low scores (85) so screening patients with low ABC scores for behavioural morbidity is warranted. At Mayo Clinic, the DHI and HADS have been used in the integrated neuro-otology program since 2008. They are included in the new patient history packet. Scores from the DHI and HADS are reported to referring clinicians along with other consultation findings. The HADS works well, but will soon be replaced by the PHQ-9/GAD-7 because the latter are now the institution's standard tools for depression and anxiety screening. The PHQ-9 and GAD-7 have been used in primary care and psychiatric research worldwide for several years. Primary care clinicians are quite familiar with them.

Treatment of behavioural morbidity in patients with vestibular disorders

No large-scale, randomized, controlled trials of therapeutic interventions for behavioural morbidity have been conducted in patients with vestibular disorders. However, a growing number of uncontrolled medication trials and modest-sized rehabilitative and psychotherapeutic investigations are being published. Table 30.3 lists seven open label trials of serotonergic antidepressants that have been conducted in the United States and Japan. These studies have focused mostly on the treatment of PPV/CSD, but their various designs included patient groups with other vestibular disorders such as vestibular migraine, peripheral vestibular deficits of various causes, traumatic brain injury, and dysautonomias. Collectively, these studies indicate that selective serotonin reuptake inhibitors (SSRIs) and serotonin norepinephrine reuptake inhibitors (SNRIs)

are safe and well tolerated by patients with vestibular symptoms. The studies showed substantial benefits for patients with PPV/CSD. Reported response rates exceed 80% for study completers (8–12 weeks of therapy) and 65% for all those who attempt treatment. Successful outcomes may not depend on the presence of comorbid anxiety or depression, though studies differ in this regard. In two US studies (59, 60), there were no differences in response rates between patients with PPV/CSD alone versus PPV/CSD plus an anxiety or depressive disorder. In two Japanese studies (80, 86), chronic vestibular symptoms did not improve in patients who had low anxiety and depression scores at study entry. For patients with PPV/CSD and vestibular migraine, response to venlafaxine was superior in the group with coexisting anxiety disorders (61). Taken together, these studies suggest that the SSRIs and SNRIs are safe and useful for two groups of patients, those with PPV/CSD and those with other vestibular disorders complicated by coexisting anxiety or depression. Medications are not effective for functional neurological disorders (33).

Table 30.4 lists clinical trials of vestibular and balance rehabilitation therapy (VBRT) and cognitive behaviour therapy (CBT) for patients with chronic dizziness. VBRT was developed with the idea of helping patients compensate for peripheral and central vestibular deficits (Chapter 17). However, the majority of clinical trials of VBRT have been conducted in subjects with chronic vestibular symptoms lasting well beyond the typical compensation period. Descriptions of subject selection methods suggest that most patients enrolled in these studies had PPV/CSD (97). A small number may have had chronic uncompensated vestibular deficits, but the majority certainly did not. Anxiety and depression were not usually measured, except in the investigation by Meli and colleagues (93) who showed that VBRT alone was an effective treatment for behavioural morbidity in patients with chronic dizziness, reducing anxiety and depression. Collectively, these studies support the efficacy of VBRT for patients with chronic vestibular symptoms, though the most likely mechanism of action is behavioural desensitization, not vestibular compensation (97).

Small controlled trials demonstrated short-term improvements in dizziness, behavioural morbidity, and related functional impairments with CBT (97). Unfortunately, the benefits seem to be lost over time as the gains recorded at the end of acute treatment (95)

Table 30.3 Serotonergic antidepressants for chronic dizziness

Authors	Medication class	Medication	Description of study
Staab et al., 2002 (59)	Selective serotonin reuptake inhibitors (SSRIs)	Various	Retrospective series of 60 patients. CSD ± comorbid psychiatric disorders
Horii et al., 2004 (80)		Paroxetine	Prospective open trial of 47 patients. Chronic dizziness ± neurotological or psychiatric comorbidity
Staab et al., 2004 (60)		Sertraline	Prospective open trial of 20 patients. CSD ± comorbid psychiatric disorders
Simon et al., 2005 (86)		Fluoxetine	Prospective open trial of 3 patients with CSD and 2 with peripheral vestibular deficits
Horii et al., 2007 (98)		Fluvoxamine	Prospective open trial of 60 patients. Chronic dizziness ± neurotological or psychiatric comorbidity
Staab, 2011 (61)	Serotonin norepinephrine reuptake inhibitors (SNRIs)	Venlafaxine	Retrospective series of 32 patients. CSD + vestibular migraine with or without comorbid anxiety disorders
Horii et al., 2008 (87)		Milnacipran	Prospective open trial of 40 patients. Chronic dizziness ± neurotological or psychiatric comorbidity

CSD, chronic subjective dizziness.

Table 30.4 Rehabilitative and behavioural treatments for chronic dizziness

Treatment	Authors	Description of study
Vestibular and balance rehabilitation therapy (VBRT)	Jacob et al., 2001 (88)	Pilot study of 9 patients treated with 2 weeks of self-exposure exercises, then 8–12 weeks of therapist-directed VBRT
	Yardley et al., 2001 (89)	Randomized study comparing 33 patients treated with self-exposure exercises to 43 untreated control subjects
	Cohen and Kimball, 2003 (90)	Comparison of 3 home-based rehabilitation programmes in 53 patients with chronic vestibular symptoms
	Pavlou et al. 2004 (91)	Parallel group study comparing 20 patients treated with VBRT to 20 patients treated with VBRT plus desensitization exercises using a visual motion simulator
	Yardley et al., 2004 (92)	Randomized trial of home-based VBRT directed by primary care nurses in 83 patients versus usual primary care in 87 patients
	Meli et al., 2007 (93)	Randomized study comparing physical and psychological outcomes in 40 patients treated with VBRT versus 40 untreated controls
Cognitive behavioural therapy (CBT)	Johansson et al., 2001 (94)	Study of 9 elderly patients treated with elements of CBT added to VBRT versus 10 patients on a waiting list
	Holmberg et al., 2006 (95)	Parallel group study comparing 16 patients treated with CBT to 15 patients treated with self-exposure exercises
	Holmberg et al., 2007 (96)	1-year follow-up of the authors' 2006 study (above)

were no longer demonstrable at 1-year follow-up (96). A possible approach is to combine elements of CBT with VBRT. The theoretical benefit is that CBT would address thinking patterns that sustain vestibular symptoms and behavioural comorbidity while VBRT would diminish physical symptoms. Small pilot studies support this idea (88, 94).

Conclusions

Behavioural factors are ubiquitous in mobile beings, including humans. The brain's threat system is tightly linked to postural and oculomotor control systems at multiple levels and exerts profound influences on balance function in health and disease. Research conducted worldwide during the last 20–30 years provides the basis for developing an integrated approach to clinical care, research, and education in neuro-otology. Numerous hurdles stand in the way of this goal, but the strongest impediment needs the fewest resources to abolish. It requires setting aside long established and oft cherished notions such as 'psychogenic dizziness' that are products of dichotomous thinking about medical-psychiatric interactions. In neuro-otology, these relics of 20th century medicine relegate some of the most common and treatable aspects of vestibular morbidity to afterthoughts or ignorance to the detriment of patients' well-being and advances in the field.

Anxiety disorders, particularly panic and generalized anxiety, may be primary causes of vestibular symptoms. Conversely, vestibular diseases may trigger new anxiety disorders or exacerbate pre-existing ones. Anxiety affects the clinical manifestations of vestibular diseases and may interfere with successful medical or surgical treatments if not recognized and incorporated into multi-modality intervention plans.

The clinical syndrome of phobic postural vertigo (PPV) was first described 25 years ago. A streamlined definition, called chronic subjective dizziness (CSD), was published in 2007, based on the results of replication and validation studies. A consensus definition of PPV/CSD is in the offing, combining the observations and expertise of German, American, and other international investigators who have studied this common entity. These efforts coupled with research studies that have described its clinical course, triggers, provoking factors, and most importantly, successful treatments should provide the impetus for greater recognition of this condition in neuro-otology centres worldwide. In institutions around the world where it is regularly considered in the diagnostic process, is it the second most common clinical problem, accounting for many patients who otherwise leave neuro-otology consultations without a diagnosis or recommendations for treatment.

References

1. Staab JP (2009). Psychological aspects of vestibular disorders. In Eggers SDZ, Zee DS (Eds) *Vertigo and Imbalance: Clinical Neurophysiology of the Vestibular System*, Handbook of Clinical Neurophysiology, Vol. 9, pp. 502–22. Philadelphia, PA: Elsevier Health Sciences.
2. Brown LA, Gage WH, Polych MA, Sleik RJ, Winder TR (2002). Central set influences on gait. Age-dependent effects of postural threat. *Exp Brain Res*, 145, 286–96.
3. Adkin AL, Frank JS, Carpenter MG (2002). Fear of falling modifies anticipatory postural control. *Exp Brain Res*, 143, 160–70.
4. Gage WH, Sleik RJ, Polych MA, McKenzie NC, Brown LA (2003). The allocation of attention during locomotion is altered by anxiety. *Exp Brain Res*, 150, 385–94.
5. Hallam RS, Hinchcliffe R (1991). Emotional stability; its relationship to confidence in maintaining balance. *J Psychosom Res*, 35(4–5), 421–30.
6. Lepicard EM, Venault P, Perez-Diaz F, *et al.* (2000). Balance control and posture differences in the anxious BALB/cByJ mice compared to the non anxious C57BL/6J mice. *Behav Brain Res*, 117, 185–95.
7. Lepicard EM, Venault P, Negroni J, *et al.* (2003). Posture and balance responses to a sensory challenge are related to anxiety in mice. *Psychiatry Res*, 118, 273–84.
8. Venault P, Rudrauf D, Lepicard EM, Berthoz A, Jouvent R, Chapouthier G (2001). Balance control and posture in anxious mice improved by SSRI treatment. *Neuroreport*, 12, 3091–4.
9. Balaban CD (2002). Neural substrates linking balance control and anxiety. *Physiol Behav*, 77, 469–75.
10. Jacob RG, Redfern MS, Furman JM (2009). Space and motion discomfort and abnormal balance control in patients with anxiety disorders. *J Neurol Neurosurg Psychiatry*, 80, 74–8.
11. Hoffman DL, O'Leary DP, Munjack DJ (1994). Autorotation test abnormalities of the horizontal and vertical vestibulo-ocular reflexes in panic disorder. *Otolaryngol Head Neck Surg*, 110, 259–69.
12. Jacob RG, Furman JM, Durrant JD, Turner SM (1996). Panic, agoraphobia, and vestibular dysfunction. *Am J Psychiatry*, 153, 503–12.

13. Jacob RG, Furman JM, Durrant JD, Turner SM (1997). Surface dependence: a balance control strategy in panic disorder with agoraphobia. *Psychosom Med*, 59, 323–30.

14. Sklare DA, Stein MB, Pikus AM, Uhde TW (1990). Dysequilibrium and audiovestibular function in panic disorder: symptom profiles and test findings. *Am J Otol*, 11, 338–41.

15. Swinson RP, Cox BJ, Rutka J, Mai M, Kerr S, Kuch K (1993). Otoneurological functioning in panic disorder patients with prominent dizziness. *Compr Psychiatry*, 34, 127–9.

16. Tecer A, Tukel R, Erdamar B, Sunay T (2004). Audiovestibular functioning in patients with panic disorder. *J Psychosom Res*, 57, 177–82.

17. Perna G, Dario A, Caldirola D, Stefania B, Cesarani A, Bellodi L (2001). Panic disorder: the role of the balance system. *J Psychiatr Res*, 35, 279–86.

18. Yardley L, Britton J, Lear S, Bird J, Luxon LM (1995). Relationship between balance system function and agoraphobic avoidance. *Behav Res Ther*, 33, 435–9.

19. Perna G, Alpini D, Caldirola D, Raponi G, Cesarani A, Bellodi L (2003). Serotonergic modulation of the balance system in panic disorder: an open study. *Depress Anxiety*, 17, 101–6.

20. Cevette MJ, Puetz B, Marion MS, Wertz ML, Muenter MD (1995). Aphysiologic performance on dynamic posturography. *Otolaryngol Head Neck Surg*, 112, 676–88.

21. Redfern MS, Furman JM, Jacob RG (2007). Visually induced postural sway in anxiety disorders. *J Anxiety Disord*, 21, 704–16.

22. Erez O, Gordon CR, Sever J, Sadeh A, Mintz M (2004). Balance dysfunction in childhood anxiety: findings and theoretical approach. *J Anxiety Disord*, 18, 341–56.

23. Mian ND, Wainwright L, Briggs-Gowan MJ, Carter AS (2011). An ecological risk model for early childhood anxiety: the importance of early child symptoms and temperament. *J Abnorm Child Psychol*, 39, 501–12.

24. Staab JP, Newman-Toker DE, Carey JP, Bisdorff AR (in press). Progress in the Development of an International Classification of Vestibular Disorders. *Otol Neurotol*

25. Eckhardt A, Tettenborn B, Krauthauser H, *et al.* (1996). Vertigo and anxiety disorders—results of interdisciplinary evaluation. *Laryngorhinootologie*, 75, 517–22.

26. Eckhardt-Henn A, Breuer P, Thomalske C, Hoffmann SO, Hopf HC (2003). Anxiety disorders and other psychiatric subgroups in patients complaining of dizziness. *J Anxiety Disord*, 17, 369–88.

27. Staab JP, Ruckenstein MJ (2003). Which comes first? Psychogenic dizziness versus otogenic anxiety. *Laryngoscope*, 113, 1714–18.

28. Staab JP, Ruckenstein MJ (2007). Expanding the differential diagnosis of dizziness. *Arch Otolaryngol Head Neck Surg*, 13, 170–6.

29. National Institutes of Mental Health Statistics. http://www.nimh.nih.gov/statistics/index.shtml (accessed 9 July, 2011).

30. Staab JP (2006). Chronic subjective dizziness: The interface between psychiatry and neuro-otology. *Curr Opin Neurol*, 19, 41–8.

31. American Psychiatric Association (2000). *The Diagnostic and Statistical Manual of Mental Disorders, 4th edition, text revision.* Washington, DC: American Psychiatric Association.

32. American Psychiatric Association. *DSM-5 Development J 03 Functional Neurological Disorder (Conversion Disorder).* http://www.dsm5.org/ProposedRevision/Pages/proposedrevision.aspx?rid=8 (accessed 9 July, 2011).

33. Honaker JA, Gilbert JM, Staab JP (2010). Chronic subjective dizziness versus conversion disorder: discussion of clinical findings and rehabilitation. *Am J Audiology*, 19, 3–8.

34. Clark DB, Hirsch BE, Smith MG, Furman JM, Jacob RG (1994). Panic in otolaryngology patients presenting with dizziness or hearing loss. *Am J Psychiatry*, 151, 1223–5.

35. Grunfeld EA, Gresty MA, Bronstein AM, Jahanshahi M (2003). Screening for depression among neuro-otology patients with and without identifiable vestibular lesions. *Int J Audiol*, 42, 161–5.

36. Persoons P, Luyckx K, Desloovere C, Vandenberghe J, Fischler B (2003). Anxiety and mood disorders in otorhinolaryngology outpatients presenting with dizziness: validation of the self-administered PRIME-MD Patient Health Questionnaire and epidemiology. *Gen Hosp Psychiatry*, 25, 316–23.

37. Ruckenstein MJ, Staab JP (2001). The Basic Symptom Inventory-53 and its use in the management of patients with psychogenic dizziness. *Otolaryngol Head Neck Surg*, 125, 533–56.

38. Evans DL, Staab JP, Petitto JM, *et al.* (1999). Depression in the medical setting: Biopsychological interactions and treatment considerations. *J Clin Psychiatry*, 60(suppl 4), 40–55.

39. Eagger S, Luxon LM, Davies RA, Coelho A, Ron MA (1992). Psychiatric morbidity in patients with peripheral vestibular disorder: a clinical and neuro-otological study. *J Neurol Neurosurg Psychiatry*, 55, 383–7.

40. Kammerlind AS, Ledin TE, Skargren EI, Odkvist LM (2005). Long-term follow-up after acute unilateral vestibular loss and comparison between subjects with and without remaining symptoms. *Acta Otolaryngol (Stockh)*, 125, 946–53.

41. Godemann F, Schabowska A, Naetebusch B, Heinz A, Strohle A (2006) The impact of cognitions on the development of panic and somatoform disorders: a prospective study in patients with vestibular neuritis. *Psychol Med*, 36, 99–108.

42. Coker NJ, Coker RR, Jenkins HA, Vincent KR (1989). Psychological profile of patients with Meniere's disease. *Arch Otolaryngol Head Neck Surg*, 115, 1355–7.

43. Celestino D, Rosini E, Carucci ML, Marconi PL, Vercillo E (2003). Meniere's disease and anxiety disorders. *Acta Otorhinolaryngol Ital*, 23, 421–7.

44. Takahashi M, Ishida K, Iida M, Yamashita H, Sugawara K (2001). Analysis of lifestyle and behavioral characteristics in Meniere's disease patients and a control population. *Acta Otolaryngol (Stockh)*, 121, 254–6.

45. Savastano M, Maron MB, Mangialaio M, Longhi P, Rizzardo R (1996). Illness behaviour, personality traits, anxiety, and depression in patients with Meniere's disease. *J Otolaryngol*, 25, 329–33.

46. Onuki J, Takahashi M, Odagiri K, Wada R, Sato R (2005). Comparative study of the daily lifestyle of patients with Meniere's disease and controls. *Ann Otol Rhinol Laryngol*, 114, 927–33.

47. Eggers SDZ, Staab JP, Neff BA, Goulson AM, Carlson ML, Shepard NT (2011). Investigation of the coherence of definite and probable vestibular migraine as distinct clinical entities. *Otol Neurotol*, 32, 1144–51.

48. Best C, Eckhardt-Henn A, Tschan R, Dieterich M (2009). Psychiatric morbidity and comorbidity in different vestibular vertigo syndromes. Results of a prospective longitudinal study over one year. *J Neurol*, 256, 58–65.

49. Boleas-Aguirre MS, Sánchez-Ferrandiz N, Guillén-Grima F, Perez N (2007). Long-term disability of class A patients with Ménière's disease after treatment with intratympanic gentamicin. *Laryngoscope*, 117, 1474–81.

50. Committee on Hearing and Equilibrium of the American Academy of Otolaryngology-Head and Neck Surgery (1995). Guidelines for the diagnosis and evaluation of therapy in Ménière's disease. *Otolaryngol Head Neck Surg*, 113, 181–5.

51. Yardley L, Masson E, Verschuur C, Luxon L, Haacke NP (1992). Symptoms, anxiety and handicap in dizzy patients: development of the Vertigo Symptom Scale. *J Psychosom Res*, 36, 731–41.

52. Jacobson GP, Newman CW (1990). The development of the Dizziness Handicap Inventory. *Arch Otolaryngol Head Neck Surg*, 116, 424–7.

53. Staab JP, Ruckenstein MJ (2005). Chronic dizziness and anxiety: Effect of course of illness on treatment outcome. *Arch Otolaryngol Head Neck Surg*, 131, 675–79.

54. Brandt T, Dieterich M (1986). Phobischer Attacken-Schwank-schwindel, ein neues Syndrom? *Munch Med Wschr*, 28, 247–250.

55. Brandt T (1996). Phobic postural vertigo. *Neurology*, 46, 1515–19.

56. Huppert D, Strupp M, Rettinger N, Hecht J, Brandt T (2005). Phobic postural vertigo—a long-term follow-up (5 to 15 years) of 106 patients. *J Neurol*, 252, 564–9.

57. Kapfhammer HP, Mayer C, Hock U, Huppert D, Dieterich M, Brandt T (1997). Course of illness in phobic postural vertigo. *Acta Neurol Scand*, 95, 23–8.

58. Staab J, Eggers S, Neff B, Shepard N, Goulson A, Carlson M (2010). Validation of a clinical syndrome of persistent dizziness and unsteadiness, *J Vest Res*, 149–268.

59. Staab JP, Ruckenstein MJ, Solomon D, Shepard NT (2002). Serotonin reuptake inhibitors for dizziness with psychiatric symptoms. *Arch Otolaryngol Head Neck Surg*, 2002, 128, 554–60.

60. Staab JP, Ruckenstein MJ, Amsterdam JD (2004). A prospective trial of sertraline for chronic subjective dizziness. *Laryngoscope*, 114, 1637–41.

61. Staab JP (2011). Clinical clues to a dizzying headache. *J Vest Res*, 21, 331–40.

62. Shepard NT, Solomon D, Ruckenstein M, Staab J (2003). Evaluation of the vestibular (balance) system. In Snow JB, Ballenger JJ (Eds) *Ballenger's Otorhinolaryngology Head and Neck Surgery* (16th ed), pp. 161–94. Hamilton, ON: BC Decker.

63. Guidetti G, Monzani D, Civiero N (2002). Head-shaking nystagmus in the follow-up of patients with vestibular diseases. *Clin Otolaryngol*, 27, 124–8.

64. Bisdorff A, von Brevern M, Lempert T, Newman-Toker, DE (2009). Classification of vestibular symptoms: towards an international classification of vestibular disorders. *J Vestib Res*, 19, 1–13.

65. Costa PT, McCrae RR (1992). *NEO Personality Inventory Revised (NEO-PI-R™)*. Lutz, FL: Psychological Assessments Resources, Inc.

66. Staab J, Rohe D, Eggers S, Shepard N (2009) Anxious, introverted personality traits in chronic subjective dizziness. Abstracts of the 56th Annual Meeting of the Academy of Psychosomatic Medicine, Las Vegas, NV, November 12, 2009, http://www.apm.org/ann-mtg/2009/index.shtml (accessed 16 July, 2011).

67. Karg K, Burmeister M, Shedden K, Sen S (2011). The serotonin transporter promoter variant (5-HTTLPR), stress, and depression meta-analysis revisited: evidence of genetic moderation, *Arch Gen Psychiatry*, 68, 444–54.

68. Pollak L, Klein C, Rafael S, Vera K, Rabey JM (2003). Anxiety in the first attack of vertigo. *Otolaryn Head Neck Surg*, 128, 829–34.

69. Carpenter MG, Frank JS, Adkin AL, Paton A, Allum JH (2004). Influence of postural anxiety on postural reactions to multi-directional surface rotations. *J Neurophysiol*, 92, 3255–65.

70. Ohno H, Wada M, Saitoh J, Sunaga N, Nagai M (2004). The effect of anxiety on postural control in humans depends on visual information processing. *Neuroscience Lett*, 364, 37–9.

71. Wada M, Sunaga N, Nagai M (2001). Anxiety affects the postural sway of the antero-posterior axis in college students. *Neurosci Lett*, 302, 157–9.

72. Viaud-Delmon I, Ivanenko YP, Berthoz A, Jouvent R (2000). Adaptation as a sensorial profile in trait anxiety: a study with virtual reality. *J Anxiety Dis*, 14, 583–601.

73. Heinrichs N, Edler C, Eskens S, Mielczarek MM, Moschner C (2007). Predicting continued dizziness after an acute peripheral vestibular disorder. *Psychosom Med*, 69, 700–7.

74. Godemann F, Siefert K, Hantschke-Bruggemann M, Neu P, Seidl R, Strohle A (2005) What accounts for vertigo one year after neuritis vestibularis—anxiety or a dysfunctional vestibular organ? *J Psychiatr Res*, 39, 529–34.

75. Monzani D, Marchioni D, Bonetti S, *et al.* (2004). Anxiety affects vestibulospinal function of labyrinthine-defective patients during horizontal optokinetic stimulation. *Acta Otorhinolaryngol Ital*, 24, 117–24.

76. Alessandrini M, D'Erme G, Bruno E, Napolitano B, Magrini A (2003). Vestibular compensation: analysis of postural re-arrangement as a control index for unilateral vestibular deficit. *NeuroReport*, 14, 1075–9.

77. Krafczyk S, Schlamp V, Dieterich M, Haberhauer P, Brandt T (1999). Increased body sway at 3.5–8 Hz in patients with phobic postural vertigo. *Neurosci Lett*, 259, 149–52.

78. Siegbert Krafczyk S, Tietze S, Swoboda W, Valković P, Brandt T (2006). Artificial neural network: A new diagnostic posturographic tool for disorders of stance. *Clin Neurophysiol*, 117, 1692–8.

79. Querner V, Krafczyk S, Dieterich M, Brandt T (2000). Patients with somatoform phobic postural vertigo: the more difficult the balance task, the better the balance performance. *Neurosci Lett*, 285, 21–4.

80. Horii A, Mitani K, Kitahara T, Uno A, Takeda N, Kubo T (2004). Paroxetine, a selective serotonin reuptake inhibitor, reduces depressive symptoms and subjective handicaps in patients with dizziness. *Otol Neurotol*, 25, 536–43.

81. Zigmond AS, Snaith RP (1983). The Hospital Anxiety And Depression Scale. *Acta Psychiatr Scand*, 67, 361–70.

82. Spitzer RL, Kroenke K, Williams JBW (1999). Validation and utility of a self-report version of PRIME- MD—The PHQ primary care study. *JAMA*, 282, 1737–44.

83. Spitzer RL, Kroenke K, Williams JBW, Lowe B (2006). A brief measure for assessing generalized anxiety disorder—The GAD-7. *Arch Intern Med*, 166, 1092–7.

84. Powell LE, Myers AM (1995). The Activities-specific Balance Confidence (ABC) scale. *J Gerontol*, 50A, M28–34.

85. Legters K, Whitney SL, Porter R, Buczek F (2005). The relationship between the Activities-specific Balance Confidence Scale and the Dynamic Gait Index in peripheral vestibular dysfunction. *Physiother Res Int*, 10, 10–22.

86. Simon NM, Parker SW, Wernick-Robinson M, *et al.* (2005). Fluoxetine for vestibular dysfunction and anxiety: a prospective pilot study. *Psychosomatics*, 46, 334–9.

87. Horii A, Kitahara T, Masumura C, Kizawa K, Maekawa C, Kubo T (2008). Effects of milnacipran, a serotonin noradrenaline reuptake inhibitor (SNRI) on subjective handicaps and posturography in dizzy patients. Abstracts from the XXVth Congress of the Barany Society, 31 March–3 April, 2008, Kyoto, Japan.

88. Jacob RG, Whitney SL, Detweiler-Shostak G, Furman JM (2001). Vestibular rehabilitation for patients with agoraphobia and vestibular dysfunction: A pilot study. *J Anxiety Disord*, 15, 131–46.

89. Yardley L, Beech S, Weinman J (2001). Influence of beliefs about the consequences of dizziness on handicap in people with dizziness, and the effect of therapy on beliefs. *J Psychosom Res*, 50, 1–6.

90. Cohen HS, Kimball KT (2003). Increased independence and decreased vertigo after vestibular rehabilitation. *Otolaryngol Head Neck Surg*, 128, 60–70.

91. Pavlou M, Lingeswaran A, Davies RA, Gresty MA, Bronstein AM (2004). Simulator based rehabilitation in refractory dizziness. *J Neurol*, 251, 983–95.

92. Yardley L, Donovan-Hall M, Smith HE, Walsh BM, Mullee M, Bronstein AM (2004). Effectiveness of primary care–based vestibular rehabilitation for chronic dizziness. *Ann Intern Med*, 141, 598–605.

93. Meli A, Zimatore G, Badaracco C, De Angelis E, Tufarelli D (2007). Effects of vestibular rehabilitation therapy on emotional aspects in chronic vestibular patients. *J Psychosom Res*, 63, 185–90.

94. Johansson M, Akerlund D, Larsen HC, Andersson G (2001). Randomized controlled trial of vestibular rehabilitation combined with cognitive-behavioral therapy for dizziness in older people. *Otolaryngol Head Neck Surg*, 125, 151–6.

95. Holmberg J, Karlberg M, Harlacher U, Rivano-Fischer M, Magnusson M (2006). Treatment of phobic postural vertigo: A controlled study of cognitive-behavioral therapy and self-controlled desensitization. *J Neurol*, 253, 500–6.

96. Holmberg J, Karlberg M, Harlacher U, Magnusson M (2007). One-year follow-up of cognitive behavioral therapy for phobic postural vertigo. *J Neurol*, 254, 1189–92.

97. Staab JP (2011). Behavioral aspects of vestibular rehabilitation. *NeuroRehabilitation*, 29, 179–83.

98. Horii A, Uno A, Kitahara T, *et al.* (2007). Effects of fluvoxamine on anxiety, depression, and subjective handicaps of chronic dizziness patients with or without neuro-otologic diseases. *J Vestib Res*, 17(1), 1–8.

Index

£90